The Companion to Specialist Surgical Practice eLibrary

Series edited by

O. James Garden and Simon Paterson-Brown

The content of all eight volumes of the Fifth Edition of the **Companion to Spe... Surgical Practice** is now available both in print and as part of an electronic library. Your purchase of this book allows you to download the fully searchable contents to your desktop, laptop, tablet or smartphone.

Your **Companion to Specialist Surgical Practice eLibrary** is portable: the titles in the series download to your device or you can access online so they are with you whenever you need them.

Your eBook is much more than just 'pictures of pages':

- customize your page views
- search in single books that you have purchased or across any volumes in the series in your collection
- highlight and take searchable notes, and even print and copy-and-paste with bibliographic support
- utilize reference lists linked where available to Medline citations (including authors, title, source, and often an abstract) to journal articles and an indication of free electronic full-text availability.

To purchase other eBooks in the **Companion to Specialist Surgical Practice eLibrary** please visit www.elsevierhealth.com/companionseries

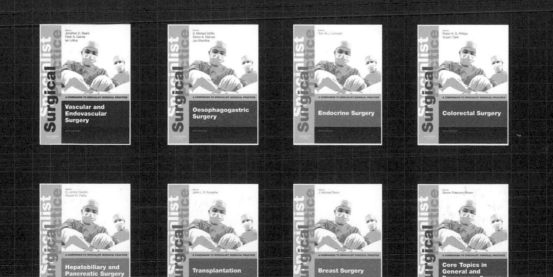

Colorectal Surgery

A COMPANION TO SPECIALIST SURGICAL PRACTICE

Series Editors
O. James Garden
Simon Paterson-Brown

Colorectal Surgery

FIFTH EDITION

Edited by

Robin K.S. Phillips
MBBS FRCS
Professor of Colorectal Surgery,
Imperial College London;
Consultant Surgeon and Clinical Director,
St Mark's Hospital,
Harrow, UK

Sue Clark
MD FRCS(Gen Surg)
Consultant Colorectal Surgeon,
St Mark's Hospital, Harrow;
Adjunct Professor of Surgery,
Imperial College,
London, UK

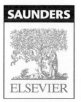

SAUNDERS

ELSEVIER

Edinburgh   London   New York   Oxford   Philadelphia   St Louis   Sydney   Toronto   2014

SAUNDERS
ELSEVIER

Fifth edition © 2014 Elsevier Limited. All rights reserved.

First edition 1997
Second edition 2001
Third edition 2005
Fourth edition 2009
Fifth edition 2014

ISBN 978-0-7020-4965-1
e-ISBN 978-0-7020-4973-6

British Library Cataloguing in Publication Data
A catalogue record for this book is available from the British Library

Library of Congress Cataloging in Publication Data
A catalog record for this book is available from the Library of Congress

Notice

ELSEVIER your source for books,
journals and multimedia
in the health sciences
www.elsevierhealth.com

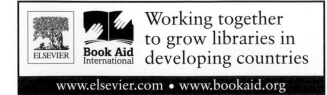

Working together
to grow libraries in
developing countries

www.elsevier.com • www.bookaid.org

The Publisher's policy is to use paper manufactured from sustainable forests

Printed in China

Commissioning Editor: Laurence Hunter
Development Editor: Lynn Watt
Project Manager: Vinod Kumar Iyyappan
Designer/Design Direction: Miles Hitchen
Illustration Manager: Jennifer Rose
Illustrator: Antbits Ltd

Contents

Contents

Contributors

Sue Clark, MD, FRCS(Gen Surg)
Consultant Colorectal Surgeon, The Polyposis
Registry, St Mark's Hospital, Harrow; Adjunct
Professor of Surgery, Imperial College, London, UK

Eric J. Dozois, MD, FACS, FASCRS
Professor of Surgery, Consultant, Division of
Colon and Rectal Surgery, Mayo Clinic, Rochester,
MN, USA

Anton V. Emmanuel, BSc, MD, FRCP
Department of Gastroenterology (GI Physiology),
University College London, London, UK

Nicola Fearnhead, BMBCh, FRCS, DM
Consultant Colorectal Surgeon, Department of
Colorectal Surgery, Addenbrooke's Hospital,
Cambridge, UK

Lester Gottesman, MD
Divison of Colon and Rectal Surgery, St Luke's/
Roosevelt Hospital; Associate Professor Clinical
Surgery, Columbia University College of Physicians
and Surgeons, New York, NY, USA

Adam Haycock, MBBS, MRCP, BSc, MD
Honorary Senior Lecturer, Imperial College;
Consultant Gastroenterologist and Endoscopy
Training Lead, Wolfson Unit for Endoscopy, St Mark's
Hospital, Harrow, UK

Ahmed Zia Janjua, MBBS, FCPS, FRCSI
Department of Colorectal Surgery, Hampshire
Hospitals Foundation Trust, Basingstoke, UK

Ian Jenkins, MD, FRCS, EBSQ(Coloproctology)
Consultant Colorectal Surgeon, Department of
Surgery, St Mark's Hospital, Harrow, UK

Scott Kelley, MD
Division of Colon and Rectal Surgery, Mayo Clinic,
Rochester, MN, USA

Robin Kennedy, MS, FRCS
Consultant Surgeon, Department of Surgery, St
Mark's Hospital, Harrow; Adjunct Professor of
Surgery, Imperial College, London, UK

Andrew Latchford, BSC (Hons),
MBBS, FRCP, MD
Consultant Gastroenterologist, Derriford Hospital,
Plymouth, UK

Paul-Antoine Lehur, MD, PhD
Professor of Digestive Surgery, Clinique de Chirurgie
Digestive et Endocrinienne, Institut Des Maladies de
l'Appareil Digestif, University Hospital de Nantes,
Nantes, France

Jit-Fong Lim, MBBS (S'pore), FRCS (Glasgow),
FAMS (S'pore)
Senior Consultant, Fortis Colorectal Hospital,
Singapore; Adjunct Assistant Professor, Duke-NUS
Graduate School of Medicine, Singapore

Peter Lunniss, MS, FRCS
Academic Surgical Unit, Barts and the London
Medical College; Consultant Colorectal Surgeon,
Academic Department of Medical and Surgical
Gastroenterology, Homerton University Hospital
(Retired), London, UK

Brendan J. Moran, MBBCh, FRCS, FRCSI, MCR
Consultant Colorectal Surgeon, Hampshire Hospitals
Foundation Trust, Basingstoke, UK

Neil J.McC. Mortensen, MBChB, MD, FRCS
Department of Colorectal Surgery, Oxford University
Hospitals, Oxford, UK

Robin K.S. Phillips, MBBS, FRCS
Professor of Colorectal Surgery, Imperial College
London; Consultant Surgeon and Clinical Director,
St Mark's Hospital, Harrow, UK

Ganesh Radhakrishna, MBChB, MRCP(UK),
FRCR
Consultant Clinical Oncologist, St James' Institute of
Oncology, St James' University Hospital, Leeds, UK

Alexis M.P. Schizas, BSc, MSc, MD(Res),
FRCS(Gen Surg)
Consultant Colorectal Surgeon, Department of
Surgery, Guy's and St Thomas' NHS Foundation
Trust, London, UK

Contributors

John H. Scholefield, MBChB, FRCS,
ChM (Distinction)
Professor of Surgery and Head of Division of
Academic Surgery, Division of GI Surgery, Queen's
Medical Centre, University Hospital, Nottingham, UK

David Sebag-Montefiore, MBBS, FRCP, FRCR
Consultant Clinical Oncologist, St James' Institute
of Oncology, St James' University Hospital,
Leeds, UK

Francis Seow-Choen, MBBS, FRCS(Ed), FAMS,
FRES
Colorectal Surgeon and Director, Seow-Choen
Colorectal Surgery PLC; Colorectal Surgeon,
Medical Director and Senior Consultant, Fortis
Colorectal Hospital, Singapore

Josef A. Shehebar, MD
Division of Colon & Rectal Surgery, Morristown
Medical Center; Assistant Professor of Surgery, Mount
Sinai School of Medicine, Morristown, NJ, USA

Robert J.C. Steele, MD, FRCS(Ed), FRCS,
FCSHK
Professor of Surgery, Head of Department of
Surgery, University of Dundee Medical School,
Ninewells Hospital, Dundee, UK

Siwan Thomas-Gibson, MD, FRCP
Consultant Gastroenterologist, Honorary Senior
Lecturer Imperial College, Endoscopy Clinical and
Training Lead, St Mark's Hospital, Harrow, UK

Mark Thompson-Fawcett, MBChB, MD, FRACS
Associate Professor of Surgery, University of Otago;
Colorectal Surgeon, Dunedin Hospital, New Zealand

Carolynne Jane Vaizey, MBChB, MD, FRCS(Gen),
FCS(SA)
Consultant Colorectal Surgeon and Chairman of
Surgery, St Mark's Hospital London; Director of the
Sir Alan Parks Physiology Unit, Lead Surgeon for the
Lennard Jones Intestinal Failure Unit, London, UK

Janindra Warusavitarne, BMed, FRACS PhD
Consultant Colorectal Surgeon, St Mark's Hospital,
Harrow, UK

Andrew B. Williams, MS, FRCS(Gen Surg)
Consultant Colorectal Surgeon, Department of
Surgery, St Thomas' Hospital, London, UK

Des Winter, MB, FRCSI, MD, FRCS(Gen)
Consultant Surgeon, Centre for Colorectal Disease,
St Vincent's University Hospital and University
College, Dublin, Ireland

Mark T.C. Wong, MBBD, FRCS
Consultant Surgeon, Department of
Colorectal Surgery, Singapore General Hospital;
Director, SGH Anorectal Ultrasound & Physiology
Laboratory; Director, SGH Pelvic Floor Disorder
Service; Adjunct Assistant-Professor,
Duke-NUS Graduate Medical School;
Clinical Senior Lecturer, YLL School of Medicine,
Singapore

Series Editors' preface

It is now some 17 years since the first edition of the *Companion to Specialist Surgical Practice* series was published. We set ourselves the task of meeting the educational needs of surgeons in the later years of specialist surgical training, as well as consultant surgeons in independent practice who wished for contemporary, evidence-based information on the subspecialist areas relevant to their general surgical practice. The series was never intended to replace the large reference surgical textbooks which, although valuable in their own way, struggle to keep pace with changing surgical practice. This Fifth Edition has also had to take due account of the increasing specialisation in 'general' surgery. The rise of minimal access surgery and therapy, and the desire of some subspecialties such as breast and vascular surgery to separate away from 'general surgery', may have proved challenging in some countries, but has also served to emphasise the importance of all surgeons being aware of current developments in their surgical field. As in previous editions, there has been increasing emphasis on evidence-based practice and contributors have endeavoured to provide key recommendations within each chapter. The eBook versions of the textbook have also allowed the technophile improved access to key data and content within each chapter.

We remain indebted to the volume editors and all the contributors of this Fifth Edition. We have endeavoured where possible to bring in new blood to freshen content. We are impressed by the enthusiasm, commitment and hard work that our contributors and editorial team have shown and this has ensured a short turnover between editions while maintaining as accurate and up-to-date content as is possible. We remain grateful for the support and encouragement of Laurence Hunter and Lynn Watt at Elsevier Ltd. We trust that our original vision of delivering an up-to-date affordable text has been met and that readers, whether in training or independent practice, will find this Fifth Edition an invaluable resource.

O. James Garden, BSc, MBChB, MD, FRCS(Glas), FRCS(Ed), FRCP(Ed), FRACS(Hon), FRCSC(Hon)
Regius Professor of Clinical Surgery, Clinical Surgery School of Clinical Sciences, The University of Edinburgh and Honorary Consultant Surgeon, Royal Infirmary of Edinburgh

Simon Paterson-Brown, MBBS, MPhil, MS, FRCS(Ed), FRCS(Engl), FCS(HK)
Honorary Senior Lecturer, Clinical Surgery School of Clinical Sciences, The University of Edinburgh and Consultant General and Upper Gastrointestinal Surgeon, Royal Infirmary of Edinburgh

Editors' preface

Colorectal surgery has continued to see many innovations and changes since the Fourth Edition. This edition has been substantially re-written and there are many new faces. Sue Clark joins as co-editor and there are new lead contributors in rectal cancer, diverticular disease, ulcerative colitis, incontinence, and sexually transmitted diseases and the anorectum. New techniques, such as percutaneous and transcutaneous tibial nerve stimulation for faecal incontinence as well as extralevator abdomino-perineal excision, are covered.

The topics have all been brought right up to date and the authors have written clearly, concisely and authoritatively. Important points are distinguished by single-tick (expert opinion) and double-tick (strong recommendation) logos and the references remain reduced in order to accommodate new material while at the same time weighty references are highlighted with a small vignette explaining their worth. Much is new.

We are confident that readers will enjoy this Fifth Edition. They will find more than enough to inform, more than enough for examinations worldwide, and more than enough to support them in active consultant practice.

Acknowledgements

We should like to thank Bharti Huda who has coordinated and chased up many contributors, followed up on queries and arranged submissions on time.

Robin K.S. Phillips
Sue Clark
Harrow

Evidence-based practice in surgery

Critical appraisal for developing evidence-based practice can be obtained from a number of sources, the most reliable being randomised controlled clinical trials, systematic literature reviews, meta-analyses and observational studies. For practical purposes three grades of evidence can be used, analogous to the levels of 'proof' required in a court of law:

1. **Beyond all reasonable doubt.** Such evidence is likely to have arisen from high-quality randomised controlled trials, systematic reviews or high-quality synthesised evidence such as decision analysis, cost-effectiveness analysis or large observational datasets. The studies need to be directly applicable to the population of concern and have clear results. The grade is analogous to burden of proof within a criminal court and may be thought of as corresponding to the usual standard of 'proof' within the medical literature (i.e. $P<0.05$).

2. **On the balance of probabilities.** In many cases a high-quality review of literature may fail to reach firm conclusions due to conflicting or inconclusive results, trials of poor methodological quality or the lack of evidence in the population to which the guidelines apply. In such cases it may still be possible to make a statement as to the best treatment on the 'balance of probabilities'. This is analogous to the decision in a civil court where all the available evidence will be weighed up and the verdict will depend upon the balance of probabilities.

3. **Not proven.** Insufficient evidence upon which to base a decision, or contradictory evidence.

Depending on the information available, three grades of recommendation can be used:

a. Strong recommendation, which should be followed unless there are compelling reasons to act otherwise.

b. A recommendation based on evidence of effectiveness, but where there may be other factors to take into account in decision-making, for example the user of the guidelines may be expected to take into account patient preferences, local facilities, local audit results or available resources.

c. A recommendation made where there is no adequate evidence as to the most effective practice, although there may be reasons for making a recommendation in order to minimise cost or reduce the chance of error through a locally agreed protocol.

✔✔ Evidence where a conclusion can be reached **'beyond all reasonable doubt'** and therefore where a **strong recommendation** can be given. This will normally be based on evidence levels:
- Ia. Meta-analysis of randomised controlled trials
- Ib. Evidence from at least one randomised controlled trial
- IIa. Evidence from at least one controlled study without randomisation
- IIb. Evidence from at least one other type of quasi-experimental study.

✔ Evidence where a conclusion might be reached **'on the balance of probabilities'** and where there may be other factors involved which influence the recommendation given. This will normally be based on less conclusive evidence than that represented by the double tick icons:
- III. Evidence from non-experimental descriptive studies, such as comparative studies and case–control studies
- IV. Evidence from expert committee reports or opinions or clinical experience of respected authorities, or both.

Evidence which is associated with either a **strong recommendation** or **expert opinion** is highlighted in the text in panels such as those shown above, and is distinguished by either a double or single tick icon, respectively. The references associated with double-tick evidence are highlighted in the reference lists at the end of each chapter along with a short summary of the paper's conclusions where applicable.

The reader is referred to Chapter 1, 'Evidence-based practice in surgery' in the volume, *Core Topics in General and Emergency Surgery* of this series, for a more detailed description of this topic.

1

Anorectal investigation

Alexis M.P. Schizas
Andrew B. Williams

Introduction

Many tests are available to investigate anorectal disorders, each only providing part of a patient's assessment, so results should be considered together and alongside the clinical picture derived from a careful history and physical examination.

Investigations provide information about structure alone, function alone, or both, and have been directed to five general areas of interest: faecal incontinence, constipation (including Hirschsprung's disease), anorectal sepsis, rectal prolapse (including solitary rectal ulcer syndrome) and anorectal malignancy.

Anatomy and physiology of the anal canal

The adult anal canal is approximately 4 cm long and begins as the rectum narrows, passing backwards between the levator ani muscles. There is in fact wide variation in length between the sexes, particularly anteriorly, and between individuals of the same sex. The canal has an upper limit at the pelvic floor and a lower limit at the anal opening. The proximal canal is lined by simple columnar epithelium, changing to stratified squamous epithelium lower in the canal via an intermediate transition zone just above the dentate line. Beneath the mucosa is the subepithelial tissue, composed of connective tissue and smooth muscle. This layer increases in thickness throughout life and forms the basis of the vascular cushions thought to aid continence.

Lateral to the subepithelial layer the caudal continuation of the circular smooth muscle of the rectum forms the internal anal sphincter, which terminates caudally with a well-defined border at a variable distance from the anal verge. Continuous with the outer layer of the rectum the longitudinal layer of the anal canal lies between the internal and external anal sphincters and forms the medial edge of the intersphincteric space. The longitudinal muscle comprises smooth muscle cells from the rectal wall, augmented with striated muscle from a variety of sources, including the levator ani, puborectalis and pubococcygeus muscles. Fibres from this layer traverse the external anal sphincter forming septa that insert into the skin of the lower anal canal and adjacent perineum as the corrugator cutis ani muscle.

The striated muscle of the external sphincter surrounds the longitudinal muscle and between these lies the intersphincteric space. The external sphincter is arranged as a tripartite structure, classically described by Holl and Thompson and later adopted by Gorsch and by Milligan and Morgan. In this system the external sphincter is divided into deep, superficial and subcutaneous portions, with the deep and subcutaneous sphincter forming rings of muscle and, between them, the elliptical fibres of the superficial sphincter running anteriorly from the perineal body to the coccyx posteriorly. Some consider the external sphincter to be a single muscle contiguous with the puborectalis muscle, while others have adopted a two-part model. The latter proposes a deep anal sphincter and a superficial anal sphincter, corresponding to the puborectalis and deep external anal sphincter combined, as well as the fused superficial and subcutaneous sphincter of the tripartite model. Anal endosonography (AES) and magnetic resonance imaging (MRI) have not resolved the dilemma, although most authors report a three-part sphincter where the puborectalis muscle is fused with the deep sphincter.[1,2] The external anal sphincter is innervated by the pudendal nerve (S2–S4), which leaves the pelvis via the lower part of the greater sciatic notch, where it passes under the pyriformis muscle. It then crosses the ischial spine and sacrospinous ligament to enter the ischiorectal fossa through the lesser sciatic notch or foramen via the pudendal (or Alcock's) canal.

The pudendal nerve has two branches: the inferior rectal nerve, which supplies the external anal sphincter and sensation to the perianal skin; and the perineal nerve, which innervates the anterior perineal muscles together with the sphincter urethrae and forms the dorsal nerve of the clitoris (penis). Although puborectalis receives its main innervation from a direct branch of the fourth sacral nerve root, it may derive some innervation via the pudendal nerve.

The autonomic supply to the anal canal and pelvic floor comes from two sources. The fifth lumbar nerve root sends sympathetic fibres to the superior and inferior hypogastric plexuses, and the parasympathetic supply is from the second to fourth sacral nerve roots via the nervi erigentes. Fibres of both systems pass obliquely across the lateral surface of the lower rectum to reach the region of the perineal body.

The internal anal sphincter has an intrinsic nerve supply from the myenteric plexus together with an additional supply from both the sympathetic and parasympathetic nervous systems. Sympathetic nervous activity is thought to enhance and parasympathetic activity to reduce internal sphincter contraction. Relaxation of the internal anal sphincter may be mediated via non-adrenergic, non-cholinergic nerve activity via the neural transmitter nitric oxide.

Anorectal physiological studies alone cannot separate the different structures of the anal canal;

instead, they provide measurements of the resting and squeeze pressures along the canal. Between 60% and 85% of resting anal pressure can be attributed to the action of the internal anal sphincter.[3] The external anal sphincter and the puborectalis muscle generate the maximal squeeze pressure.[3] Symptoms of passive anal leakage (where the patient is unaware that episodes are happening) are attributed to internal sphincter dysfunction, whereas urge symptoms and frank incontinence of faeces are due to external sphincter problems.[4]

Faecal continence is maintained by the complex interaction of many different variables. Stool must be delivered at a suitable rate from the colon into a compliant rectum of adequate volume. The consistency of this stool should be appropriate and accurately sensed by the sampling mechanism. Sphincters should be intact and able to contract adequately to produce pressures sufficient to prevent leakage of flatus, liquid and solid stool. For effective defecation there needs to be coordinated relaxation of the striated muscle components with an increase in intra-abdominal pressure to expel the rectal contents. The structure of the anorectal region should prevent herniation or prolapse of elements of the anal canal and rectum during defecation.

As a result of the complex interplay between the factors involved in continence and faecal evacuation, a wide range of investigations is needed for full assessment. A defect in any one element of the system in isolation is unlikely to have great functional significance and so in most clinical situations there is more than one contributing factor.

Rectoanal inhibitory reflex

Increasing rectal distension is associated with transient reflex relaxation of the internal anal sphincter and contraction of the external anal sphincter, known as the rectoanal inhibitory reflex (**Fig. 1.1**).[5] The exact neurological pathway for this reflex is unknown, although it may be mediated via the myenteric plexus and stretch receptors in the pelvic floor. Patients with rectal hyposensitivity have higher thresholds for rectoanal inhibitory reflex; it is absent in patients with Hirschsprung's disease, progressive systemic sclerosis, Chagas' disease, and initially absent after a coloanal anastomosis, although it rapidly recovers.

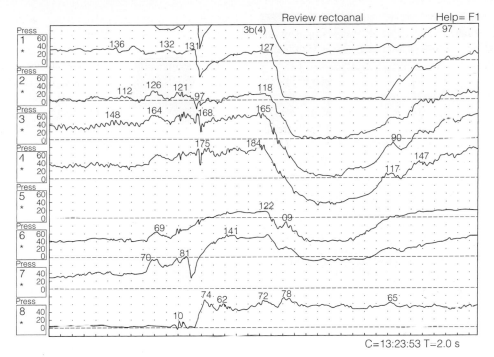

Figure 1.1 • Normal rectoanal inhibitory reflex.

> ✅ The rectoanal inhibitory reflex may enable rectal contents to be sampled by the transition zone mucosa to enable discrimination between solid, liquid and flatus. The rate of recovery of sphincter tone after this relaxation differs for the proximal and distal canal, which may be important in maintaining continence.[6]

Further studies investigating the role of the rectoanal inhibitory reflex in incontinent patients show that as rectal volume increases greater sphincter relaxation is seen, whereas constipated patients have a greater recovery velocity of the resting anal pressure in the proximal anal canal.

Manometry

A variety of different catheter systems exist to measure anal pressure and it is important to note that measurements differ depending on the system employed. Systems include microballoons filled with air or water, microtransducers and water-perfused catheters. These may be hand-held or automated. Hand-held systems are withdrawn in a measured stepwise fashion with recordings made after each step (usually of 0.5–1.0 cm intervals); this is called

a station pull-through. Automated withdrawal devices allow continuous data recording (vector manometry).

Water-perfused catheters use hydraulic capillary infusers to perfuse catheter channels, which are arranged either radially or obliquely staggered. Each catheter channel is then linked to a pressure transducer (**Fig. 1.2**). Infusion rates of perfusate (sterile water) vary between 0.25 and 0.5 mL/min per channel. Systems need to be free from air bubbles, which may lead to inaccurate recordings, and must avoid leakage of perfusate onto the perianal skin, which may lead to falsely high resting pressures due to reflex external sphincter action. Perfusion rates should remain constant, because faster rates are associated with higher resting pressures, while larger diameter catheters lead to greater recorded pressure.[7]

Balloon systems may be used to overcome some of these problems and may be more representative of pressure generated within a hollow viscus than recordings using a perfusion system. They are not subject to the same problems as a perfusion system when canal pressures are radially asymmetrical.[7] Balloons can be filled with either air or water. Over the range of balloon sizes used (diameter 2–10 mm), diameter appears to have less of an effect on the

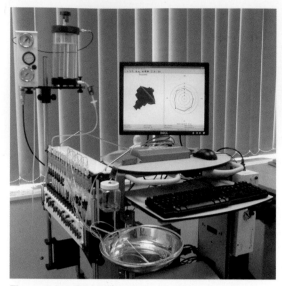

Figure 1.2 • Perfusion system used for anorectal manometry. Standard water perfusion set-up plus computer interface for anorectal manometry. The screen shows a vector volume profile.

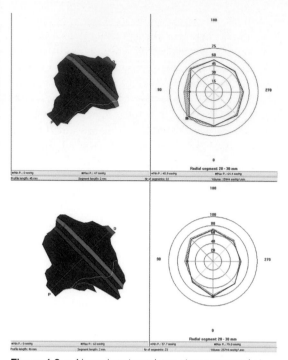

Figure 1.3 • Normal vector volume at squeeze and at rest. Note that asymmetry of the sphincter contour can be normal.

pressures recorded than it does with water-perfused catheter systems.

Microtransducers have been developed that can accurately measure canal pressure. However, they are expensive and fragile and more prone to inaccuracies when radial pressure asymmetry is present. They have been validated against water-filled balloon systems and may be useful in the performance of ambulatory studies.

Vector volume manometry utilises a radially arranged eight-channel catheter that is automatically withdrawn from the anal canal during rest and squeeze, and computer software that produces a three-dimensional reconstruction of the anal canal (**Fig. 1.3**).[8] This system is able to assess radial asymmetry or vector symmetry index (i.e. how far the radial symmetry of the anal canal differs from a perfect circle, which has a radial asymentry of 0% or vector symmetry index of 1). Sphincter defects are associated with symmetry indices of 0.6 or less.

Vector volume manometry may differentiate between idiopathic and traumatic faecal incontinence by showing global external sphincter weakness rather than a localised area of scarred sphincter indicated by an asymmetrical vectogram.[8,9] Anal vector manometry has been extensively used to assess obstetric anal sphincter injury. Following caesarean section no change in anal pressures is

seen; however, after vaginal delivery a fall in rest and squeeze pressures occurs.[10] The reduction in pressures has been shown to be greatest after a third or fourth degree tear confirmed on anal endosonography (AES). Functional anal sphincter length and vector volumes have been shown to decrease both at rest and during contraction after obstetric anal sphincter injury.[11] Vector volumes decrease further in women with persistent flatus incontinence.

High-definition manometry uses closely spaced solid-state sensors simultaneously to measure circumferential pressures in the rectum and throughout the anal canal, so there is no need to perform a station pull-through manoeuvre.[12]

Pressure changes in the anal canal can be measured in a number of ways and each method has been validated for its repeatability and reproducibility, although individual methods are not interchangeable.[13] Although the correlation between measurements made using different systems and catheters is good, the absolute values are different, so that when comparing the results of different studies it is essential to consider the method used to obtain the pressure measurements.

Significant variation exists in the results of anorectal manometry in normal asymptomatic subjects. Men have higher mean resting and squeeze pressures.[14] Pressures decline after the age of 60 years, changes most marked in women.[15] These facts must be considered when selecting appropriate control subjects for clinical studies. Normal mean anal canal resting tone in healthy adults is 50–100 mmHg. Resting tone increases in a cranial to caudal direction along the canal such that the maximal resting pressure is found 5–20 mm from the anal verge.[3,16] The high-pressure zone (the part of the anal canal where the resting pressure is >50% of the maximum resting or squeeze pressure) is similar at rest between men and women (20 mm in length) but longer in men than women when squeezing (31 mm vs. 23 mm).[16] In a normal individual the rise in pressure on maximal squeezing should be at least 50–100% of the resting pressure (usually 100–180 mmHg).[17] Reflex contraction of the external sphincter should occur when the rectum is distended, on coughing, or with any rise in intra-abdominal pressure.

✔✔ In the assessment of patients with faecal incontinence, both resting and maximal squeeze pressures are significantly lower in patients with incontinence than in matched controls,[18] but there is considerable crossover between the pressures recorded in patients and controls.[19]

Ambulatory manometry

The use of continuous ambulatory manometry to record rectal and anal canal pressures[20] has provided information on the functioning of the sphincter mechanism in a more physiological situation. The generation of giant waves of pressure in the rectum or neorectum may relate to episodes of incontinence in patients after restorative proctocolectomy. Ambulatory manometry has also identified patients in whom episodes of internal sphincter relaxation are not accompanied by reflex external sphincter contraction,[21] a finding that may prove useful in selecting patients likely to benefit from biofeedback treatment.

Anal and rectal sensation

The anal canal is rich in sensory receptors,[22] including those for pain, temperature and movement, with the somatic sensation of the anal transitional mucosa being more sensitive than that of the perianal skin. In contrast, the rectum is relatively

insensitive to pain, although crude sensation may be transmitted via the nervi erigentes of the parasympathetic nervous system.[23]

A variety of methods have been used to measure anal sensation. Initial assessment of anal sensation used a stiff bristle to detect light touch in the anal canal and hot and cold metal rods to detect temperature sensation.[22] Thermal sensation has been assessed with water-perfused thermodes;[24] normal subjects can detect a change in temperature of 0.92 °C.[24] The ability of the mucosa to detect a small electrical current can be assessed by the use of a double platinum electrode and a signal generator providing a square wave impulse at 5 Hz of 100 μs duration. The lowest recorded current of three readings at the point at which the subject feels a tingling or pricking sensation in the anal canal is noted as the sensation threshold. Normal electrical sensation for the most sensitive area of the anal canal (the transition zone) is 4 mA (2–7 mA). Rectal mucosal electrical sensation may also be measured using the same technique as that used for anal mucosal electrical sensation measurement, with slight modification of the stimulus (500 μs duration at a frequency of 10 Hz).[23]

The sensation of rectal filling is measured by progressively inflating a balloon placed within the rectum or by intrarectal saline infusion.[23] Normal perception of rectal filling occurs after inflation of 10–20 mL, the sensation of the urge to defecate occurs after 60 mL, and normally up to 230 mL is tolerated in total before discomfort occurs.[23]

✔ The clinical use of these measurements may be limited due to the large inter- and intrasubject variation in values and the wide normal range, reducing the discriminatory value of this technique as a clinical investigation.[25]

Temperature sensation may be vital in the discrimination of solid stool from liquid and flatus,[24] and is reduced in patients with faecal incontinence. It is thought that this sensation is important in the sampling reflex, although this is brought into question by the fact that the sensitivity of the anal mucosa to temperature change is not great enough to detect the very slight temperature gradient between the rectum and anal canal.

Anal mucosal electrical sensation threshold increases with age and thickness of the subepithelial layer of the anal canal. Anal canal electrical sensation is reduced in idiopathic faecal incontinence,[26] diabetic neuropathy, descending perineum syndrome and haemorrhoids.[26] There are differing reports on whether there is any correlation between electrical sensation and measurement of motor function of the sphincters (pudendal terminal motor latency and single-fibre electromyography).

The sampling mechanism and maintenance of faecal continence are complex multifactorial processes, as seen by the fact that the application of local anaesthetic to the sensitive anal mucosa does not lead to incontinence and in some individuals actually improves continence.

Rectal compliance

The relation between changes in rectal volume and the associated pressure changes is termed compliance, which is calculated by dividing the change in volume by the change in pressure. Compliance is measured by inflating a rectal balloon with saline or air or by directly infusing saline at physiological temperature into the rectum. In the former method, the filling of the rectal balloon can be either incremental or continuous. When continuous inflation of the rectal balloon is used, the rate of inflation should be 70–240 mL/min.[25] Mean rectal compliance is about 4–14 mL/cmH$_2$O, with pressures of 18–90 cmH$_2$O at the maximum tolerated volume.[27] Reports on the reproducibility of the measurement of rectal compliance are varied and many have found great variation within the same subject;[25,27] the most reproducible measurement is usually the maximum tolerated volume. The use of the barostat to measure rectal compliance has been shown to be reproducible at pressures of between 36 and 48 mmHg. The compliance of the rectum does not differ between men and women up to the age of 60 years, but after this age women have more compliant rectums. It is reduced in Behçet's disease and Crohn's disease and after radiotherapy in a dose-related fashion. It is also reduced in irritable bowel syndrome.

> ✔ The association between changes in rectal compliance and faecal incontinence is less clear. Some state that compliance is normal in incontinence whereas others have found a reduction in compliance associated with faecal incontinence,[18] although changes in compliance may be secondary to the incontinence and not causative. Altered compliance may play a role in soiling and constipation associated with megarectum.

Pelvic floor descent

Parks et al. first described the association between excessive descent of the perineum and anorectal dysfunction, and subsequently it has been described in a number of conditions: faecal incontinence, severe constipation, solitary rectal ulcer syndrome, and anterior mucosal and full-thickness rectal prolapse. The presumption in all these conditions is that abnormal perineal descent, especially during straining, causes traction and damage to the pudendal and pelvic floor nerves, leading to progressive neuropathy and muscular atrophy. Irreversible pudendal nerve damage occurs after a stretch of 12% of its length, and often the descent of the perineum in these patients is of the order of 2 cm, which is estimated to cause pudendal nerve stretching of 20%.

Descent of the perineum was initially measured using the St Mark's perineometer. The perineometer is placed on the ischial tuberosities and a movable latex cylinder is positioned on the perineal skin. The distance between the level of the perineum and the ischial tuberosities is measured at rest and during straining.[28] Negative readings indicate that the plane of the perineum is above the tuberosities and a positive value indicates descent below this level. In normal asymptomatic adults the plane of the perineum at rest should be −2.5±0.6 cm, descending to +0.9±1.0 cm on straining. When measured using dynamic proctography, similar measurements of pelvic floor descent are obtained. The anorectal angle normally lies on a line drawn between the coccyx and the most anterior part of the pubis, and descends by 2±0.3 cm on straining.

Excessive perineal descent is found in 75% of subjects who chronically strain during defecation. The degree of descent correlates with age and is greater in women. Although increased perineal descent on straining has been shown to be associated with features of neuropathy, namely decreased anal mucosal electrical sensitivity and increased pudendal nerve terminal motor latency, not all patients with abnormal descent have abnormal neurology.[29] Perineal descent is also associated with faecal incontinence, although the degree of incontinence and the results of anorectal manometry do not correlate with the extent of pelvic floor laxity.[30]

Electrophysiology

Neurophysiological assessment of the anorectum includes assessment of the conduction of the pudendal and spinal nerves, and electromyography (EMG) of the sphincter.

Electromyography

Electromyographic traces can be recorded from the separate components of the sphincter complex both at rest and during active contraction of the striated components. Initially, EMG was used to map sphincter defects before surgery, but AES is now so superior in its ability to map defects and is so much better tolerated by patients[31] that EMG has largely become a research tool. Broadly, two techniques of EMG are used: concentric needle studies and single-fibre studies.

Concentric needle EMG records the activity of up to 30 muscle fibres from around the area of the needle both at rest and during voluntary squeeze. The amplitude of the signal recorded correlates with the maximal squeeze pressure,[32] polyphasic long-duration action potentials indicating reinnervation subsequent to denervation injury. The main use of this technique has been in the confirmation and mapping of sphincter defects. Examination of puborectalis EMG may be more sensitive than cinedefecography in the detection of paradoxical puborectalis contraction in obstructed defecation,[33] although paradoxical puborectalis contraction is also present in normal subjects.

The use of an anal plug or sponge can record global electrical activity from the anal sphincters,[32] EMG amplitudes recorded in this way correlating with voluntary squeeze pressure. In the future, sponge electrode EMG may have a role in directing biofeedback retraining for anismus.

When EMG is performed using a needle with a smaller recording area (25 µm diameter) the action potential from individual motor units is recorded. Denervated muscle fibres can regain innervation from branching of adjacent axons, leading to an increase in the number of muscle fibres supplied by a single axon. With multiple readings (an average of 20) using this small-diameter needle, the mean fibre density (MFD) for an area of sphincter can be calculated (i.e. the mean number of muscle action potentials per unit area or axon). Denervation and subsequent reinnervation are also indicated by neuromuscular 'jitter', which is caused by variation in the timing of triggering and non-triggering potentials.[34] An increase in sphincter MFD is often found in cases of idiopathic incontinence and is associated with recognised histological changes in sphincter structure. Atrophic sphincter muscle shows a loss of the characteristic mosaic pattern of distribution of type 1 and type 2 muscle fibres. There is also selective muscle fibre hypertrophy together with fibro-fatty fibre degeneration. These changes predominantly affect the external anal sphincter but the puborectalis and levators are also affected to a lesser extent.

MFD correlates inversely with squeeze pressure and is increased in patients with excessive perineal descent.[35] The correlation with direct assessment of the integrity of sphincter innervation (pudendal nerve terminal motor latency) is less clear.

Pudendal nerve terminal motor latency

Pudendal nerve conduction can be assessed by stimulating as the nerve enters the ischio-rectal fossa at the ischial spines. This investigation only examines the fastest conducting fibres of the pudendal nerve and so can still be normal even in the presence of abnormal sphincter innervation. The normal value for pudendal nerve terminal motor latency (PNTML) is 2.0 ± 0.5 ms.[36]

Prolongation of PNTML is associated with idiopathic faecal incontinence, rectal prolapse, solitary rectal ulcer syndrome, severe constipation and sphincter defects. Nerve latency is delayed with increasing age and is prolonged in 24% of all faecally incontinent patients and 31% of those presenting with constipation.[36]

✓ PNTML is operator dependent and has a poor correlation with clinical symptoms and histological findings. The American Gastroenterology Association does not recommend the use of this test for the evaluation of patients with faecal incontinence.[37]

Spinal motor latency

Transcutaneous stimulation of the sacral motor nerve roots provides further information on the innervation of the pelvic floor. The motor response from stimulation at the level of the first and fourth lumbar vertebrae can be recorded using standard

EMG needles inserted into the puborectalis and external sphincter. By comparing the latency times between the two levels, the latency of the motor component of the cauda equina can be assessed. Up to 23% of patients with idiopathic faecal incontinence will have cauda equina delay.[38]

Defecography/evacuation proctography

Defecography or evacuation proctography involves video fluoroscopy of the patient evacuating barium paste of stool consistency. Barium-soaked gauze may also be inserted into the vagina and barium paste may be applied to the perineum to aid in assessing the anorectal angle and perineal descent.[39] Opacification of the small bowel with an orally ingested contrast medium or injection of contrast into the peritoneum (peritoneography) will reveal enteroceles in 18% of patients with pelvic floor weakness,[40] with only half filling with bowel.[41] Defecography is a dynamic examination; it not only provides information on anorectal structural changes during defecation, but it also assesses function. While anatomical changes during evacuation (namely rectocele, enterocele, rectoanal intussusception, rectal prolapse and changes in anorectal angle) may be evident, the extent and duration of emptying is of more clinical significance.[42]

> ✅ Anatomical abnormalities demonstrated on proctography are of poor discriminatory value in determining patients from controls. The only measurements that can discriminate between normal subjects and those with severe constipation are the time taken to evacuate and the completeness of evacuation.[43]

During normal evacuation the anorectal angle increases because of relaxation of puborectalis. Normal evacuation should be 90% complete (and 60% complete with a pouch). Rectoceles are significant if they are greater than 3 cm or require perianal/vaginal digitation to empty.

Dynamic pelvic MRI

Using a modified T2-weighted single-shot fast spin-echo imaging sequence or a T2-weighted fast imaging with steady-state precession MRI sequence,

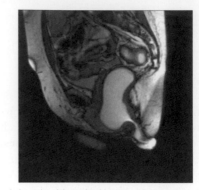

Figure 1.4 • A mid-sagittal image of the anal canal and rectum using MRI proctography, showing an anterior rectocele.

anorectal and pelvic floor motion can be imaged at 1.2- to 2-second intervals. During dynamic MRI, proctography provides pelvic images at rest and when the subject strains. This gives an overview of pelvic floor movement and organ prolapse, and rectal dynamics are assessed during evacuation after adding 150 mL of ultrasound gel to the rectum[44] (**Fig. 1.4**). There are few differences in the detection of clinically relevant findings between supine MRI and seated MRI, with the exception of detecting rectal intussusceptions, for which seated MRI is superior.[45]

> ✅ MRI defecography has been shown to alter the surgical approach in 67% of patients who underwent surgery for faecal incontinence.[46] It has also been shown that interobserver agreement for assessing anorectal motion by MRI proctography is better than with barium defecography.

Dynamic transperineal and three-dimensional pelvic floor ultrasound

Developments in diagnostic ultrasound imaging can contribute to the diagnostic work-up of female patients with obstructed defecation, rectal intussusception, rectal prolapse and rectoceles. Dynamic pelvic floor scanning has been found to correlate well with defecating proctography. MRI and three-dimensional ultrasonography can accurately diagnose puborectalis avulsion off its insertion on the os pubis.[47] Pelvic floor ultrasound has advantages, as it is better tolerated and is cheaper.

Scintigraphy

Scintigraphy using technetium-labelled sulphur colloid mixed with dilute veegum powder may also be used for defecography.[48] The advantages of this technique are that a quantitative result is obtained and a lower dose of radiation is used. However, the study is not dynamic and does not correlate with patient symptoms or manometric assessment. Radioisotope testing may also be used to assess colonic transit time to diagnose idiopathic slow transit constipation. Colonic transit time is measured more easily by tracking the progress of ingested sets of radio-opaque markers with plain abdominal radiography. Standard protocol takes a single plain abdominal radiograph 5 days after commencing ingestion of the markers (usually different-shaped markers are taken daily over the first 3 days).

Imaging the rectum and anal sphincters

The indications for anorectal imaging may be divided into three broad clinical areas: sepsis and fistula disease, malignancy, and faecal incontinence. The available techniques include surface scanning techniques, namely computed tomography (CT) and body coil MRI, and endoanal imaging, namely anal endosonography (AES), with or without subsequent multiplanar (three-dimensional) reconstruction, and endocoil MRI (largely unavailable now).

Anal endosonography/endorectal ultrasound

The two-dimensional endoluminal ultrasound of the rectum utilises a transducer that rotates through 360° within a water-filled balloon in order to provide acoustic coupling. The newer three-dimensional endoluminal ultrasound uses a double-crystal design with 6–16 MHz frequency range encased in a cylindrical transducer shaft. The transducer is then used with a specially designed rectosigmoidoscope and water-filled condom covering the transducer. This allows rectal scanning without moving or replacing the probe. The ultrasonic anatomy has been described in detail as a result of scanning dissected specimens and comprises alternating bands of reflection created by the interfaces between the different anatomical structures present.[49] An alternating bright and dark pattern of rings is seen corresponding to the layers of the rectal wall.

To enable examination of the anal sphincters, the water-filled condom is removed from the three-dimensional transducer and for the two-dimensional endorectal ultrasound (EUS) the water-filled balloon has to be replaced with a water-filled plastic cone (**Fig. 1.5a**). The anal canal mucosa is generally not seen on AES; the subepithelial tissue is highly reflective and surrounded by the low reflection from the internal anal sphincter. The width of the internal sphincter increases with age: the normal width for a patient aged 55 years or younger is 2.4–2.7 mm, whereas in an older patient the normal range is 2.8–3.4 mm. As the width of the sphincter increases it becomes progressively more reflective and more indistinct; this may be due to a relative increase in the fibroelastic content of this muscle as a consequence of ageing. Both the external anal sphincter and the longitudinal muscle are of moderate reflectivity. The intersphincteric space often returns a bright reflection (**Fig. 1.5b**).[50]

The development of high-resolution three-dimensional AES constructed from a synthesis of standard two-dimensional cross-sectional images produces a digital volume that may be reviewed and can be used to perform measurements in any plane, yielding more information on the anal sphincter complex. This provides more reliable measurements, and volume measurements can also be performed.[51] Another development in the use of three-dimensional AES is the volume render mode. This allows analysis of information inside a three-dimensional volume by digitally enhancing individual voxels. The volume-rendered image provides better visualisation performance when there are not large differences in the signal levels of pathological structures compared with surrounding tissues.

Endocoil receiver MRI

MRI provides images with excellent tissue differentiation, although spatial resolution of the anal sphincters using a body coil receiver is poor. When an endoanal receiver coil is used, spatial resolution is vastly improved locally around the coil (within about 4 cm), enabling the acquisition of images of the anal sphincters with both excellent tissue differentiation and spatial resolution. Endocoils have either rectangular or saddle geometry and measure 6–10 cm in length and 7–12 mm in diameter. This increases to 17–19 mm after encasement in an acetal homopolymer (Delrin) former. The coil is inserted in the left lateral position and then se-

cured with sandbags or with a purpose-built holder to avoid movement artefact.[50,52,53]

On T2-weighted images, the external sphincter and longitudinal muscle return a relatively low signal. The internal sphincter returns a relatively high signal and enhances with gadolinium (an intravenous contrast agent used in MRI). The subepithelial tissue has a signal intensity value between that of the internal and external sphincters (**Fig. 1.6**).

Imaging in rectal cancer

CT has an accuracy of 89% in assessing rectal tumours with extensive spread beyond the serosal layer; however, when only cases of moderate tumour spread are assessed, the accuracy is much lower (55%).[54] The accuracy of CT has been improved by the advent of multislice technique CT and further improvement is expected from modern scanners with up to 64 detector rows. CT is also used to assess metastatic disease involving the liver and lungs.

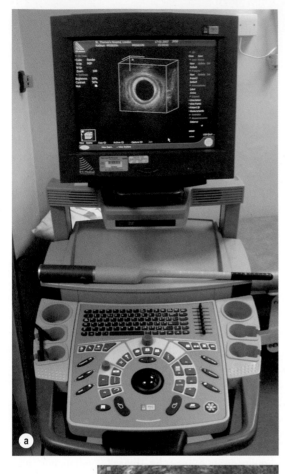

Subepithelium

Internal sphincter

Longitudinal muscle

External sphincter

(b)

Figure 1.5 • **(a)** BK Medical three-dimensional endoanal ultrasound machine and 2050 probe. **(b)** The layers of the sphincter are depicted by the three-dimensional endoanal ultrasound probe.

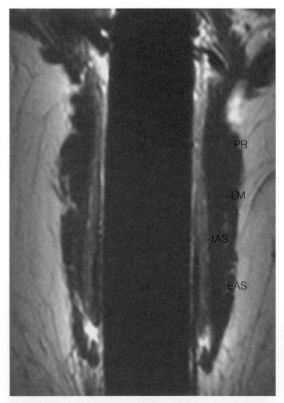

PR

-LM

-IAS

EAS

Figure 1.6 • A mid-coronal image of the anal canal using endocoil MRI. EAS, external anal sphincter; IAS, internal anal sphincter; LM, longitudinal muscle; PR, puborectalis.

The development of positron emission tomography (PET) combined with CT has improved the detection of recurrent rectal carcinoma.[55] PET/CT can also yield additional pretreatment staging information in patients with low rectal cancer.[56] EUS, by comparison, can correctly detect T-stage rectal cancers in 75–87% of cases, with a trend to over-stage in 22%.[57] Three-dimensional EUS has improved accuracy in T-staging of tumours when compared to two-dimensional EUS (accuracy 87% vs. 82%). Perirectal lymph nodes involved with tumour are seen on EUS as well-defined areas of low reflectivity, although malignant nodal status has also been associated with a degree of inhomogeneity on EUS. EUS is superior to CT and has a positive predictive value for tumour invasion beyond the muscularis propria of 98%. If a lymph node measures greater than 5 mm in diameter on EUS, there is a 45–70% chance that it is involved with tumour.[58]

Body coil MRI has been used to assess the stage of rectal tumours and it would appear to give comparable results to EUS,[59] with an accuracy of 88% at detecting transmural spread, 87% anal sphincter infiltration,[56,60] and an accuracy of T-staging of 75% and a 94% accuracy in detecting circumferential resection margin involvement.[61] A meta-analysis of 84 studies showed EUS to be slightly superior to MRI in assessing nodal status.[62] Unfortunately, none of the investigations enables reliable detection of nodal spread. Body coil MRI has the advantage over EUS in that it can be performed even in the presence of stenotic tumours. Furthermore, after radiotherapy EUS will tend to over-stage tumours, leading to a marked reduction in its diagnostic accuracy, especially in the differentiation between T2 and T3 tumours. The other area where MRI is superior to EUS is in the assessment of recurrent tumours. The appearances of fibrosis after surgery and recurrent tumour in the pelvis are very similar using either EUS or CT, which makes assessment for recurrent disease very difficult. On MRI the signals from these two tissue types (especially on T2-weighted images) are quite different, allowing greater tissue differentiation.

✔✔ EUS appears better at estimating the stage of T0, T1, T2 rectal tumours[63] and nodal staging.[62] However, the main determinant of local recurrence is circumferential resection margin and EUS is poor at assessing this, whereas MRI has been shown to be much more accurate.[62]

Imaging in anal sepsis and anal fistulas

Both surface imaging and endoanal imaging have been employed in the assessment of perianal sepsis. CT is unsatisfactory for the assessment of fistulas because of the poor definition of tracks, which is largely due to volume averaging. AES may be used to assess anal fistulas and has been shown to be accurate for the definition of the anatomy of anal sepsis, especially horseshoe collections and the anatomy of complex fistulas.[64] Endosonography is also able to detect and assess sphincter damage caused by chronic sepsis.

Endosonography is less accurate in the assessment of suprasphincteric sepsis and it is often difficult to differentiate between supralevator and infralevator collections, leading to inaccuracy in up to 20% of cases.[65] The internal opening on AES is identified by penetration of the internal anal sphincter by the track because of the lack of definition of the mucosa and is of limited value close to the anal margin. The diagnostic accuracy of AES is increased with the use of hydrogen peroxide injected into fistulous tracks to act as a contrast medium.[66] The use of three-dimensional AES and volume rendering improves the accuracy of AES further.[67] MRI has the most to offer in the assessment of perianal sepsis. Anal sepsis appears on MRI as areas of very high signal, which enhance with the administration of the intravenous contrast agent gadolinium. Definition is further increased with the use of STIR (short tau inversion recovery) sequences to suppress the signal returned by fat (**Fig. 1.7**).

✔✔ The use of dynamic contrast-enhanced MRI has been reported to provide better delineation of fistulas than AES, which is better than examination under anaesthetic (EUA). Correct classification with clinical examination has been achieved in 61% of cases using EUA, 81% using AES and 90% using MRI. AES predicts accurately the site of the internal opening in 91% of cases compared with 97% for MRI.[68]

Imaging in faecal incontinence

AES has revealed that many patients who were thought to have idiopathic faecal incontinence in fact have a surgically remediable sphincter defect.

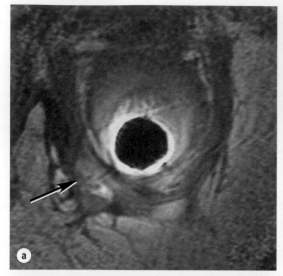
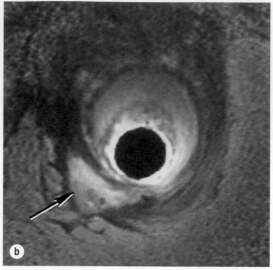
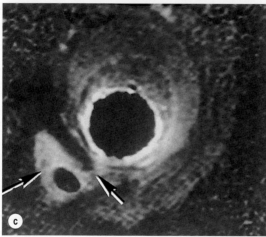

Figure 1.7 • Examples of complex perirectal sepsis as shown by the endoanal magnetic resonance probe. **(a,b)** T1-weighted images of an intersphincteric collection prior to and following gadolinium–DTPA contrast (arrow). **(c)** Short tau inversion recovery (STIR) image of the abscess cavity showing a central gas-containing cavity (long arrow) and a fistula at the 7 o'clock position (short arrow).

It has also been shown that a much higher proportion of women sustain sphincter damage during childbirth than is suspected by clinical assessment alone.[69] While the true incidence of sphincter tears may be lower than initially thought,[70] many women sustain important morphological changes to the sphincter following delivery.[71] The ability of AES to diagnose and correctly assess the extent of external sphincter damage has been validated by comparison with EMG studies and findings at surgery.[72] AES is superior in the differentiation between those patients with idiopathic faecal incontinence and those with a sphincter defect when compared with either simple manometric assessment or vector volume studies.

MRI is also used to assess patients with faecal incontinence and the diagnosis of sphincter defects

using endocoil MRI has been validated with surgical confirmation of defect presence and extent. Endocoil MRI may be superior to AES in the detection and assessment of external sphincter defects as a result of better sphincter definition using MRI, although it is more important that the clinician is familiar with the imaging technique used.[73]

MRI has multiplanar capability (i.e. axial, sagittal and coronal images can be acquired), whereas standard AES provides only axially oriented images. The acquisition of volume ultrasound data has overcome this problem, and using three-dimensional AES has led to a better understanding of sphincter injury. A direct correlation exists between the length of a defect and the arc of displacement of the two ends of the sphincter.[74]

The use of endocoil MRI has shown that incontinence in the absence of a sphincter defect may be due to atrophy, where the sphincter has been replaced by fat and fibrous tissue.[53,75] The presence of external anal sphincter atrophy on endocoil MRI has been associated with poor results from anterior sphincteroplasty.

Summary

A wide variety of physiological and morphological tests is available for the assessment of the anus and rectum. Although there is no clear correlation between manometric/neurophysiological testing and clinical symptomatology in patients with idiopathic faecal incontinence, there is considerable value in performing these tests before surgery in order to predict long-term outcome. Anorectal investigation has revealed a large group of parous women who have occult sphincter trauma that may have a clinical impact as the women get older.

Anorectal physiological assessment is essential as an objective measure in patients with faecal incontinence and for the diagnosis of Hirschsprung's disease, and may help select those patients who will have acceptable function after colo-anal anastomosis or an ileo-anal pouch.

Endoanal imaging is becoming the gold standard in the preoperative determination of sphincter integrity and defines those patients most likely to benefit from surgical intervention. Endorectal imaging of rectal tumours correlates well with histological assessment of tumour depth and is accurate for the diagnosis of recurrent tumour after anterior resection (especially when using MRI).

In patients with primary evacuatory disorders, neurophysiological testing and defecography assist in the demonstration of unsuspected rectoanal intussusception or rectocele who may benefit from surgery and those who may be suitable candidates for biofeedback therapy.

Anorectal investigation continues to have a major role in clinical research and has helped outline the anatomy of the component parts of the sphincter complex as well as to define the physiology of both defecation and anal continence. The understanding of these processes is vital to the correct management of patients with anorectal disorders.

Key points

- Normal pelvic floor function relies on a complex interplay between various mechanisms.
- Sphincter function may be assessed using anal manometry and electrophysiology.
- Sphincter anatomy may be assessed using AES and MRI, the former being the standard for the diagnosis of sphincter trauma.
- Dynamic MRI evacuation proctography and dynamic pelvic floor scans are useful in the assessment of patients with evacuatory disorders.
- Pelvic MRI or three-dimensional AES may be used to assess anorectal sepsis and can predict recurrence of anal fistulas after surgery.
- Preoperative staging of early rectal cancer is superior with EUS. Circumferential resection margin prediction is most accurate when using MRI.

References

1. Guo M, Gao C, Li D, et al. MRI anatomy of the anal region. Dis Colon Rectum 2010;53(11):1542–8.
2. Desouza NM, Kmiot WA, Puni R, et al. High resolution magnetic resonance imaging of the anal sphincter using an internal coil. Gut 1995;37(2):284–7.
3. Williams AB, Cheetham MJ, Bartram CI, et al. Gender differences in the longitudinal pressure profile of the anal canal related to anatomical structure as demonstrated on three-dimensional anal endosonography. Br J Surg 2000;87(12):1674–9.
4. Engel AF, Kamm MA, Bartram CI, et al. Relationship of symptoms in faecal incontinence to specific sphincter abnormalities. Int J Colorectal Dis 1995;10(3):152–5.
5. Gowers WR. The automatic action of the sphincter ani. Proc R Soc Lond 1877;26:77–84.
6. Goes RN, Simons AJ, Masri L, et al. Gradient of pressure and time between proximal anal canal and high-pressure zone during internal anal sphincter relaxation. Its role in the fecal continence mechanism. Dis Colon Rectum 1995;38(10):1043–6.

7. Taylor BM, Beart RW, Phillips SF. Longitudinal and radial variations of pressure in the human anal sphincter. Gastroenterology 1984;86:693–7.

8. Braun JC, Treutner KH, Dreuw B, et al. Vector manometry for differential diagnosis of fecal incontinence. Dis Colon Rectum 1994;37(10):989–96.

9. Samarasekera DN, Wright Y, Lowndes RH, et al. Comparison of vector symmetry index and endoanal ultrasonography in the diagnosis of anal sphincter disruption. Tech Coloproctol 2008;12(3):211–5.

10. Donnelly VS, O'Herlihy C, Campbell DM, et al. Postpartum fecal incontinence is more common in women with irritable bowel syndrome. Dis Colon Rectum 1998;41(5):586–9.

11. Willis S, Faridi A, Schelzig S, et al. Childbirth and incontinence: a prospective study on anal sphincter morphology and function before and early after vaginal delivery. Langenbecks Arch Surg 2002;387(2):101–7.

12. Jones MP, Post J, Crowell MD. High-resolution manometry in the evaluation of anorectal disorders: a simultaneous comparison with water-perfused manometry. Am J Gastroenterol 2007;102(4):850–5.

13. Schizas AM, Emmanuel AV, Williams AB. Anal canal vector volume manometry. Dis Colon Rectum 2011;54(6):759–68.

14. Enck P, Kuhlbusch R, Lubke H, et al. Age and sex and anorectal manometry in incontinence. Dis Colon Rectum 1989;32:1026–30.

15. Sun WM, Read NW. Anorectal function in normal human subjects: effect of gender. Int J Colorectal Dis 1989;4(3):188–96.

16. Schizas AM, Emmanuel AV, Williams AB. Vector volume manometry – methods and normal values. Neurogastroenterol Motil 2011;23(9):886-e393.

17. Jorge JM, Wexner SD. Anorectal manometry: techniques and clinical applications. Southern Med J 1993;86(8):924–31.

18. Bharucha AE, Fletcher JG, Harper CM, et al. Relationship between symptoms and disordered continence mechanisms in women with idiopathic faecal incontinence. Gut 2005;54(4):546–55.
In this study 35% of patients with faecal incontinence had reduced resting pressure and 73% of faecal incontinence patients had reduced squeeze pressures, which was a higher percentage than the control group. This study also found that volume and pressure thresholds for desired defecation were lower in faecal incontinence patients.

19. McHugh SM, Diamant NE. Effect of age, gender, and parity on anal canal pressures. Contribution of impaired anal sphincter function to fecal incontinence. Dig Dis Sci 1987;32(7):726–36.
McHugh and Diamant found that in faecally incontinent patients, 39% of women and 44% of men had normal resting and squeeze pressures, and 9% of asymptomatic normal individuals were unable to generate an appreciable pressure on maximal squeeze.

20. Kumar D, Waldron D, Williams NS, et al. Prolonged anorectal manometry and external anal sphincter electromyography in ambulant human subjects. Dig Dis Sci 1990;35(5):641–8.

21. Sun WM, Read NW, Miner PB, et al. The role of transient internal sphincter relaxation in faecal incontinence? Int J Colorectal Dis 1990;5(1):31–6.

22. Duthie HL, Gairns FW. Sensory nerve-endings and sensation in the anal region of man. Br J Surg 1960;47:585–95.

23. Kamm MA, Lennard-Jones JE. Rectal mucosal electrosensory testing – evidence for a rectal sensory neuropathy in idiopathic constipation. Dis Colon Rectum 1990;33(5):419–23.

24. Miller R, Bartolo DCC, Cervero F, et al. Anorectal temperature sensation: a comparison of normal and incontinence patients. Br J Surg 1987;74(6):511–5.

25. Kendall GPN, Thompson DG, Day SJ, et al. Inter- and intraindividual variation in pressure–volume relations of the rectum in normal subjects and patients with irritable bowel syndrome. Gut 1990;31:1062–8.

26. Roe AM, Bartolo DC, Mortensen NJ. New method for assessment of anal sensation in various anorectal disorders. Br J Surg 1986;73:310–2.

27. Sorensen M, Rasmussen OO, Tetzschner T, et al. Physiological variation in rectal compliance. Br J Surg 1992;79(10):1106–8.

28. Lubowski DZ, Swash M, Nicholls RJ, et al. Increase in pudendal nerve terminal motor latency with defaecation straining. Br J Surg 1988;75(11):1095–7.

29. Engel AF, Kamm MA. The acute effect of straining on pelvic floor neurological function. Int J Colorectal Dis 1994;9(1):8–12.

30. Read NW, Bartolo DC, Read MG, et al. Differences in anorectal manometry between patients with haemorrhoids and patients with descending perineum syndrome: implications for management. Br J Surg 1983;70(11):656–9.

31. Law PJ, Kamm MA, Bartram CI. A comparison between electromyography and anal endosonography in mapping external anal sphincter defects. Dis Colon Rectum 1990;33(5):370–3.

32. Sorensen M, Tetzschner T, Rasmussen OO, et al. Relation between electromyography and anal manometry of the external anal sphincter. Gut 1991;32(9):1031–4.

33. Karlbom U, Edebol Eeg-Olofsson K, Graf W, et al. Paradoxical puborectalis contraction is associated with impaired rectal evacuation. Int J Colorectal Dis 1998;13(3):141–7.

34. Wexner SD, Marchetti F, Salanga VD, et al. Neurophysiologic assessment of the anal sphincters. Dis Colon Rectum 1991;34(7):606–12.

35. Womack NR, Morrison JF, Williams NS. The role of pelvic floor denervation in the aetiology of idiopathic faecal incontinence. Br J Surg 1986;73(5):404–7.

36. Kiff ES, Swash M. Slowed conduction in the pudendal nerves in idiopathic (neurogenic) faecal incontinence. Br J Surg 1984;71(8):614–6.

37. Barnett JL, Hasler WL, Camilleri M. American Gastroenterological Association medical position statement on anorectal testing techniques. American Gastroenterological Association. Gastroenterology 1999;116(3):732–60.

38. Snooks SJ, Swash M, Henry MM. Abnormalities in central and peripheral nerve conduction in patients with anorectal incontinence. J R Soc Med 1985;78(4):294–300.

39. Delemarre JB, Kruyt RH, Doornbos J, et al. Anterior rectocele: assessment with radiographic defecography, dynamic magnetic resonance imaging, and physical examination. Dis Colon Rectum 1994;37(3):249–59.

40. Kelvin FM, Maglinte DD, Benson JT. Evacuation proctography (defecography): an aid to the investigation of pelvic floor disorders. Obstet Gynecol 1994;83(2):307–14.

41. Halligan S, Bartram CI. Evacuation proctography combined with positive contrast peritoneography to demonstrate pelvic floor hernias. Abdom Imaging 1995;20(5):442–5.

42. Halligan S, Bartram CI. Is barium trapping in rectoceles significant? Dis Colon Rectum 1995;38(7):764–8.

43. Turnbull GK, Bartram CI, Lennard-Jones JE. Radiologic studies of rectal evacuation in adults with idiopathic constipation. Dis Colon Rectum 1988;31(3):190–7.

44. Bertschinger KM, Hetzer FH, Roos JE, et al. Dynamic MR imaging of the pelvic floor performed with patient sitting in an open-magnet unit versus with patient supine in a closed-magnet unit. Radiology 2002;223(2):501–8.

45. Bharucha AE. Update of tests of colon and rectal structure and function. J Clin Gastroenterol 2006;40(2):96–103.

46. Hetzer FH, Andreisek G, Tsagari C, et al. MR defecography in patients with fecal incontinence: imaging findings and their effect on surgical management. Radiology 2006;240(2):449–57.

47. Dietz HP, Bernardo MJ, Kirby A, et al. Minimal criteria for the diagnosis of avulsion of the puborectalis muscle by tomographic ultrasound. Int Urogynecol J 2011;22(6):699–704.

48. McLean RG, King DW, Talley NA, et al. The utilization of colon transit scintigraphy in the diagnostic algorithm for patients with chronic constipation. Dig Dis Sci 1999;44(1):41–7.

49. Beynon J, Foy DM, Temple LN, et al. The endosonic appearances of normal colon and rectum. Dis Colon Rectum 1986;29(12):810–3.

50. Williams AB, Bartram CI, Halligan S, et al. Endosonographic anatomy of the normal anal canal compared with endocoil magnetic resonance imaging. Dis Colon Rectum 2002;45(2):176–83.

51. West RL, Felt-Bersma RJ, Hansen BE, et al. Volume measurements of the anal sphincter complex in healthy controls and fecal-incontinent patients with a three-dimensional reconstruction of endoanal ultrasonography images. Dis Colon Rectum 2005;48(3):540–8.

52. Desouza NM, Hall AS, Puni R, et al. High resolution magnetic resonance imaging of the anal sphincter using a dedicated endoanal coil. Comparison of magnetic resonance imaging with surgical findings. Dis Colon Rectum 1996;39(8):926–34.

53. Stoker J, Rociu E, Zwamborn AW, et al. Endoluminal MR imaging of the rectum and anus: technique, applications, and pitfalls. Radiographics 1999;19(2):383–98.

54. Nicholls RJ, Mason AY, Morson BC, et al. The clinical staging of rectal cancer. Br J Surg 1982;69(7):404–9.

55. Even-Sapir E, Parag Y, Lerman H, et al. Detection of recurrence in patients with rectal cancer: PET/CT after abdominoperineal or anterior resection. Radiology 2004;232(3):815–22.

56. Gearhart SL, Frassica D, Rosen R, et al. Improved staging with pretreatment positron emission tomography/computed tomography in low rectal cancer. Ann Surg Oncol 2006;13(3):397–404.

57. Orrom WJ, Wong WD, Rothenberger DA, et al. Endorectal ultrasound in the preoperative staging of rectal tumors. A learning experience. Dis Colon Rectum 1990;33(8):654–9.

58. Beynon J, Mortensen NJ, Foy DM, et al. Preoperative assessment of mesorectal lymph node involvement in rectal cancer. Br J Surg 1989;76(3):276–9.

59. McNicholas MM, Joyce WP, Dolan J, et al. Magnetic resonance imaging of rectal carcinoma: a prospective study. Br J Surg 1994;81(6):911–4.

60. Brown G, Radcliffe AG, Newcombe RG, et al. Preoperative assessment of prognostic factors in rectal cancer using high-resolution magnetic resonance imaging. Br J Surg 2003;90(3):355–64.

61. Al-Sukhni E, Milot L, Fruitman M, et al. Diagnostic accuracy of MRI for assessment of T category, lymph node metastases, and circumferential resection margin involvement in patients with rectal cancer: a systematic review and meta-analysis. Ann Surg Oncol 2012;Jan 20, online.

62. Lahaye MJ, Engelen SM, Nelemans PJ, et al. Imaging for predicting the risk factors – the circumferential resection margin and nodal disease – of local recurrence in rectal cancer: a meta-analysis. Semin Ultrasound CT MR 2005;26(4):259–68.
This meta-analysis on the accuracy of preoperative imaging includes studies between 1985 and 2004. It showed that MRI is the only investigation accurate at predicting circumferential resection margin. EUS is slightly but not significantly superior at predicting nodal status.

63. Bipat S, Glas AS, Slors FJ, et al. Rectal cancer: local staging and assessment of lymph node involvement with endoluminal US, CT, and MR imaging – a meta-analysis. Radiology 2004;232(3):773–83.

A meta-analysis of 90 articles showed that for muscularis propria invasion, EUS and MRI had similar sensitivities but the specificity of EUS (86%) was significantly higher than that of MRI (69%). For perirectal tissue invasion, sensitivity of EUS (90%) was significantly higher than that of CT (79%) and MRI (82%). EUS was more accurate than CT and MRI at diagnosing perirectal tissue invasion and there was no difference in diagnosis of lymph node involvement.

64. Deen KI, Williams JG, Hutchinson R, et al. Fistulas in ano: endoanal ultrasonographic assessment assists decision making for surgery. Gut 1994;35(3):391–4.

65. Choen S, Burnett S, Bartram CI, et al. Comparison between anal endosonography and digital examination in the evaluation of anal fistulae. Br J Surg 1991;78(4):445–7.

66. West RL, Dwarkasing S, Felt-Bersma RJ, et al. Hydrogen peroxide-enhanced three-dimensional endoanal ultrasonography and endoanal magnetic resonance imaging in evaluating perianal fistulas: agreement and patient preference. Eur J Gastroenterol Hepatol 2004;16(12): 1319–24.

67. Sudol-Szopinska I, Kolodziejczak M, Szopinski TR. The accuracy of a postprocessing technique – volume render mode – in three-dimensional endoanal ultrasonography of anal abscesses and fistulas. Dis Colon Rectum 2011;54(2):238–44.

68. Buchanan GN, Halligan S, Bartram CI, et al. Clinical examination, endosonography, and MR imaging in preoperative assessment of fistula in ano: comparison with outcome-based reference standard. Radiology 2004;233(3):674–81.

This prospective trial of 104 patients with anal fistulas showed that AES with a high-frequency transducer is superior to digital examination but MRI is superior to AES.

69. Donnelly V, Fynes M, Campbell D, et al. Obstetric events leading to anal sphincter damage. Obstet Gynecol 1998;92(6):955–61.

70. Williams AB, Bartram CI, Halligan S, et al. Anal sphincter damage after vaginal delivery using three-dimensional endosonography. Obstet Gynecol 2001;97(5 Pt 1):770–5.

71. Williams AB, Bartram CI, Halligan S, et al. Alteration of anal sphincter morphology following vaginal delivery revealed by multiplanar anal endosonography. BJOG 2002;109(8):942–6.

72. Tjandra JJ, Milsom JW, Schroeder T, et al. Endoluminal ultrasound is preferable to electromyography in mapping anal sphincteric defects. Dis Colon Rectum 1993;36(7):689–92.

73. Malouf AJ, Williams AB, Halligan S, et al. Prospective assessment of accuracy of endoanal MR imaging and endosonography in patients with fecal incontinence. Am J Roentgenol 2000;175(3):741–5.

74. Gold DM, Bartram CI, Halligan S, et al. Three-dimensional endoanal sonography in assessing anal canal injury. Br J Surg 1999;86(3):365–70.

75. Williams AB, Bartram CI, Modhwadia D, et al. Endocoil magnetic resonance imaging quantification of external anal sphincter atrophy. Br J Surg 2001;88(6):853–9.

2

Colonoscopy and flexible sigmoidoscopy

Siwan Thomas-Gibson
Adam Haycock

Introduction

Since flexible endoscopy of the colon was introduced in 1963 it has become the gold-standard diagnostic test for evaluation of colonic disease. Improvements in technique and technology have also led to advances in therapeutic procedures, and the boundary between endoscopic, laparoscopic and open procedures is becoming increasingly blurred. A good understanding of both the technique and technology is essential for an endoscopist to perform high-quality, safe endoscopy. This chapter gives an insight into how colonoscopy is influencing the practice of colorectal surgery.

Indications and contraindications

Flexible sigmoidoscopy vs. colonoscopy

Indications for colonoscopy or flexible sigmoidoscopy must be weighed against the risk/benefit profile. Diagnostic colonoscopy has a significantly higher risk of complications relating to sedation and bowel preparation than flexible sigmoidoscopy. Flexible sigmoidoscopy is also quicker, cheaper and easier to perform. The British Society of Gastroenterology (BSG) recommendations are that flexible sigmoidoscopy should be performed with a colonoscope (**Fig. 2.1**). However, studies have shown that in up to a quarter of cases, full examinination of the sigmoid colon is not achieved and the splenic flexure is reached only in a minority of cases.[1]

Contraindications

The only absolute contraindications to endoscopic examination of the colon are a competent patient who is unwilling to give consent or a known free colonic perforation. Relative contraindications include: acute diverticulitis, immediately postoperative patients, patients with a recent myocardial infarction (within 30 days), pulmonary embolism, severe coagulopathy (particularly for therapeutic procedures) or haemodynamic instability. In fulminant colitis, a limited examination with flexible sigmoidoscopy to ascertain extent of disease and acquire confirmatory biopsies is often helpful. In general, colonoscopy or flexible sigmoidoscopy is considered to be safe in pregnancy, but should probably be deferred in most cases if the indication does not require immediate examination.[2]

Sedation

Sedation during colonoscopy continues to be the subject of much debate and research. A recent large multicentre European audit of current practice[3] showed that most colonoscopies were done using moderate (conscious) sedation, and that although deep sedation was associated with shorter procedure times and fewer technical difficulties, it was also

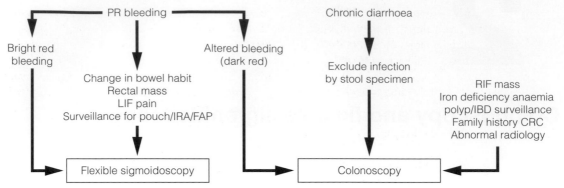

Figure 2.1 • Algorithm for determining colonoscopy or flexible sigmoidoscopy as the initial investigation of choice.

more resource intensive and required more hospitalisations for complications. Flexible sigmoidoscopy is most often performed unsedated as the use of intravenous sedation would negate many of the potential benefits of the procedure. Unsedated colonoscopy is certainly possible and practical in a subset of patients with few complications and good acceptability.[4]

> ✓ As the practice and evidence varies widely, current recommendations are to use the minimum amount of drugs within the manufacturers' guidelines to ensure patient comfort and the success of the endoscopy.[5]

Insertion technique

Insertion technique varies greatly even amongst expert colonoscopists. Technique will depend on the local circumstances, sedation practice, endoscopist preference and equipment available. However, there are some basic principles that are recognised to contribute to safe, efficient colonoscopy.

Handling and scope control

Most skilled colonoscopists now adopt the one-person, single-handed approach where the right hand is used to manipulate the shaft and the left hand operates the angulation controls. Tip control is gained by a combination of up/down angulation with the large wheel and clockwise/anticlockwise torque applied with the right hand.

Insertion and steering

A digital rectal examination should be performed to lubricate the anal canal, relax the sphincters, and detect any anal and distal rectal pathology prior to insertion. The initial view is usually a 'red-out' due to the lens pressing against the rectal mucosa. Gentle insufflation, slow withdrawal and small amounts of tip angulation are used to gain a view of the lumen.

Tips for insertion and steering

- **Pull back more, push in less.** The first rule of expert colonoscopy is to keep the shaft straight. This allows for accurate tip control, prevents stretching of the mesentery, minimises discomfort and shortens the colon by a 'concertina' effect of telescoping the bowel wall over the shaft. Pulling back often reduces acute angles of bends, disimpacts the tip of the scope and improves the view. In contrast, excessive pushing of the scope often results in formation of large loops, excessive pain, loss of one-to-one tip control and increases the risk of iatrogenic perforation.[6]
- **Insufflate little and suction frequently.** Pain or discomfort during colonoscopy is often due to stretching of the bowel wall by excessive gas insufflation. Pneumatic perforation of the right colon from over-insufflation has been reported.[7] Frequent suctioning of gas prevents this and may often allow progression of the tip through the colon by the concertina effect. The use of carbon dioxide rather than air has been shown to cause less discomfort and is widely recommended.[8]
- **Use torque frequently.** Twisting clockwise or counter-clockwise with the right hand applies torque to the shaft of the scope. With a straight shaft and bent tip, use of torque will provide lateral movement at the tip and help to stiffen the scope to prevent looping during advancement. Application of torque is also essential for loop resolution. Without the use of image guidance such as ScopeGuide, the application of torque will be determined

both by frequency of loop type and 'feel' of the instrument. The majority of sigmoid loops (N-loops, 80%; alpha loops, 10%) require clockwise torque and pull back to resolve; atypical loops (reverse sigmoid N-spiral, 1%; reverse-alpha, 5%) require anticlockwise torque.

Patient position change

Moving the patient's position from the left lateral position during both insertion and withdrawal can shift both fluid away from and air into the uppermost segment of bowel, preventing unnecessary suctioning of fluid and insufflation of gas. It can provide mechanical advantage by opening up acute bends, especially at the rectosigmoid junction, splenic and hepatic flexures. The effective use of gravity to assist the passage of the endoscope is a simple, cost-neutral, effective technique that is easily learnt. It has been shown to be effective in promoting endoscope tip advancement in two-thirds of cases.[9] However, it does require cooperation from the patient and can be difficult if heavy sedation or general anaesthesia is used (**Fig. 2.2**).

Abdominal hand pressure

The use of abdominal hand pressure aims to prevent the shaft of the endoscope looping by opposing pressure close to the anterior abdominal wall. Pressure is best used to prevent a loop from forming rather than applying it to an already formed loop, which is unlikely to be successful and may increase

the discomfort felt by the patient. Specific pressure on anterior-protruding loops is more likely to be helpful as intubation progresses than non-specific pressure.[10] Efficacy in promoting tip advancement is less than for patient position change,[9] as many loops do not protrude anteriorly. However, physicians in a recent audit unanimously advocated its use as a technique during colonoscopy.[11]

Three-dimensional imager

A non-invasive magnetic imaging system (ScopeGuide, Olympus Optical Company) has been commercially available since 2002. It uses low-voltage magnetic fields to produce a real-time, three-dimensional image of the entire colonoscope shaft in both anteroposterior and lateral views, allowing the colonoscopist to visualise the configuration of the scope within the patient (see **Fig. 2.3**). This can help determine if there is an anterior component to the loop and so assist with loop resolution, as well as aiding accurate tip location. A sensor can assist with accurate hand-pressure placement.

Two randomised controlled trials have shown improvement in caecal intubation rate and pain scores for both experts and trainees using the imager,[12,13] one trial showing a benefit in localising lesions[14] with no significant impact on completion rate or length of procedure.

Withdrawal technique

It should be remembered that the aim of colonoscopy is to visualise the whole of the colonic mucosa in order to identify pathology. A systematic review of back-to-back studies[15] has shown a polyp miss rate at colonoscopy of 22% even in expert hands, although most missed polyps were small (<1 cm). All studies investigating miss rates have shown a variation in performance between endoscopists, but this can be wide even with expert examiners (>10 000 procedures), with sensitivities ranging from 17% to 48% in one large study.[16] This implies that there is a link between individual technical skill and outcome measures.

Withdrawal time

Recent publications have stressed the importance of spending sufficient time inspecting the colonic mucosa on withdrawal as a key marker for the adequacy of the examination.

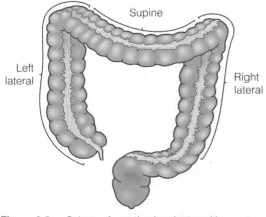

Figure 2.2 • Schema for optimal patient position change.

Supine

Left lateral

Right lateral

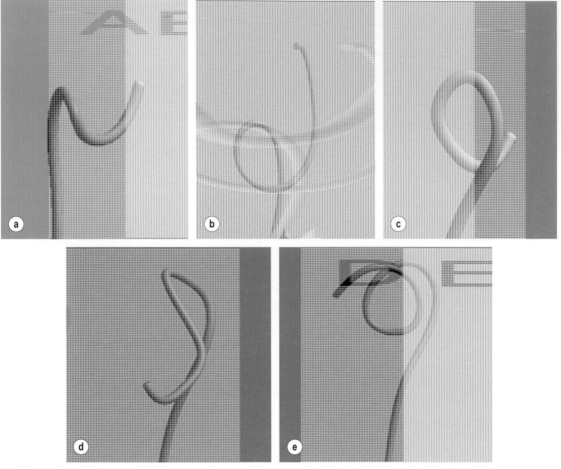

Figure 2.3 • ScopeGuide images of: **(a)** Sigmoid N-loop; **(b)** alpha loop; **(c)** reverse alpha loop; **(d)** deep transverse loop; **(e)** gamma loop.

✅✅ The current recommendation is that colonoscopists should spend 6–10 minutes during withdrawal inspecting the colonic mucosa.[17] A landmark study[18] looking specifically at withdrawal time found that endoscopists who spent longer than 6 minutes on withdrawal in a negative colonoscopy had significantly higher adenoma detection rates (ADR) than their quicker colleagues.

Optimal examination technique

Although there is little direct evidence, it seems logical that those colonoscopists who take longer to withdraw also use techniques that increase visualisation of abnormalities. In one study looking at differences in technique between two colonoscopists with different polyp miss rates,[19] a lower miss rate was judged by independent experts to have a superior withdrawal technique for each of the following examination criteria: (1) examining the proximal sides of flexures, folds and valves; (2) cleaning and suctioning; (3) adequacy of distension; and (4) adequacy of time spent viewing. A study looking at the quality of inspection at flexible sigmoidoscopy[20] has included similar criteria: (1) time spent viewing the mucosa; (2) re-examination of poorly viewed areas; (3) suctioning of fluid pools; (4) distension of the lumen; and (5) lower rectal examination.

The following continuous quality improvement targets regarding withdrawal (adapted from Rex et al.[17]) aim to standardise withdrawal technique to maximise detection rates:

1. Mean examination times during withdrawal should average at least 6–10 minutes.

2. Adenoma prevalence rates detected during colonoscopy in persons over 50 years of age undergoing first-time examination should be ≥25% in men and ≥15% in women.
3. Documentation of quality of bowel preparation in all cases.

Bowel preparation

It is self-evident that pools of fluid or faeces will obscure good visualisation of the mucosa, and many studies have looked at the effectiveness of various bowel preparations for clearing the colon prior to colonoscopy.

✔✔ Evidence-based recommendations on bowel preparation for colonoscopy have been published following an American Task Force review of the literature.[21]

It has been shown that better quality preparation at flexible sigmoidoscopy results in a higher ADR,[22] but crucially important, endoscopists with a higher ADR are more likely to be critical of the quality of bowel preparation.

Position change

The use of position change has been shown in a randomised controlled trial to improve luminal distension between the hepatic flexure and sigmoid-descending junction during colonoscope withdrawal.[23] The same schema can be used for each segment as previously illustrated for insertion (Fig. 2.2). A single-centre trial has shown that the improved visualisation that results can also improve polyp and adenoma detection rates.[24] These data require replication in large multicentre studies and may have a significant impact on technical performance for those colonoscopists who are used to using moderate or deep sedation for their examinations.

Antispasmodics

Premedication with an antispasmodic such as hyoscine N-butyl bromide (Buscopan) has been used for colonoscopy to decrease the amount of muscular spasm caused by peristalsis. Small randomised studies have shown that it can shorten the total procedure time for flexible sigmoidoscopy as compared with placebo,[25] and that it may be beneficial in terms of ease of insertion[26] and the time required for caecal intubation, total procedure time, adequacy of sedation and scales of patient comfort during colonoscopy.[27] Caution must be taken in patients with known cardiac history as it can produce a sinus tachycardia. Other antispasmodics such as glucagon and the use of warm water irrigation may be used in patients in whom anticholinergics are contraindicated, although currently there are no data showing any significant benefit.[28]

Rectal retroflexion

Colorectal cancer is most common in the distal colon, and most experts routinely perform retroflexion in the rectum. Although the evidence that this significantly improves detection rates is still being debated,[29,30] it probably allows clearer views of the proximal sides of rectal valves and the top of the anal canal. If the rectal lumen is narrow, a paediatric colonoscope or thin upper gastrointestinal (GI) endoscope can be used.

Quality assurance

There are now detailed guidelines for quality standards in colonoscopy, which include key performance indicators, measurable outcomes and minimum standards.[8,31] These aim to ensure a high-quality, effective and patient-centred service by setting benchmarks for both individual endoscopists and unit performance. Development of these guidelines has in a large measure been driven by the implementation of bowel cancer screening programmes, which involve asymptomatic individuals choosing to undergo invasive investigations. It is imperative to minimise risk for this group by provision of a safe, high-quality service. This has had the benefit of improving quality assurance standards for the whole of endoscopy.

Endoscopy training in the UK

The largest prospective study of colonoscopy practice in the UK in 2004[32] revealed poor outcomes in terms of completion and perforation rates, as well as deficiencies in almost all aspects of training. Guidelines on training have been published both in the UK and USA.[33,34] Accredited national courses in endoscopy have been developed to provide more readily available and structured training, and have now become essential components of gastroenterology training. Focus has also been placed on ensuring that those endoscopists responsible for training or performing screening procedures on healthy populations are themselves competent to do so. 'Training the Trainers' courses teach experienced endoscopists adult education theory and its application to skills training in endoscopy. Accreditation for colonoscopists wishing to undertake colorectal cancer screening is now mandatory in England and Wales. Both initiatives are aimed at maximising the provision of high-quality endoscopy and training on a national basis and not just in teaching centres. A national audit in 2011 of all colonoscopies done in England has demonstrated improvements in virtually all aspects of colonoscopy (unpublished data), including training, validating the rigorous quality assurance process undertaken in recent years.

The use of both computer and animal endoscopic simulation has now been shown to be of value in the early phase of colonoscopy training, with transfer of skills to live patients,[35] and in the management of gastrointestinal bleeding.[36] New computer simulators have been developed (Olympus Colonoscopy Simulator Endo TS-1, Olympus Optical Company) that more accurately model real-life colonoscopy and are currently undergoing evaluation.

✓ Current European recommendations are that endoscopy simulators, where available, should be used to allow training to occur in a safe, controlled environment.[37]

New optical techniques in endoscopy

There are many new developments in colonoscopic technique that may improve polyp detection and identification of pathology. These range from simple additions to the standard procedure such as the use of dye-spray, through to advanced endoscope technology such as narrow band imaging (NBI) and confocal endomicroscopy.

Chromoendoscopy

Chromoendoscopy is a technique that uses a surface dye such as indigo carmine to make irregularities in the colonic mucosa more readily apparent to the endoscopist (**Fig. 2.4**).

✓✓ The use of chromoendoscopy has been shown to significantly improve adenoma detection during surveillance of high-risk groups such as ulcerative colitis[38–40] and familial colorectal cancer syndromes.[41,42]

It has also been shown to aid identification of flat or depressed adenomas,[43] which are much more prevalent than was previously thought and have a high risk of malignant transformation. It can, however, be time-consuming and currently there is no substantive evidence for its use during routine colonoscopy.

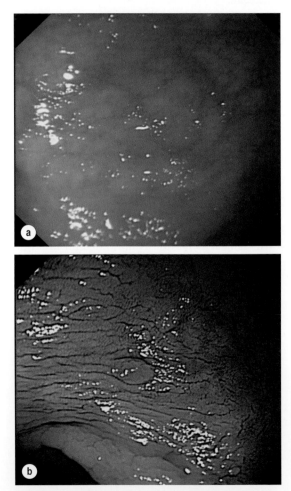

Figure 2.4 • (a) Polyp in white light. **(b)** With indigo carmine dye-spray.

Narrow band imaging (NBI)

An increased microvascular density is one of the early histological features of colonic adenoma development. NBI uses optical filters to narrow the bandwidth of white light, picking out the central spectrum to enhance the visualisation of the capillary network, thus enabling an adenoma to become more visible against the surrounding mucosa (**Fig. 2.5**). It is activated by the push of a button on enabled scopes, which has clear advantages over the use of dye-spray. NBI may have utility in high-risk groups where spotting even diminutive adenomas is important for risk stratification. In some high-risk conditions, for example hereditary non-polyposis colorectal cancer (HNPCC) patients, the use of NBI has significantly increased the ADR in back-to-back studies.[44,45] Using a classification system of vascular intensity, NBI has good sensitivity and specificity in distinguishing neoplastic and non-neoplastic polyps,[46] and can aid in prediction of histology using pit-pattern recognition (see below). Recent randomised trials have not shown significant benefit in routine endoscopy.[47,48]

High-magnification endoscopy

High-magnification endoscopes can magnify the image up to 100 times, and newer high-definition scopes have a much greater pixel density and ability to improve detail discrimination. In conjunction with dye-spray or NBI their use permits identification of a polyp's surface 'pit pattern' to assist in distinguishing between cancerous, adenomatous and non-adenomatous polyps. A classification system devised by Kudo et al. in 1994[49] has been shown to have a reasonable diagnostic accuracy (overall 86.1%, sensitivity 90.8%, specificity 72.7%) when compared to histological findings[50] (**Fig. 2.6**). There is a learning curve in identification of the patterns, however, so for inexperienced endoscopists it does not significantly reduce the number of histological samples taken. Further work is being conducted to confirm its real-world utility and establish simple classification systems.[51]

Retrograde viewing devices

New developments to augment current colonoscopy include the use of an auxiliary imaging device that is inserted into the working channel and extends

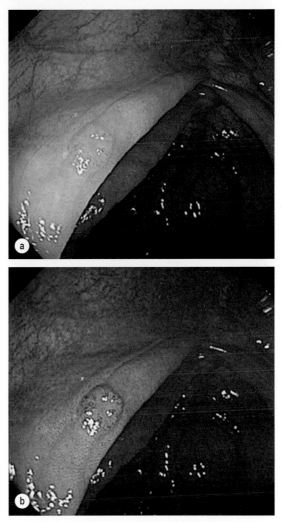

Figure 2.5 • **(a)** Polyp in white light. **(b)** With narrow band imaging.

beyond the colonoscope tip. It then retroflexes, providing a continuous retrograde view during withdrawal to detect lesions missed by the forward-viewing colonoscope. One such, the Third Eye Retroscope™ (Avantis Medical Systems Inc.), has been shown in a randomised clinical trial to increase adenoma detection rate by up to 23% compared to conventional colonoscopy.[52]

Confocal laser endomicroscopy

Confocal laser endomicroscopy combines a standard video endoscope with a miniaturised laser microscope. Using intravenous sodium fluorescein as a contrast agent, 'virtual histology' can be created, allowing visualisation of both the surface epithelium

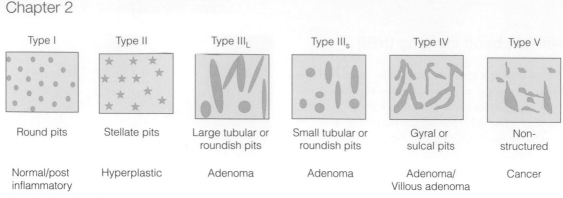

Figure 2.6 • Classification of pit pattern at high-magnification chromoendoscopy (after Kudo et al.).

and some of the lamina propria, including the micro-vasculature. Confocal endomicroscopy may have major implications in the future of colonoscopy as it can allow in vivo visualisation of cellular structures, potentially providing accurate identification of colonic intra-epithelial neoplasia and carcinoma. This may enable 'smart' biopsy targeting, increasing detection rates and decreasing histopathological workload.

Endoscopic therapy

One of the exciting benefits of improving endoscopic skills and technology is the increasingly successful application of novel therapeutic techniques. Therapy that previously required open invasive procedures can now be performed in a minimally invasive way.

Basic therapy

Polypectomy

The ability to remove adenomatous tissue endoscopically forms the basis of all cancer prevention and surveillance programmes. The resectability of a polyp depends on its size, characteristics and accessibility. Polyps that are unlikely to be removable endoscopically are those with submucosal invasion, large sessile polyps extending beyond 50% of the bowel wall circumference, large rectal polyps extending beyond the dentate line, or lesions encircling the appendix orifice.[53]

Small polyps less than 4 mm in size can be removed by hot biopsy, cold forceps or cold snare. Good hot biopsy technique is essential and involves tenting of the mucosa to concentrate a short burst of current through a pseudo-stalk, thereby heating directly below the polyp, but not across the bowel wall.[54] However, hot biopsy is falling out of favour due to increased (and perhaps unnecessary) risk of diathermy injury causing delayed bleeding or even perforation, and in general should be employed only distal to the splenic flexure, if at all. Cold snare is a safe alternative for such diminutive polyps. Larger stalked polyps are best removed using a conventional large or mini-snare. The stalk should be transected approximately halfway between the polyp and the bowel wall. This ensures a clear resection margin whilst leaving sufficient stalk in situ to facilitate endoscopic treatment should post-polypectomy bleeding occur. Diathermy unit settings should be chosen to ensure enough coagulating current is applied to allow adequate haemostasis of the blood vessels within the polyp stalk. A validated Direct Observation of Polypectomy Skills (DOPyS) assessment tool has been developed to assist with the training and evaluation of polypectomy technique,[55] and is now in clinical use for competency assessment of trainees and in the Bowel Cancer Screening accreditation process in England.

Retrieval of the polyp is important to determine the histology and grade of dysplasia. Small polyps can be sucked through the scope into a polyp trap, while larger polyps can be grasped or snared and withdrawn with the scope. Retrieval baskets or Roth nets are particularly useful for retrieving more than one piece of tissue or multiple polyps.

Endoscopic mucosal resection (EMR)

EMR involves injection of fluid into the submucosal space to lift the mucosa (and the polyp) away from the muscle layer of the bowel wall (**Fig. 2.7**). This facilitates removal of sessile or flat lesions, reducing the risk of thermal injury to the bowel wall.[56] The authors found the addition of adrenaline(1:200 000)

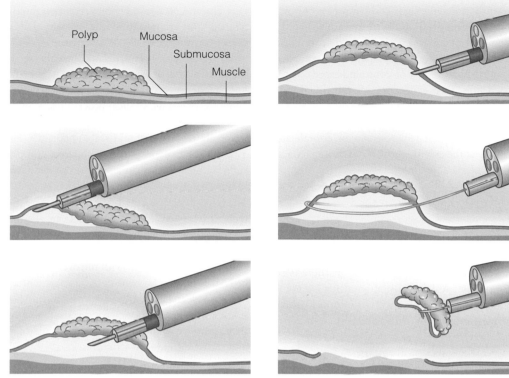

Figure 2.7 • Technique for endoscopic mucosal resection.

to improve haemostasis and a few drops of methylene blue to help differentiate the submucosal plane helpful. Large lesions (>2 cm) can be removed in a piecemeal fashion safely using a submucosal lift.

✔✔ Polyp recurrence may be reduced following piecemeal resection by the judicious use of argon plasma coagulation (APC) to destroy small areas of residual polyp around the resected margin.[57]

The 'non-lifting' sign, when a 'de novo' polyp fails to lift with a submucosal injection, should raise a suspicion of malignant invasion of the submucosa. Lesions that do not lift should be biopsied, tattooed and referred for surgical resection (see Chapter 17 for tattoo protocol).

Lower gastrointestinal (GI) bleeding investigation

The lower GI tract accounts for a quarter to a third of all hospitalised cases of GI bleeding,[58] with diverticular disease being by far the most common cause. Colitis, cancer, polyps and angiodysplasia account for the majority of the rest. Most lower GI bleeding stops spontaneously and in those cases an elective colonoscopy with standard bowel preparation is appropriate. In the uncommon case of continued bleeding, endoscopic therapy is the treatment of choice as it is currently considered safer, with a greater diagnostic yield, than urgent angiography and embolisation.[59] An urgent therapeutic colonoscopy after rapid purge can decrease both the recurrence of bleeding and the need for surgical intervention.[60] Surgery is reserved for cases of recurrent, uncontrolled or massive bleeding.

Colonic decompression

The three main causes of bowel obstruction are cancer, diverticular disease and a sigmoid volvulus. Flexible sigmoidoscopy with placement of a decompression tube is the initial treatment of choice for a volvulus. It has a high initial success rate (78%) but is only a temporising measure as recurrence is common and elective surgery is therefore still considered the definitive treatment. Emergency surgery is reserved for a volvulus unresponsive to endoscopic therapy or for patients with bowel ischaemia or peritonitis.

Acute colonic pseudo-obstruction (Ogilvie's syndrome) may mimic the signs and symptoms of bowel obstruction. It may be initially treated conservatively with removal of any triggering factor(s), mobilisation and the use of a parasympathomimetic agent such as neostigmine (if not contraindicated). If this approach fails, then endoscopic placement of a decompression tube is generally accepted as the first invasive therapeutic manoeuvre.[58] Emergency surgery is again only indicated in resistant or complicated cases, such as those with perforation or ischaemia.

Advanced therapy

Endoscopic submucosal dissection (ESD)

ESD is a technique that has been developed for 'en-bloc' resection of large lesions in the gastrointestinal tract. A deep, submucosal lift is created using a viscous solution such as sodium hyaluronate or 10% glycerine. Mucosal and submucosal incisions are made using a modified needle knife to dissect the mucosa from the submucosa. A transparent hood is attached to the endoscope tip to help retract tissue and maintain the submucosal field of view. The benefit of this technique is that it produces excellent specimens for histological analysis, but the technique itself is difficult and success depends on excellent endoscopic and haemostatic skills. It is also quite time-consuming, usually taking between 2 and 3 hours in expert hands, and should be performed only when surgical backup is available. It has only recently been applied in the colon, and the current data are limited to small case–control studies.[61–63] Successful en-bloc resection has been reported in 74–98.6% of cases, with a perforation risk in the colon of around 5% in expert hands. However, there is a steep learning curve, with poorer results and higher complication rates in less expert hands.[64,65]

Stricture dilatation and stenting

The dilatation of colonic strictures is generally reserved for benign disease, whereas the use of self-expandable metal stents (SEMS) is usually indicated for malignant disease.

Through-the-scope (TTS) balloon dilatators have been used in the management of strictures associated with inflammatory bowel disease, non-steroidal anti-inflammatory drug (NSAID)-induced colonic strictures and diverticular strictures. Success rates vary (around 50%), sometimes requiring multiple attempts,[66] but complication rates remain high, with a risk of perforation or bleeding between 4% and 11%.

SEMS are usually inserted through the scope and can be deployed as far as the proximal ascending colon. Preoperative stenting of malignant strictures can allow for one-stage surgical procedures, allowing en-bloc resection of both the stent and tumour in theatre in a fully resuscitated and stable patient.[67] This has a favourable patient outcome and cost compared to surgical intervention alone, and no adverse effect on tumour recurrence rates or survival has been shown.[68] The overall success rate of preoperative stent placement is over 85%. Covered stents can also be used for palliation of malignant strictures, with patency established up to a year,[69] although the risk of stent migration is higher than with uncovered stents.

SEMS can also be considered as a potential therapy for selected benign strictures and has been reported with anastomotic strictures unresponsive to dilatation,[70] Crohn's disease,[71] diverticular disease[67] and radiation-induced strictures.[72]

Natural orifice transluminal endoscopic surgery (NOTES)

As technology and endoscopic skill evolve, the lines between what is possible endoscopically, laparoscopically and traditionally have become increasingly blurred. NOTES involves the intentional puncture of one of the viscera (e.g. stomach, rectum, vagina, urinary bladder) with an endoscope to access the abdominal cavity and perform an intra-abdominal operation. It is currently in the early stages of development and although there are now many published clinical case series demonstrating feasibility,[73] most studies have concluded that there is a need to develop new endoscopic instruments to improve outcomes prior to wider application.

Competing technologies

Currently, optical colonoscopy remains the gold-standard test for examination of the colon due to its relatively high pathology detection rate and the ability to perform therapy. However, newer techniques are emerging that may be considered as 'disruptive technologies' that will undoubtedly change the current position.

Computed tomography colonography (or virtual colonoscopy)

Computed tomography colonography (CTC), also known as virtual colonoscopy (VC; or 'CT pneumocolon'), is now an established technique for detecting colon cancer and colonic polyps.[74] VC comprises two low-dose CT scans of the abdomen and pelvis, and is less invasive than optical colonoscopy, requires no conscious sedation and is better tolerated by patients. The diagnostic performance characteristics are potentially comparable to expert optical colonoscopy with large polyp (>10 mm in maximal diameter) sensitivity exceeding 90% and cancer sensitivity of 96%,[75] but it lacks the facility for mucosal biopsy or polyp removal. It has, however, now superseded barium enema as the radiological test of choice for the colon.

Self-propelling colonoscopes

One disadvantage of traditional optical colonoscopy is the prolonged training required for expertise. There would be significant advantages to providing the same examination and potential for therapy without the need for an experienced operator. A disposable, self-propelling and self-navigating colonoscope (Aer-O-Scope, GI View Ltd., Ramat Gan, Israel) has been developed. It advances through the colon by means of CO_2 introduction between a rectal balloon and a balloon at the tip of the endoscope. It has been shown in porcine models to provide a sensitive inspection of the colonic mucosa without the need for tip manipulation[76] and to be safe in initial human testing.[77] Further evaluation is ongoing.

Colon capsule

Wireless capsule endoscopy (WCE) is a safe, minimally invasive, non-sedation requiring, patient-friendly modality to visualise the bowel, and is now considered first line for investigation of small bowel disease. The development of the PillCam colon capsule (Given Imaging Ltd, Yoqneam, Israel) aims to widen the application to investigation of colonic disease. It is attractive for similar reasons and, unlike optical colonoscopy, only requires expertise in image interpretation. Initial studies with the original PillCam Colon 1[78,79] found that for patients with positive findings, the rates of detection were similar to those obtained with conventional colonoscopy, with no serious adverse events reported. The second-generation PillCam Colon Capsule 2 has a wider field of view and adaptive frame rate, and a multicentre feasibility study has demonstrated sensitivity and specificity of 89% and 76%, respectively, for polyps >6 mm.[80]

Conclusions

This chapter has given an overview of the role of flexible sigmoidoscopy and colonoscopy in the diagnosis, treatment and prevention of colorectal disease. Traditional optical endoscopy is becoming more refined and new technologies are emerging that will impact on the need for open or laparoscopic surgery. A focus on training and continual skill development is essential for all those endoscopists wishing to perform high-quality, safe endoscopy.

Key points

- Good technique is vital for high-quality safe endoscopy.
- Sedation practice should be standardised and use the minimum amount of drug required for patient comfort.
- Withdrawal times should be in excess of 6 minutes in normal colonoscopies.
- Advanced imaging techniques are now becoming more widely available and may impact on current practice.
- All endoscopists should be familiar with basic therapeutic techniques (polypectomy, diathermy, decompression) and consider referral for advanced therapy (EMR, ESD, stenting).
- Competing technologies are evolving and need to be evaluated for their utility in clinical practice.

References

1. Painter J, Saunders DB, Bell GD, et al. Depth of insertion at flexible sigmoidoscopy: implications for colorectal cancer screening and instrument design. Endoscopy 1999;31(3):227–31.

2. Siddiqui U, Proctor D. Flexible sigmoidoscopy and colonoscopy during pregnancy. Gastrointest Endosc Clin N Am 2006;16(1):59–69.

3. Froehlich F, Harris JK, Wietlisbach V, et al. Current sedation and monitoring practice for colonoscopy: an International Observational Study (EPAGE). Endoscopy 2006;38(5):461–9.

4. Takahashi Y, Tanaka H, Kinjo M, et al. Sedation-free colonoscopy. Dis Colon Rectum 2005;48(4):855–9.

5. Teague R. Safety and sedation during endoscopic procedures. British Society of Gastroenterology; 2003.

6. Waye J, Rex D, Williams C. Colonoscopy principles and practice. Blackwell; 2003.

7. Luchette FA, Doerr RJ, Kelly K, et al. Colonoscopic impaction in left colon strictures resulting in right colon pneumatic perforation. Surg Endosc 1992;6(6):273–6.

8. Segnan N, Patnick J, von Karsa L. European guidelines for quality assurance in colorectal cancer screening and diagnosis. 1st ed. European Commission; 2009.

9. Shah SG, Saunders BP, Brooker JC, et al. Magnetic imaging of colonoscopy: an audit of looping, accuracy and ancillary maneuvers. Gastrointest Endosc 2000;52(1):1–8.

10. Waye JD, Yessayan SA, Lewis BS, et al. The technique of abdominal pressure in total colonoscopy. Gastrointest Endosc 1991;37(2):147–51.

11. Prechel JA, Young CJ, Hucke R, et al. The importance of abdominal pressure during colonoscopy: techniques to assist the physician and to minimize injury to the patient and assistant. Gastroenterol Nurs 2005;28(3):232–6.

12. Hoff G, Bretthauer M, Dahler S, et al. Improvement in caecal intubation rate and pain reduction by using 3-dimensional magnetic imaging for unsedated colonoscopy: a randomized trial of patients referred for colonoscopy. Scand J Gastroenterol 2007;42(7):885–9.

13. Shah SG, Brooker JC, Williams CB, et al. Effect of magnetic endoscope imaging on colonoscopy performance: a randomised controlled trial. Lancet 2000;356(9243):1718–22.

14. Cheung HY, Chung CC, Kwok SY, et al. Improvement in colonoscopy performance with adjunctive magnetic endoscope imaging: a randomized controlled trial. Endoscopy 2006;38(3):214–7.

15. van Rijn JC, Reitsma JB, Stoker J, et al. Polyp miss rate determined by tandem colonoscopy: a systematic review. Am J Gastroenterol 2006;101(2):343–50.

16. Rex DK, Cutler CS, Lemmel GT, et al. Colonoscopic miss rates of adenomas determined by back-to-back colonoscopies. Gastroenterology 1997;112(1):24–8.

17. Rex DK, Bond JH, Winawer S, et al. Quality in the technical performance of colonoscopy and the continuous quality improvement process for colonoscopy: recommendations of the U.S. Multi-Society Task Force on Colorectal Cancer. Am J Gastroenterol 2002;97(6):1296–308.
Guidelines on technical performance and quality improvement for colonoscopy produced by the American Task Force.

18. Barclay RL, Vicari JJ, Doughty AS, et al. Colonoscopic withdrawal times and adenoma detection during screening colonoscopy. N Engl J Med 2006;355(24):2533–41.
Observational study of 12 experienced colonoscopists over 7882 colonoscopies showing a 10-fold difference in ADR between endoscopists and a significant difference in those who spend more or less than 6 minutes during withdrawal in normal colonoscopies.

19. Rex DK. Colonoscopic withdrawal technique is associated with adenoma miss rates. Gastrointest Endosc 2000;51(1):33–6.

20. Thomas-Gibson S, Rogers PA, Suzuki N, et al. Development of a video assessment scoring method to determine the accuracy of endoscopist performance at screening flexible sigmoidoscopy. Endoscopy 2006;38(3):218–25.

21. Wexner SD, Beck DE, Baron TH, et al. A consensus document on bowel preparation before colonoscopy: prepared by a Task Force from the American Society of Colon and Rectal Surgeons (ASCRS), the American Society for Gastrointestinal Endoscopy (ASGE), and the Society of American Gastrointestinal and Endoscopic Surgeons (SAGES). Dis Colon Rectum 2006;49(6):792–809.
Comprehensive literature review and recommendations from the American Task Force.

22. Thomas-Gibson S, Rogers P, Cooper S, et al. Judgement of the quality of bowel preparation at screening flexible sigmoidoscopy is associated with variability in adenoma detection rates. Endoscopy 2006;38(5):456–60.

23. East JE, Suzuki N, Arebi N, et al. Position changes improve visibility during colonoscope withdrawal: a randomized, blinded, crossover trial. Gastrointest Endosc 2007;65(2):263–9.

24. East JE, Bassett P, Arebi N, et al. Dynamic patient position changes during colonoscope withdrawal increase adenoma detection: a randomized, crossover trial. Gastrointest Endosc 2011;73(3):456–63.

25. Saunders BP, Elsby B, Boswell AM, et al. Intravenous antispasmodic and patient-controlled analgesia are of benefit for screening flexible sigmoidoscopy. Gastrointest Endosc 1995;42(2):123–7.

26. Saunders BP, Williams CB. Premedication with intravenous antispasmodic speeds colonoscope insertion. Gastrointest Endosc 1996;43(3):209–11.

27. Marshall JB, Patel M, Mahajan RJ, et al. Benefit of intravenous antispasmodic (hyoscyamine sulfate) as premedication for colonoscopy. Gastrointest Endosc 1999;49(6):720–6.

28. Cutler CS, Rex DK, Hawes RH, et al. Does routine intravenous glucagon administration facilitate colonoscopy? A randomized trial. Gastrointest Endosc 1995;42(4):346–50.

29. Chu Q, Petros JG. Extraperitoneal rectal perforation due to retroflexion fiberoptic proctoscopy. Am Surg 1999;65(1):81–5.

30. Hanson JM, Atkin WS, Cunliffe WJ, et al. Rectal retroflexion: an essential part of lower gastrointestinal endoscopic examination. Dis Colon Rectum 2001;44(11):1706–8.

31. Quality assurance guidelines for colonoscopy. NHS Cancer Screening Programmes; 2011.

32. Bowles CJ, Leicester R, Romaya C, et al. A prospective study of colonoscopy practice in the UK today: are we adequately prepared for national colorectal cancer screening tomorrow? Gut 2004;53(2):277–83.

33. ASGE, American Society for Gastrointestinal Endoscopy. Principles of training in gastrointestinal endoscopy. Gastrointest Endosc 1999;49(6):845–53.

34. Guidelines for the Training, Appraisal and Assessment of Trainees in Gastrointestinal Endoscopy. accessed at http://www.thejag.org.uk/JAG_2004.pdf; 2004.

35. Park J, MacRae H, Musselman LJ, et al. Randomized controlled trial of virtual reality simulator training: transfer to live patients. Am J Surg 2007;194(2):205–11.

36. Hochberger J, Matthes K, Maiss J, et al. Training with the compactEASIE biologic endoscopy simulator significantly improves hemostatic technical skill of gastroenterology fellows: a randomized controlled comparison with clinical endoscopy training alone. Gastrointest Endosc 2005;61(2):204–15.

37. Axon AT, Aabakken L, Malfertheiner P, et al. Recommendations of the ESGE workshop on Ethics in Teaching and Learning Endoscopy. First European Symposium on Ethics in Gastroenterology and Digestive Endoscopy, Kos, Greece, June 2003. Endoscopy 2003;35(9):761–4.

38. Hurlstone DP, Sanders DS, McAlindon ME, et al. High-magnification chromoscopic colonoscopy in ulcerative colitis: a valid tool for in vivo optical biopsy and assessment of disease extent. Endoscopy 2006;38(12):1213–7.
    Biphasic examination with 1000 images from 300 patients obtained via conventional or magnification imaging. Magnification imaging was significantly better than conventional colonoscopy for predicting disease extent in vivo ($P < 0.0001$).

39. Kiesslich R, Fritsch J, Holtmann M, et al. Methylene blue-aided chromoendoscopy for the detection of intraepithelial neoplasia and colon cancer in ulcerative colitis. Gastroenterology 2003;124(4):880–8.
    Randomised controlled trial of 165 patients showing a significantly better correlation between the endoscopic assessment of degree ($P=0.0002$) and extent (89% vs. 52%; $P < 0.0001$) of colonic inflammation and the histopathological findings in the chromoendoscopy group compared with the conventional colonoscopy group. More targeted biopsies were possible and significantly more neoplasias were detected (32 vs. 10; $P = 0.003$).

40. Rutter MD, Saunders BP, Schofield G, et al. Pancolonic indigo carmine dye spraying for the detection of dysplasia in ulcerative colitis. Gut 2004;53(2):256–60.
    Back-to-back colonoscopies in 100 patients showing significantly more dysplasia detection with chromoendoscopy and targeted biopsies ($P=0.02$). Chromoendoscopy required fewer biopsies (157 vs. 2904) yet detected nine dysplastic lesions, seven of which were only visible after indigo carmine application.

41. Hurlstone DP, Karajeh M, Cross SS, et al. The role of high-magnification-chromoscopic colonoscopy in hereditary nonpolyposis colorectal cancer screening: a prospective "back-to-back" endoscopic study. Am J Gastroenterol 2005;100(10):2167–73.
    Back-to-back colonoscopies in 25 asymptomatic HNPCC patients. Pan-chromoscopy identified significantly more adenomas than conventional colonoscopy ($P=0.001$) and a significantly higher number of flat adenomas ($P=0.004$).

42. Lecomte T, Cellier C, Meatchi T, et al. Chromoendoscopic colonoscopy for detecting preneoplastic lesions in hereditary nonpolyposis colorectal cancer syndrome. Clin Gastroenterol Hepatol 2005;3(9):897–902.
    Back-to-back colonoscopies in 36 asymptomatic HNPCC patients. The use of chromoendoscopy significantly increased the detection rate of adenomas in the proximal colon, from 3 of 33 patients to 10 of 33 patients ($P=0.045$).

43. Hurlstone DP, Cross SS, Adam I, et al. Efficacy of high magnification chromoscopic colonoscopy for the diagnosis of neoplasia in flat and depressed lesions of the colorectum: a prospective analysis. Gut 2004;53(2):284–90.

44. East JE, Suzuki N, Bassett P, et al. Narrow band imaging with magnification for the characterization of small and diminutive colonic polyps: pit pattern and vascular pattern intensity. Endoscopy 2008;40(10):811–7.

45. East JE, Suzuki N, Saunders BP. Comparison of magnified pit pattern interpretation with narrow band imaging versus chromoendoscopy for diminutive colonic polyps: a pilot study. Gastrointest Endosc 2007;66(2):310–6.

46. Tischendorf JJ, Wasmuth HE, Koch A, et al. Value of magnifying chromoendoscopy and narrow band imaging (NBI) in classifying colorectal polyps: a prospective controlled study. Endoscopy 2007;39(12):1092–6.

47. Adler A, Pohl H, Papanikolaou IS, et al. A prospective randomized study on narrow-band imaging versus conventional colonoscopy for adenoma detection: does NBI induce a learning effect? Gut 2007;57(1):59–64.

48. Rex DK, Helbig CC. High yields of small and flat adenomas with high-definition colonoscopes using either white light or narrow band imaging. Gastroenterology 2007;133(1):42–7.

49. Kudo S, Hirota S, Nakajima T, et al. Colorectal tumours and pit pattern. J Clin Pathol 1994;47(10):880–5.

50. Liu HH, Kudo SE, Juch JP. Pit pattern analysis by magnifying chromoendoscopy for the diagnosis of colorectal polyps. J Formos Med Assoc 2003;102(3):178–82.

51. Tanaka S, Sano Y. Aim to unify the narrow band imaging (NBI) magnifying classification for colorectal tumors: current status in Japan from a summary of the consensus symposium in the 79th Annual Meeting of the Japan Gastroenterological Endoscopy Society. Dig Endosc 2011;23(Suppl. 1):131–9.

52. Leufkens AM, DeMarco DC, Rastogi A, et al. Effect of a retrograde-viewing device on adenoma detection rate during colonoscopy: the TERRACE study. Gastrointest Endosc 2011;73(3):480–9.

53. Waye JD. New methods of polypectomy. Gastrointest Endosc Clin N Am 1997;7(3):413–22.

54. Williams CB. Small polyps: the virtues and the dangers of hot biopsy. Gastrointest Endosc 1991;37(3):394–5.

55. Gupta S, Anderson J, Bhandari P, et al. Development and validation of a novel method for assessing competency in polypectomy: direct observation of polypectomy skills. Gastrointest Endosc 2011;73(6):1232–9 e2.

56. Waye JD. Endoscopic mucosal resection of colon polyps. Gastrointest Endosc Clin N Am 2001;11(3):537–48, vii.

57. Brooker JC, Saunders BP, Shah SG, et al. Treatment with argon plasma coagulation reduces recurrence after piecemeal resection of large sessile colonic polyps: a randomized trial and recommendations. Gastrointest Endosc 2002;55(3):371–5.
Patients with apparent complete excision of adenomatous polyps were randomised to application of APC to the margins or not. Postpolypectomy application of APC reduced recurrence at 3 months (1/10 APC, 7/11 no APC; $P = 0.02$).

58. Peura DA, Lanza FL, Gostout CJ, et al. The American College of Gastroenterology Bleeding Registry: preliminary findings. Am J Gastroenterol 1997;92(6):924–8.

59. Zuckerman GR, Prakash C. Acute lower intestinal bleeding. Part II: Etiology, therapy, and outcomes. Gastrointest Endosc 1999;49(2):228–38.

60. Jensen DM, Machicado GA, Jutabha R, et al. Urgent colonoscopy for the diagnosis and treatment of severe diverticular hemorrhage. N Engl J Med 2000;342(2):78–82.

61. Hurlstone DP, Atkinson R, Sanders DS, et al. Achieving R0 resection in the colorectum using endoscopic submucosal dissection. Br J Surg 2007;94(12):1536–42.

62. Tamegai Y, Saito Y, Masaki N, et al. Endoscopic submucosal dissection: a safe technique for colorectal tumors. Endoscopy 2007;39(5):418–22.

63. Onozato Y, Kakizaki S, Ishihara H, et al. Endoscopic submucosal dissection for rectal tumors. Endoscopy 2007;39(5):423–7.

64. Farhat S, Chaussade S, Ponchon T, et al. Endoscopic submucosal dissection in a European setting. A multi-institutional report of a technique in development. Endoscopy 2011;43(8):664–70.

65. Kim ES, Cho KB, Park KS, et al. Factors predictive of perforation during endoscopic submucosal dissection for the treatment of colorectal tumors. Endoscopy 2011;43(7):573–8.

66. Saunders BP, Brown GJ, Lemann M, et al. Balloon dilation of ileocolonic strictures in Crohn's disease. Endoscopy 2004;36(11):1001–7.

67. Baron TH, Harewood GC. Enteral self-expandable stents. Gastrointest Endosc 2003;58(3):421–33.

68. Carne PW, Frye JN, Robertson GM, et al. Stents or open operation for palliation of colorectal cancer: a retrospective, cohort study of perioperative outcome and long-term survival. Dis Colon Rectum 2004;47(9):1455–61.

69. Spinelli P, Mancini A. Use of self-expanding metal stents for palliation of rectosigmoid cancer. Gastrointest Endosc 2001;53(2):203–6.

70. Guan YS, Sun L, Li X, et al. Successful management of a benign anastomotic colonic stricture with self-expanding metallic stents: a case report. World J Gastroenterol 2004;10(23):3534–6.

71. Matsuhashi N, Nakajima A, Suzuki A, et al. Long-term outcome of non-surgical strictureplasty using metallic stents for intestinal strictures in Crohn's disease. Gastrointest Endosc 2000;51(3):343–5.

72. Yates 3rd MR, Baron TH. Treatment of a radiation-induced sigmoid stricture with an expandable metal stent. Gastrointest Endosc 1999;50(3):422–6.

73. Moris DN, Bramis KJ, Mantonakis EI, et al. Surgery via natural orifices in human beings: yesterday, today, tomorrow. Am J Surg 2011;Dec 27. Epub ahead of print.

74. Burling D, Taylor SA, Halligan S. Virtual colonoscopy: current status and future directions. Gastrointest Endosc Clin N Am 2005;15(4):773–95.

75. Halligan S, Taylor SA. CT colonography: results and limitations. Eur J Radiol 2007;61(3):400–8.

76. Arber N, Grinshpon R, Pfeffer J, et al. Proof-of-concept study of the Aer-O-Scope omnidirectional colonoscopic viewing system in ex vivo and in vivo porcine models. Endoscopy 2007;39(5):412–7.

77. Vucelic B, Rex D, Pulanic R, et al. The Aer-O-Scope: proof of concept of a pneumatic, skill-independent, self-propelling, self-navigating colonoscope. Gastroenterology 2006;130(3):672–7.

78. Eliakim R, Fireman Z, Gralnek IM, et al. Evaluation of the PillCam Colon capsule in the detection of colonic pathology: results of the first multicenter, prospective, comparative study. Endoscopy 2006;38(10):963–70.

79. Schoofs N, Deviere J, Van Gossum A. PillCam colon capsule endoscopy compared with colonoscopy for colorectal tumor diagnosis: a prospective pilot study. Endoscopy 2006;38(10):971–7.

80. Eliakim R, Yassin K, Niv Y, et al. Prospective multicenter performance evaluation of the second-generation colon capsule compared with colonoscopy. Endoscopy 2009;41(12):1026–31.

3

Inherited bowel cancer

Sue Clark
Andrew Latchford

Introduction

Individuals develop colorectal cancer as a result of interaction between genotype and the environment to which they are exposed. The lifetime risk of colorectal cancer in the UK population is about 5%. As it is common, many people by chance alone have at least one affected relative;[1] as the number of affected relatives increases, so does the risk of developing the disease.[2] As far as genetic factors are concerned, there is a spectrum of risk: at one end are those with no particular genetic predisposition, and at the other those who will inevitably develop bowel cancer. Between the extremes lie those whose genetic constitution plays some role. While open to error, it is possible to divide the population into three broad categories of risk for colorectal cancer: low, moderate and high risk.

In the high-risk group, the contribution of inheritance (genotype) is overwhelming, though environmental influences may modify disease severity (phenotype). It is this minority (accounting for less than 5% of large bowel cancer) that is traditionally described as being at risk of 'inherited bowel cancer'.

In the low- and moderate-risk groups, genotype may still contribute to risk but less markedly, and is thought to play a part in about 30% of colorectal cancers.[3] This may be due to low penetrance genes that influence dietary carcinogen metabolism.

This chapter deals predominantly with those in the high-risk group. Although these individuals comprise a minority of those at risk overall, there is sufficient knowledge about the specific syndromes that fall within this category to provide important opportunities for cancer prevention.

Assessment of risk

The crucial step in allocating individuals to one of these risk categories is the documentation of an accurate family history, which in turn allows an empirical assessment of risk.[2] It should focus on the site and age at diagnosis of all cancers in family members, as well as the presence of related features such as colorectal adenomas. This can be time-consuming, especially when the information needs to be verified. Few surgeons are able to devote the necessary time or skill to do this satisfactorily, and it is here that family cancer clinics or registries for inherited bowel cancer have an important role.[4]

A full personal history should also be taken, with particular attention focused on:

- symptoms (e.g. rectal bleeding, change in bowel habit) that should be investigated as usual;
- previous large bowel polyps;
- previous large bowel cancers;
- cancers at other sites;
- other risk factors for colorectal cancer (inflammatory bowel disease, ureterosigmoidostomy, acromegaly); these conditions are not discussed further in this chapter, but may warrant surveillance of the large bowel.

The family history has many limitations, particularly in small families. Other difficulties arise because of incorrect information or early death of individuals before they develop cancers. A vast range of complex pedigrees arise, and rather than try to devise guidelines to cover all of them, common sense is needed. If a family seems to fall between risk groups it is safest to manage the family as if in the higher risk group. Despite this, some families will appear to be at high risk simply because of chance clustering of truly sporadic cancer while some, particularly small families with Lynch syndrome, will be inadvertently assigned to the low- or moderate-risk groups. Even in families affected with an autosomal dominant condition, 50% of family members will not have inherited the causative mutation and will therefore not be at any increased risk of developing cancer.

Family histories evolve, so that the allocation of an individual to a particular risk group may change if further family members develop tumours. It is important that patients are informed of this, particularly if they are in the low- or moderate-risk groups and therefore not undergoing regular surveillance.

Low-risk group

Individuals in this group have:

1. no personal history of bowel cancer; no confirmed family history of bowel cancer; or
2. no first-degree relative (i.e. parent, sibling or child) with bowel cancer; or
3. one first-degree relative with bowel cancer diagnosed at age 50 years or older.

Moderate-risk group

This has been divided into high and lower risk subgroups.

Low-moderate risk

This group comprises:

1. those with one affected relative diagnosed under 50 years; or
2. two affected first-degree relatives diagnosed at age 60 years or older.

High-moderate risk

This group comprises those with:

1. three or more affected relatives in a first-degree kinship (none under 50 years); or
2. two affected relatives diagnosed under 60 years (or with a mean age at diagnosis under 60 years) in a first-degree kinship.

High-risk group

This category encompasses Lynch syndrome and the various polyposis syndromes. Criteria for inclusion include:

1. member of a family with known familial adenomatous polyposis (FAP) or other polyposis syndrome; or
2. member of a family with known Lynch syndrome; or
3. pedigree suggestive of autosomal dominantly inherited colorectal (or other Lynch syndrome-associated) cancer; or
4. pedigree indicative of autosomal recessive inheritance, suggestive of MYH-associated polyposis (MAP).

Diagnosis of the polyposis syndromes is comparatively straightforward as there is a recognisable phenotype in each. Lynch syndrome is much more difficult as there is no such characteristic phenotype, other than the occurrence of cancers.

Management

Low-risk group

The risk of bowel cancer even in these individuals may be up to twice the average risk,[2] although this tends to be expressed after the sixth decade of life.

> ✔ There is no evidence to support invasive surveillance in this group.[5]

It is important to explain to these individuals that they are at only marginally increased risk of developing colorectal cancer, and that this risk is not sufficient to outweigh the disadvantages of colonoscopy. They should be aware of the symptoms of colorectal cancer, and the importance of reporting if further members of the family develop tumours. Population screening for colorectal cancer has recently been introduced in the UK, and individuals in this risk category should be encouraged to take part.

Moderate-risk group

✅ There is a three- to sixfold relative risk for individuals in this category,[2] but probably only a marginal benefit from surveillance.[5]

Part of the reason for this is that the incidence of colorectal cancer is very low in the young and rises markedly in the elderly. Even those aged 50 who have a sixfold relative risk by virtue of their family history are less likely to develop colorectal cancer in the following 10 years than are 60-year-olds at average risk.[6]

✅ Current recommendations[5] are that individuals at high-moderate risk should be offered colonoscopy 5-yearly starting at 50 years of age; those in the low-moderate risk group should be offered a one-off colonoscopy aged 55 years.

If polyps are found, follow-up is modified accordingly. Flexible sigmoidoscopy is not sufficient, as neoplasms in individuals with a strong family history are often proximal; if the caecum is not reached, virtual colonoscopy should be performed.

Again, these individuals should be informed of the symptoms of colorectal cancer, the importance of reporting changes in family history and that they should take part in population screening when they reach the appropriate age.

High-risk group

There is up to a 1 in 2 chance of inheriting a lifetime risk that can be in excess of 50% of developing bowel cancer in this group, and referral to a clinical genetics service is essential. The polyposis syndromes are usually diagnosed from the phenotype, supplemented by genetic testing. Diagnostic confusion can arise, particularly in cases where there are adenomatous polyps insufficient to be diagnostic of FAP. This may occur in MAP, FAP with an attenuated phenotype, or Lynch syndrome. A careful search for extracolonic features, mismatch repair

immunohistochemistry and microsatellite instability assessment of tumour tissue, and germline mutation detection can sometimes help. Despite this, the diagnosis in some families remains in doubt. In these circumstances the family members should be offered thorough surveillance.

Lynch syndrome

Lynch syndrome is inherited in an autosomal dominant fashion, is responsible for about 2% of colorectal cancers and is the commonest of the inherited bowel cancer syndromes. The terminology in this area is extremely confusing and has recently been revised.[7] Labelled first as the 'cancer family syndrome', the name was changed to hereditary non-polyposis colorectal cancer (HNPCC) to distinguish it from the polyposis syndromes and to highlight the absence of the large numbers of colorectal adenomas found in FAP. However, scanty adenomatous polyps are a feature of Lynch syndrome.

Various different diagnostic criteria have been used, including different definitions based on family history. Mutations in mismatch repair (MMR) genes were identified in some, but not all, families with an apparent dominantly inherited cancer syndrome. It has been suggested that the term Lynch syndrome be used where there is evidence of mismatch repair mutation. For those families where there is a strong family history fulfilling the Amsterdam criteria (see below), but MMR mutation has been excluded, the term 'familial colorectal cancer type X' should be used. HNPCC has been used to cover both of these groups but is largely obsolete.

Clinical features

Lynch syndrome is characterised by early onset of colorectal cancer, the average age at diagnosis being 45 years. These tumours have certain distinguishing pathological features. There is a predilection for the proximal colon, and tumours are frequently multiple (synchronous and metachronous). They tend to be mucinous, poorly differentiated and of 'signet-ring' appearance, with marked infiltration by lymphocytes and lymphoid aggregation at their margins. The associated cancers and their frequencies are detailed in Table 3.1.[8] The prognosis of these cancers tends to be better than in the same tumours arising sporadically.

Table 3.1 • Cancers associated with Lynch syndrome

Site	Frequency (%)
Large bowel	30–75
Endometrium	30–70 (of women)
Stomach	5–10
Ovary	5–10 (of women)
Urothelium (renal pelvis, ureter, bladder)	5
Other (small bowel, pancreas, brain)	<5

Genetics

Lynch syndrome is due to germline mutations in MMR genes, whose role is to correct errors in base-pair matching during replication of DNA or to initiate apoptosis when DNA damage is beyond repair. The vast majority of cases are due to mutations in the MMR genes (*hMLH1*, *hMSH2*, *hMSH6*, *hPMS2*). Recently, transmissible epimutations in the non-MMR gene *EPCAM* have been identified as a cause of Lynch syndrome. Other MMR gene mutations (*hMLH3*, *hMSH3*, *hPMS1*) have been reported in some families with Lynch syndrome but their clinical significance is not established.

The MMR genes are tumour-suppressor genes: patients with Lynch syndrome inherit a defective copy from one parent and tumorigenesis is triggered when the solitary normal gene in a cell becomes mutated or lost, so that DNA mismatches are no longer repaired in that cell. Defective MMR results in the accumulation of mutations in a host of other genes, leading to tumour formation.

A hallmark of tumours with defective MMR is microsatellite instability (MSI). Microsatellites are regions where a short DNA sequence (up to five nucleotides) is repeated. There are large numbers of such sequences in the human genome, the majority in non-coding DNA. Base-pair mismatches occurring during DNA replication are normally repaired by the MMR proteins. In tumours with a deficiency of these proteins this mechanism fails and microsatellites become mutated, resulting in a change in the number of sequence repeats and hence the length of the microsatellite (microsatellite instability). Typically in such a tumour over half of all microsatellites will exhibit this phenomenon.

About 15% of sporadic colorectal cancers show MSI. Most occur in older patients and are due to inactivation of MMR genes by promoter methylation, which is not, as far as we know, related to any inherited factor.

Diagnosis

Pedigree

Over the years a confusing range of 'criteria' have emerged. The International Collaborative Group on HNPCC (ICG-HNPCC) proposed the Amsterdam criteria in 1990 (Box 3.1). These were not intended as a diagnostic definition but rather to target genetic research by identifying families very likely to have a dominantly inherited cancer predisposition. The Amsterdam criteria were modified by the ICG-HNPCC in 1999 (Box 3.2) to include Lynch syndrome-associated cancers other than colorectal cancer (Amsterdam II criteria).[9] Subsequent studies have shown that approximately half the families that meet these criteria have Lynch syndrome (i.e. an MMR mutation is identified), and a similar proportion of individuals with Lynch syndrome come from families not meeting these criteria (i.e. 50% of Lynch syndrome families do not meet the Amsterdam criteria).

Therefore, although family history alone may be used to highlight high-risk families, it is insufficient to make a diagnosis of Lynch syndrome, and a combination of

Box 3.1 • Amsterdam criteria I

- At least three relatives with colorectal cancer, one of whom should be a first-degree relative of the other two
- At least two successive generations should be affected
- At least one colorectal cancer should be diagnosed before age 50 years
- FAP should be excluded
- Tumours should be verified by pathological examination

Box 3.2 • Amsterdam criteria II

- At least three relatives with a Lynch syndrome-associated cancer (colorectal, endometrial, small bowel, ureter, renal pelvis), one of whom should be a first-degree relative of the other two
- At least two successive generations should be affected
- At least one colorectal cancer should be diagnosed before age 50 years
- FAP should be excluded
- Tumours should be verified by pathological examination

tumour analysis and/or genetic testing is used in addition to family history to make the diagnosis.

Analysis of tumour tissue

A reference panel of five microsatellite markers is used to detect MSI; if two of the markers show instability, the tumour is designated 'MSI-high'. The value of MSI testing is that Lynch syndrome is due to MMR mutation and therefore virtually all colorectal cancers arising as a result of Lynch syndrome will be MSI-high. The Bethesda guidelines[10] (Box 3.3) were proposed to determine whether tumour tissue from an individual should be tested for MSI. The aim was to provide a sensitive set of guidelines that would encompass nearly all Lynch syndrome-associated colorectal cancers but also many 'sporadic cancers', and to use MSI testing to exclude those individuals lacking MSI-high, whose cancers are extremely unlikely to be caused by Lynch syndrome. Those designated MSI-high can then be further investigated using immunohistochemistry and genetic testing. Using this approach, approximately 90% of individuals with colorectal cancer due to Lynch syndrome can be identified.

MSI testing is expensive and requires DNA extraction. A simpler approach is to use standard immunohistochemical techniques to identify MMR proteins.[11] This technique has the benefit of identifying the gene that is likely to be mutated and therefore can be used to direct further genetic testing. However, it is not 100% sensitive, particularly in benign adenomatous colonic polyps and endometrial cancer, and so care is needed in interpreting the results.

Box 3.3 • Bethesda criteria for determining whether the tumour tissue from an individual with colorectal cancer should be tested for microsatellite instability

- Colorectal cancer diagnosed at age <50 years
- Multiple colorectal or other Lynch syndrome-associated tumours, either at the same time (synchronous) or occurring over a period of time (metachronous)
- Individuals diagnosed with colorectal cancer at <60 years, in whom the tumour has microscopic characteristics indicative of microsatellite instability
- Individuals with colorectal cancer who have one or more first-degree relatives diagnosed with a Lynch syndrome-related tumour at age 50 years or younger
- Individuals with colorectal cancer who have two or more first- or second-degree relatives diagnosed with a Lynch syndrome-related tumour at any age

Genetic testing

The decision whether to perform germline genetic testing on a blood sample from an at-risk or affected person takes the features of the patient, family and tumour into account. This cautious approach is currently justified on the grounds of cost, since genetic testing for MMR genes in the first member of the family (mutation detection) costs around £1000. Once a mutation has been detected in a family, testing other at-risk family members to determine whether they too carry the abnormal gene (predictive testing) is much more straightforward, and allows those without the mutation to be discharged from further surveillance.

As with the other syndromes described in this chapter, testing should be undertaken only after the patient has been counselled appropriately and given informed consent. The consent process should include an offer to provide written information, including a frank discussion of the benefits and risks (e.g. to employment, insurance) of genetic testing. A multidisciplinary clinic where counselling is available is ideal.[12] However, not every individual will accept an offer of genetic testing. Significant predictors of test uptake by individuals include an increased perception of risk, greater confidence in the ability to cope with unfavourable genetic news, more frequent thoughts of cancer and having had at least one colonoscopy.[13]

Germline gene testing may have several outcomes (Box 3.4) and the results should be relayed via the multidisciplinary clinic, where counselling is available.[14] There are also complexities of interpretation of results that mandate this (missense mutations, genetic heterogeneity).[15] Unregulated genetic testing for cancer risk has led to errors and adverse outcomes for individuals. Failure to detect a mutation may be due to a variety of factors: some cases may be due to mutation in regulatory genes rather than the MMR genes themselves; there may be other genes involved that have not yet been

Box 3.4 • Outcomes of genetic testing

Mutation detected
Test at-risk family members (predictive testing): if positive, surveillance and/or other management (e.g. surgery); if negative, no surveillance required

Mutation not detected
Keep all at-risk members under surveillance

identified; there may be a technical failure to identify a mutation that is present; or the family history may be a cluster of sporadic tumours. When this happens, the at-risk family members should continue to be screened.

> ✓ Familial colorectal cancer type X, i.e. families meeting the Amsterdam criteria but with MSI-negative tumours, are at lower risk, so that 3- to 5-yearly colonoscopy is sufficient.[16]

Surveillance

> ✓✓ Colonoscopic surveillance reduces the risk of colorectal cancer in Lynch syndrome patients by 63%.[17]

Colonoscopy must be meticulous, because tiny cancers may be present,[18] and frequent as interval cancers are common. Chromoendoscopy increases the pick-up of neoplastic lesions in Lynch syndrome and is recommended.

> ✓ Colonoscopy every 1–2 years from age 25 years (or 5 years younger than the youngest affected relative, whichever is the earlier)[11] is recommended for at-risk individuals. Surveillance should continue until about 75 years or until the causative mutation in that family has been excluded.[11]

Screening for extracolonic cancers is available, but there is currently little evidence of benefit. Recommendations vary from centre to centre, but surveillance is generally advised where there is a family history of cancers at a particular site. Box 3.5 shows the options for extracolonic surveillance.[11]

Box 3.5 • Extracolonic surveillance in Lynch syndrome (some centres)

- Annual transvaginal ultrasound±colour flow Doppler imaging±endometrial sampling
- Annual CA125 level and clinical examination (pelvic and abdominal)
- Upper gastrointestinal endoscopy every 2 years
- Annual urinalysis/cytology
- Annual abdominal ultrasound of renal tracts, pelvis, pancreas
- Annual liver function tests, CA19-9, CEA

Intervention

Surgery
Prophylactic

The option of prophylactic colectomy rather than colonoscopic surveillance should be discussed with mutation carriers, because of the high risk of colorectal cancer. A similar situation pertains to prophylactic hysterectomy and bilateral salpingo-oophorectomy in women who have completed their families.

Colectomy might be subtotal, with an ileorectal anastomosis, or might take the form of a restorative proctocolectomy. The risk of metachronous cancer in the retained rectum after ileorectal anastomosis has been estimated to be about 12% at 12 years.[19] Regular endoscopy via the anus should be carried out postoperatively, at intervals no greater than 12 months.

> ✓ Use of a decision analysis model indicates large gains in life expectancy for carriers of MMR mutation when offered some intervention. Benefits were quantified as 13.5 years from surveillance, 15.6 years from proctocolectomy and 15.3 years from subtotal colectomy compared with no intervention.[20]

Adjusting for quality of life showed that surveillance led to the greatest quality-adjusted life expectancy benefit. This study provides a mathematically based indication of benefit only: individual circumstances need to be incorporated into the decision-making process when making recommendations.

Treatment

> ✓ There is a risk of metachronous bowel tumour of 16% after 10 years of follow-up.[21]

For those with colonic tumours, the main choice lies between segmental colectomy and colectomy with ileorectal anastomosis (IRA). Segmental resection leads to better function but an increased risk of metachronous cancers and full colonoscopic surveillance. Colectomy and IRA has a prophylactic element in that the entire colon is removed, but without the additional morbidity of proctectomy, reducing metachronous cancer risk; furthermore, ongoing surveillance is much easier and more acceptable. Proctocolectomy (with or without ileo-anal pouch reconstruction) is the option of choice in patients who present with rectal cancer.

Medical

Studies of colorectal cancer cell lines deficient in MMR genes have shown that MSI is reduced in cells exposed to non-steroidal anti-inflammatory drugs (NSAIDs).[22] This provides some theoretical support for the CAPP2 (Colorectal Adenoma/Carcinoma Prevention Programme 2) study,[23] recently completed in Lynch syndrome patients, using aspirin and resistant starch as chemopreventive agents. This study reported reduced colorectal cancer rates in those treated with 600 mg aspirin daily. Further studies are needed before firm advice can be given regarding the optimum dose and duration of treatment.

The benefit of cytotoxic chemotherapy (notably 5-fluorouracil) for cancers in the setting of Lynch syndrome has been questioned.[11] This may be because some agents act by damaging DNA, which results in apoptosis. MMR proteins are thought to play a part in signalling the presence of irreversible DNA damage and initiating apoptosis, a pathway absent in these tumours. Prospective clinical trials are required before it can be determined what, if any, benefit there is from cytotoxic chemotherapy in the treatment of colorectal cancer in Lynch syndrome.

Familial adenomatous polyposis

Less common than Lynch syndrome, the risk of colorectal cancer in patients with FAP is nearly 100%. FAP is usually characterised by:

- hundreds of colorectal adenomatous polyps at a young age (second or third decade of life) (**Fig. 3.1**);

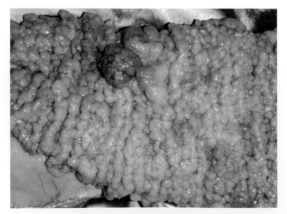

Figure 3.1 • Colectomy specimen from a patient with FAP.

- duodenal adenomatous polyps;
- multiple extraintestinal manifestations (Box 3.6);
- mutation in the tumour-suppressor adenomatous polyposis coli (*APC*) gene on chromosome 5q;
- autosomal dominant inheritance (offspring of affected individuals have a 1 in 2 chance of inheriting FAP).

Diagnosis

FAP was originally defined by the presence of over 100 colorectal adenomas. This clinical definition is still useful, as a mutation in the *APC* gene can only be identified in up to 80% of affected individuals. The majority of new cases come from families with a known history of the disease, but confusion can arise as approximately 20% are due to a new mutation.[24] In these circumstances there will be no family history of colorectal cancers at a young age or of multiple polyps. Further potential sources of confusion are the recent discovery of MAP (see later) and the well-documented existence of attenuated FAP characterised by a relative paucity of polyps (10–100) and a later age of developing colorectal cancer.[25]

Inadequate colonoscopy may lead to a false diagnosis of attenuation, an error that can be avoided by the use of dye-spray (chromoendoscopy).[26]

Box 3.6 • Extracolonic manifestations in FAP

Ectodermal origin
- Epidermoid cysts
- Pilomatrixoma
- Tumours of central nervous system
- Congenital hypertrophy of the retinal pigment epithelium

Mesodermal origin
- Connective tissue: desmoid tumours, excessive adhesions
- Bone: osteoma, exostosis, sclerosis
- Dental: dentigerous cyst, odontoma, supernumerary teeth, unerupted teeth

Endodermal origin
- Adenomas and carcinomas of duodenum, stomach, small intestine, biliary tract, thyroid, adrenal cortex
- Fundic gland polyps
- Hepatoblastoma

A further point that should be borne in mind is that some individuals with Lynch syndrome have a number of adenomatous polyps. Where the diagnosis requires confirmation, the use of dye-spray and random biopsies looking for microadenomas (a hallmark of FAP and MAP, but not seen in Lynch syndrome) are helpful, as is upper gastrointestinal (GI) endoscopy (up to 80% of FAP patients have gastric fundic gland polyps and the lifetime risk of duodenal adenomas is over 90%), as are testing for MSI and immunohistochemistry of tumours.

Genetic testing

✔ The issue of genetic testing is a useful paradigm highlighting the fundamental role played by registries. Identification of at-risk family members who might be offered gene testing is critical and is usually made possible by the comprehensive collation of family pedigrees that such registries are uniquely positioned to obtain and update.

An uncontrolled approach to testing and the release of results can lead to inadequate counselling and the provision of incorrect information to patients.[27]

An affected family member should be tested first. The mutation can be located in approximately 80% of affected individuals. Once the mutation has been identified, at-risk members of the family can be offered simple blood testing. Should the known family mutation not be found in the at-risk individual, that person can be discharged from further surveillance[28] but should be informed that he or she remains at the same risk of sporadic colorectal cancer as any member of the general population. Such an approach eliminates unnecessary colonic examination and costs less than conventional clinical screening.[29]

Genotype–phenotype correlation

The site of the mutation in the *APC* gene can influence the expression of FAP.[30] Genotype–phenotype correlation is seen in the association between certain mutations and severe FAP (dense colorectal polyposis with relatively early colorectal cancer development), and between other mutations and less severe FAP ('attenuated' polyposis).[31] However, individuals with identical mutations can display differences in phenotypic expression, suggesting that other modifier genes and the environment play a role in disease expression.[32]

Some of the multiple extracolonic manifestations of FAP (see Box 3.6),[33] such as desmoid disease, also show some correlation with the mutation site; others, notably duodenal polyposis and malignancy, do not.

These genotype–phenotype correlations have led to suggestions that the findings of molecular analysis might guide both surveillance and treatment.[31,34,35] At present, however, it is important to emphasise that prophylactic colectomy or proctocolectomy (almost always with a pouch) remain the management options of choice for the large bowel in all patients with proven FAP.

Surveillance

If the family mutation is known, at-risk family members are usually offered predictive genetic testing in their early teens. If this is not possible, then clinical surveillance is required. It is very unusual for significant colorectal polyps to develop before the teenage years and while cancers have been described in children, they are exceptionally rare. If an individual has symptoms attributable to the large bowel (anaemia, rectal bleeding or change in bowel habit), colonoscopy should be performed. Otherwise annual flexible sigmoidoscopy starting at 13–15 years of age is recommended. If no polyps are detected, 5-yearly colonoscopy should be started at the age of about 20 years, with annual flexible sigmoidoscopy in the intervening years.

The large bowel

Surgery
Prophylactic

Once the diagnosis has been made, either by predictive genetic testing or by the detection of adenomatous polyposis during surveillance of an at-risk family member, the aim is to offer prophylactic surgery before a cancer develops. If the diagnosis has been made on the basis of flexible sigmoidoscopy, colonoscopy should be performed to assess the colonic polyp burden. If the individual is symptomatic or the polyps are dense or large, surgery should be undertaken as soon as is practical. In other cases it is usual to defer surgery until a time when its social and educational impact will be minimised, usually a long summer vacation or 'gap' after leaving school.

As the surgical options have increased, so has the controversy surrounding the choice between them. Increasingly, laparoscopically assisted surgery is becoming available and has great attractions in this group, where a good cosmetic result makes surgery more acceptable. The available operations are:

- colectomy and ileorectal anastomosis (IRA);
- restorative proctocolectomy (RPC) with an ileal pouch–anal anastomosis;
- total proctocolectomy and end ileostomy (almost exclusively for those with very low rectal cancer).

Most young people facing prophylactic colectomy want to avoid a permanent ileostomy, so the choice really lies between the first two options. The biggest attraction of RPC is that the entire large bowel is removed, so that there is no risk of polyps or cancer developing in a retained rectum. However, a cuff of rectal mucosa is retained when a stapled anastomosis is performed, and cancers at this site have been reported.[36] A mucosectomy can be done to remove this area and a handsewn pouch anal anastomosis created, but this is a more technically demanding technique, which probably also results in poorer functional outcome. Furthermore, follow-up studies have shown adenoma formation within ileo-anal pouches[37] and the development of cancer has been reported.

The advantages of IRA are that it is a one-stage procedure (whereas RPC often involves a temporary defunctioning ileostomy) with lower morbidity and mortality.

> ✅ The functional results in terms of defecatory frequency and leakage are generally slightly better with IRA than after RPC.[38]

Sexual and reproductive function can both be compromised by proctectomy. There is a small but definite risk of erectile and ejaculatory dysfunction in men undergoing proctectomy. In addition there is a pouch failure rate of about 10%, resulting in the need for a permanent ileostomy. These potential complications are particularly difficult to accept for essentially healthy young people undergoing surgery for prophylaxis rather than treatment.

> ✅ Recent studies have shown that RPC for both FAP[39] and ulcerative colitis adversely affects fertility in women.

It is known that some groups are at particular risk of developing rectal cancer after IRA. These are individuals with numerous rectal polyps and carriers of certain mutations (such as at codon 1309). Historical data show a cumulative rectal cancer risk of up to 30% by 60 years of age, but at the time many of these patients underwent IRA, RPC was not available. IRA was the only option to avoid a permanent ileostomy, and thus was done in circumstances when it would not now be recommended.

> ✅ In selected cases the risk of rectal cancer is low and IRA is a reasonable option.[40]

Many patients will have experience of one or both operations from other family members who have undergone them, which may affect their choice. Ultimately, they need to be informed about the advantages and disadvantages of both procedures, as well as the implications of their genotype (if identified) so that their decision can be as informed as possible.

Treatment

In the presence of a colonic cancer, the surgical decision-making is essentially the same as in prophylactic surgery. In individuals with severe rectal polyposis or in those carrying a mutation at codon 1309 of the *APC* gene, the risks of subsequent uncontrollable rectal polyposis requiring completion proctectomy, or of rectal cancer itself, are high and outweigh the disadvantages of RPC. In those with few rectal polyps, mutations at other sites and the few patients with a genuine attenuated phenotype, IRA may represent a better option. Ultimately, it remains for the informed patient to make a choice.

When rectal cancer is present, the choice is between RPC and proctocolectomy and ileostomy. As in any case of rectal cancer, a very low tumour precludes sphincter preservation. Careful local staging and multidisciplinary management are crucial in these cases.

Surveillance after surgery

Follow-up is required after all procedures. After IRA or RPC, peranal digital and flexible endoscopic examination are mandatory at intervals of up to 12 months, depending on findings. The NSAID sulindac has been used to control rectal adenomas[41] and pouch adenomas,[42] but sulindac must be used with caution in view of earlier reports of cancer despite chemoprevention and surveillance in this setting. The selective cyclo-oxygenase (COX)-2 inhibitor celecoxib showed a moderate reduction in large bowel polyps in treated patients[43] but no longer has a licence and can no longer be recommended in FAP. More recently the use of omega 3 fish oil supplements has been shown to have a similar beneficial effect to these NSAIDs in control of colorectal polyps.[44] Aspirin has not been shown to have a significant effect in reduction of polyp burden.[45] Following colectomy, the major causes of mortality and morbidity are duodenal cancers and desmoid tumours. This knowledge guides postoperative management.[46]

Upper gastrointestinal tract polyps

Non-adenomatous gastric polyps (fundic gland polyps) occur in up to 80% of patients with FAP. It is doubted whether these lesions have malignant potential, which at most is extremely low.[47]

> ✅ Duodenal adenomas occur in nearly all patients with FAP but are severe in only 10%, with malignant change occurring in 5%.[48]

Surveillance of the upper gastrointestinal tract

Surveillance usually begins in the third decade of life (in the asymptomatic patient), with endoscopies at intervals of between 6 months and 5 years depending on the severity of duodenal polyposis.[49] A staging system for duodenal polyposis has been developed (Table 3.2) to allow surveillance to be tailored to disease severity and to identify individuals at high risk of developing malignancy.[50]

> ✅ Duodenal surveillance is beneficial. Duodenal cancer detected at surveillance endoscopy has a significantly improved overall survival compared to symptomatic cancers.[51]

The ampulla and periampullary area must be examined, being at particularly high risk, so a side-viewing as well as end-viewing scope should be used in the examination. If the ampulla is abnormal due to the development of an adenoma the frequency of endoscopic surveillance may need to be altered according to the severity of the ampullary disease.[52]

Management of duodenal polyposis

> ✅✅ Management of severe duodenal polyposis is difficult. No chemopreventive options are available and endoscopic therapy does not have robust data to support its use. Referral to a specialist centre is wise.

Open duodenotomy and polypectomy is associated with high recurrence rates and is not recommended.[53] The role of advanced endoscopic techniques, often under general anaesthesia, is not established but may be used to manage those with more severe disease and delay the need for definitive surgery.

While prophylactic pancreatico-duodenectomy or pylorus-preserving pancreatico-duodenectomy has been described with good outcomes, associated morbidity and mortality are substantial.[54] However, the poor prognosis once invasive disease is present and the high rate of progression to cancer of advanced polyposis (36% over 10 years in one series) means that this aggressive approach can be justified

Table 3.2 • Spigelman staging of severity of duodenal polyposis in FAP

	Points allocated		
	1	2	3
Number of polyps	1–4	5–20	>20
Polyp size (mm)	1–4	5–10	>10
Histological type	Tubular	Tubulovillous	Villous
Degree of dysplasia	Mild	Moderate	Severe

Total points	Spigelman stage	Recommended follow-up interval
0	0	5 years
1–4	I	5 years
5–6	II	3 years
7–8	III	1 year and consider endoscopic therapy
9–12	IV	Consider prophylactic duodenectomy

in some cases with Spigelman stage IV disease. Cancer risk and hence the need for intervention is minimal in patients with stage 0–II disease.

Desmoid tumours

Desmoid tumours are fibromatous lesions consisting of clonal proliferations of myofibroblasts (**Fig. 3.2**). They occur in approximately 15% of individuals with FAP, with a mortality rate of about 10%.[55] Most exhibit cycles of growth and resolution and, while causing discomfort and being unsightly, may not cause significant problems. Most desmoids associated with FAP arise either intra-abdominally (usually within the small bowel mesentery) or on the abdominal wall, although they can appear in the extremities and trunk. They are histologically benign, but within the abdomen can cause small bowel and ureteric obstruction, intestinal ischaemia or perforation, all of which can be fatal. A model of desmoid tumour development, based on the appearance of a precursor plaque-like lesion, has been proposed, offering a possibility for prevention or early treatment.[56]

The aetiology of desmoid tumours is multifactorial, with contributions from trauma (e.g. operative), oestrogens, specific *APC* gene mutations and modifier genes.

Management

The challenge in the management of these bizarre tumours is to identify the minority that are rapidly and relentlessly progressive and to avoid harming patients with unnecessarily aggressive attempts to treat the rest. Ureteric obstruction is not infrequent, and as the consequences can be obviated by

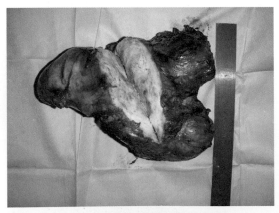

Figure 3.2 • A desmoid tumour excised from the abdominal wall.

ureteric stenting it is wise to perform regular renal tract imaging (usually with ultrasound) in patients otherwise being managed non-operatively every 6 months.

Computed tomography (CT) provides the best imaging with respect to size and relationship to surrounding structures, but T2-weighted magnetic resonance imaging (MRI) sequences may provide useful information about cellularity and growth potential. Ultrasound can be used to monitor the ureters.

> ✔ Treatment options include NSAIDs, antioestrogens, surgical excision and cytotoxic chemotherapy.[57]

Anecdotal successes with a variety of NSAIDs and antioestrogens abound (e.g. sulindac 150–200 mg twice daily alone or in combination with very-high-dose tamoxifen 80–120 mg daily), although good evidence of efficacy is lacking. Evaluation of these treatments is further hampered by the natural history of desmoids, which have been documented to regress spontaneously and exhibit relentless growth in only a small minority of patients.

> ✔ Evidence[55] supports the use of surgery as first-line treatment for abdominal wall and extra-abdominal desmoids, although the recurrence rate is high.

There is no evidence to support the concern that this might be increased by the use of prosthetic materials to repair any resulting defect. Historical evidence of significant morbidity and mortality has led to the recommendation that surgery should usually be avoided where possible for intra-abdominal desmoids. If such surgery is required, because of progressive disease or desmoid-related complications, then careful patient selection and a referral to a specialist centre may lead to good outcomes with low morbidity and mortality, although recurrence remains a problem.[58]

MYH-associated polyposis (MAP)

Recent study of patients with the phenotype of FAP but no identifiable *APC* mutation has led to the discovery of this form of adenomatous polyposis, which has considerable clinical overlap with FAP, but is genetically distinct.[59]

Clinical features

The large bowel

As in FAP, the most consistent feature of MAP is the development of colonic adenomas and carcinomas. The number of polyps is very variable,[60] with about half the patients in one series having a phenotype consistent with classical FAP (hundreds of polyps) and half having an attenuated phenotype with fewer than 100 polyps. Some cases of cancer have been reported in individuals with a definite genetic diagnosis of MAP, but very few polyps indeed, and the lifetime risk of colorectal cancer is almost 100% by the age of 60. The distribution differs from FAP in that there is a greater proportion of right-sided cancers, which also develop slightly later, at an average of 47 years.

The upper gastrointestinal tract

Gastric fundic gland polyps and duodenal adenomas occur in MAP, but less commonly, with 20–30% having duodenal polyps.[61]

Other manifestations

It has been suggested that there is an increased frequency of breast cancer in MAP, up to 18% in one series.[62] Osteomas and dental cysts have also been documented. To date no MAP patient with desmoid has been reported.

Genetics

This condition is due to biallelic mutation of the mutY human homologue (*MYH*) gene on chromosome 1p. Thus, for the first time, autosomal recessive inheritance has been described in the context of inherited bowel cancer. The frequency of mutation carriage (heterozygosity) in the general population may be as high as 1 in 200, but individuals who are heterozygotes appear to be at most only at minimally increased risk of colorectal cancer.

Genetic testing is available, and should be considered in individuals with a clinical diagnosis of FAP, but no detectable *APC* mutation, as well as patients presenting with fewer adenomas. The recessive inheritance means that there will often be no family history of colorectal cancer or polyps. This mode of inheritance also poses challenges in terms of genetic counselling and family testing strategies.

Management

The management of an affected individual is essentially the same as for FAP, although as a higher proportion has an attenuated phenotype, and the age of onset may be a little later, it may be that more patients can be managed, at least initially, by annual colonoscopy and polypectomy. Upper gastrointestinal tract surveillance is started at around the age of 25.

There is insufficient evidence currently to support breast screening, but female patients should be informed of the potentially increased risk. Breast self-examination and participation in population-based breast cancer screening should be encouraged.

The lifetime risk of a heterozygote carrier developing colorectal cancer has not yet been fully clarified, but studies to date indicate that any increase in risk is modest (in the range 1.5–2 times). Thus surveillance is not currently recommended.

Peutz–Jeghers syndrome

Peutz–Jeghers syndrome is an autosomal dominant condition characterised by mucocutaneous pigmentation (**Fig. 3.3**) together with multiple gastrointestinal hamartomatous polyps. The gene responsible in some patients is *STK11* (*LKB1*) on chromosome 19p13, although there is evidence of genetic heterogeneity as mutation at this site has been excluded in some families.

A 78-year follow-up of the original family described by Peutz is instructive.[63] Survival of affected family members was found to be reduced as a result of bowel obstruction and the development of a range of cancers.

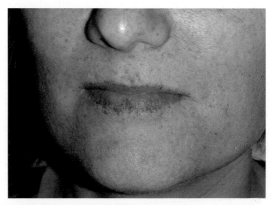

Figure 3.3 • Peutz–Jeghers pigmentation.

Bowel obstruction

The commonest polyp-related complication is small bowel obstruction, often caused by intussusception with a polyp at the apex. Repeated episodes result in increasingly difficult laparotomies and loss of bowel length.

> ✔ The incidence of subsequent small bowel obstruction can be reduced by adequate intraoperative small bowel enteroscopy, allowing identification and removal of all polyps at the time of initial laparotomy.[64]

Cancer risk

Individuals with Peutz–Jeghers syndrome are at significantly increased risk of gastrointestinal malignancy, although the risk has not been well defined. Other areas at increased risk include the breasts (female), ovaries, cervix, pancreas and testes.[65]

Surveillance and management

Up-to-date surveillance protocols are best obtained from local registries. Most involve annual review with physical examination and measurement of haemoglobin. Upper and lower gastrointestinal endoscopies (with polypectomy) and capsule endoscopy or MRI enterography are performed every 2–3 years. Endoscopic surveillance and polypectomy may reduce the risk of cancer development but further data are required.[66] Surveillance also identifies polyps that may become symptomatic; if large polyps are seen in the small bowel or symptoms suggesting intermittent small bowel obstruction occur, or if there are small-bowel polyps with anaemia, a double-balloon enteroscopy or laparotomy with intraoperative enteroscopy and polypectomy is recommended to clear the small bowel of polyps and prevent frank obstruction.

As far as malignancy at other sites is concerned, where surveillance programmes have been shown to be useful in the general population they should be used. Annual breast surveillance with MRI or ultrasonography is recommended from 25 to 50 years of age and thereafter mammography substituted, due to the very high risk of breast cancer.[67] It is important to stress that females should remain up to date with cervical smears and self-examine their breasts and that men should self-examine their testes. There is no evidence to support ovarian and pancreatic surveillance in Peutz–Jeghers syndrome.[67,68]

Juvenile polyposis

Not to be confused with the finding of an isolated juvenile polyp (which has very low, if any, malignant potential), juvenile polyposis is an autosomal dominant condition where multiple characteristic hamartomatous juvenile polyps occur, mostly in the colon but also in the upper gastrointestinal tract. Other features sometimes associated are macrocephaly, hereditary haemorrhagic telangiectasia and congenital heart disease. Some affected individuals harbour germline mutations in the *SMAD4* gene,[67] while others have germline mutations in the *BMPR1A* gene.

There is a risk of colorectal cancer approaching 40% and an increased risk of gastric cancer, particularly in those with an *SMAD4* germline mutation. Regular endoscopic screening[69] by oesophago-gastroduodenoscopy and colonoscopy, with polypectomy for large polyps, is mandatory. Occasionally prophylactic colectomy or gastrectomy is required.

Cowden disease

The *PTEN* gene on chromosome 10q22 is associated with this syndrome, which consists of gastrointestinal hamartomas and cancers, plus a high risk of cancer of the female breast, thyroid, uterus and cervix, benign fibrocystic breast disease, non-toxic goitre and varied benign mucocutaneous lesions, particularly trichilemmomas. Targeted screening seems sensible, but there is little evidence to support it.

Other inherited colorectal cancer syndromes

Multiple hyperplastic polyps that have adenomatous features (mixed polyposis syndromes) are associated with a high risk for colorectal cancer,[70] as is serrated polyposis.[71] Both conditions can be inherited. Endoscopy and even timely colectomy may be necessary. Large (>1 cm) multiple and right-sided hyperplastic or serrated polyps (as opposed to the much more common, though frequently multiple, diminutive rectal and sigmoid ones) should alert the surgeon to potential future risk.

A variant mutation of the *APC* gene on chromosome 5q (E1317Q) has been associated with an increased risk of colorectal cancer without any of the syndromes described above, particularly in the Ashkenazi Jewish population.[72] Research into the same population has provided evidence for the existence of another colorectal cancer susceptibility gene on chromosome 15q.[73] Caution should therefore be exercised in discharging Ashkenazi Jewish kindreds on the basis of a negative gene test, as mutations in the other colorectal cancer genes found in this population may be present.[74]

Summary

The emerging complexity of inherited bowel cancer, coupled with rapid advances in knowledge, reinforce the need for the availability of experienced, informed and up-to-date opinion in the areas of diagnosis and management. Individual surgeons will rarely be able to meet all of these needs. Patients and their families are best served by the existence of good working relationships between managing clinicians, family cancer clinics and registries based in expert centres.

Key points

- Genetic factors make a significant contribution to colorectal cancer.
- High-risk families should be referred to special interest registries, genetics units or clinical groups.
- Lynch syndrome and FAP are the main autosomal dominant conditions involved.
- An understanding of these conditions is required to recognise and diagnose them.
- Individuals with these conditions are at risk of a range of extracolonic tumours, so need specialised follow-up.

References

1. Fuchs CS, Giovannucci EL, Colditz GA, et al. A prospective study of family history and the risk of colorectal cancer. N Engl J Med 1994;331:1669–74.

2. Houlston RS, Murday V, Harocopos C, et al. Screening and genetic counselling for relatives of patients with colorectal cancer in a family cancer clinic. Br Med J 1990;301:366–8.

3. Lichtenstein P, Holm NV, Verkasalo PK, et al. Environmental and heritable factors in the causation of cancer: analyses of cohorts of twins from Sweden, Denmark, and Finland. N Engl J Med 2000;343:78–85.

4. Lips CJ. Registers for patients with familial tumours: from controversial areas to common guidelines. Br J Surg 1998;85:1316–8.

5. Cairns SR, Scholefield JH, Steele RJ, et al. Guidelines for colorectal cancer screening and surveillance in moderate and high risk groups (update from 2002). Gut 2010;59:666–89.

6. Dunlop M, Campbell H. Screening for people with a family history of colorectal cancer. Br Med J 1997;314:1779–80.

7. Jass JR. Hereditary non-polyposis colorectal cancer: the rise and fall of a confusing term. World J Gastroenterol 2006;12:4943–50.

8. Aarnio M, Sankila R, Pukkala E, et al. Cancer risk in mutation carriers of DNA-mismatch-repair genes. Int J Cancer 1999;81:214–8.

9. Vasen HF, Watson P, Mecklin JP, et al. New clinical criteria for hereditary nonpolyposis colorectal cancer (HNPCC, Lynch syndrome) proposed by the International Collaborative group on HNPCC. Gastroenterology 1999;116:1453–6.

10. Umar A, Boland CR, Terdiman JP, et al. Revised Bethesda Guidelines for hereditary nonpolyposis colorectal cancer (Lynch syndrome) and microsatellite instability. J Natl Cancer Inst 2004;96:261–8.

11. Vasen HF, Moslein G, Alonso A, et al. Guidelines for the clinical management of Lynch syndrome (hereditary non-polyposis cancer). J Med Genet 2007;44:353–62.

12. Scholefield JH, Johnson AG, Shorthouse AJ. Current surgical practice in screening for colorectal cancer based on family history criteria. Br J Surg 1998;85:1543–6.

13. Esplen MJ, Madlensky L, Butler K, et al. Motivations and psychosocial impact of genetic testing for HNPCC. Am J Med Genet 2001;103:9–15.

14. Burke W, Petersen G, Lynch P, et al. Recommendations for follow-up care of individuals with an inherited predisposition to cancer. I. Hereditary nonpolyposis colon cancer. Cancer Genetics Studies Consortium. JAMA 1997;277:915–9.

15. Syngal S, Fox EA, Li C, et al. Interpretation of genetic test results for hereditary nonpolyposis colorectal cancer: implications for clinical predisposition testing. JAMA 1999;282:247–53.

16. Dove-Edwin I, de Jong AE, Adams J, et al. Prospective results of surveillance colonoscopy in dominant familial colorectal cancer with and without Lynch syndrome. Gastroenterology 2006;130:1995–2000.

17. Jarvinen HJ, Aarnio M, Mustonen H, et al. Controlled 15-year trial on screening for colorectal cancer in families with hereditary nonpolyposis colorectal cancer. Gastroenterology 2000;118:829–34.
    A prospective controlled trial showing that colonoscopic surveillance in Lynch syndrome led to a 63% reduction in colorectal cancer and a significant decrease in mortality.

18. Church J. Hereditary colon cancers can be tiny: a cautionary case report of the results of colonoscopic surveillance. Am J Gastroenterol 1998;93:2289–90.

19. Rodriguez-Bigas MA, Vasen HF, Pekka-Mecklin J, et al. Rectal cancer risk in hereditary nonpolyposis colorectal cancer after abdominal colectomy. International Collaborative Group on HNPCC. Ann Surg 1997;225:202–7.

20. Syngal S, Weeks JC, Schrag D, et al. Benefits of colonoscopic surveillance and prophylactic colectomy in patients with hereditary nonpolyposis colorectal cancer mutations. Ann Intern Med 1998;129:787–96.

21. de Vos tot Nederveen Cappel WH, Nagengast FM, Griffioen G, et al. Surveillance for hereditary nonpolyposis colorectal cancer: a long-term study on 114 families. Dis Colon Rectum 2002;45:1588–94.

22. Ruschoff J, Wallinger S, Dietmaier W, et al. Aspirin suppresses the mutator phenotype associated with hereditary nonpolyposis colorectal cancer by genetic selection. Proc Natl Acad Sci U S A 1998;95:11301–6.

23. Burn J, Gerdes AM, Macrae F, et al. Long-term effect of aspirin on cancer risk in carriers of hereditary colorectal cancer: an analysis from the CAPP2 randomised controlled trial. Lancet 2011;378(9809):2081–7.
    A prospective, randomised trial whose primary endpoint was colorectal cancer development in patients with Lynch syndrome. It showed that taking 600 mg aspirin for 25 months significantly reduced risk of both colorectal and all Lynch syndrome-associated cancers after a period of 55 months.

24. Bisgaard ML, Fenger K, Bulow S, et al. Familial adenomatous polyposis (FAP): frequency, penetrance, and mutation rate. Hum Mutat 1994;3:121–5.

25. Hernegger GS, Moore HG, Guillem JG. Attenuated familial adenomatous polyposis: an evolving and poorly understood entity. Dis Colon Rectum 2002;45:127–34.

26. Wallace MH, Frayling IM, Clark SK, et al. Attenuated adenomatous polyposis coli: the role of ascertainment bias through failure to dye-spray at colonoscopy. Dis Colon Rectum 1999;42:1078–80.

27. Giardiello FM, Brensinger JD, Petersen GM, et al. The use and interpretation of commercial APC gene testing for familial adenomatous polyposis. N Engl J Med 1997;336:823–7.

28. Berk T, Cohen Z, Bapat B, et al. Negative genetic test result in familial adenomatous polyposis: clinical screening implications. Dis Colon Rectum 1999;42:307–10.

29. Bapat B, Noorani H, Cohen Z, et al. Cost comparison of predictive genetic testing versus conventional clinical screening for familial adenomatous polyposis. Gut 1999;44:698–703.

30. Wu JS, Paul P, McGannon EA, et al. APC genotype, polyp number, and surgical options in familial adenomatous polyposis. Ann Surg 1998;227:57–62.

31. Vasen HF, van der Luijt RB, Slors JF, et al. Molecular genetic tests as a guide to surgical management of familial adenomatous polyposis. Lancet 1996;348:433–5.

32. Crabtree MD, Tomlinson IP, Hodgson SV, et al. Explaining variation in familial adenomatous polyposis: relationship between genotype and phenotype and evidence for modifier genes. Gut 2002;51:420–3.

33. Brett M, Hershman M, Glazer G. Other manifestations of familial adenomatous polyposis. In: Phillips RKS, Spigelman AD, Thomson JPS, editors. Familial adenomatous polyposis and other polyposis syndromes. London: Edward Arnold; 1994. p. 142–58.

34. Soravia C, Berk T, Madlensky L, et al. Genotype–phenotype correlations in attenuated adenomatous polyposis coli. Am J Hum Genet 1998;62:1290–301.

35. Bertario L, Russo A, Radice P, et al. Genotype and phenotype factors as determinants for rectal stump cancer in patients with familial adenomatous polyposis. Ann Surg 2000;231:538–43.

36. Van Duijvendijk P, Vasen HF, Bertario L, et al. Cumulative risk of developing polyps or malignancy at the ileal pouch-anal anastomosis in patients with familial adenomatous polyposis. J Gastrointest Surg 1999;3:325–30.

37. Parc YR, Olschwang S, Desaint B, et al. Familial adenomatous polyposis: prevalence of adenomas in the ileal pouch after restorative proctocolectomy. Ann Surg 2001;233:360–4.

38. Aziz O, Athanasiou T, Fazio VW, et al. Meta-analysis of observational studies of ileorectal versus ileal pouch-anal anastomosis for familial adenomatous polyposis. Br J Surg 2006;93:407–17.

39. Olsen KO, Juul S, Bulow S, et al. Female fecundity before and after operation for familial adenomatous polyposis. Br J Surg 2003;90:227–31.

40. Church J, Burke C, McGannon E, et al. Risk of rectal cancer in patients after colectomy and ileorectal anastomosis for familial adenomatous polyposis: a function of available surgical options. Dis Colon Rectum 2003;46:1175–81.

41. Giardiello FM, Offerhaus JA, Tersmette AC, et al. Sulindac induced regression of colorectal adenomas in familial adenomatous polyposis: evaluation of predictive factors. Gut 1996;38:578–81.

42. Ho JW, Yuen ST, Chung LP, et al. The role of sulindac in familial adenomatous polyposis patients with ileal pouch polyposis. Aust N Z J Surg 1999;69:756–8.

43. Steinbach G, Lynch PM, Phillips RK, et al. The effect of celecoxib, a cyclooxygenase-2 inhibitor, in familial adenomatous polyposis. N Engl J Med 2000;342:1946–52.

44. West NJ, Clark SK, Phillips RK, et al. Eicosapentaenoic acid reduces rectal polyp number and size in familial adenomatous polyposis. Gut 2010;59:918–25.

45. Burn J, Bishop DT, Chapman PD, et al. A randomized placebo-controlled prevention trial of aspirin and/or resistant starch in young people with familial adenomatous polyposis. Cancer Prev Res (Phila) 2011;4:655–65.

46. Vasen H, Bulow S, Leeds Castle Polyposis Group. Guidelines for the surveillance and management of familial adenomatous polyposis (FAP): a world wide survey among 41 registries. Colorectal Dis 1999;1:214–21.

47. Hofgartner WT, Thorp M, Ramus MW, et al. Gastric adenocarcinoma associated with fundic gland polyps in a patient with attenuated familial adenomatous polyposis. Am J Gastroenterol 1999;94:2275–81.

48. Groves CJ, Saunders BP, Spigelman AD, et al. Duodenal cancer in patients with familial adenomatous polyposis (FAP): results of a 10 year prospective study. Gut 2002;50:636–41.

49. Burke CA, Beck GJ, Church JM, et al. The natural history of untreated duodenal and ampullary adenomas in patients with familial adenomatous polyposis followed in an endoscopic surveillance program. Gastrointest Endosc 1999;49:358–64.

50. Spigelman AD, Williams CB, Talbot IC, et al. Upper gastrointestinal cancer in patients with familial adenomatous polyposis. Lancet 1989;2:783–5.

51. Bülow S, Christensen IJ, Højen H, et al. Duodenal surveillance improves the prognosis after duodenal cancer in familial adenomatous polyposis. Colorectal Dis 2011; Oct 4. Epub ahead of print.
Patients from a previous study (*n*=304) were followed up. This is the first study to show a survival benefit from surveillance of the duodenum in FAP. Survival after a surveillance detected cancer was significantly better than after a symptomatic cancer (8 years vs. 0.8 years; *P*<0.0001).

52. Latchford AR, Neale KF, Spigelman AD, et al. Features of duodenal cancer in patients with familial adenomatous polyposis. Clin Gastroenterol Hepatol 2009;7:659–63.

53. Penna C, Phillips RK, Tiret E, et al. Surgical polypectomy of duodenal adenomas in familial adenomatous polyposis: experience of two European centres. Br J Surg 1993;80:1027–9.

54. Skipworth JR, Morkane C, Raptis DA, et al. Pancreaticoduodenectomy for advanced duodenal and ampullary adenomatosis in familial adenomatous polyposis. HPB (Oxford) 2011;13:342–9.

55. Clark SK, Neale KF, Landgrebe JC, et al. Desmoid tumours complicating familial adenomatous polyposis. Br J Surg 1999;86:1185–9.

56. Clark SK, Smith TG, Katz DE, et al. Identification and progression of a desmoid precursor lesion in patients with familial adenomatous polyposis. Br J Surg 1998;85:970–3.

57. Sturt NJ, Clark SK. Current ideas in desmoid tumours. Fam Cancer 2006;5:275–85.

58. Latchford AR, Sturt NJ, Neale K, et al. A 10-year review of surgery for desmoid disease associated with familial adenomatous polyposis. Br J Surg 2006;93:1258–64.

59. Al-Tassan N, Chmiel NH, Maynard J, et al. Inherited variants of MYH associated with somatic G:C→T:A mutations in colorectal tumors. Nat Genet 2002;30:227–32.

60. Sieber OM, Lipton L, Crabtree M, et al. Multiple colorectal adenomas, classic adenomatous polyposis, and germ-line mutations in MYH. N Engl J Med 2003;348:791–9.

61. Kanter-Smoler G, Bjork J, Fritzell K, et al. Novel findings in Swedish patients with MYH-associated polyposis: mutation detection and clinical characterization. Clin Gastroenterol Hepatol 2006;4:499–506.

62. Nielsen M, Franken PF, Reinards TH, et al. Multiplicity in polyp count and extracolonic manifestations in 40 Dutch patients with MYH associated polyposis coli (MAP). J Med Genet 2005;42:e54.

63. Westerman AM, Entius MM, de Baar E, et al. Peutz–Jeghers syndrome: 78-year follow-up of the original family. Lancet 1999;353:1211–5.

64. Edwards DP, Khosraviani K, Stafferton R, et al. Long-term results of polyp clearance by intraoperative enteroscopy in the Peutz–Jeghers syndrome. Dis Colon Rectum 2003;46:48–50.

65. Hearle N, Schumacher V, Menko FH, et al. Frequency and spectrum of cancers in the Peutz–Jeghers syndrome. Clin Cancer Res 2006;12:3209–15.

66. Latchford AR, Neale K, Phillips RK, et al. Peutz–Jeghers syndrome: intriguing suggestion of gastrointestinal cancer prevention from surveillance. Dis Colon Rectum 2011;54:1547–51.

67. Beggs AD, Latchford AR, Vasen HF, et al. Peutz–Jeghers syndrome: a systematic review and recommendations for management. Gut 2010;59:975–86.

68. Latchford A, Greenhalf W, Vitone LJ, et al. Peutz–Jeghers syndrome and screening for pancreatic cancer. Br J Surg 2006;93:1446–55.

69. Brosens LA, van Hattem A, Hylind LM, et al. Risk of colorectal cancer in juvenile polyposis. Gut 2007;56:965–7.

70. Ilyas M, Straub J, Tomlinson IP, et al. Genetic pathways in colorectal and other cancers. Eur J Cancer 1999;35:335–51.

71. Boparai KS, Mathus-Vliegen EM, Koornstra JJ, et al. Increased colorectal cancer risk during follow-up in patients with hyperplastic polyposis syndrome: a multicentre cohort study. Gut 2010;59:1094–100.

72. Lamlum H, Al Tassan N, Jaeger E, et al. Germline APC variants in patients with multiple colorectal adenomas, with evidence for the particular importance of E1317Q. Hum Mol Genet 2000;9:2215–21.

73. Tomlinson I, Rahman N, Frayling I, et al. Inherited susceptibility to colorectal adenomas and carcinomas: evidence for a new predisposition gene on 15q14-q22. Gastroenterology 1999;116:789–95.

74. Yuan ZQ, Wong N, Foulkes WD, et al. A missense mutation in both hMSH2 and APC in an Ashkenazi Jewish HNPCC kindred: implications for clinical screening. J Med Genet 1999;36:790–3.

4

Colonic cancer

Robert J.C. Steele

Introduction

Colorectal cancer is a major health problem. In the UK, it is the second most common cause of cancer death, accounting for some 16 000 deaths in 2004. In 2002 there were approximately 35 000 new cases, of which about 13 000 were rectal and 22 000 colonic.[1] Although the overall numbers in men and women are similar, the incidence of rectal cancer is higher in men and that of colonic cancer is higher in women. The 5-year relative survival rate is currently in the region of 50% and has improved over the last 30 years from a figure of around 20% in 1971–75.[1]

Surprisingly, there is no precise definition of colonic cancer. Although the colon comprises the large bowel proximal to the rectum, the definition of the rectum is unclear. Anatomical texts describe the top of the rectum as the point where the sigmoid mesocolon ends or that part of the large bowel level with the third sacral vertebra.[2] Surgeons, on the other hand, prefer to think of the rectum as the segment of large bowel lying within the true pelvis. As far as rectal cancer is concerned, the UK definition is a tumour within 15 cm of the anal verge on rigid sigmoidoscopy,[3] whereas authorities from the USA have preferred 11 or 12 cm.[4] Perhaps the simplest definition is the intraoperative identification of the fusion of the two antemesenteric taenia into an amorphous area where the true rectum begins.

These distinctions are important for two reasons. First, radiotherapy is not appropriate for colonic tumours and, secondly, comparisons between outcomes for colorectal cancer surgery are impossible unless uniform definitions are adopted. This problem has yet to be addressed by international consensus.

Natural history

Within the colon, about 50% of cancers arise in the left side and 25% in the right (**Fig. 4.1**); in 4–5% of cases there are synchronous lesions. It is now widely accepted that the majority of colonic cancers arise from pre-existing adenomatous polyps, the supporting evidence being as follows:[5]

1. The prevalence of adenomas correlates well with that of carcinomas, the average age of adenoma patients being around 5 years younger than patients with carcinomas.
2. Adenomatous tissue often accompanies cancer, and it is unusual to find small cancers with no contiguous adenomatous tissue.
3. Sporadic adenomas are identical histologically to the adenomas of familial adenomatous polyposis (FAP), and this condition is unequivocally premalignant.
4. Large adenomas are more likely to display cellular atypia and genetic abnormalities than small lesions.

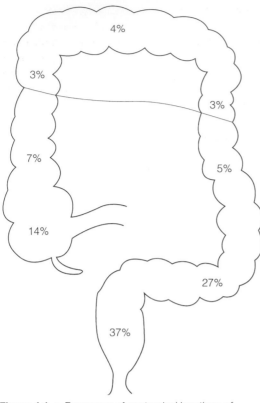

Figure 4.1 • Frequency of anatomical locations of colorectal cancer. Based on data from the Royal College of Surgeons audit in Trent Region and Wales.

5. The distribution of adenomas throughout the colon is similar to that for carcinomas.
6. Adenomas are found in up to one-third of all surgical specimens resected for colorectal cancer.
7. The incidence of colorectal cancer has been shown to fall with a long-term screening programme involving colonoscopy and polypectomy.

✔✔ Although the majority of adenomas diagnosed in the West are polypoid or exophytic, the flat adenoma, defined as an adenoma where the depth of the dysplastic tissue is no more than twice that of the mucosa, is now a recognised entity.[6] There is good evidence that these lesions are premalignant, and may indeed have a greater tendency towards malignant transformation than polypoid adenomas. They are difficult to find, but may account for up to 40% of all adenomas.[6] Reliable diagnosis requires a skilful, experienced colonoscopist and the use of dye sprayed on to the colonic mucosa to highlight the contours of the abnormal tissue.

When invasion has taken place, colonic cancer can spread directly and via the lymphatic, blood and transcoelomic routes.

Direct spread

Direct spread occurs longitudinally, transversely and radially, but as adequate proximal and distal clearance is technically feasible in the majority of colonic cancers, it is radial spread that is of most importance. In a retroperitoneal colonic cancer, radial spread may involve the ureter, duodenum and muscles of the posterior abdominal wall; the intraperitoneal tumour may involve small intestine, stomach, pelvic organs or the anterior abdominal wall.

Lymphatic spread

In general, the lymphatic spread of colonic cancer progresses from the paracolic nodes along the main colonic vessels to the nodes associated with either cephalad or caudal vessels, eventually reaching the para-aortic glands in advanced disease. This orderly process does not always occur, however, and in about 30% of cases nodal involvement can skip a tier of glands.[7] In contrast to rectal disease, it is rare for a colonic cancer that has not breached the muscle wall to exhibit lymph node metastases[7] (overall, about 15% of cases confined to the bowel wall will be found to have lymph node metastases).

Blood-borne spread

The most common site for blood-borne spread of colorectal cancer is the liver, presumably arriving by the portal venous system. Up to 37% of patients may have detectable liver metastases at the time of operation, and around 50% of patients may be expected to develop overt disease at some time. The lung is the next most common site, with around 10% of patients developing lung metastases at some stage; other reported sites include ovary, adrenal, bone, brain and kidney.

Transcoelomic spread

Colonic cancer may spread throughout the peritoneum, either via the subperitoneal lymphatics or by virtue of viable cells being shed from the serosal surface of a tumour, giving rise to malignant ascites, which is relatively rare.

Aetiology

Knowledge of molecular genetics in sporadic colorectal cancer has increased rapidly in recent years, but the stimuli that lead to these carcinogenic changes are still obscure.

Genetic factors

The genetic changes associated with colorectal cancer have been widely studied, and the molecular background to inherited colorectal cancer is dealt with in Chapter 3. However, the genetic events in sporadic colorectal cancer are also quite well understood. Mutations of the adenomatous polyposis coli (APC) gene, which is central to ordered cell motility, are thought to occur early as they are found in 60% of all adenomas and carcinomas.[8]K-ras mutations, which induce cell growth by activating growth factor signal transduction, similarly occur in both adenomas and carcinomas. However, as they are more common in large adenomas than

in small adenomas they are thought to represent a later event.[9] Mutation of the p53 gene is common in invasive colonic cancers but rare in adenomas and is therefore deemed to be a late event that accompanies the development of invasion.[10] This is thought to be important as the p53 protein has roles in the repair of DNA and the induction of programmed cell death.[11]

The sequence of events described above is depicted in **Fig. 4.2**, but it must be stressed that this merely illustrates one possible multistep process; indeed, there is now good evidence that K-ras and p53 mutations very rarely occur in the same tumour, suggesting alternative pathways to carcinogenesis.[12] Many other genetic events have been observed in sporadic colorectal cancer, and no single event has been seen in all cancers. Thus the range of mutations, inactivations and deletions is wide, and it is likely that no single pattern will be applicable to every tumour. Nevertheless, knowledge of specific genetic events that take place in colorectal carcinogenesis may well have implications for diagnosis, prognosis and ultimately for gene therapy. For example, there is now evidence that K-ras mutations are not only associated with advanced stage at presentation, but also with poor prognosis in node-negative disease.[13]

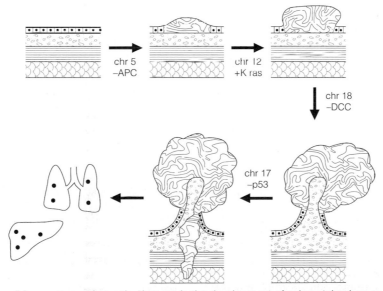

Figure 4.2 • A possible sequence of genetic changes in the development of colorectal polyps and invasive cancer.

Diet and lifestyle

✔✔ In 2007, the World Cancer Research Fund (WCRF) published its report on Food, Nutrition, Physical Activity and the Prevention of Cancer based on a systematic review of the world literature.[14] With respect to colon cancer, evidence for decreased risk was found for physical exercise, dietary fibre, calcium, garlic, non-starchy vegetables and pulses. Evidence for increased risk was uncovered for obesity, red meat, processed meat, alcohol, animal fat and sugar. It is clear that being overweight and underactive stand out as major risk factors, and governments worldwide have recognised this as an area for action. Smoking is also important and long-term smoking is associated with relative risks of between 1.5 and 3.0.[15]

Predisposing conditions

Long-standing inflammatory bowel disease, both ulcerative colitis and Crohn's disease, increases the risk of colorectal cancer. Previous gastric surgery has also been implicated, and although the association is controversial, the risk may be about twofold. Altered bile acid metabolism may play a role in this process, both after gastrectomy and after vagotomy. The risk after ureterosigmoidostomy is well established, although this operation has now been largely superseded by the use of an isolated ileal conduit for urinary diversion.

Presentation

Colon cancer can present as an emergency or with chronic symptoms that are well recognised. Right-sided cancer typically presents with anaemia, as the liquid nature of the faeces and the wider diameter of the colon make obstructive symptoms unusual. When the tumour is situated in the descending or sigmoid colon, change of bowel habit, colicky abdominal pain and blood in the stool are the commonest symptoms. Occasionally, the patient may notice the primary tumour as a mass and even more rarely a sigmoid cancer may cause pneumaturia and urinary infection by fistulation into the bladder, and a gastrocolic fistula may cause faecal vomiting or severe diarrhoea.

Unfortunately, many of the symptoms of colon cancer are common and non-specific, and there has been a good deal of recent work attempting to refine the indications for investigation. Guidelines have been developed to classify those at high risk warranting urgent investigation based on change in bowel habit, rectal bleeding in the absence of anal symptoms, palpable abdominal or rectal masses and anaemia (Box 4.1).[16] These guidelines are not particularly discriminatory, however, and weighted scoring systems may be more accurate.

Investigation

Currently, investigative techniques include barium enema, sigmoidoscopy, colonoscopy and computed tomography (CT) colography.

Barium enema usually demonstrates a colonic cancer as an irregular polypoid lesion or an 'apple

Box 4.1 • UK Department of Health criteria for high and low risk of colorectal cancer

Higher risk
- Rectal bleeding with a change in bowel habit to looser stools or increased frequency of defecation persisting for 6 weeks (all ages)
- Change in bowel habit as above without rectal bleeding and persisting for 6 weeks (>60 years)
- Persistent rectal bleeding without anal symptoms* (>60 years)
- Palpable right-sided abdominal mass (all ages)
- Palpable rectal mass (not pelvic) (all ages)
- Unexplained iron deficiency anaemia (all ages)

Low risk
Patients with no iron deficiency anaemia, no palpable rectal or abdominal mass
- Rectal bleeding with anal symptoms and no persistent change in bowel habit (all ages)
- Rectal bleeding with an obvious external cause, e.g. anal fissure (all ages)
- Change in bowel habit without rectal bleeding (<60 years)
- Transient changes in bowel habit, particularly to harder or decreased frequency of defecation (all ages)
- Abdominal pain as a single symptom without signs and symptoms of intestinal obstruction (all ages)

*Soreness, discomfort, itching, lumps, prolapse or pain. Reproduced from Thompson MR, Heath I, Ellis BG et al. Identifying and managing patients at low risk of bowel cancer in general practice. Br Med J 2003; 327:263–5. With permission from BMJ Publishing Group Ltd.

core' stricture with destruction of the mucosal pattern; benign polyps may also be seen as typical filling defects. It must be stressed, however, that false-positive and false-negative results may occur in up to 1% and 7% of cases, respectively, with errors usually occurring in the sigmoid colon and caecum.[17]

Although rigid sigmoidoscopy may provide satisfactory rectal visualisation, it has been largely superseded by flexible sigmoidoscopy. This provides useful supplementary information, and neoplasia may be detected in the sigmoid colon in 25% of cases with 'normal' barium enemas, especially if there is coexisting diverticular disease. It may therefore be argued that colonoscopy should be the investigation of choice, but it carries a risk of perforation (much greater than barium enema), and even in good hands failure to achieve caecal intubation can be expected in 10% of cases. In addition, precise localisation of a tumour seen at colonoscopy is difficult as the only reliable landmarks are the anus and the terminal ileum.

Preoperative histological confirmation of a colonic cancer is ideal, but this can be achieved only by performing endoscopy in every case. If imaging demonstrates an unequivocal carcinoma, then biopsy may be deemed unnecessary, but where there is any reasonable doubt regarding the nature of a stricture or other lesion, then endoscopic visualisation and biopsy are mandatory.

✅ CT as a primary investigative modality is now coming to the fore with the development of CT colography or 'virtual colonoscopy', which is effective in detecting polypoid lesions down to 6 mm in diameter. This is fast becoming a standard investigation and is replacing the barium enema as the radiological investigation of choice.

When the diagnosis has been made, staging of the primary tumour, liver and lungs is now considered mandatory in the majority of cases. A fit patient with metastatic disease may be suitable for active treatment, whereas an elderly patient with a relatively asymptomatic primary and evidence of widespread dissemination may escape resection. CT of the chest and abdomen is now regarded as the staging modality of choice, supplanting chest X-ray and ultrasound.[18] Until recently, magnetic resonance imaging (MRI) scanning was considered to be less useful because of the long image acquisition time, but with ultrafast scanning MRI may become the investigation of choice for both distant and local disease.

Screening

Colon cancer is a suitable candidate for screening. Prognosis after treatment is much better in early stage disease and the polyp–carcinoma sequence offers an opportunity to prevent cancer by treating premalignant disease. The ideal screening test should detect the majority of tumours without a large number of false positives, i.e. it should have high sensitivity and specificity. In addition, it must be safe and acceptable to the population offered screening. In colorectal cancer, the most widely studied test is Haemoccult, a guaiac-based test that detects the peroxidase-like activity of haematin in faeces. Because this activity is diminished as haemoglobin travels through the gastrointestinal tract,[19] upper gastrointestinal bleeding is less likely to be detected than colonic bleeding. On the other hand, false-positive results may be produced by ingestion of animal haemoglobin or vegetables containing peroxidase, and because of the intermittent nature of bleeding from tumours, the sensitivity of Haemoccult is only about 50–70%.[20]

Screen-detected tumours are much more likely to be at an early stage than symptomatic disease, but this does not prove that screening is beneficial. Even improved survival in patients whose tumours are detected by screening is not conclusive because of the biases inherent in screening. These biases are threefold, and comprise selection bias, length bias and lead-time bias.

Selection bias arises from the tendency of people who accept screening to be particularly health conscious and therefore atypical of the population as a whole. Length bias indicates the tendency for screening to detect a disproportionate number of cancers that are slow growing, and thereby have a good prognosis. Lead-time bias results from the time between the date of detection of a cancer by screening and the date when it would have been diagnosed had the subject not been screened. As survival is measured from the time of diagnosis, screening advances the date at which diagnosis is made, thus lengthening the survival time without necessarily altering the date of death.

✔✔ Because of these biases, effectiveness can be assessed only by comparing disease-specific mortality in a population offered screening with that in an identical population not offered screening. This has to be done in the context of a well-designed randomised controlled trial, and for colorectal cancer three trials using faecal occult blood (FOB) have reported mortality data.[21–23] The first of these was carried out in Minnesota,[21] and showed a significant 33% reduction in colorectal cancer-specific mortality with annual FOB testing and a significant 21% reduction in a group offered biennial screening. In Nottingham, a trial of biennial FOB testing demonstrated a 15% reduction in cumulative mortality[22] and an almost identical study carried out in Funen, Denmark, showed an 18% reduction in mortality.[23]

There seems little doubt that FOB screening can reduce mortality from colorectal cancer, when applied to unselected populations, and the challenges for the future are to increase uptake and to improve the sensitivity and specificity of the screening test. Worldwide there is increasing interest in using faecal immunological testing (FIT) for blood, which appears to be more accurate than the indirect guaiac test.[24]

Another approach is to use endoscopy as a primary screening test. As 70% of cancers and large adenomas are found in the distal 60 cm of the large bowel, flexible sigmoidoscopy has been proposed as a screening test, and there is good evidence that it is more sensitive than FOB testing. Once-only flexible sigmoidoscopy between the ages of 55 and 64 has been investigated as a screening modality in a multicentre randomised study,[25] and has been shown to reduce colorectal cancer mortality *and* incidence, particularly in the rectum and left colon; the incidence reduction is undoubtedly due to adenoma removal at the time of flexible sigmoidoscopy. A commitment has been made by the UK government to introduce flexible sigmoidoscopy into the national screening programme, although adequate uptake in the general population remains a concern.

Surveillance after adenoma detection

Surveillance of patients diagnosed as having adenomatous polyps poses a significant challenge in terms of the use of colonoscopy resources, particularly with the introduction of population screening. For this reason, guidelines have been developed that classify patients as being at low, intermediate or high risk for adenoma recurrence.[26] The low-risk category includes those with one or two adenomas less than 1 cm in diameter, and either no follow-up or a repeat colonoscopy at 5 years is recommended. For those at intermediate risk, defined as three to four adenomas or at least one adenoma greater than 1 cm in diameter, colonoscopy at 3 years is recommended. High-risk patients, those with five or more small adenomas or three or more where at least one is greater than 1 cm in diameter, should have another colonoscopy at 1 year. While the evidence upon which these guidelines is based is not very strong, they represent a sensible approach, and one that has been adopted widely in the UK.

Elective surgery

Given that a patient is fit for surgery, and does not have advanced disseminated disease, resection of a colonic cancer is the primary treatment.

Preparation for surgery

✔ The first priority is to obtain informed consent, and the surgeon must be prepared to discuss the risks of death, complications such as anastomotic dehiscence, venous thromboembolism and wound infection, and disease recurrence. The patient must also be assessed for fitness for operation. This implies obtaining a full history and examination, full blood count, urea and electrolyte examination, and electrocardiogram (ECG) where indicated. In addition, investigations for disseminated disease should be performed as outlined above.

Blood transfusion

The patient must have blood taken for crossmatch, but the amount of blood requested will depend on the individual procedure. Group and save alone will be suitable for most hemicolectomies, although it may be prudent to have two units of blood available if operative difficulties are anticipated.

There is still some debate as to the effects of blood transfusion on prognosis in colorectal cancer. Since the report by Burrows and Tartter[27] that blood transfusion may be associated with an increased likelihood of recurrence, there have been many reports, some making allowance for case mix, which have reached conflicting conclusions.

✔✔ A randomised trial comparing the use of predeposited autologous and allogeneic blood in patients undergoing resection for colorectal cancer has shown no difference in prognosis.[28] For this reason, observed effects of blood transfusion on recurrence must be treated with caution.

Bowel preparation

✔ Immediately before surgery, many surgeons require the patient to undergo some form of mechanical bowel preparation.

A wide variety of washouts, enemas and purgatives have been used, and one of the most popular regimens uses Picolax®. This combines a senna compound (10 mg sodium picosulphate), which is activated by colonic bacteria and causes vigorous mass contraction, with magnesium citrate, which reduces water and sodium reabsorption, so that a large hyperosmolar fluid load reaches the caecum.

A popular alternative is polyethylene glycol salt solution, which can achieve preparation within 3 hours. It does, however, necessitate 4–5 L of oral intake, and many elderly patients find this difficult. Nasogastric whole-gut irrigation with an electrolyte solution obtains excellent results, but patients find it very unpleasant.

Care must be taken not to attempt preoperative preparation in the presence of obstruction. If a patient experiences excessive pain or abdominal distension during preparation, it should be stopped. In such cases, the use of intraoperative preparation should be considered (see below).

✔✔ It is by no means certain that bowel preparation is essential to prevent anastomotic leakage or its consequences. Most anastomotic leaks are caused by technical error (such as poor knotting/suturing or too much tension) or biological failure (usually from ischaemia), neither of which will be influenced by bowel preparation. The effects of an early leak (usually due to poor technique) would probably be obviated by bowel preparation, but most leaks occur late after the patient has recommenced oral feeding so that any value of preoperative bowel preparation will have been lost. For this reason there is an increasing tendency for surgeons to omit bowel preparation altogether and, indeed, the results of several randomised trials support this view.[29] However, it remains sensible to prepare the bowel if a proximal stoma is likely in order to prevent a column of stool feeding an anastomotic leak, should one occur.

Thromboembolism prophylaxis

✔✔ Although there have been no studies confined to patients with colorectal cancer, a meta-analysis of appropriate randomised trials has shown that rates of deep vein thrombosis (DVT), pulmonary embolism and death from pulmonary embolism can all be significantly reduced by the use of subcutaneous heparin in general surgical patients.[30]

Offset against the advantages are the problems of increased bleeding, particularly when performing pelvic surgery, so that there still remains room for surgeons to choose. Low-molecular-weight heparin has received attention recently, and a large randomised trial of patients undergoing abdominal surgery has shown that it is less likely to cause bleeding-related complications than standard heparin.[31]

Other measures include graduated compression stockings, intravenous dextran and intermittent pneumatic calf compression. Stockings alone are less effective than other methods, and dextran is not as effective as heparin, but there is at least one trial indicating that intermittent compression is equivalent to heparin in reducing the incidence of DVT.

Antibiotic prophylaxis

✔✔ All patients should receive antibiotic prophylaxis, as there is good evidence from several randomised trials that systemic antibiotics reduce the risk of sepsis after colorectal surgery.[32]

The choice of antibiotic and the route of administration are still open to debate, but in the UK the intravenous use of metronidazole for Bacteroides fragilis combined with broad-spectrum cover against gut anaerobes is favoured.

✔✔ A single dose of cephalosporin plus metronidazole is just as effective as a three-dose regimen in preventing wound infection.[33]

If there is significant contamination at the time of surgery, then prolonging antibiotic therapy for 3–5 days may be appropriate. Whatever regimen is used, it is important that the antibiotics are given immediately before the inoculation of bacteria into the wound, and the ideal timing is immediately after induction of anaesthesia.

Chapter 4

Bladder catheterisation

This is usually done after the patient has been anaesthetised to monitor urine output per- and postoperatively. The urethral route is most commonly used, although there is evidence that suprapubic catheterisation may be preferable.[34]

Resection

Radical excision of a colonic tumour along with the appropriate vascular pedicle and accompanying lymphatic drainage is the most appropriate operation to obtain local control. Occasionally, a very limited resection may be appropriate in an unfit patient or one with widespread disease.

Classical resection removes the lymphatic drainage that lies along the named arterial blood supply, thereby rendering the associated colon ischaemic; thus, right hemicolectomy removes the ileocolic and right colic arteries, transverse colectomy removes the middle colic artery and left hemicolectomy removes the left colic artery. However, transverse colectomy has fallen out of favour owing to a perception that anastomotic leakage is unacceptably high, and the distinction between left hemicolectomy and sigmoid colectomy is irrelevant if the principle of radical excision of the vascular pedicle is accepted. Thus, many surgeons would now hold that the decision as to type of operation lies between right hemicolectomy and left hemicolectomy, with the extent of bowel resection dependent on site of tumour.

A standard right hemicolectomy involves division of the ileocolic and right colic arteries at their origins from the superior mesenteric artery (**Fig. 4.3**). The marginal artery or the right branch of the middle colic artery will also need division to complete vascular isolation. For tumours of the descending colon and sigmoid colon, a formal left hemicolectomy involves division of the inferior mesenteric artery at its origin from the aorta (**Fig. 4.4**).

Splenic flexure carcinoma

The main controversy arises with tumours in the region of the splenic flexure, and here there are two options. One is to regard the tumour as left

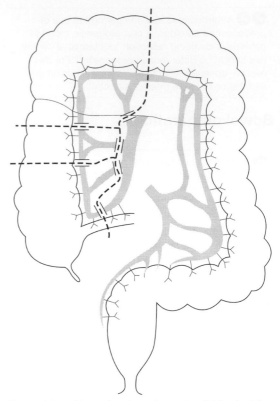

Figure 4.3 • Alternative sites of vascular division in right hemicolectomy.

sided, and to carry out a left hemicolectomy, dividing the inferior mesenteric artery at its origin and dividing the left branch of the middle colic artery. A more conservative approach to this operation is to preserve the inferior mesenteric trunk, but this is essentially a segmental resection. The other approach is to carry out an extended right hemicolectomy, dividing the middle colic artery and the ascending branch of the left colic artery.

Expert opinion is divided as to which approach to take, but left hemicolectomy will necessitate anastomosis between right colon and rectum, which may be difficult to achieve without tension in some patients. Furthermore, the blood supply of the colon is inconstant. In 6% of cases there is no left colic artery and the blood supply of the splenic flexure is from the middle colic artery. In 22% of cases the middle colic artery is absent and the blood supply of the splenic flexure comes from both the left and right colic arteries. A cancer operation involves removing the tumour with its associated lymphatic drainage, and as the lymphatic drainage

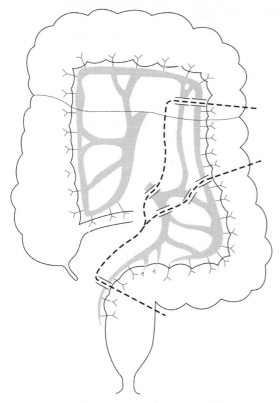

Figure 4.4 • Alternative sites of vascular division in left hemicolectomy.

follows the arterial blood supply, it would seem sensible to ligate the right colic, middle colic and left colic arteries, making extended right hemicolectomy necessary.

For these reasons, I prefer extended right hemicolectomy, with an anastomosis between sigmoid colon and mobile well-vascularised ileum. It must be stressed, however, that the ideal operation will be dictated by individual anatomy, the most important criteria being lack of tension and good blood supply as evidenced by brisk bleeding and good colour at the cut bowel ends.

The Large Bowel Cancer Project found a high local recurrence rate and poor survival for patients with splenic flexure carcinoma, regardless of stage and presentation, which may reflect surgical inadequacy of primary treatment.[35]

Advanced tumours

When a tumour is locally advanced, it may still be possible to achieve a curative resection if the surgeon is prepared to resect adjacent involved organs, such as ureter, duodenum, stomach, spleen, small bowel, bladder and uterus (Rupert Turnbull at the Cleveland Clinic classified tumours that involved other organs as Dukes' D, for which he achieved a number of cures). In addition, about 5% of women will have macroscopic ovarian metastases and a further 2% will have microscopic disease. For this reason, a few surgeons carry out routine oophorectomy in all women with colorectal cancer.

In a patient with a truly inoperable tumour of the colon an ileocolonic bypass may be appropriate for lesions of the right side, whereas for tumours of the distal colon a defunctioning colostomy may be preferable. With multiple colonic tumours, a subtotal or total colectomy should be considered.

Operative technique

✓ The descriptions of operative technique given here refer to open surgery only, as the laparoscopic approach is dealt with elsewhere. For all colonic resections, it is my preference to have the patient in the legs apart position using a split-leg table, even if access to the anus or pelvis is not required, as this facilitates distribution of surgeon, scrub nurse and assistants around the table. The use of a multicomponent self-retaining retractor such as the 'Omnitract®' is also advised.

Right hemicolectomy

I prefer midline incisions for all colonic resections, as there is no muscle damage and access is gained to all parts of the abdomen and pelvis. For a right hemicolectomy it is useful to have two-thirds of the incision above the umbilicus to facilitate mobilisation of the hepatic flexure.

With the surgeon standing on the patient's right, the right colon is retracted towards the midline by the assistant, and the peritoneum in the right paracolic gutter is divided. This extends from the caecal pole to the hepatic flexure, and cephalad to this point the lesser sac is entered and the greater omentum divided below the gastroepiploic arcade up to the point of intended division of the transverse colon. The right colon is then retracted firmly towards the midline, and the plane between the colonic mesentery and the posterior abdominal wall is carefully developed with diathermy, taking care not to damage the duodenum. As this is done, the ureter and gonadal vessels will fall away safely. This is done until the superior mesenteric vessels are clearly identified so that the right colic and ileocolic vessels can be ligated and divided very close to their origins. The bowel wall is then cleared at the sites of transection and single crushing clamps are applied. Soft clamps may be applied on proximal small bowel and distal large bowel, and the bowel is divided on the crushing clamps, leaving them on the specimen.

Left hemicolectomy

A long midline incision is employed, extending from above the umbilicus to the symphysis pubis. The operator stands on the patient's left side, and the assistant retracts the sigmoid colon medially. The peritoneum lateral to the sigmoid and descending colon is divided close to the 'white line' of fusion using diathermy. It should then be possible to see the plane between the mesentery and the retroperitoneal structures, which can be further developed using a combination of firm medial traction of the bowel by the assistant and countertraction applied by the operator on the retroperitoneum using a swab or forceps.

This manoeuvre will ensure that ureter and gonadal vessels are swept away. Care must be taken to identify the hypogastric nerves, and these should be separated from the mesentery or they may be damaged as the upper rectum is prepared for anastomosis. The splenic flexure should then be mobilised, and this is best done by dissecting the greater omentum off the transverse colon and continuing laterally towards the flexure. If the tumour is in the region of the splenic flexure, however, it is advisable to divide the gastrocolic ligament and take the omentum with the specimen. In either event, the spleen is at risk from tears caused by traction on its peritoneal attachments and, despite extreme care, splenectomy is sometimes necessary. For minor tears, however, application of a haemostatic agent such as oxycellulose is sufficient.

Once the left colon has been mobilised, the origin of the inferior mesenteric artery is identified by dividing the peritoneum over the aorta close to the fourth part of the duodenum, ligated and divided. To obtain full mobility it is then necessary to divide the inferior mesenteric vein just below the inferior border of the pancreas. The colon is then divided as described for right hemicolectomy at a convenient point in the transverse colon and at the rectosigmoid junction.

Anastomosis

For anastomosis after resection of a colonic cancer, I prefer to use hand suturing, although it is appreciated that stapling may produce excellent results.

Appositional serosubmucosal anastomosis

This method, initially described by Matheson et al.,[36] utilises a single layer of interrupted 3/0 braided polyamide. For mobile anastomoses (usually ileocolic) the first step is to ensure that the ends to be anastomosed are roughly equal in circumference. This is usually achieved by making an incision on the antemesenteric aspect of the small bowel, although some surgeons prefer to use an end-to-side technique. One side of the anastomosis is performed on the serosal aspect of the bowel between the mesenteric and antemesenteric borders, placing the sutures 4 mm apart and 4 mm deep, ensuring that the muscle layer and the submucosa but not the mucosa have been included (**Fig. 4.5**). The sutures are left untied until they have all been inserted (**Fig. 4.6**), and each knot is then tied by hand to ensure a snug but non-constrictive result. The half-completed anastomosis is then turned over and the process repeated. Mesenteric defects are not closed.

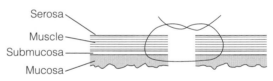

Figure 4.5 • Placement of the appositional serosubmucosal suture.

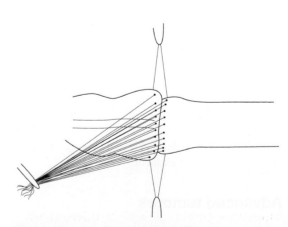

Figure 4.6 • Ileocolic anastomosis. The sutures are left untied until they have all been inserted.

For colorectal or ileorectal anastomoses, the posterior row of sutures is inserted first, holding each suture with a specially designed suture clamp or individual artery forceps. If artery forceps are used, they should be threaded on to a forceps holder to avoid tangling. Again, the sutures are tied by hand after insertion of the whole row, the knots being tied on the luminal side of the anastomosis after the proximal bowel has been 'parachuted' down the sutures to the upper rectum (**Fig. 4.7**). The knot tails are then cut so that they are covered by the cut edges of the undisturbed mucosal layers. On completion of the posterior aspect of the anastomosis, the anterior part is performed in a similar fashion, but with the knots tied on the extraluminal side. This type of anastomosis is greatly facilitated by the use of curved 'Heaney' needle holders, with the needle mounted facing out from the convex side of the tip.

Stapled anastomoses

After right hemicolectomy the most widely employed stapled anastomosis is the 'functional end-to-end'. Here, the ends of the colon and ileum are stapled closed at the time of specimen excision, and two small enterotomies are made to permit insertion of the limbs of a linear cutting stapler. The anastomosis is then performed by firing the stapler, taking care not to include mesentery (**Fig. 4.8**), and after checking the staple line for bleeding the remaining defect is closed with a linear stapler. After left hemicolectomy, a true end-to-end anastomosis can be performed using a circular anastomosing stapler introduced per anum (**Fig. 4.9**), but in some male patients the intact rectum can be difficult to negotiate.

Results of anastomotic techniques

The interrupted serosubmucosal technique is recommended for its adaptability to any anastomosis

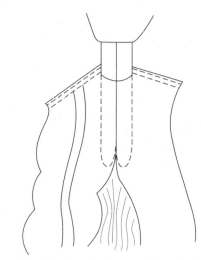

Figure 4.8 • 'Functional end-to-end' ileocolonic stapled anastomosis.

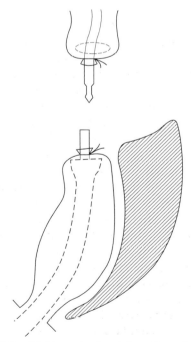

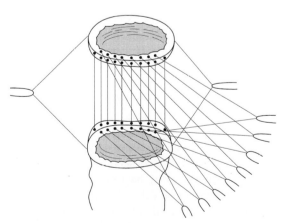

Figure 4.7 • Colorectal anastomosis. The sutures are held in individual forceps and the colon slid down to the rectum before tying.

Figure 4.9 • End-to-end colorectal anastomosis using a circular stapling device.

involving the colon, but it is also associated with the best results in the literature, with leak rates of 0.5–3% in sizeable series.[37,38]

✓✓ Stapling has been compared with hand suturing in several randomised trials and, although the results vary, there seems to be no consistent difference in colonic anastomotic dehiscence between the two approaches. In one trial there was evidence that tumour recurrence was less in the stapled group, but no distinction between rectal and colonic resections was made.[39]

Drains

✓✓ After the anastomosis is complete, many surgeons will leave a drain in the peritoneal cavity either to minimise the consequences of an anastomotic leak or to prevent the accumulation of fluid that might be infected. There is no evidence to support this practice, and three randomised trials have shown there to be no advantage associated with drainage of colonic or colorectal anastomoses.[40–42]

Postoperative care/complications

✓✓ After colectomy, postoperative care is similar to that of any patient undergoing major abdominal surgery, and there is now increasing interest in 'fast-track' or enhanced recovery. This involves a multimodal approach to postoperative recovery that is based on early feeding, early mobilisation, i.v. fluid and sodium restriction, and avoidance of both drains and nasogastric intubation; initial epidural analgesia with avoidance of parenteral opiates may also be employed. A median hospital stay (including readmissions) after open colonic surgery of 3 days can be achieved if this policy is pursued, but it involves considerable commitment, not only from the patient, but also from anaesthetic staff, nursing staff and community healthcare.[43]

Anastomotic dehiscence

Although patients undergoing colectomy may suffer any of the complications associated with major abdominal surgery, anastomotic breakdown is the major source of morbidity specific to this type of operation. Subclinical leaks occur more frequently than clinically obvious leaks, but after resection of a colonic tumour the overall significant leak rate should currently be no more than 4%.[18]

A leak may present in a variety of ways, and the onset of symptoms may be quite insidious. Warning signs are pyrexia, increasing pulse rate and abdominal distension due to paralytic ileus, as well as unexplained cardiorespiratory disturbance. The patient may then go on to develop localised or generalised peritonitis, or a faecal fistula, usually through the wound. Occasionally a patient will develop sudden generalised peritonitis and septicaemic shock as a result of rapid faecal contamination of the peritoneal cavity.

Because of the heterogeneous nature of the symptoms, a leak should be suspected in any patient with an anastomosis who is not progressing as well as expected. Investigations that may prove useful in a doubtful case include a full blood count, abdominal and chest radiographs, and a water-soluble contrast enema (increasingly CT is employed). The white cell count is usually raised, although not inevitably. Plain radiographs will frequently demonstrate distended loops of bowel and gas may be seen under the diaphragm, although both of these may be seen after any laparotomy in the absence of a leak. The most useful investigation is a water-soluble contrast enema (often now CT), and in the patient with clinical signs consistent with a leak, extravasation of contrast at the anastomosis secures the diagnosis.

The treatment of an anastomotic dehiscence depends on the specific mode of presentation. The patient with general peritonitis requires laparotomy after appropriate resuscitation. With a major disruption, the anastomosis should be taken down and the two ends exteriorised if possible; primary repair of the anastomotic dehiscence should not be attempted. After dealing with the anastomosis, careful peritoneal toilet must be performed using copious quantities of warm saline with or without antibiotic, and the patient will require at least 5 days of intravenous antibiotic therapy.

In the patient with localised peritonitis who remains otherwise well, a conservative approach with systemic antibiotics may be appropriate, but laparotomy should not be delayed if there is any deterioration. A faecal fistula can also be treated in this way, but care must be taken with the surrounding skin, and nutritional support may be required if drainage is prolonged.

Management of the polyp cancer

In the colon, unlike the rectum, small invasive cancers are not amenable to formal intraluminal resection. However, after colonoscopic polypectomy subsequent histological examination of the specimen may reveal a focus of invasive cancer. A relatively rare situation in the past, this has rapidly become a common occurrence with the introduction of colorectal population screening and it poses the problem of what to do next. Clearly, if there is a risk of residual tumour, either in the colonic wall or in the regional lymph nodes, then completion colectomy is advisable, but quantifying this risk is by no means simple. Evidence from cohort studies, such as it is, suggests that further surgery is not required unless there is histological evidence of tumour within 1 mm of the resection margin, lymphovascular invasion or poor differentiation of the tumour.[44] It is to be hoped, however, that the wealth of experience that is accumulating from the UK National Colorectal Screening Programme will help to refine these criteria.

When a completion colectomy is required, one difficulty that can be encountered by the surgeon is identifying the section of colon that is to be removed. Colonoscopic localisation of a lesion is notoriously unreliable, and polypectomy scars heal very quickly. For these reasons, if an endoscopist has any reason to suspect that a polyp may be harbouring invasive malignancy (over 2 cm, ulcerated or hard), then the polypectomy site should be marked with an injection of submucosal ink in order to guide the surgeon in the event of further intervention.

Emergency management

In the UK, about 20% of patients with colonic cancer will present as an emergency and 16% will present with obstruction. Bleeding and perforation are less common modes of emergency presentation; when perforation occurs, it is often in the caecum as a result of distal obstruction in the face of a competent ileocaecal valve. Obstruction is thus the most likely reason for emergency or urgent operation.

Investigation

The patient with obstruction will usually present with colicky abdominal pain and abdominal distension, with a variable degree of vomiting and change of bowel habit. Paradoxically, the obstructed patient may complain of diarrhoea rather than constipation, owing to overflow. The first specific investigation in this case will be a plain abdominal radiograph, which will demonstrate the typical features of large or, in the case of an obstructing caecal cancer, small bowel obstruction.

Particular attention should be paid to the size of the caecum on the radiograph, and whether or not gas is present in small bowel loops. If the caecum is 12 cm or more in diameter and there is no evidence of decompression into the small bowel, then there is significant risk of caecal perforation and urgent intervention is required. The same applies when the caecum is tender to palpation.

Before committing the patient to laparotomy, however, it is important to identify the site of obstruction, as colonic pseudo-obstruction can mimic the clinical and radiological signs of mechanical obstruction. Increasingly, the water-soluble contrast enema is being replaced by an abdominal CT with contrast. Barium should not be used as it can become inspissated in the segment of colon distal to the obstruction, and if there is a perforation barium can enter the peritoneal cavity with disastrous consequences.

Management of obstruction

Once mechanical obstruction is diagnosed and the patient resuscitated, laparotomy should proceed with experienced surgical and anaesthetic staff in attendance, preferably during daylight hours. The first task at laparotomy is usually to decompress the gaseous distension of the large bowel, and this can be achieved by inserting a 19-gauge (white) needle attached to suction into the lumen through a convenient taenia. If a larger tube is required to evacuate large amounts of liquid faeces, this should be inserted into the caecum via an enterotomy in the terminal ileum.

When the bowel can be safely handled, a decision must be made as to the type of operation required. If the obstruction is due to a right-sided lesion, it is usually easy and safe to carry out a standard right hemicolectomy. If, however, the cancer is on the left side, several options are available.

Traditionally, obstructing left-sided cancers were treated by a three-stage approach, starting with a defunctioning loop colostomy, followed by resection and anastomosis, and then by closure of the defunctioning stoma. This gradually gave way to a two-stage procedure, with primary resection of the tumour in the form of a Hartmann operation, where the proximal colon is brought out as an end colostomy and the distal segment either closed off or brought out as a mucous fistula.[45]

Recently, however, there has been a move towards one-stage procedures, and here the choice lies between a subtotal colectomy with ileocolic or ileorectal anastomosis and a left hemicolectomy after on-table colonic irrigation.[46] For tumours in the region of the splenic flexure, the former approach is often sensible, especially if there is doubt about the viability of the caecum.

> ✔✔ There is also an argument for subtotal colectomy for tumours in the more distal colon, but a randomised trial comparing both strategies found that patients treated by left hemicolectomy had more acceptable postoperative bowel function.[47]

If a decision is made to perform a left hemicolectomy, then many surgeons irrigate the colon proximal to the site of obstruction using the technique described by Dudley et al.[48] This is illustrated in **Fig. 4.10**, and although anaesthetic scavenging tubing inserted proximal to the tumour and a large Foley catheter inserted into the caecum by means of an enterotomy in the appendix or the terminal ileum were originally described, a number of dedicated devices are now available.

Clearly the choice of operation will depend on individual circumstances, and few surgeons would attempt an anastomosis in the presence of severe intra-abdominal sepsis or in a severely ill patient. In these cases, a Hartmann resection is acceptable, and in some situations a defunctioning stoma may be the best option. Increasingly, expanding metal stents are being used in obstructing left-sided colonic tumours. Although most experience has been palliative in intent, more lesions are now being treated in this way to allow decompression followed by bowel preparation and elective resection of the tumour.[49] Whether or not this is the optimal method for treating obstructing colonic tumours will depend on the results of ongoing randomised trials.

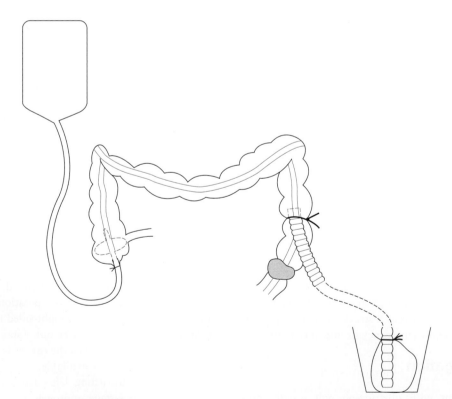

Figure 4.10 • On-table colonic irrigation.

Management of perforation

In the patient who is found to have a perforated caecum as a result of an obstructing distal cancer, an extended right hemicolectomy or subtotal colectomy is the treatment of choice. Whether or not an anastomosis is fashioned will depend on the degree of peritoneal contamination. For the cancer that has perforated primarily, it is important to resect the lesion itself to eliminate not only the malignancy but also the source of sepsis. This can be technically demanding, and for left-sided lesions will almost always necessitate a Hartmann procedure.

Management of advanced disease

The surgical management of the advanced primary tumour is covered in the section on elective surgery. In colonic cancer, local recurrence usually occurs at the suture line and, in the absence of disseminated disease, re-resection should be attempted, although palliative bypass may be all that can be achieved. The patient with distant metastases poses different challenges.

Operable metastases

Hepatic resection for colorectal cancer metastases is now widely practised, but it has never been tested by a randomised trial, and all comparative studies have used retrospective data from historical controls.[50]

> ✅ With careful patient selection, hepatectomy for colorectal metastases can be associated with a 5-year survival of around 33%,[50] and although the most widely accepted criterion for resection is one to three resectable metastases in one lobe of the liver, many surgeons are now extending their indications.

The role of preoperative chemotherapy in these patients is currently unclear, and the results of a phase III multicentre international trial are awaited. There is, however, some non-randomised evidence that preoperative treatment with 5-fluorouracil plus folinic acid (FUFA) and oxaliplatin may improve both resectability and long-term survival.

> ✅ In a proportion of patients with liver disease that is not amenable to resection, in situ ablation using radiofrequency energy may be employed.[51] This may prolong survival, but as yet must be regarded as palliative.

Pulmonary metastases may also be amenable to resection, but as only 10% of patients develop such metastases and only 10% of these have disease confined to the lung, very few patients will be suitable. Nonetheless, segmental resection of the lung may be associated with 5-year survival rates of 20–40%.[52]

Inoperable disseminated disease

> ✅✅ In the patient with widespread disease, chemotherapy containing 5-fluorouracil (5-FU) is the only established therapeutic option, but this can only be regarded as palliative. Few studies have compared chemotherapy with supportive treatment only, and the survival benefits, although significant, are not great. Based on a recent meta-analysis, patients with ECOG scores of 2, 1 and 0 treated with this type of chemotherapy have median survival times of 4, 10 and 14 months, respectively.[53]
>
> Recently, the oral 5-FU prodrugs UFT and capecitabine have come into use, and as they have been found to offer equivalent survival with the advantage of increased ease of delivery they are now regarded as suitable single agents for first-line use. Even more recently, combination chemotherapy with intravenous 5-FU and either irinotecan or oxaliplatin has been demonstrated to enhance survival as both first- and second-line therapy.[54] Both of these strategies have been approved in the UK by the National Institute for Clinical Excellence (NICE).[55]

Monclonal antibody treatment either in the form of bevacizumab (an antibody against vascular endothelial growth factor)[56] or cetuximab (an antibody against epidermal growth factor receptor)[57] has been shown to confer survival advantages in combination with conventional chemotherapy. However, although cetuximab along with combination chemotherapy has been recommended by NICE to downstage liver metastases in patients fit for liver surgery, bevacizumab has not been recommended on the grounds that it is not cost-effective.[55]

Pathological staging

Accurate, detailed and consistent pathology reporting for colorectal cancer is important for estimating prognosis and planning further treatment in terms of adjuvant therapy (see Chapter 6). Both macroscopic and histological appearances must be described in some detail, and the following information should be available.

Microscopic description

1. Size of the tumour (greatest dimension).
2. Site of the tumour in relation to the resection margins.
3. Any abnormalities of the background bowel.

Microscopic description

1. Histological type.
2. Differentiation of the tumour, based on the predominant grade within the tumour.[58]

3. Maximum extent of invasion into/through the bowel wall (submucosa, muscularis propria, extramural).
4. Serosal involvement by tumour, if present.[59]
5. A statement on the completeness of excision at the cut ends (including the 'doughnuts' from stapling devices) and at any radial margin.
6. The number of lymph nodes examined, the number containing metastases, and whether or not the apical node is involved.
7. Extramural vascular invasion if present.[60]
8. Pathological staging of the tumour according to Dukes' classification.[61,62]

Dukes' staging is simple, reproducible and widely recognised, but TNM staging is becoming increasingly recognised as the international standard; the two systems are described in Table 4.1. Some pathologists use the Jass classification,[63] although its usefulness may be limited by observer variation in

Table 4.1 • Clinicopathological staging of colorectal cancer

Dukes' staging* (based on histological examination of the resection specimen)	
A	Invasive carcinoma not breaching the muscularis propria
B	Invasive carcinoma breaching the muscularis propria, but not involving regional lymph nodes
C1	Invasive carcinoma involving the regional lymph nodes (apical node negative)
C2	Invasive carcinoma involving the regional lymph nodes (apical node positive)
TNM staging[†]	
T	Primary tumour
TX	Primary tumour cannot be assessed
T0	No evidence of primary tumour
Tis	Carcinoma in situ
T1	Tumour invades submucosa
T2	Tumour invades muscularis propria
T3	Tumour invades through muscularis propria into subserosa or into non-peritonealised pericolic or perirectal tissues
T4	Tumour perforates the visceral peritoneum or directly invades other organs or structures[‡]
N	Regional lymph nodes
NX	Regional lymph nodes cannot be assessed
N0	No regional lymph node metastasis
N1	Metastasis in 1–3 pericolic or perirectal lymph nodes
N2	Metastasis in 4 or more pericolic or perirectal lymph nodes
M	Distant metastasis
M0	No distant metastases
M1	Distant metastases

*Dukes' stage D has come to mean the presence of distant metastases.
[†]UT, ultrasound depth; yT, following neoadjuvant therapy.
[‡]Direct invasion in T4 includes invasion of other segments of the colorectum by way of the serosa, e.g. invasion of the sigmoid colon by a carcinoma of the caecum.

the degree of lymphocytic infiltration at the advancing margin of the tumour (one of the four parameters that contribute to the classification) and the fact that its prognostic value appears to be confined to rectal tumours.

After curative resection, cancer registry data indicate that age-adjusted 5-year survival for Dukes' stage A colonic cancer is 85%, for stage B 67% and for stage C 37%. These results can be improved on as evidenced by individual series,[64] and the 'Will Rogers' effect (stage migration owing to variable quality of pathology reporting) may play a role in this respect.

Recommendations for best practice

These recommendations summarise the evidence-based guidelines from the Association of Coloproctology and the Scottish Intercollegiate Guidelines Network for the management of colorectal cancer as they apply to colonic tumours.[18,65]

Investigation

1. Patients with suspicious symptoms or proven colorectal cancer should be investigated with either endoscopic visualisation of the whole rectum plus a high-quality double-contrast barium enema or a total colonoscopy or CT colography.
2. Unless it cannot alter management, all patients should have screening (preoperative where possible) for lung and liver metastases by CT scanning.

Preparation for surgery

1. All patients undergoing surgery for colon cancer should give informed consent. This implies being given information about the likely benefits and risks of the proposed treatment and details of any alternatives.
2. Mechanical bowel preparation before surgery is no longer recommended (except where an upstream stoma is planned – rare with colonic tumours and more applicable to total mesorectal excision surgery).
3. Subcutaneous heparin or intermittent compression should be employed as thromboembolism prophylaxis in surgery for colorectal cancer unless there is a specific contraindication.

4. All patients undergoing surgery for colorectal cancer should have antibiotic prophylaxis. It is impossible to be dogmatic as regards the precise regimen, but a single dose of appropriate intravenous antibiotics appears to be effective.

Elective surgical treatment

1. Any tumour with a distal margin at 15 cm or less from the anal verge using a rigid sigmoidoscope should be classified as rectal.
2. Although no definite recommendations can be made regarding anastomotic technique, the interrupted serosubmucosal method is adaptable to all colonic anastomoses and has the lowest reported leak rate in the literature.
3. Laparoscopic surgery for colorectal cancer should be performed only by experienced laparoscopic surgeons who have been properly trained in colorectal surgery, and who are prepared to audit their results very carefully.

Emergency treatment

1. Emergency surgery should be carried out during daytime hours as far as possible by experienced surgeons and anaesthetists.
2. In patients presenting with obstruction, steps should be taken to exclude pseudo-obstruction before operation.
3. Stoma formation should be carried out in the patient's interests only, and not as a result of lack of experienced surgical staff or appropraite stenting facilities.
4. The overall mortality for emergency/urgent surgery should be 20% or less.

Treatment of advanced disease

1. It is recommended that effective palliation with optimal quality of remaining life should be the main aim of therapy in advanced disease.
2. Consideration should be given to palliative chemotherapy in patients with local advanced and metastatic disease. Thus, patients with advanced disease who remain in good general condition should have the opportunity to discuss the possible benefits of palliative therapy with an oncologist.
3. Consideration should be given to surgical treatment in selected patients with locally advanced and metastatic disease. In particular,

the patient with limited hepatic involvement should be considered for partial hepatectomy by an experienced liver surgeon.

Outcomes

Surgeons should carefully audit the outcome of their colorectal cancer surgery.

1. They should expect to achieve an operative mortality of less than 20% for emergency surgery and 5% for elective surgery for colorectal cancer.
2. Wound infection rates after surgery for colorectal cancer should be less than 10%.

3. Surgeons should expect to achieve an overall leak rate below 4% for colonic resection.
4. Surgeons should examine carefully their practice with a view to meeting or improving on targets set by national long-term mortality statistics.

Pathology

All resected colorectal tumours should be submitted for histological examination. The report should reach an acceptable standard, providing information that will be useful in assessing prognosis, planning treatment and carrying out audit.

Key points

- It is now accepted that most if not all colon cancers arise from pre-existing adenomas. Flat adenomas, which are difficult to detect without special endoscopic techniques, may be a significant precursor lesion.
- The main lifestyle factors that predispose to colon cancer are currently recognised as obesity, lack of exercise, red and processed meat, a low-fibre diet, alcohol and smoking.
- Colonoscopy is the gold standard investigative technique, but CT colography is playing an increasingly important role. CT scanning is the optimal method of preoperative staging.
- Faecal occult blood screening can reduce colon cancer mortality, and is currently being introduced throughout the UK and in many other countries. The evidence to support flexible sigmoidoscopy in this context is awaited.
- Enhanced recovery programmes after colonic resection are effective in reducing hospital stay.
- Colon cancer patients presenting as emergencies, particularly obstruction, should be treated by colorectal specialists, and stenting facilities should be available.
- The range of agents available for treating advanced disease is rapidly expanding and, although many will not be suitable, all patients with metastases should be considered for surgical treatment.

References

1. Cancer Research UK Statistics on Colorectal Cancer. http://www.cancerresearchuk.org/ aboutcancer/statistics/ statstables/colorectalcancer.
2. Williams PL, Warwick R. Gray's anatomy. Edinburgh: Churchill Livingstone; 1980.
3. UKCCCR. Handbook for the clinicopathological assessment and staging of colorectal cancer. UKCCCR;1989.
4. Bass BL, Enker WE, Lightdale CJ. Advances in colorectal carcinoma surgery. New York: World Medical Press; 1993.
5. Leslie A, Carey FA, Pratt NR, et al. The colorectal adenoma–carcinoma sequence. Br J Surg 2002;89:845–60.
6. Rembacken BJ, Fujii T, Cairns A, et al. Flat and depressed colonic neoplasms: a prospective study of 1000 colonoscopies in the UK. Lancet 2000;355:1211–4.
7. Jinnai D. In: Goligher JC, editor. Surgery of the anus, rectum and colon. 4th ed. London: Baillière Tindall; 1982. p. 447.
8. Powell SM, Zilz N, Beazer-Barclay Y, et al. APC mutations occur early during colorectal tumorigenesis. Nature 1992;359:235–7.
9. Scott N, Bell SM, Sagar P, et al. p53 expression and K-ras mutation in colorectal adenomas. Gut 1993;34:621–4.
10. Kikuchi-Yanoshita R, Konishi M, Ito S, et al. Genetic changes of both p53 alleles associated with the conversion from colorectal adenoma to early carcinoma in familial adenomatous polyposis and non-familial adenomatous polyposis patients. Cancer Res 1992;52:3965–71.
11. Kastan MB, Onyekwere O, Sidransky D, et al. Participation of p53 protein in the cellular response to DNA damage. Cancer Res 1991;51:6304–11.
12. Smith G, Carey FA, Beattie J, et al. Mutations in APC, Kirsten-ras, and p53 – alternative genetic

pathways to colorectal cancer. Proc Natl Acad Sci U S A 2002;99:9433–8.

13. Conlin A, Smith G, Carey FA, et al. The prognostic significance of K-ras, p53, and APC mutations in colorectal cancer. Gut 2005;54:1283–6.

14. World Cancer Research Fund. Food, nutrition, physical activity and the prevention of cancer; a global perspective. Washington, DC: AICR; 2007.

15. Giovannucci E. An updated review of the epidemiological evidence that cigarette smoking increases risk of colorectal cancer. Cancer Epidemiol Biomarkers Prev 2001;10:725–31.

16. Thompson MR, Heath I, Ellis BG, et al. Identifying and managing patients at low risk of bowel cancer in general practice. Br Med J 2003;327:263–5.

17. Anderson N, Cook HB, Coates R. Colonoscopically detected colorectal cancer missed on barium enema. Gastrointest Radiol 1991;16:123–7.

18. Association of Coloproctology of Great Britain and Ireland. Guidelines for the management of colorectal cancer. 3rd ed. Association of Coloproctology of Great Britain and Ireland; 2007.

19. Burton RM, Landreth KS, Barrows GH, et al. Appearance, properties and origin of altered human haemoglobin in faeces. Lab Invest 1976;35:111–5.

20. Bennett DH, Hardcastle JD. Early diagnosis and screening. In: Williams NS, editor. Colorectal cancer (Clinical Surgery International, Vol. 20). Edinburgh: Churchill Livingstone; 1996. p. 21–37.

21. Mandel JS, Church TR, Ederer F, et al. Colorectal cancer mortality: effectiveness of biennial screening for fecal occult blood. J Natl Cancer Inst 1999;91:434–7.

22. Hardcastle JD, Robinson MHE, Moss SM, et al. Randomised controlled trial of faecal occult blood screening for colorectal cancer. Lancet 1996;348:1472–7.

23. Kronborg O, Fenger C, Olsen J, et al. A randomized study of screening for colorectal cancer with fecal occult blood test at Funen in Denmark. Lancet 1996;348:1467–71.

These three randomised trials (Refs 21–23) provide evidence that disease-specific mortality can be reduced by faecal occult blood screening for colorectal cancer, and form the basis for current debates regarding the introduction of national screening programmes in several countries.

24. Allison JE, Sakoda LC, Levin TR, et al. Screening for colorectal neoplasms with new fecal occult blood tests: update on performance characteristics. J Natl Cancer Inst 2007;99:1462–70.

25. Atkin WS, Edwards R, Kralj-Hans I, et al. Once-only flexible sigmoidoscopy screening in prevention of colorectal cancer: a multicentre randomised controlled trial. Lancet 2010;375:1624–33.

26. Atkin WS, Saunders BP. Surveillance guidelines after removal of colorectal adenomatous polyps. Gut 2002;51(Suppl. v):v6–vv979.

27. Burrows L, Tartter P. Effect of blood transfusions on colonic malignancy recurrence rate. Lancet 1982;ii:662.

28. Busch ORC, Hop WCJ, Hoynck van Papendrecht MAW, et al. Blood transfusions and prognosis in colorectal cancer. N Engl J Med 1993;328:1372–6.

29. Guanega K, Attallah AN, Castro AA, et al. Mechanical bowel preparation for elective colorectal surgery. Cochrane Database Syst Rev 2006;(2).

30. Collins R, Scrimgeour A, Yusuf S, et al. Reduction in fatal pulmonary embolism and venous thrombosis by perioperative administration of subcutaneous heparin. N Engl J Med 1988;318:1162–73.

This important meta-analysis established the use of low-dose subcutaneous heparin as a prophylactic measure in abdominal surgery.

31. Kakkar VV, Cohen AT, Edmonson RA, et al. Low molecular weight versus standard heparin for prevention of venous thromboembolism after major abdominal surgery. Lancet 1993;341:259–65.

32. Keighley MRB, Williams NS. Perioperative care. In: Keighley MRB, Williams NS, editors. Surgery of the anus, rectum and colon. 3rd ed. Elsevier Saunders; 2008.

33. Rowe-Jones DC, Peel ALG, Kingston RD, et al. Single dose cefotaxime plus metronidazole versus three dose cefotaxime plus metronidazole as prophylaxis against wound infection in colorectal surgery: multicentre prospective randomised study. Br Med J 1990;300:18–22.

As a result of several trials, the place of prophylactic antibiotics in colorectal surgery is now firmly established, and a single dose is as effective as multiple doses.

34. O'Kelly TJ, Mathew A, Ross S, et al. Optimum method for urinary drainage in major abdominal surgery: a prospective randomised trial of suprapubic versus urethral catheterisation. Br J Surg 1995;82:1367–8.

35. Aldridge MC, Phillips RKS, Hittinger R, et al. Influence of tumour site on presentation, management and subsequent outcome in large bowel cancer. Br J Surg 1986;73:663–70.

36. Matheson NA, McIntosh CA, Krukowski ZH. Continuing experience with single layer appositional anastomosis in the large bowel. Br J Surg 1985;72:S104–6.

These results have yet to be bettered, and form a persuasive argument for the use of the serosubmucosal anastomotic technique.

37. Carty NJ, Keating J, Campbell J, et al. Prospective audit of an extramucosal technique for intestinal anastomosis. Br J Surg 1991;78:1439–41.

38. Leslie A, Steele RJC. The interrupted serosubmucosal anastomosis – still the gold standard. Colorectal Dis 2003;5:362–6.

39. Docherty JG, McGregor JR, Akyol AM, et al. Comparison of manually constructed and stapled anastomoses in colorectal surgery. Ann Surg 1995;221:176–84.

40. Hoffmann J, Shoukouh-Amiri MH, Damm P, et al. A prospective, controlled study of prophylactic drainage after colonic anastomoses. Dis Colon Rectum 1987;30:449–52.

41. Johnson CD, Lamont PM, Orr N, et al. Is a drain necessary after colonic anastomosis? J R Soc Med 1989;82:661–4.

42. Sagar PM, Couse N, Kerin M, et al. Randomised trial of drainage of colorectal anastomosis. Br J Surg 1993;80:769–71.

43. Wind J, Polle SW, Fung Kon Jin PH, et al. Systematic review of enhanced recovery programmes in colonic surgery. Br J Surg 2006;93:800–9.

44. Ruiz-Tovar J, Jimenez-Miramon J, Valle A, et al. Endoscopic resection as unique treatment for early colorectal cancer. Rev Esp Enferm Dig 2010;102:435–41.

45. Rothenberger DA, Mayoral J, Deen K. Obstruction and perforation. In: Williams NS, editor. Colorectal cancer (Clinical Surgery International, Vol. 20). Edinburgh: Churchill Livingstone; 1996. p. 123–33.

46. Koruth NM, Krukowski ZH, Youngson GG, et al. Intra-operative colonic irrigation in the management of left-sided large bowel emergencies. Br J Surg 1985;72:708–11.

47. SCOTIA Study Group. Single-state treatment for malignant left-sided colonic obstruction: a prospective randomised trial comparing subtotal colectomy with segmental resection following intraoperative irrigation. Br J Surg 1996;82:1622–7.
One of the few randomised trials of surgical technique in emergency colonic surgery, this study indicates that segmental resection of obstructed colon cancer provides better long-term results than subtotal colectomy.

48. Dudley HAF, Radcliffe AG, McGeehan D. Intraoperative irrigation of the colon to permit primary anastomosis. Br J Surg 1980;67:80.

49. Watson AJ, Shanmugam V, Mackay I, et al. Outcomes after placements of colorectal stents. Colorectal Dis 2005;7:70–3.

50. Garden OJ, Rees M, Poston GJ, et al. Guidelines for resection of colorectal liver metastases. Gut 2006;55(Suppl. III):iii1–8.

51. Hompes D, Prevoo W, Ruers T. Radiofrequency ablation as a treatment tool for liver metastases of colorectal origin. Cancer Imaging 2011;11:23–30.

52. Shirouzu K, Isomoto H, Hayashi A, et al. Surgical treatment for patients with pulmonary metastases after resection of primary colorectal carcinoma. Cancer 1995;76:393–8.

53. Thirion P, Wolmark N, Haddad E, et al. Impact of chemotherapy in patients with colorectal metastases confined to the liver: a re-analysis of 1,458 non-operable patients randomised in 22 trials and 4 meta-analyses. Proc Am Soc Clin Oncol 1999;10:1317–20.

54. Grothley A, Sarjent D. Overall survival of patients with advanced colorectal cancer correlates with availability of fluorouracil, irinotecan and oxaliplatin regardless of whether doublet or singlet agent therapy is used first line. J Clin Oncol 2005;23:9441–2.

55. National Institute for Clinical Excellence (NICE). Clinical guidline: the diagnosis and management of colorectal cancer. NICE; 2011.

56. Hurwitz H, Fechrenbacher L, Novotny W, et al. Bevacizumab plus irinotecan, fluorouracil and leucovorin for metastatic colorectal cancer. N Engl J Med 2004;350:2335–42.

57. Cunningham D, Humblet Y, Siena S, et al. Cetuximab monotherapy and cetuximab plus irinotecan in irinotecan refractory metastatic colorectal cancer. N Engl J Med 2004;351:337–45.

58. Halvorsen TB, Seim E. Degree of differentiation in colorectal adenocarcinomas: a multivariate analysis of the influence on survival. J Clin Pathol 1988;41:532–7.

59. Shepherd NA, Baxter KJ, Love SB. Influence of local peritoneal involvement on pelvic recurrence and prognosis in rectal cancer. J Clin Pathol 1995;48:849–55.

60. Talbot IC, Ritchie S, Leighton M, et al. Invasion of veins by carcinoma of the rectum: method of detection, histological features and significance. Histopathology 1981;5:141–63.

61. Dukes CE, Bussey HJR. The spread of rectal cancer and its effect on prognosis. Br J Cancer 1958;12:309–20.

62. UICC. TNM classification of malignant tumours. 7th ed. Wiley-Liss; 2010.

63. Jass JR, Love SB, Northover JMA. A new prognostic classification of rectal cancer. Lancet 1987;i:1303–6.

64. Hawley PR. In: Goligher JC, editor. Surgery of the anus, rectum and colon. 4th ed. London: Baillière Tindall; 1984. p. 549.

65. Scottish Intercollegiate Guidelines Network. Diagnosis and management of colorectal cancer. : A national clinical guideline SIGN; 2011.

5

Rectal cancer

A. Zia Janjua
Brendan J. Moran

Introduction

Cancer of the rectum, defined as a tumour within 15 cm from the anal verge, accounts for approximately 30% of all colorectal malignancies. There were 14 440 new cases of rectal cancer registered in the UK in 2008.[1]

Treatment is predominantly surgical excision with addition of neoadjuvant therapy (radiotherapy or chemoradiotherapy administered preoperatively) in selected cases. Total mesorectal excision (TME) is now considered the gold standard, with fewer local recurrences and better overall survival.[2-6] Major resectional surgery is technically challenging due to relative inaccessibility within the confines of the bony pelvis, difficulty in reconstruction, risk of anastomotic leakage and local recurrence.

Major surgery is associated with significant morbidity, mortality and may be inappropriate in some cases. Availability of a range of treatments, both surgical and non-surgical, for management of rectal cancer makes it critical that patient assessment, cancer staging (Box 5.1), perioperative optimisation (Box 5.2) and selection of appropriate therapy be carried out in a multidisciplinary team (MDT) setting.

Objectives of surgery

The aims of rectal cancer surgery are to cure the patient and if possible preserve normal bowel,

bladder and sexual function. Mechanisms to achieve these aims encompass two key treatment modalities, namely surgical technique[2,3,7] and neoadjuvant therapy, both of which have been shown to reduce local recurrence.[4,5] Optimal surgery, in the form of TME, reduces local recurrence and improves survival.[2-6,8,9] Evidence from randomised trials has reported the reduction in local recurrence with neoadjuvant radiotherapy,[2,5,10] though to date only one trial has reported improved survival.[11] Preoperative radiotherapy can 'downstage' the primary tumour, but caution is warranted. The original histology provides an estimate of the likelihood of occult hepatic and other systemic metastases already present at the time of resection. Neoadjuvant radiotherapy has no effect on this original estimate: even if the primary tumour shrinks or disappears completely (pathologically complete response, pCR) in a subset (approximately 10–20% after chemoradiotherapy), a tumour that is truly local will be cured by adequate locoregional therapy; inadequate locoregional therapy will lead to local recurrence. In the presence of occult metastases, the outcome will be determined by the metastases.

The rectal cancer surgeon can impact on:

1. in-hospital mortality;
2. local recurrence;
3. quality of life.

History
- Altered bowel habit
- Bleeding/mucus PR
- Tenesmus, urgency
- Constant anal pain
- Continence issues

Digital rectal examination/rigid sigmoidoscopy
- Extent and position of neoplasm
- Mobility/fixity
- Sphincter assessment
- Accurate measurement of tumour distance from anal verge and dentate line

Colonoscopy and biopsy
- Synchronous polyps in 13–36%
- Synchronous cancers 3–5%

CT thorax/abdomen and pelvis MRI/EUS
- Staging local extent, predicting status of resection margin
- Carcinoembryonic antigen (CEA)
- Preoperative discussion at MDT

Box 5.2 • Perioperative optimisation

- Assessment and optimisation of comorbidities
- Plan for enhanced recovery protocol/fast track surgery
- Antibiotic prophylaxis
- Deep vein thrombosis prophylaxis

In-hospital mortality

Postoperative deaths in hospital involve patient, tumour and surgeon-related factors. Clearly, in an elderly patient with comorbidity who presents in an emergency with an obstructing tumour, the risks of death are much higher than in a younger patient undergoing elective surgery. Elective surgery under the age of 80 years has an overall in-hospital mortality of 1–8% compared with 6–16% mortality in those over 80.[8,12] A patient over 80 with malignant large bowel obstruction has a 1 in 3 chance of in-hospital mortality.[13] Similarly, the in-hospital mortality in the presence of an anastomotic leak is much higher.[14] Anastomotic leak rates vary between surgeons. Whilst a low anastomosis, preoperative radiotherapy and other factors increase the risk of leakage, the one major consistent mechanism to reduce the rate and consequences of leakage is a defunctioning

stoma. This surgical decision to defunction or not is crucial and increasingly most authorities agree that defunctioning should be considered in all patients who have had a TME for rectal cancer. From time to time the decision to adopt a local approach, particularly for early tumours, may be optimal for a patient. Thus, a decision for local excision, trans-anal endoscopic microsurgery (TEMS) or even local radiotherapy will be influenced by weighing up the likely benefit of the alternative and fitness of the patient for a major resection.

Local recurrence

Local recurrence after rectal surgery is defined as disease in the pelvis, including recurrence at the site of anastomosis and in the perineum.[15] Local recurrence is for the most part incurable and results in major morbidity with debilitating symptoms of pelvic pain, ureteric obstruction, intestinal and urinary tract fistulation, and poor bowel and urinary function. Increasingly local recurrence is recognised as failure of complete tumour excision at primary surgery. Thus, local 'recurrence' may, in many cases, represent persistent and progressive disease, rather than true recurrence. There are a number of predictors of risk of local recurrence (Box 5.3). Practically all are associated with both locally advanced tumours and frequently metastatic disease at presentation. Additionally, they predict for a high risk of subsequent postoperative systemic recurrence. Fortunately, some of these factors can be predicted preoperatively, which helps in planning the appropriate management in an MDT setting, employing appropriate neoadjuvant treatments in selective cases.

Box 5.3 • Risk factors for local recurrence

- Size of the primary[16]
- Involvement of the circumferential resection margin (CRM)[10]
- Distal location of the tumour/nearness to anal verge[12,16]
- Extramural vascular invasion[8,9]
- Tumour differentiation[8,9]
- Nodal status[8–10]
- Extent of extramural spread[8–10]
- Peritoneal involvement by tumour[7,8,17]

Reported local recurrence rates vary from 2.6% to 32% and are probably most influenced by surgical technique.[18,19] The lowest recurrence rates and best survival have been consistently reported with TME.[2,3,6,18–20]

Magnetic resonance imaging in assessment of circumferential resection margin and the role of preoperative radiotherapy

Rectal cancer spreads by local extension, via the lymphatics and via the bloodstream. Lymphatic drainage is associated with the arterial pedicle and is generally addressed by a combination of TME and high ligation of the inferior mesenteric artery. Local spread of a rectal cancer in the confines of the narrow pelvis results in a risk of involvement of the mesorectal fascia, the circumferential resection margin (CRM) in TME. Involvement of the CRM on the resected specimen appears to be the main determinant of adverse risk of local recurrence. A positive CRM, defined as tumour within 1 mm of the margin of the resected specimen, and depth of extramural invasion are independent predictors of local recurrence and poor prognosis.[10,16] These observations are supported by studies from Norway[21] and the Netherlands.[22]

The CRM may also be involved due to metastatic nodal disease. There is debate as to whether involved nodes, in their own right, increase local recurrence even if not directly involving the CRM. It has been reported that patients with positive lymph nodes have a higher risk of local recurrence.[23] However, others found that lymph node involvement was not associated with higher local recurrence, provided optimal TME is performed.[21,24] While other risk factors, such as vascular invasion, differentiation, etc., are undoubtedly major determinants of long-term survival, the single main factor that can be manipulated by optimal treatment is the CRM.

Debate persists as to the merits of routine or selective neoadjuvant therapy for patients with rectal cancer. However, there has been a recent shift towards selective use due to the adverse risks of radiotherapy and reports showing no long-term survival benefit in operable rectal cancer.[4,25] Indeed, many neoadjuvant trials have been conducted against an unacceptably high rate of local recurrence in the control arm,[26] as well as inconvenience and costs associated with radiotherapy.

Complications of preoperative radiotherapy

While a detailed discussion about radiotherapy is provided elsewhere (Chapter 6), a few issues with regard to early and later complications are noteworthy. Early complications include perineal wound breakdown, diarrhoea, proctitis, urinary tract infection, small bowel obstruction, leucopenia and venous thrombosis.

In addition, radiotherapy has been shown to have adverse effects on anal function and on the function and integrity of a coloanal anastomosis with or without formation of a colonic pouch.[27]

Comparing the pre- and postoperative situations, a German study[28] reported Grade 3 or 4 acute toxicity in 27% of patients with preoperative chemoradiotherapy versus 40% in the postoperative group ($P = 0.001$); the corresponding rates of long-term toxic effects were 14% and 24%, respectively ($P = 0.01$).

Downstaging rectal cancer with preoperative radiotherapy

The 15 cm rectum has been arbitrarily divided into three parts, with the lower rectum 0–6 cm, the middle rectum 7–11 cm and the upper rectum 12–15 cm from the anal verge. There is little debate as to whether a T3 middle or upper rectal cancer (that is, above 7 cm) is particularly at high risk of local recurrence, providing surgery is adequate and that a TME has resulted in an intact cover of mesorectal fat and fascia. However, in the lower rectum a T3 tumour has, by definition, gone through the wall of the bowel and commonly will have an involved margin at the level of the sphincter complex unless the rectum is excised 'en bloc' with the sphincter. Endoanal ultrasound appears to be particularly good at estimating the T stage.[29] Correlations with pathology indicate accuracy of endoluminal ultrasound (EUS), particularly in T staging, though less so in N staging.[29] EUS is particularly helpful in selecting patients who may be suitable for local excision, generally agreed to be early T1 tumours. However, the main determinant of local recurrence is undoubtedly a positive CRM and EUS is poor at assessment of the CRM. Magnetic resonance imaging (MRI) has been particularly useful in the ability to visualise the CRM and to accurately predict either involved, threatened or clear margins and thus direct treatment strategy.[30,31] A patient with an obviously involved margin on MRI should be considered for neoadjuvant therapy to reduce margin involvement at subsequent surgery by 'downstaging' and perhaps 'downsizing' the tumour. All patients with a threatened margin (which really includes most very low tumours) should also be considered for preoperative treatment, whereas patients with clear margins can be treated by optimal surgery alone.

Increasingly, neoadjuvant therapy includes a combination of chemotherapy and radiotherapy. Frykholm et al.[32] published a small randomised controlled trial in 2001 wherein patients with fixed rectal carcinomas were randomised to preoperative radiotherapy or chemo-radiotherapy (CRT). This trial showed a significant improvement in resectability and reduction in local failure with the use of CRT.[32] With preoperative irradiation of clinically mobile lesions, pathological complete response (PCR) rates of 10–20% have been reported, and with preoperative chemo-radiation, higher PCR rates of 30–35% have been reported.[33]

The delay following neoadjuvant treatment may be important. A dose of 25 cGy in five fractions (short-course radiotherapy) is usually combined with surgery within 1 week, with minimal downstaging or downsizing. Interim results from the ongoing Stockholm-III trial, which compared outcomes of timing of surgery after short-course radiotherapy (SCRT) with immediate surgery, SCRT and surgery >6 weeks later, and conventional long-course radiotherapy (RT), which traditionally has involved surgery >6 weeks after completion of RT, have been reported.[34] SCRT was associated with more complications and more mortality in the elderly if surgery was delayed by more than 10 days after completion of RT therapy, unless surgery was delayed for 6 weeks when results were comparable to those after conventional long-course radiotherapy (LCRT). The recommendation was that surgery after SCRT should be done either within 5 days or delayed for more than 4 weeks.

There has been debate as to the optimal delay even in long-course regimens. The Lyon R90-01 trial reported that long-course radiotherapy with a delay of 6–8 weeks for surgery results in a significantly better tumour response and pathological downstaging of rectal cancer compared to an interval of 3 weeks.[35]

MRI can predict T stage and CRM status

Recent reports suggests that a CRM at risk of tumour involvement can be reliably seen at preoperative MRI, with correlated histology of the resected specimen.[30,31,36] Data from the prospective, multicentred MRI and Rectal Cancer European Equivalence Study (MERCURY) confirm accurate prediction both of the T staging and CRM clearance of 1 mm of the resection margin. When the CRM was predicted free of tumour and the patient had surgery alone, a histologically clear CRM was achieved in 91%. Furthermore, the extramural depth of penetration was accurately predicted to within 0.5 mm in 95% of 295 patients who had surgery alone. Thus, it is possible to classify tumours preoperatively into T3a (extramural tumour extension less than 5 mm) and T3b (extramural tumour extension greater than 5 mm) subgroups and thus consider neoadjuvant therapy in advanced tumours. Vascular invasion and lymph node involvement can also be predicted, though sensitivity and specificity for nodal status remains problematic.

Previous studies reported a varying accuracy for T staging between 67% and 83%, with a considerable interobserver variability.[36]

However, it is the distance to the CRM that is the most powerful predictor of local recurrence, rather than T stage. In a large series of MRI evaluations of CRM, there was higher accuracy for predicting tumour-free resection margins (95%) than for prediction of T stage.[31]

Tumour disruption

Cutting into a primary tumour while mobilising the rectum will run a very high risk of spilling viable cancer cells. The occasions when this may happen in rectal cancer surgery include the following:

1. When an adherent loop of intestine is thought to be stuck onto the tumour by 'inflammatory' adhesions. The loop should be resected en bloc with the primary tumour rather than pinched off.[37]

2. Fragmentation of the envelope of the mesorectum. Heald has shown the importance of maintaining the integrity of the mesorectal envelope.[26] Rough traction, blunt dissection, and failure to identify and follow the mesorectal fascia will contribute to disruption of the mesorectal envelope, which on removal will look ragged and shredded. Precise surgery using sharp or diathermy dissection under vision will reduce this problem.

3. Injudicious exploration of the anterior plane in a man with an anterior encroaching tumour (**Fig. 5.1**).

An anterior encroaching tumour in the male rarely penetrates through Denonvillier's fascia to involve the seminal vesicles, prostate or base of bladder. However, all surgeons have experienced cases where this has occurred. Anterior tumours in females are less problematic as the uterus and vagina act as a barrier to involvement of the bladder and an en-bloc hysterectomy can be performed when the uterus or posterior vagina is involved.

An extensive anterior tumour may require neoadjuvant therapy and on occasions pelvic exenteration with total cystectomy and may require cooperation with a urological team. Attention to detail and appropriate experience and radiological training result in very accurate MRI images clearly demonstrating the mesorectal fascia (Fig. 5.1).

Extent of excision – TME versus mesorectal transection, pelvic lymphadenectomy and level of vascular ligation

The extent of resection relates to the necessity for a total mesorectal excision, the management of involved pelvic side-wall nodes and the role of lateral pelvic lymphadenectomy (LPLD)[38–40] and high versus low vascular ligation.[41,42]

TME

It is now generally accepted that TME is optimal therapy for low or mid-rectal cancer. The need for TME for upper rectal cancer is debatable and now considered unnecessary for oncological reasons. The key aspect is the extent of mesorectal spread distally, which has recently been reported to be up 3 cm below the distal margin of the tumour.[43] Heald et al. described distal mesorectal deposits up to 4 cm.[44] Thus, a mesorectal clearance of 5 cm below the lower edge of the tumour by mesorectal transection (which should be carefully performed tangentially to the mesorectum and muscle tube) would seem adequate and thus would not always warrant TME for upper rectal cancer. The reasons to consider mesorectal transection revolve around a probable reduction in anastomotic leakage and

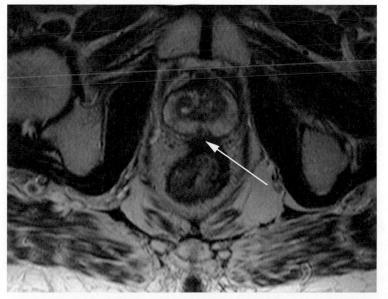

Figure 5.1 • An anterior tumour invading into the prostate can be seen (arrow).

better neorectal function when part of the meso-rectum and some of the distal rectum is preserved.

Lateral pelvic lymph nodal involvement

There is ongoing debate as to the incidence, man-agement and relevance of lateral pelvic side-wall nodes both in the East (in particular Japan) and the West, and a recent review provides an up-to-date analysis of many of the issues.[40] In essence, the incidence may be similar, mainly an issue with low rectal cancer and involved nodes increasingly sus-pected at preoperative MRI.[40]

In a retrospective review by Ueno and colleagues of 237 patients with T3/4 low rectal cancer who underwent R0 resection, including lateral pelvic lymphadenectomy (LPLD), the incidence of lateral nodal involvement increased with decreasing tu-mour height.[45] Lateral nodes were involved in 17% when the tumour was 8 cm or less from the anal verge. On subset analysis this varied from 42% for tumours below 2 cm to 10.5% for tumours between 6 and 8 cm. A multicentre retrospective review from 12 leading Japanese hospitals of 2916 patients with T3/4 low rectal cancer reported lateral nodal in-volvement in 20.1% with tumours below the peri-toneal reflection compared with 8.8% in those with upper rectal cancer.[46] Similarly, 20% involvement in low cancers has been reported in Brazil.[47]

Factors predicting an increased risk of involved lateral nodes include involved mesorectal nodes, female patients, advanced T stage, poor tumour differentiation, lymphovascular invasion and low rectal cancer.

There is undoubtedly a subset of patients with involved pelvic side-wall nodes who might benefit from LPLD, though it is of interest that neoadju-vant CRT may be as effective as nodal removal.[40] A more selective approach and modified surgi-cal techniques such as pelvic autonomic nerve preserving dissection reduce the morbidity of LPLD.[40,48–50]

High versus low inferior mesenteric artery ligation

The inferior mesenteric artery (IMA) can be divided either flush on the aorta, although 1–2 cm distally from its origin is now recommended to reduce au-tonomic nerve injury (high ligation), or below the take-off of the left colic artery (low ligation). There

has been no reported difference in terms of cancer survival.[41]

General opinion has always supported using the descending colon instead of the sigmoid when performing an anastomosis to the anal canal. Not only does the sigmoid colon generate fairly high pressures, which could therefore lead to relatively poor function, but more importantly the marginal artery may be minimal, or absent, in the sigmoid, which is thus prone to ischaemia if used for anas-tomosis. However, the descending colon will not generally reach the anal canal unless the splenic flexure is mobilised in all cases, and there is a high tie of the inferior mesenteric artery, as the left colic artery is too short and will not permit the descend-ing colon to reach (**Fig. 5.2**). Hence a low anasto-mosis will almost always need a high ligation, but for technical rather than cancer-specific reasons. A high anastomosis can usually be achieved quite easily with either a high or low ligation. A system-atic review of published data in 2008 did not find any oncological or colonic perfusion advantage in high ligation.[51]

Similarly, in a randomised controlled trial compar-ing colonic pouches with straight coloanal anasto-mosis employed in the sigmoid colon, 42% of cases had no adverse complications or functional effects compared with use of the descending colon.[52]

Implantation of viable cells

There is experimental evidence, supported by clini-cal observations, that colorectal cancer cells are shed into the bowel lumen and that viable clones of cells can implant and grow.[53] A 'triple stapling' technique, where a linear stapler is placed below a cancer prior to peranal washout and a second linear stapler is placed distally across the washed muscle tube, facilitates distal washout and elimi-nates clamp slippage and faecal spillage and im-proves access to the distal rectum for ultra-low anastomosis.[54]

Quality of life

Increasingly, quality of life (QoL) has been recog-nised as an important aspect of cancer care. In rectal cancer surgery QoL issues include preservation of

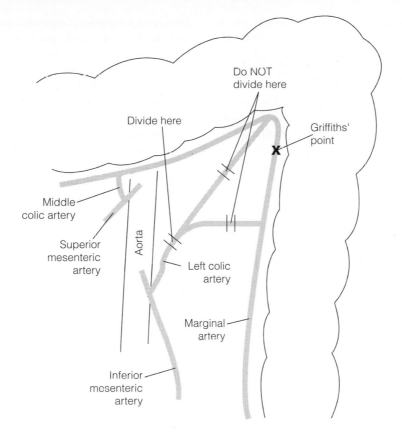

Figure 5.2 • When mobilising the vascular supply to the splenic flexure, do not divide the terminal branches of the left colic artery but rather leave them to support the marginal artery at the splenic flexure and divide the main trunk of the left colic as indicated. Frequently, the inferior mesenteric vein has to be mobilised below the inferior border of the pancreas to gain further length.

continence, reasonable bowel frequency and avoidance, as far as possible, of permanent sexual and urinary disturbance.

Preservation of continence by restorative resection

Despite an increasing proportion of patients undergoing restorative resection, some still require an abdominoperineal excision (APE) with a permanent stoma. An APE may be required for the following:

1. Cancer involving the sphincter or so near to it that attempts to preserve the sphincter complex are unjustified.
2. The functional result of restorative surgery is likely to be so poor that a colostomy would provide better QoL.

3. The potential complications of attempts to restore intestinal continuity are prohibitive, particularly in the frail and elderly.

Distal clearance margin

The literature is unclear on the definition of the distal margin. A distance of 5 cm of anorectal muscle tube at rigid sigmoidoscopy in a preoperative setting may expand to 8 cm after rectal mobilisation, and then shrink to 3 cm after specimen removal, simply because of contraction of the longitudinal muscle. If an attempt is then made to pin out the specimen, a margin of 4–5 cm may be achieved after fixation, but without pinning out the final margin may measure only 2 cm.[55]

Against this background, it is very uncommon for rectal cancer to spread more than 1 cm below the distal palpable margin of the tumour. An exception is when the tumour is poorly differentiated, when distances up to 4.5 cm have occasionally been reported.[56] Of course, the preoperative biopsy may not accurately represent the final tumour histology, but given this caveat it is usually advised that a 5-cm distal clearance margin should still be considered for a poorly differentiated tumour, whereas a 2-cm margin should suffice otherwise. This distal muscle tube margin should not be confused with the recommended 5 cm of distal mesorectum recommended for higher tumours. For very low tumours the mesorectum has tapered out and is no longer an issue. In these cases distal muscle tube excision is the issue.

For cancer in the lower third of the rectum, provided a tumour is not poorly differentiated, being able to apply a right-angled clamp, or staple line, below the lower margin of the tumour is generally considered sufficient clearance.[57] From time to time, the histology report will describe the tumour abutting the distal margin (i.e. being within 1 cm or less of the margin) but not involving it. Studies of resected specimens have shown that so long as the margin itself is uninvolved then the risk of recurrence is not increased,[37] provided that adequate circumferential clearance has been achieved.

Tumour height – the importance of rectal palpation (PR)

It is common to measure the height of the lower border of the tumour from the anal verge, which is often a variable point, for example being much further from the dentate line in patients with a funnel anus.

The dentate line can usually be felt with the examining finger. The mucosa above is more slippery to the examining finger than is the skin of the pecten. What actually matters in the critical case is not the measured height of the lower border of the tumour to the dentate line, but rather whether there is a sufficient margin either for a clamp or stapler to be placed below the tumour and above the dentate line or for the dentate line to be divided transanally without going too close to any palpably indurated tongue of tumour projecting downwards towards the dentate line. Added to this is a general assessment of the bulk of the tumour, the accessibility of the pelvis, the functional quality of the anus and the potential for improving tumour characteristics by the application of preoperative radiotherapy.

Quality of the anal function

A woman with a prior history of multiple vaginal deliveries, particularly if there has been a forceps delivery or a complication of episiotomy, has a fairly high chance of an occult sphincter injury, detectable by anal ultrasonography. In practice, one is usually guided to the quality of anal function by a history of flatus continence and an absence of episodes of faecal incontinence in the past. In a patient in more recent times, the tumour itself may have contributed to a sense of urgency and thereby may lead to unreasonable pessimism as to the true state of the anal function.

Nevertheless, a patient with an undoubtedly poor quality anal function will not be well served by an ultra-low anastomosis and would be very much better off with an end colostomy. When the tumour itself is reasonably high in the rectum, then a low Hartmann operation or better still an intersphincteric resection of the short Hartmann stump will avoid the complications of a perineal wound, but with a lower tumour an abdominoperineal excision would seem safest.

Abdominoperineal excision

Surgeons familiar with deep pelvic dissection and total mesorectal excision are now far less familiar with the bottom end of an abdominoperineal excision (APE), particularly in males. The scope for technical error is high as there is no clear anatomical plane from below, except anteriorly, where the plane, though present, can be exceedingly difficult. Pathologists report 'coning' or 'waisting' of the specimen, especially at the level of the levators (**Fig. 5.3**).

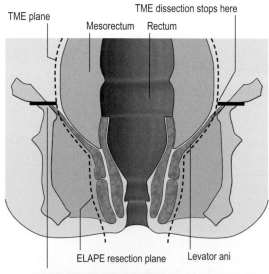

Figure 5.3 • TME and extralevator abdominoperineal (ELAPE) resection planes.

To some extent this is to be expected, as any cut voluntary muscle will contract and naturally give some impression of 'coning', but it is probable that surgeons are not excising the pelvic floor widely enough. Unless tumour is in the distal anal canal, when there will be a threat of inguinal lymphatic spread, wide excision of ischiorectal fat is probably unnecessary, although it is important to excise widely at the level of the pelvic floor, particularly as this is the point where any cancer is likely to be situated (if it were not, then TME and restorative resection might be feasible).

> ✅ Extralevator APE (ELAPE) is recommended for advanced low rectal cancer and the prone position is increasingly favoured.[58]

The risk of local recurrence can be reduced by considering neoadjuvant therapy in all cases that require an APE. However, this risks over-treatment with increased early and long-term complications. It is likely that a selective neoadjuvant policy, even for very low tumours, will be the norm in the future.

Reconstruction (colonic pouch, end-to-side or end-to-end anastomosis)

Straight coloanal anastomosis may result in poor function, certainly for a number of months and on occasion for a year or two. In a study of 84 cases treated at St Mark's Hospital by proctectomy with coloanal anastomosis, 8% went on to have a permanent colostomy constructed.[59] Increasingly, a neorectal reservoir is recommended, with most favouring a colonic 'J' pouch 5–6 cm in length.[60] Several reports confirm that early function with a colonic pouch is superior to a straight coloanal anastomosis.[60–63] This is particularly important in elderly patients, in those with a slightly compromised anal function and in those with a relatively short life expectancy.

Additionally, a colonic pouch may result in a lower anastomotic leak rate compared with an end-to-end anastomosis.[52] General opinion now favours routine use of a pouch or a side-to-end anastomosis after TME.

Sexual and urinary disturbance

The pelvic autonomic nerves are responsible for normal urinary and sexual function (particularly in the male). The presacral nerves lie like a wishbone,

joined at the sacral promontory and parting as they run distally on either pelvic side wall and are responsible for ejaculation in the male. The nerves can be identified at the start of the posterior dissection and preserved in most cases.

The nervi erigentes lie anterolaterally in the angle between the seminal vesicles and the prostate and are responsible for male erection. Attempts to control bleeding by diathermy, clamping or suturing in this area may result in erectile failure, even when injury has been unilateral. With a posteriorly situated tumour early division of Denonvillier's fascia helps to protect the nerves, but in an anterior tumour Denonvillier's fascia should be removed as it acts as a barrier to tumour penetration, and in these circumstances the nerves are at higher risk.[64]

There have been suggestions that laparoscopic rectal mobilisation may be associated with more nerve injury, though this may be a learning curve phenomenon.[65,66]

> ✅ Patients should be warned that urinary and sexual dysfunction may follow rectal excision, whether for benign or malignant disease.

Temporary defunctioning stomas

Anastomotic leakage after ultra-low anastomosis is common, with reports of an incidence ranging from 10% to 28%. A recent excellent Swedish trial comparing patients after TME randomised to a defunctioning stoma or no stoma reported a reduction in leak rate from 28% to 10.3% in patients randomised to a stoma.[67] A meta-analysis and systematic review of the literature in 2008 also found that a diverting stoma is associated with fewer clinical leaks and recommended a diverting stoma in all low rectal anastomoses.[68] Similar findings were reported from pooled data from major multicentre European trials.[69]

Follow-up

There are three issues that need to be considered during follow-up:

1. Was a synchronous tumour overlooked preoperatively?
2. How should metachronous tumours be looked for?
3. Is there benefit in follow-up?

Synchronous tumours

There is approximately a 4% risk of a synchronous cancer at the time of the original resection and a 10–20% chance of a synchronous polyp. Preoperative barium enema, computerised tomography colography (CTC) or colonoscopy is recommended to identify cases where surgical management might involve more extensive, or even an additional, resection. If a complete preoperative colonic assessment was not performed, postoperative colonoscopy at about 6 months is recommended.

Metachronous tumours

The risk of a metachronous tumour is about 4%. It would seem sensible to screen the colon at intervals of 1, 3 and 5 years, and then every 5 years, with a final screen at the age of 75, which should protect the patient until at least the age of 80 years, when the risks of routine surveillance colonoscopy may start to outweigh benefit.

Surveillance for local and distant recurrence

Overall, 60–80% of recurrences of rectal cancer present within 2 years of surgery and more than 90% within 5 years. Recurrence may be a misnomer as it may represent progression of disease not detected initially while locoregional recurrence may be a result of inadequate local treatment.

A meta-analysis in 2007 concluded that intensive follow-up after curative resection of colorectal cancer improved overall survival and re-resection rates for recurrent disease.[70] A Cochrane review in 2008 came to the same conclusion, advocating intensive follow-up for patients after curative treatment for colorectal cancer.[71] Detection and resection of liver metastases is associated with 25–51% 5-year survival.[72] It is also generally agreed that chemotherapy for advanced unresectable disease may improve quality of life and is more effective when applied early.

> ✓✓ Two meta-analyses of all randomised trials of follow-up have shown improved survival with intensive follow-up.[73,74]

The way forward

- Optimal imaging is crucial and may involve functional imaging such as PETCT in combination with pelvic MRI.
- More accurate imaging will allow more selective use of neoadjuvant radiotherapy, which is a local treatment with little impact on systemic disease.
- Neoadjuvant chemotherapy (omitting radiotherapy) may improve outcome in patients detected at imaging to have a high risk of systemic metastases.

Key points

- MRI assesses the status of the mesorectal fascia (the potential CRM), aiding selection for neoadjuvant treatment.
- Optimal outcome for rectal cancer requires adequate TME.
- Consider defunctioning stoma in low anterior resection.
- Extralevator APE is optimal management of advanced low rectal cancer involving sphincters.
- Evidence suggests benefit of intensive follow-up.

References

1. Cancer Research UK. info.cancerresearchuk.org/cancerstats/types/bowel/incidence; 2011.
2. Enker WE. Total mesorectal excision – the new golden standard of surgery for rectal cancer. Ann Med 1997;29(2):127–33.
3. Heald RJ, Moran BJ, Ryall RDH, et al. Rectal cancer: the Basingstoke experience of total mesorectal excision, 1978–1997. Arch Surg 1998;133(8):894–9.
4. Kapiteijn E, Marijnen CAM, Nagtegaal ID, et al. Preoperative radiotherapy combined with total mesorectal excision for resectable rectal cancer. N Engl J Med 2001;345:638–46.

5. Martling AL, Holm T, Rutqvist LE, et al. Effect of surgical training programme on outcome of rectal cancer in the County of Stockholm. Stockholm Colorectal Cancer Study Group, Basingstoke Bowel Cancer Research Project. Lancet 2000;356(9224):93–6.

6. Kapiteijn E, Putter H, Van de Velde CJ. Impact of the introduction and training of total mesorectal excision on recurrence and survival in rectal cancer in the Netherlands. Br J Surg 2002;89(9):1142–9.

7. Croxford M, Salerno G, Watson M, et al. Colorectal 23–28. Br J Surg 2004;91(SI):63–5.

8. Hermanek P. Current aspects of a new staging classification of colorectal cancer and its clinical consequences. Chirug 1989;60(2):78–82.

9. Hermanek P. International documentation system for colorectal cancer – reporting pathological findings. Verth Dtsch Ges Pathol 1991;75:386–8.

10. Quirke P, Dixon MF, Durdey P, et al. Local recurrence of rectal adenocarcinoma due to inadequate surgical resection. Histopathological study of lateral tumour spread and surgical excision. Lancet 1986;328(8514):996–9.

11. Swedish Rectal Cancer Trial. Improved survival with preoperative radiotherapy in resectable rectal cancer. N Engl J Med 1997;336(14):980–7.

12. Waddah B, Al-Refaie M, Parsons HM, et al. Operative outcomes beyond 30 day mortality. Ann Surg 2011;253:947–52.

13. Fielding LP, Fry JS, Phillips RKS, et al. Prediction of outcome after curative surgery for large bowel cancer. Lancet 1986;328(8512):904–6.

14. Fielding LP, Stewart-Brown S, Blesovsky L, et al. Anastomotic integrity after operations for large bowel cancer: a multicentre study. Br Med J 1980;281:411–4.

15. Marsh PJ, James RD, Schofield PF. Definition of local recurrence after surgery for rectal carcinoma. Br J Surg 1995;82(4):465–8.

16. Birbeck KF, Macklin CP, Tiffin NJ, et al. Rates of circumferential resection margin involvement vary between surgeons and predict outcomes in rectal cancer surgery. Ann Surg 2002;235(4):449–57.

17. Shephard NA, Baxter KJ, Love SB. Influence of local peritoneal involvement on pelvic recurrence and prognosis in rectal cancer. J Clin Pathol 1995;48(9):849–55.

18. Scholefield JH. How does surgical technique affect outcome in rectal cancer? J Gastroenterol 2000;35(Suppl. 12):126–9.

19. Docherty JG, McGregor JR, O'Dwyer PJ, et al. Local recurrence of colorectal cancer: the problems, mechanisms, management and adjuvant therapy. Br J Surg 1994;81(7):1082.

20. Nicholls RJ, Hall C. Treatment of non-disseminated cancer of the lower rectum. Br J Surg 1996;83(1):15–8.

21. Wibe A, Rendedal PR, Svensson E, et al. Prognostic significance of the circumferential resection margin following total mesorectal excision for rectal cancer. Br J Surg 2002;89(3):327–34.

22. Nagtegaal ID, Marijnen CAM, Kranenbarg EK, et al. Circumferential margin involvement is still an important predictor of local recurrence in rectal carcinoma: not one millimeter but two millimeters is the limit. Am J Surg Path 2002;26(3):350–7.

23. Jatzko GR, Jagoditsch M, Lisoberg PH, et al. Long-term results of radical surgery for rectal cancer: multivariate analysis of prognostic factors influencing survival and local recurrence. Eur J Surg Oncol 1999;25(3):284–91.

24. Simunovic M, Sexton R, Moran BJ, et al. Optimal pre-operative assessment and surgery for rectal cancer may greatly limit the need for radiotherapy. Br J Surg 2003;90(8):999–1003.

25. Sebag-Montefiore D, Stephens RJ. Steele R, et al. Preoperative Radiotherapy versus Selective postoperative chemoradiotherapy in patients with rectal cancer (MRC CR07 NCIG-CTG C016) - a multi-center randomized trial. Lancet 2009 Mar 7;373(9666):811–20.

26. McFarlane JK, Ryall RDH, Heald RJ. Mesorectal excision for rectal cancer. Lancet 1993;341:457–60.

27. Da Silva GM, Berho M, Wexner SD, et al. Histologic analysis of the irradiated anal sphincter. Dis Colon Rectum 2003;46(11):1492–7.

28. Sauer R, Becker H, Hohenberger W, et al. Preoperative versus postoperative chemoradiotherapy for rectal cancer. N Engl J Med 2004;351:1731–40.

29. Pijl MEJ, Chaoui AS, Wahl RL, et al. Radiology of colorectal cancer. Eur J Cancer 2002;38:887–98.

30. Brown G, Radcliffe AG, Newcombe RG, et al. Preoperative assessment of prognostic factors in rectal cancer using high-resolution magnetic resonance imaging. Br J Surg 2003;90(3):355–64.

31. Beets-Tan RG. MRI in rectal cancer: the T stage and circumferential resection margin. Colorectal Dis 2003;5(5):392–5.

32. Frykholm GJ, Påhlman L, Glimelius B. Combined chemo- and radiotherapy vs. radiotherapy alone in the treatment of primary, nonresectable adenocarcinoma of the rectum. Int J Radiat Oncol Biol Phys 2001;50(2):427–34.

33. Sebag-Montefiore D. Treatment of T4 tumours: the role of radiotherapy. Colorectal Dis 2003;5(5):432–5.

34. Pettersson D, Cedermark B, Holm T, et al. Interim analysis of the Stockholm III trial of preoperative radiotherapy regimens for rectal cancer. Br J Surg 2010;97(4):580–7.

35. Gerard J-P, Chapet O, Nemoz C, et al. Improved sphincter preservation in low rectal cancer with high-dose preoperative radiotherapy: the Lyon R96-02 randomized trial. J Clin Oncol 2004;22(12):2404–9.

36. Blomqvist L, Holm T, Rubio C, et al. Rectal tumours – MR imaging with endorectal and/or phased-array coils, and histopathological staging on giant sections. A comparative study. Acta Radiol 1997;38(3):437–44.

37. Phillips RKS, Hittinger R, Blesovsky L, et al. Local recurrence after 'curative' surgery for large bowel cancer. The overall picture. Br J Surg 1984;71:12–6.

38. Enker WE, Philipshen S, Heilwell ML, et al. En bloc pelvic lymphadenectomy and sphincter preservation in the surgical management of rectal cancer. Ann Surg 1986;293:426–33.

39. Moriya Y, Hojo K, Sawada T, et al. Significance of lateral node dissection for advanced rectal carcinoma at or below the peritoneal reflection. Dis Colon Rectum 1989;32:307–15.

40. Yano H, Moran BJ. The incidence of lateral pelvic side-wall nodal involvement in low rectal cancer may be similar in Japan and the West. Br J Surg 2008;95(1):33–49.

41. Surtees P, Ritchie J, Phillips RKS. High versus low ligation of the inferior mesenteric artery in rectal cancer. Br J Surg 1990;77:618–21.

42. Corder AP, Karanjia ND, Williams JD, et al. Flush aortic tie versus selective preservation of the ascending left colic artery in low anterior resection for rectal carcinoma. Br J Surg 1992;79:680–2.

43. Scott N, Jackson P, Al-Jaberi T, et al. Total mesorectal excision and local recurrence: a study of tumour spread in the mesorectum distal to rectal cancer. Br J Surg 1995;82:1031–3.

44. Heald RJ, Husband EM, Ryall D. The mesorectum in rectal cancer surgery: the clue to recurrence? Br J Surg 1982;69:613–6.

45. Ueno M, Oya M, Azekura K, et al. Incidence and prognostic significance of lateral lymph node metastasis in patients with advanced low rectal cancer. Br J Surg 2005;92(6):756–63.

46. Sugihara K, Kobayashi H, Kato T, et al. Indication and benefit of pelvic sidewall dissection for rectal cancer. Dis Colon Rectum 2006;49(11):1663–72.

47. Almeida Quadros C, Lopes A, Araújo I, et al. Retroperitoneal and lateral pelvic lymphadenectomy mapped by lymphoscintigraphy and blue dye for rectal adenocarcinoma staging: preliminary results. Ann Surg Oncol 2006;13(12):1617–21.

48. Moriya Y, Sugihara K, Akasu T, et al. Nerve-sparing surgery with lateral node dissection for advanced lower rectal cancer. Eur J Cancer 1995;31A(7–8):1229–32.

49. Sugihara K, Moriya Y, Akasu T, et al. Pelvic autonomic nerve preservation for patients with rectal carcinoma. Oncologic and functional outcome. Cancer 1996;78(9):1871–80.

50. Mori T, Takahashi K, Yasuno M. Radical resection with autonomic nerve preservation and lymph node dissection techniques in lower rectal cancer surgery and its results: the impact of lateral lymph node dissection. Langenbecks Arch Surg 1998;383(6):409–15.

51. Lange M, Buunen M, van de Velde C, et al. Level of arterial ligation in rectal cancer surgery: low tie preferred over high tie. A review. Dis Colon Rectum 2008;51(7):1139–45.

52. Hallbook O, Paholman L, Krog M, et al. Randomized comparison of straight and colonic J pouch anastomosis after low rectal excision. Ann Surg 1996;224:58–65.

53. Umpleby HC, Fermor B, Symes MO, et al. Viability of exfoliated colorectal carcinoma cells. Br J Surg 1984;71:659–63.

54. Edwards DP, Sexton R, Heald RJ, et al. Long-term results show triple stapling facilitates safe low colorectal and coloanal anastomosis and is associated with low rates of local recurrence after anterior resection for rectal cancer. Tech Coloproctol 2007;11(1):17–21.Epub 2007 Feb 16.

55. Phillips RKS. Adequate distal margin of resection for adenocarcinoma of the rectum. World J Surg 1992;16:463–6.

56. Williams NS, Dixon M, Johnston D. Reappraisal of the 5 cm rule of distal excision for carcinoma of the rectum: a study of distal intramural spread and of patients' survival. Br J Surg 1983;70:150–4.

57. Karanjia ND, Schache DJ, North WRS, et al. 'Close shave' in anterior resection. Br J Surg 1990;77:510–2.

58. Holm T, Ljung A, Haggmark T, et al. Extended abdominoperineal resection with gluteus maximus flap reconstruction of the pelvic floor for rectal cancer. Br J Surg 2007;94:232–8.

59. Sweeney JL, Ritchie JK, Hawley PR. Resection and sutured peranal anastomosis for carcinoma of the rectum. Dis Colon Rectum 1989;32:103–6.

60. Seow-Choen F, Goh HS. Prospective randomised trial comparing J colonic pouch–anal anastomosis and straight coloanal reconstruction. Br J Surg 1995;82:608–10.

61. Lazorthes F, Fages P, Chiotasso P, et al. Resection of the rectum with construction of a colonic reservoir and colo-anal anastomosis for carcinoma of the rectum. Br J Surg 1986;73:136–8.

62. Nicholls RJ, Lubowski DZ, Donaldson DR. Comparison of colonic reservoir and straight colo-anal reconstruction after rectal excision. Br J Surg 1988;75:318–20.

63. Mortensen NJM, Ramirez JM, Takeuchi N, et al. Colonic J pouch–anal anastomosis after rectal excision for carcinoma: functional outcome. Br J Surg 1995;82:611–3.

64. Heald RJ, Moran BJ, Brown G, et al. Optimal total mesorectal excision for rectal cancer is by dissection in front of Denonvilliers' fascia. Br J Surg 2004;91:121–3.

65. Quah HM, Jayne DG, Eu KW, et al. Bladder and sexual dysfunction following laparoscopically assisted and conventional open mesorectal resection for cancer. Br J Surg 2002;89:1551–6.

66. Jayne DG, Brown JM, Thorpe H, et al. Bladder and sexual function following resection for rectal cancer in a randomized clinical trial of laparoscopic versus open technique. Br J Surg 2005;92:1124–32.

67. Matthiessen PMDP, Hallbook OMDP, Rutegard JMDP, et al. Defunctioning stoma reduces symptomatic anastomotic leakage after low anterior resection of the rectum for cancer: a randomized multicenter trial. Ann Surg 2007;246(2): 207–14.

68. Huser N, Michalski CW, Erkan M, et al. Systematic review and meta-analysis of the role of defunctioning stoma in low rectal cancer surgery. Ann Surg 2008;248(1):52–60.

69. den Dulk M, Marijnen CA, Collette L, et al. Multicentre analysis of oncological and survival outcomes following anastomotic leakage after rectal cancer surgery. Br J Surg 2009;96(9):1066–75.

70. Tjandra J, Chan M. Follow-up after curative resection of colorectal cancer: a meta-analysis. Dis Colon Rectum 2007;50(11):1783–99.

71. Jeffery GM, Hickey BE, Hider PN. Follow-up strategies for patients treated for non-metastatic colorectal cancer. Cochrane Database Syst Rev 2008;2008(1).

72. Misiakos EP, Karidis NP, Kouraklis G. Current treatment for colorectal liver metastases. World J Gastroenterol 2011;17(36):4067–75.

73. Renehan AG, Egger M, Saunders MP, et al. Impact on survival of intensive follow-up after curative resection for colorectal cancer: systematic review and meta-analysis of randomised trials. Br Med J 2002;324:813. This meta-analysis has readdressed the value of intensive follow-up and finds significant benefit.

74. Jeffrey GM, Hickey BE, Hider P. Follow-up strategies for patients treated for non-metastatic colorectal cancer. Cochrane Library, IssueRef611. Oxford: Update Software; 2002.

6

Adjuvant therapy for colorectal cancer

Ganesh Radhakrishna
David Sebag-Montefiore

Introduction

Colorectal cancer is the third most common cancer in the UK, with approximately 40 000 cases diagnosed each year. Colorectal cancer is a disease where close multidisciplinary management is of key importance to successfully integrate the various medical and surgical disciplines to improve the outcome of the patient.

Recent statistics from Cancer Research UK[1] demonstrate a steady improvement in overall survival for both colon and rectal cancer. Over the last 30 years, the age-standardised 5-year survival has increased from 22% to 50% for colon cancer and from 26% to 53% for rectal cancer. It is likely that improved staging, perioperative care, surgical technique and adjuvant therapy have all played a role in this improvement.

This chapter will discuss the role of adjuvant chemotherapy in both colon and rectal cancer, and the role of radiotherapy in rectal cancer.

Adjuvant chemotherapy for colorectal cancer

The majority of trials have explored the role of adjuvant chemotherapy in colon cancer. Historically, high rates of local recurrence after rectal cancer resection meant that clinical trials could more easily determine the benefit of adjuvant chemotherapy on survival in colon cancer without the confounding effect of local recurrence that was present with rectal cancer.

Clinical trials performed in the 1980s demonstrated an improvement in overall survival with the addition of 5-fluorouracil (5-FU)-based chemotherapy after resection of stage III colon cancer.[2] A consensus statement was published by the National Institutes of Health in 1990[3] recommending 5-FU-based adjuvant chemotherapy for medically fit patients with completely resected stage III colon cancer.

Refining the role of fluoropyrimidine chemotherapy

Research in the 1990s included clinical trials that compared high- and low-dose leucovorin (LV) modulation of 5-FU and that assessed the role of levamisole and the duration of therapy. The large international QUASAR (Quick and Simple and Reliable) trial demonstrated no difference in disease-free (DFS) and overall survival (OS) between low- and high-dose leucovorin and no evidence of any benefit from the addition of levamisole to 5-FU/LV.[4] Other studies demonstrated similar outcomes for 6-month therapy compared with 1 year.[5] The combined results of these studies confirmed a 6-month course of low-dose LV combined with bolus 5-FU as standard treatment.

A number of different intravenous 5-FU regimens were used, including the 'Mayo' clinic schedule that delivered five daily injections over 1 week, repeated on a monthly basis and a once weekly schedule. In the QUASAR trial clinicians were allowed to choose either schedule. Although these two approaches were not directly compared by randomisation, similar long-term outcomes were observed with both approaches, although the once weekly schedule had significantly lower acute toxicity.

Oral fluoropyrimidine therapy

Oral 5-FU has very variable bioavailability, limiting its use in routine clinical practice. However, oral fluoropyrimidines were developed and initially compared against the Mayo clinic schedule in patients with metastatic disease before trials were performed in the adjuvant setting.

Examples of oral fluoropyrimidines include capecitabine, UFT (tegafur/uracil)/LV and S1. Initially, two large phase III trials established the non-inferiority of capecitabine when compared with the Mayo clinic schedule as first-line treatment of metastatic disease.[6,7] The subsequent adjuvant chemotherapy trial (X-ACT) randomised 1987 patients with stage III colon cancer to receive oral capecitabine or the Mayo clinic schedule, demonstrating at least equivalent outcomes for the oral therapy.[8] The long-term follow-up of this trial confirms oral capecitabine as an effective alternative to 5-FU/LV.

It is worth noting that although capecitabine was associated with less grade 3–4 toxicity and fewer hospital admissions, the control arm consisted of the Mayo clinic regimen.

In UK practice, fluoropyrimidine chemotherapy is usually offered either in the form of oral capecitabine or weekly intravenous 5-FU/LV. A small randomised study[9] explored patient preference between these two options by randomly allocating patients to 6 weeks of either oral capecitabine or weekly 5-FU followed by a further 6 weeks of the other approach. At 12 weeks, the majority of patients preferred weekly 5-FU/LV. This study also demonstrated a substantially higher rate of acute toxicity for the sequence of 5-FU/LV followed by oral capecitabine. The authors suggest caution regarding initial capecitabine dosing if patients switch over to this therapy from 5-FU/LV.

✓✓ Oral capecitabine is at least equivalent to intravenous 5-FU as adjuvant chemotherapy for colon cancer.[8]

Doublet chemotherapy

The next phase of clinical trials of adjuvant chemotherapy tested the addition of either oxaliplatin or irinotecan to fluoropyrimidine chemotherapy. Both agents when combined with a fluoropyrimidine had demonstrated improved response rates and progression-free survival when compared with a fluoropyrimidine alone in patients with metastatic colorectal cancer.[10,11] Both doublet approaches had similar efficacy and overall rates of grade 3 or 4 toxicity. A subsequent randomised trial showed similar outcomes when the sequence of oxaliplatin and irinotecan doublets was compared.[12] A series of trials then tested the role of either oxaliplatin- or irinotecan-based doublet chemotherapy in the adjuvant setting.

The addition of oxaliplatin demonstrated improved outcome. Two large trials, the MOSAIC[13] and the NSABP C07[14] studies, compared the addition of oxaliplatin to 5-FU/LV as an infusion and 5-FU/LV as a bolus, respectively (Table 6.1). The MOSAIC trial[15] randomised 2246 patients with high-risk stage II (40%) and stage III (60%) colon cancer. The 5-year disease free survival was 73.3% and 67.4% and the 6-year overall survival 78.5% versus 76% in favour of the oxaliplatin doublet. When the stage III subset is analysed separately, the 6-year OS is 72.9% versus 68.7% ($P = 0.02$) in favour of the oxaliplatin doublet.

The NSABP C07 trial[14] compared a 5-FU/high-dose leucovorin schedule given as an i.v. bolus for 6 weeks in an 8-weekly cycle with the addition of oxaliplatin 85 mg/m^2 on days 1, 15 and 29 of the same 5-FU/LV schedule. Overall, 2409 patients were randomised, with 29% stage II and 71% stage III patients. The 5-year disease-free survival was 69.4% versus 64.2% and 5-year overall survival was 80.2% versus 78.4% in favour of the oxaliplatin doublet. When the stage III subset is analysed separately, the 5-year OS is 76.5% versus 73.8% in favour of the oxaliplatin doublet.

A further trial compared the combination of oxaliplatin and capecitabine against intravenous 5-FU/LV using either the Mayo clinic or Roswell Park schedules;[16] 1886 patients with stage III colon cancer were randomised and reported 3-year disease-free survival

Table 6.1 • Disease free and Overall Survival from trials testing the addition of oxaliplatin or irinotecan to fluoropyrimidine chemotherapy

	Oxaliplatin + 5FU	5FU	Irinotecan + 5FU	
MOSAIC				
All patients n = 2246				
5 yr DFS	73.3	67.4%	–	HR 0.80 (0.68–0.93)
6 yr OS	78.5%	76.0%	–	HR 0.84 (0.71–1.00)
Stage III n = 1347				
5 yr DFS	66.4%	58.9%	–	HR 0.78 (0.65–0.93)
6 yr OS	72.9%	68.7%	–	HR 0.80 (0.65–0.97)
Stage II n = 899				
5 yr DFS	83.7%	79.9%	–	HR 0.84 (0.62–1.14)
5 yr OS	86.9%	86.8%	–	HR 1.00 (0.70–1.41)
NSABP C07				
All patients				
n = 2,409				
5 yr DFS	69.4%	64.2%	–	HR 0.82 (0.72–0.93)
5 yr OS	80.2%	78.4%	–	HR 0.88 (0.75–1.02)
Stage III				
5 yr DFS	64.4%	57.8%	–	Not stated
5 yr OS	76.5%	73.8%	–	Not stated
Stage II				
5 yr DFS	82.1%	80.1%	–	Not stated
5 yr OS	89.7%	89.6%	–	Not stated
NO16968				
n = 1886				
5 yr DFS	66.1%	59.8%	–	HR 0.80 (0.69–0.93)
5 yr OS*	77.6%	74.2%		Not stated
PETACC-03				
Stage 3				
n = 2094				
5 yr DFS	–	54.3%	56.7%	HR 0.90 (0.79–1.02)
5 yr OS	–	71.3%	73.6%	P = 0.094
CALGB 8903				
n = 1264				
5 yr DFS	–	61%	59%	Not stated
5 yr OS	–	71%	68%	Not stated

*- after 57 months follow up only. Further longer term follow up data awaited.

of 70.9% versus 66.5% in favour of the doublet schedule. Further follow-up of this trial is awaited.

✓✓ Two pivotal adjuvant chemotherapy trials demonstrated improved cancer-related outcomes when oxaliplatin is added to fluoropyrimidine chemotherapy as adjuvant therapy of colon cancer.[14,15]

However, somewhat unexpectedly, there was no evidence of any improvement in survival from the addition of irinotecan. Two large phase III trials tested the addition of irinotecan to a 5-FU platform as adjuvant therapy. The PETACC-3 trial[17] randomised 3278 patients with resected stage II (28%) and stage III (72%) colon to receive infusional 5-FU/LV with or without irinotecan. The principal survival analyses were performed for the stage III patient group. The CALGB 89803 trial[18] randomised 1264 patients with stage III colon cancer to receive weekly bolus 5-FU/LV with or without irinotecan. Both trials failed to demonstrate a significant improvement in either disease-free or overall survival (data presented in Table 6.1).

The results of these trials established that the combination of oxaliplatin combined with a fluoropyrimidine improved outcome in stage III disease. Areas of controversy include the benefit of this approach in patients over the age of 65 and in high-risk stage II colon cancer, and will be discussed later in this chapter.

Addition of 'targeted' therapy to chemotherapy

Clinical trials have shown benefit from the addition of molecular targeted agents, particularly anti-vascular endothelial growth factor (anti-VEGF) and epidermal growth factor receptor (EGFR) targeted therapy in patients with metastatic disease. The latter approach only appears to be of benefit in patients with kras wild-type tumours. This supported trials testing the addition of targeted therapies to combination chemotherapy as adjuvant therapy.

The initial experience has been very disappointing. The NSABP C08[19] trial randomised 2672 patients with stage II and III colon cancer to receive FOLFOX with or without bevacizumab and did not demonstrate any difference in 3-year disease-free survival (3-year DFS 77.4% vs. 75.5% for FOLFOX plus bevacizumab versus FOLFOX alone, respectively). The NO147 trial randomised 1760 patients with kras wild-type stage colon cancer to receive FOLFOX with or without cetuximab. Preliminary data presented at ASCO in 2010[20] reported a 3-year DFS in favour of the FOLFOX control arm (hazard ratio 1.18 (0.92–1.52)).

✔✔ There is no evidence to support the addition of targeted therapy to adjuvant chemotherapy. Two trials (one testing bevacizumab and the other cetuximab) both failed to show any impact on overall survival.[19,20]

At present none of the reported phase III trials support the addition of targeted agents to double chemotherapy as adjuvant therapy. Further research is under way to try and explain these findings.

Patient selection for adjuvant chemotherapy

The clinician is faced with a number of challenges when discussing the role of adjuvant chemotherapy with patients after colon cancer resection. In stage III disease, there is a strong evidence base that supports adjuvant chemotherapy. Although the addition of oxaliplatin improves survival, the improvement is modest and the increased acute and subsequent risks of neurotoxicity must also be considered. There is less evidence of a survival benefit in patients over the age of 65 and in patients with significant medical and surgical comorbidity who are at higher risk of death from a non-cancer-related cause.

In patients with stage II disease there are a number of risk factors that increase the risk of relapse, including T4 disease, the presence of extramural vascular invasion and poorly differentiated histology. In the MOSAIC trial the absolute improvement in overall survival for high-risk stage II disease was 1.7% compared with 0.1% in low-risk stage II and 4.2% for stage III, respectively. The QUASAR trial[21] estimated a 3.6% absolute improvement in overall survival for stage II disease (2963 patients) when 5-FU/LV chemotherapy was compared against no chemotherapy.

✔✔ The QUASAR trial demonstrated a 3.6% improvement in overall survival for stage II colorectal cancer when 5-FU/LV was compared against no chemotherapy.[4]

Acute and long-term toxicity

The acute toxicity associated with fluoropyrimidine chemotherapy is very regimen specific, with the lowest acute toxicity seen with weekly bolus 5-FU/LV and greater toxicity with capecitabine and the Mayo Clinic schedule. Capecitabine is associated with a higher incidence of palmar plantar erythema and diarrhoea compared with weekly 5-FU/I.V. In contrast, the overall grade 3–4 toxicity in the phase III trial that compared oxaliplatin capecitabine with the Mayo Clinic/Roswell Park 5-FU/LV schedules showed a relatively small but significant difference (55% vs. 47%, respectively).

In general, fluoropyrimidine chemotherapy is associated with lethargy, mucositis, and diarrhoea and hand-foot syndrome. Watery eyes, minor nosebleeds and taste alterations are common but usually reversible. The risk of neutropenic sepsis is uncommon, although a very small proportion of patients (<1%) are relatively deficient in the enzyme dihydropyrimidine dehydrogenase (DPD) that is needed to metabolise 5-FU. In this small group of patients severe toxicity is seen within the first 3 weeks of treatment, with neutropenic sepsis, grade 4 mucositis, diarrhoea and alopecia, and is associated with a significant risk of treatment-related mortality. Early identification of such patients with full supportive measures led by the oncology team is essential to maximise the successful treatment of this rare condition. At present there is no validated test to reliably identify this group of patients or to guide prospective alterations of treatment.

The addition of oxaliplatin is associated with an increased risk of diarrhoea and neutropenia. The most significant toxicity, however, is neurotoxicity. This is seen during treatment, with paraesthesia and cold sensitivity of the extremities and larynx/upper oesophagus. Sensory neuropathy may develop either during or after completion of adjuvant chemotherapy. The incidence and severity of this peripheral sensory neuropathy (PNS) reduces over time. In the MOSAIC trial, grade 3 PNS (functional impairment) reduced from 12.5% during treatment to 0.7% by 10 months. The incidence of grade 3 PNS remained at 0.7% at 48 months post-treatment.

Timing and duration of chemotherapy

When should adjuvant chemotherapy be commenced after surgical resection? Most but not all clinical trials determine a 6- to 8-week time point for the commencement of adjuvant chemotherapy. A recent meta-analysis[22] of 15 410 patients in 10 trials concluded that an increase of 4 weeks in the time to start adjuvant chemotherapy was associated with a significant decrease in overall survival. Although this may support the view that chemotherapy should start soon after surgery, the authors acknowledge that a benefit for chemotherapy may still exist when chemotherapy is commenced after significant delay (i.e. 12 weeks).

Previous trials have demonstrated that 6-month chemotherapy is as effective as a 12-month course of treatment. Further trials are under way internationally that compare a 3- versus 6-month duration of combination chemotherapy. It is anticipated that a shorter duration of chemotherapy will be associated with less neurotoxicity. However, randomised trials are required to determine non-inferior cancer and overall survival outcomes for the shorter duration of therapy.

Adjuvant therapy for rectal cancer

The approach in the development of adjuvant therapy for rectal cancer differs from colon cancer. Until the last two decades, prior to the adoption of improved surgical technique using total mesorectal excision, local recurrence was the predominant component of failure after resection of primary rectal cancer. Local recurrence can cause very distressing uncontrolled pelvic symptoms that are very difficult to palliate and are rarely eradicated. Fortunately, improvements in surgery[23,24] and an increased use of adjuvant radiotherapy have significantly altered this pattern, with local recurrence being less frequently seen. However, distant metastasis remains a significant problem and adjuvant chemotherapy is used to reduce the risk of distant failure. The supportive evidence is mainly an extrapolation of the evidence from colon cancer adjuvant chemotherapy trials applied to rectal cancer.

Radiotherapy

Radiotherapy uses ionising radiation to eliminate cancer cells. In modern practice it is usually delivered with linear accelerators (**Fig. 6.1**) that can target tumours with great accuracy (**Fig. 6.2**). Due to the dose-limiting effects of the small bowel in the abdominal cavity, and the problems that can arise treating more mobile targets outside the pelvis, radiotherapy is used almost exclusively for the treatment of rectal cancer, rather than colon cancer. Over the last three decades there has been a considerable effort to define the role of radiotherapy. Until the mid-1990s randomised controlled trials included a standard arm of surgery alone.

The established indications for adjuvant radiation in rectal cancer include:

- to reduce the risk of local recurrence;
- to shrink locally advanced rectal cancer to facilitate successful resection.

There is considerable debate regarding the use of radiotherapy to increase the rate of sphincter-preserving surgery or as organ conservation (to delay or avoid surgical resection altogether).

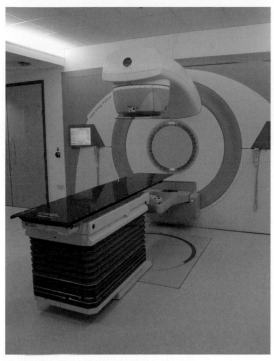

Figure 6.1 • A modern linear accelerator.

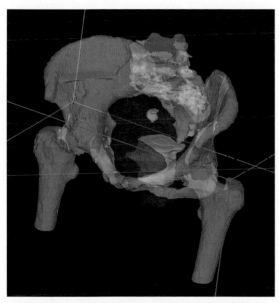

Figure 6.2 • Modem radiotherapy. Target volumes (e.g. macroscopic tumour, in primary and mesorectal nodes – orange; planning target volume, including surrounding areas at risk – red) and organs at risk (e.g. bladder – blue) can be outlined on a series of computed tomography (CT) scan slices to build up composite three-dimensional volumes. This facilitates more accurate treatment planning.

Evidence base for the use of adjuvant radiotherapy in resectable rectal cancer

A recent Cochrane overview[25] and other overviews[26,27] have all concluded that both preoperative and postoperative radiotherapy reduce the risk of local recurrence compared with surgery alone. Although cancer-specific survival was also improved there was no definite evidence of any impact on overall survival. Both preoperative radiotherapy and the use of a biological equivalent dose of >30 Gy were associated with the greatest treatment effect.

In North America, clinical trials initially focused on the benefit of postoperative radiotherapy and its integration with systemic chemotherapy for patients with both stage II and stage III rectal cancer. The NIH consensus statement in 1990[3] led to a recommendation that patients with stage II and stage III rectal cancer should receive both systemic chemotherapy and concurrent chemoradiotherapy.

In contrast, clinical trials in northern Europe evaluated radiotherapy alone in the preoperative setting and with a major interest in the use of a short accelerated schedule using 5 Gy per fraction. A sequence of randomised controlled trials, mainly in Scandinavia, refined the use of 'short-course radiotherapy' delivering 25 Gy in five daily fractions of 5 Gy with immediate surgery.[28–30] The Swedish rectal cancer trial[30] of 1168 patients was the first to report an improvement in overall survival (without the use of systemic chemotherapy). This trial also overcame the increase in early operative mortality that was seen in previous trials through the use of radiotherapy by reducing the size of the radiotherapy fields and using a multifield (three or four) technique.

However, lower local recurrence rates associated with the increasing use of total mesorectal excision (TME)[23] in individual surgical series and population-based studies require clinical trials to further evaluate the role of preoperative radiotherapy combined with TME.

Short-course radiotherapy and TME

Two trials, the Dutch TME and the MRC CR07 trials, then addressed the role of preoperative short-course radiotherapy followed by TME compared with a highly selective approach to postoperative radiotherapy restricted to patients with involvement of the circumferential resection margin. In the Dutch trial[31,32] highly selective postoperative treatment used radiotherapy alone and no systemic chemotherapy was allowed postoperatively. The CR07 trial[33] used concurrent 5-FU chemoradiotherapy (CRT) when postoperative radiotherapy was indicated and a predetermined adjuvant systemic chemotherapy policy for each centre was applied to both treatment arms.

The Dutch trial recruited 1861 patients and the MRC CR07 1350 patients. Both have demonstrated very similar findings where the risk of local recurrence was reduced from 11% with surgery first to 4–5% with the routine use of short-course preoperative radiotherapy. There was no evidence of a difference in operative mortality or anastomotic leak between the treatment arms.

No evidence of a difference in overall survival is seen between treatment arms in either trial, although a recent report from the Dutch trial has shown an improvement in overall survival in the circumferential resection margin (CRM)-negative stage III subset.[32] This is an exploratory analysis and long-term follow-up of the CR07 trial is awaited. The reduction in local recurrence is seen across the subsites of the rectum and the absolute difference between the treatment arms is seen with increasing tumour and nodal stage.

> ✓✓ The Dutch TME and MRC CR07 trials both show that short-course radiotherapy halves the risk of local recurrence when combined with TME, but there is no difference in overall survival.[32,33]

Similar findings have been reported recently in a population-based study from Sweden, where 6878 patients were studied.[34] In this study a survival advantage was reported for patients under 75 with the use of short-course radiotherapy. This finding needs confirmation in similar datasets.

Preoperative concurrent chemoradiotherapy

Two phase III trials tested the addition of concurrent 5-FU/LV to radiotherapy compared to long-course radiotherapy alone. The EORTC 22921 trial[35] recruited 1011 patients and used a factorial 2 × 2 design to compare radiotherapy 45 Gy with or without concurrent 5-FU/LV and a second randomisation of adjuvant postoperative 5-FU/LV versus no chemotherapy. The FFCD 9203 trial[36] recruited 762 patients and compared radiotherapy 45 Gy with or without concurrent 5-FU/LV with all patients recommended to receive postoperative adjuvant 5-FU/LV.

The two trials reported very similar findings. The acute toxicity was increased but acceptable with the addition of concurrent chemotherapy (CRT) and the risk of local recurrence was reduced from 15% to 8–10% in favour of CRT. No evidence of a difference in disease-free or overall survival was seen.

> ✓✓ The addition of 5-FU/LV to long-course radiotherapy halved the risk of local recurrence but had no impact on overall survival in two large European phase III trials.[35,36]

The German Rectal Cancer Group,[37] at a similar time, compared preoperative CRT versus postoperative CRT, recruiting 823 patients. This trial demonstrated a lower rate of local recurrence (6% vs. 12%), reduced acute and late toxicity in favour of preoperative CRT, but without any evidence of a difference in disease-free or overall survival.

The three trials were highly influential and led to a significant shift from the use of postoperative CRT to preoperative CRT.

Short-course radiotherapy or preoperative CRT?

Two trials have directly compared short-course radiotherapy with preoperative CRT. The Polish trial[38] was designed to test whether preoperative CRT would increase the rate of sphincter-preserving surgery and randomised 312 patients. The comparison of local recurrence and toxicity were secondary end-points and the trial was not statistically powered for these specific questions. The Trans Tasman Radiation Oncology Group[39] randomised 326 patients with local recurrence as the primary end-point. In both trials there is no evidence of a difference in local recurrence or survival.

Short-course radiotherapy and delay to surgery

Although there is clear evidence that short-course preoperative radiotherapy (SCPRT) reduces the risk of local recurrence, there is limited information regarding its efficacy in downstaging locally advanced disease where a delay prior to surgery is required. However, evidence is now emerging. Small series of patients from Sweden[40] and Leeds[41] have reported acceptable toxicity and a complete pathological response (pCR) rate of 8–15% when this approach is used in elderly and poor performance status patients. The ongoing Stockholm III trial compares SCPRT and immediate surgery with SCPRT and delay with long-course radiotherapy prior to surgery. An interim analysis of 120 patients treated with SCPRT and delay reported a pCR rate of 12.5%.[42] This approach warrants wider evaluation and offers an alternative treatment when preoperative CRT is not feasible (comorbidity, relative contraindications to 5-FU).

Late toxicity and second malignancy

Although preoperative radiotherapy and CRT reduce the risk of local recurrence, there is no evidence of an improvement in survival. The benefit in the reduction in local recurrence must be compared with the risks of late toxicity. Recognised long-term side-effects of pelvic radiotherapy for rectal cancer include faecal incontinence, sexual and urinary dysfunction, and sterility.[43–45] The Swedish[46] and Dutch[32] trials also report an increase in the risk of second malignancy. Quality-of-life data from the CR07 trial demonstrate a significant impairment in sexual function attributable to surgery and a further detriment due to radiotherapy.[43] Both the Dutch and CR07 trials show a similar pattern for faecal incontinence.[43,44] The Polish and TROG trials[38,39] have not shown a difference in quality of life when short-course radiotherapy was compared with preoperative CRT. A recent study has confirmed the detrimental effects of preoperative CRT.[47]

Patient selection

The wider use of a preoperative approach increases the importance of imaging in patient selection. The routine use of preoperative radiotherapy cannot be justified when combined with TME. For example, if the risk of local recurrence is reduced from 11% to 5% in favour of preoperative radiotherapy then approximately 16 patients need to be treated to prevent one local recurrence. It is therefore important to try and identify patients who do not require radiotherapy.

The MERCURY international phase II observational study established the role of pelvic magnetic resonance resonance imaging (MRI) in the staging of rectal cancer.[48] This study demonstrated equivalence between the measured extramural spread of tumour seen on high-resolution MRI and the same measurement on histopathology whole mounts after surgery alone. Further reports have described a good prognosis group of patients in whom the risk of local recurrence is very low without radiotherapy.[49] MRI can also identify when the primary tumour extends to or within 1 mm of the mesorectal fascia[50] (**Fig. 6.3**), a situation where downstaging with preoperative CRT is indicated (**Fig. 6.4**).

Many centres have adopted a risk-stratified approach. In the UK the recent NICE guidelines have defined three risk groups for local recurrence. In the low-risk group, radiotherapy is not given and preoperative CRT is recommended in the high-risk group (Table 6.2). In the medium-risk group SCPRT or preoperative CRT may be used as there is evidence to support both approaches and no clear evidence that one is superior to the other. The choice between SCPRT and CRT remains controversial and has recently been reviewed.[51]

Sphincter preservation

There is very little evidence to support the view that preoperative CRT increases the chance of a sphincter-preserving resection. In the majority of patients with a mid and upper rectal cancer, an anterior resection is feasible without tumour shrinkage. Very low tumours less than 4 cm from the anal verge require an abdomino-perineal excision. Therefore, it is only in a very small group of patients whose distal tumour extent is 4–6 cm from the anal verge where preoperative CRT may play a role in achieving a sphincter-preserving procedure.[52]

Organ preservation

There is increasing interest in the role of non-surgical therapy to avoid major resectional surgery.

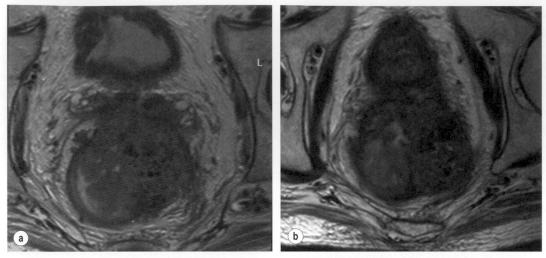

Figure 6.3 • MRI staging of rectal cancer. MRI is now a standard preoperative technique to identify tumours that either **(a)** extend beyond the expected CRM or **(b)** threaten it. Such patients can then be selected for more aggressive preoperative treatment to try and downsize the tumour and facilitate complete resection.

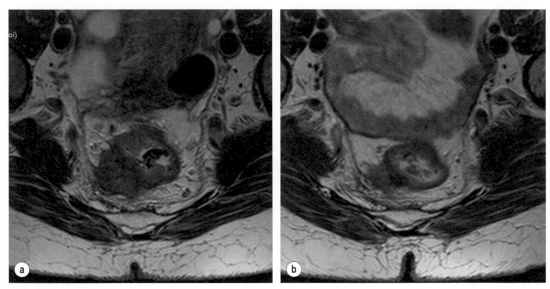

Figure 6.4 • Response to neoadjuvant chemoradiotherapy. **(a)** A bulky tumour threatens the expected CRM. **(b)** Following neoadjuvant CRT a small tumour residuum remains, although this no longer involves the CRM. The mesorectal envelope has also contracted as the tumour has reduced in size.

This approach has been pioneered by Habra-Gama, where patients with complete clinical response after chemoradiotherapy undergo intensive follow-up, with surgery reserved for locoregional failure. Approximately 20–30% of patients have sustained local control without radical surgery.[53-55]

A recent publication from a Dutch group describes similar results.[56] However, only 10% of the patients treated with CRT achieved a complete clinical response and entered the study. The definition of CCR was rigorous, consisting of negative biopsy, complete clinical resolution, and no suspicious findings on flexible sigmoidoscopy and no evidence of residual tumour on pelvic MRI.

An alternative strategy is to use transanal excisional microsurgery (TEM)[57] to accurately assess the impact of a good clinical response to preoperative treatment to determine which patients can undergo

Table 6.2 • Key trials comparing outcomes following Short-Course Pre-operative and Radiotherapy and Chemoradiation

Trial	Pat Nos	Randomisation	Nos	1 endpoint	LR	OS	DFS
Short course pre-operative radiotherapy trials							
Dutch Trial CKVO 95-04 (2011) **SCPRT**	1861	25 Gy in 5 fractions + surgery	897	LR	**10 years** 5%	**10 years** 48%	Not stated
		Surgery + highly selective RT	908		11%	49%	
CR07 (2008) **SCPRT**	1350	25 Gy in 5 fractions + surgery	674	LR	**3 years** 5%	**3 years** 80%	**3 years** 78%
		Surgery + highly selective CRT	676		11%	79%	72%
Pre-op long course RT+/− chemotherapy trials							
EORTC 22921 (2006)	1011	*45 Gy in 25 fractions* vs.	505	OS	**5 years** 17%	**5 years** 65%	**5 years** 54%
		5-FU/FA + 45 Gy	506		vs. 9%	vs. 66%	vs. 56%
FFCD 9203 (2006)	762	*45 Gy in 25 fractions* vs.	367	OS	**5 years** 17%	**5 years** 68%	No data
		FUFA + 45 GY	375		vs. 8%	vs. 67%	
Pre-op CRT vs. post-op CRT trial							
CAA/ARO/ AIO-94 (2004)	823	Preop 50.4 Gy + 5FU vs.	421	OS	**5 years** 6%	**5 years** 76%	**5 years** 68%
		Postop 55.8 Gy + 5FU	402		vs 13%	vs 74%	vs 65%

CRT, chemoradiotherapy; DFS, disease-free survival; FA, folinic acid; 5-FU, 5-fluorouracil; LR, local recurrence; OS, overall survival; RT, radiotherapy; SCPRT, short-course preoperative radiotherapy.

intensive follow-up and those who require a formal resection based on histopathological findings.

Prospective multicentre studies are required to determine the benefits of both of the above strategies. It is likely that the patients most likely to benefit from a non-surgical approach are those with early stage disease. In the UK, this group of patients is not normally treated with preoperative radiotherapy at all. Therefore, prospective data regarding the proportion of patients who have organ conservation, the rate of locoregional failure, and subsequent salvage surgery and long-term cancer outcomes are essential to determine the value of this approach.

Conclusion

There is a strong evidence base for the use of adjuvant chemotherapy in colorectal cancer and for the use of preoperative radiotherapy in rectal cancer. Appropriate patient selection is determined preoperatively by high-quality cross-sectional imaging and postoperatively by histopathology. There is a defined role for both short-course preoperative radiotherapy and concurrent chemoradiotherapy in patients with rectal cancer. The increasing interest in organ preservation requires further study in prospective multicentre studies.

Key points

- In 1990 the NIH consensus conference recommended 5-FU-based adjuvant chemotherapy for stage III colon cancer.
- Two large trials show that the addition of oxaliplatin to 5-FU improves survival in stage III colon cancer.
- There is no evidence to support the use of targeted agents as adjuvant therapy.

- There is a strong evidence base demonstrating that preoperative radiotherapy reduces the risk of local recurrence after resection of rectal cancer.
- The addition of concurrent 5-FU to long-course radiotherapy reduces the risk of local recurrence.
- A risk-adapted policy for the use of preoperative radiotherapy balances the benefit and risks.
- Strategies to achieve organ preservation require prospective multicentre study.

References

1. Rachet B, Maringe C, Nur U, et al. Population-based cancer survival trends in England and Wales up to 2007: an assessment of the NHS cancer plan for England. Lancet Oncol 2009;10(4):351–69.

2. Haydon A. Adjuvant chemotherapy in colon cancer: what is the evidence? Intern Med J 2003;33(3):119–24.

3. NIH Consensus Conference. Adjuvant therapy for patients with colon and rectal cancer. JAMA 1990;264(11):1444–50.

4. QUASAR Collaborative Group. Comparison of flourouracil with additional levamisole, higher-dose folinic acid, or both, as adjuvant chemotherapy for colorectal cancer: a randomised trial. Lancet 2000;355(9215):1588–96.

   The QUASAR trial showed that low-dose lecovorin was as effective as high-dose and that the addition of levamisole did not improve cancer outcomes. A small benefit in absolute survival from 5-FU and folinic acid for stage II colorectal cancer of 3.6% was seen.

5. O'Connell MJ, Kahn MJ, Erlichman C, et al. Optimal duration of fluorouracil plus levamisole colon cancer surgical adjuvant therapy. J Clin Oncol 1996;14(10):2887.

6. Hoff PM, Ansari R, Batist G, et al. Comparison of oral capecitabine versus intravenous fluorouracil plus leucovorin as first-line treatment in 605 patients with metastatic colorectal cancer: results of a randomized phase III study. J Clin Oncol 2001;19(8):2282–92.

7. Van Cutsem E, Twelves C, Cassidy J, et al. Oral capecitabine compared with intravenous fluorouracil plus leucovorin in patients with metastatic colorectal cancer: results of a large phase III study. J Clin Oncol 2001;19(21):4097–106.

8. Twelves C, Wong A, Nowacki MP, et al. Capecitabine as adjuvant treatment for stage III colon cancer. N Engl J Med 2005;352(26):2696–704.

   The X-ACT study showed equivalence between bolus 5-FU and folinic acid and oral fluoropyrimidine capecitabine after 6.9 years of follow-up.

9. Hennig IM, Naik JD, Brown S, et al. Severe sequence-specific toxicity when capecitabine is given after fluorouracil and leucovorin. J Clin Oncol 2008;26(20):3411–7.

10. Douillard JY, Cunningham D, Roth AD, et al. Irinotecan combined with fluorouracil compared with fluorouracil alone as first-line treatment for metastatic colorectal cancer: a multicentre randomised trial. Lancet 2000;355(9209):1041–7.

11. de Gramont A, Figer A, Seymour M, et al. Leucovorin and fluorouracil with or without oxaliplatin as first-line treatment in advanced colorectal cancer. J Clin Oncol 2000;18(16):2938–47.

12. Tournigand C, Andre T, Achille E, et al. FOLFIRI followed by FOLFOX6 or the reverse sequence in advanced colorectal cancer: a randomized GERCOR study. J Clin Oncol 2004;22(2):229–37.

13. Andre T, Boni C, Mounedji-Boudiaf L, et al. Oxaliplatin, fluorouracil, and leucovorin as adjuvant treatment for colon cancer. N Engl J Med 2004;350(23):2343–51.

14. Yothers G, O'Connell MJ, Allegra CJ, et al. Oxaliplatin as adjuvant therapy for colon cancer: updated results of NSABP C-07 trial, including survival and subset analyses. J Clin Oncol 2011;29(28):3768–74.

    The NSABP C07 study demonstrated that the addition of oxaliplatin to infusional 5-FU/LV resulted in a better 5-year disease-free survival and overall survival. This benefit was at the expense of increased acute toxicity, including neurotoxicity.

15. Andre T, Boni C, Navarro M, et al. Improved overall survival with oxaliplatin, fluorouracil, and leucovorin as adjuvant treatment in stage II or III colon cancer in the MOSAIC trial. J Clin Oncol 2009;27(19):3109–16.

    The MOSAIC study demonstrated that the addition of oxaliplatin to infusional 5-FU/LV resulted in a better 5-year disease-free survival and overall survival. This benefit was at the expense of increased acute toxicity, including neurotoxicity.

16. Haller DG, Tabernero J, Maroun J, et al. Capecitabine plus oxaliplatin compared with fluorouracil and folinic acid as adjuvant therapy for stage III colon cancer. J Clin Oncol 2011;29(11):1465–71.

17. Van Cutsem E, Labianca R, Bodoky G, et al. Randomized phase III trial comparing biweekly infusional fluorouracil/leucovorin alone or with irinotecan in the adjuvant treatment of stage III colon cancer: PETACC-3. J Clin Oncol 2009;27(19):3117–25.

18. Saltz LB, Niedzwiecki D, Hollis D, et al. Irinotecan fluorouracil plus leucovorin is not superior to fluorouracil plus leucovorin alone as adjuvant treatment for stage III colon cancer: results of CALGB 89803. J Clin Oncol 2007;25(23):3456–61.

19. Allegra CJ, Yothers G, O'Connell MJ, et al. Phase III trial assessing bevacizumab in stages II and III carcinoma of the colon: results of NSABP protocol C-08. J Clin Oncol 2011;29(1):11–6.

The C08 trial showed no difference in disease-free or overall survival when bevacizumab was added to FOLFOX chemotherapy.

20. Alberts S, Sargent D, Smyrk T, et al. Adjuvant mFOLFOX6 with or without cetuximab (Cmab) in KRAS wild type patients with resected colon cancer: results from NCCTG Intergroup Trial NO0147. J Clin Oncol 2010;28(18s):CRA3507.
The preliminary results of the N00147 trial do not show any evidence of improvement in disease-free or overall survival when cetuximab is added to FOLFOX chemotherapy.

21. Gray R, Barnwell J, McConkey C, et al. Adjuvant chemotherapy versus observation in patients with colorectal cancer: a randomised study. Lancet 2007;370(9604):2020–9.

22. Biagi JJ, Raphael MJ, Mackillop WJ, et al. Association between time to initiation of adjuvant chemotherapy and survival in colorectal cancer: a systematic review and meta-analysis. JAMA 2011;305(22):2335–42.

23. MacFarlane JK, Ryall RD, Heald RJ. Mesorectal excision for rectal cancer. Lancet 1993;341(8843):457–60.

24. Enker WE. Total mesorectal excision – the new golden standard of surgery for rectal cancer. Ann Med 1997;29(2):127–33.

25. Wong RK, Tandan V, De Silva S, et al. Pre-operative radiotherapy and curative surgery for the management of localized rectal carcinoma. Cochrane Database Syst Rev 2007;(2):CD002102.

26. Camma C, Giunta M, Fiorica F, et al. Preoperative radiotherapy for resectable rectal cancer: a meta analysis. JAMA 2000;284(8):1008–15.

27. Glimelius B, Gronberg H, Jarhult J, et al. A systematic overview of radiation therapy effects in rectal cancer. Acta Oncol 2003;42(5–6):476–92.

28. Cedermark B, Johansson H, Rutqvist LE. The Stockholm I trial of preoperative short term radiotherapy in operable rectal carcinoma. A prospective randomized trial. Stockholm Colorectal Cancer Study Group. Cancer 1995;75(9):2269–75.

29. Martling A, Holm T, Johansson H, et al. The Stockholm II trial on preoperative radiotherapy in rectal carcinoma: long-term follow-up of a population-based study. Cancer 2001;92(4):896–902.

30. Swedish Rectal Cancer Trial. Improved survival with preoperative radiotherapy in resectable rectal cancer. N Engl J Med 1997;336(14):980–7.

31. Kapiteijn E, Marijnen CA, Nagtegaal ID, et al. Preoperative radiotherapy combined with total mesorectal excision for resectable rectal cancer. N Engl J Med 2001;345(9):638–46.

32. van Gijn W, Marijnen CA, Nagtegaal ID, et al. Preoperative radiotherapy combined with total mesorectal excision for resectable rectal cancer: 12-year follow-up of the multicentre, randomised controlled TME trial. Lancet Oncol 2011;12(6):575–82.

The Dutch TME trial demonstrated that the addition of short-course preoperative radiotherapy halved the risk of local recurrence but with no evidence of en effect on overall survival.

33. Sebag-Montefiore D, Stephens RJ, Steele R, et al. Preoperative radiotherapy versus selective postoperative chemoradiotherapy in patients with rectal cancer (MRC CR07 and NCIC-CTG C016): a multicentre, randomised trial. Lancet 2009;373(9666);811–20.
The MRC CR07 trial demonstrated that the addition of short-course preoperative radiotherapy halved the risk of local recurrence but with no evidence of an effect on overall survival.

34. Tiefenthal M, Nilsson PJ, Johansson R, et al. The effects of short course preoperative irradiation on local recurrence rate and survival in rectal cancer: a population-based nationwide study. Dis Colon Rectum 2011;54(6):672–80.

35. Bosset JF, Collette L, Calais G, et al. Chemotherapy with preoperative radiotherapy in rectal cancer. N Engl J Med 2006;355(11):1114–23.
The EORTC 22921 trial showed that the addition of 5-FU/LV to long-course radiotherapy halved the risk of local recurrence but without any difference in overall survival.

36. Gérard JP, Conroy T, Bonnetain F, et al. Preoperative radiotherapy with or without concurrent fluorouracil and leucovorin in T3–4 rectal cancers: results of FFCD 9203. J Clin Oncol 2006;24(28):4620–5.
The FFCD 9203 trial showed that the addition of 5-FU/LV to long-course radiotherapy halved the risk of local recurrence but without any difference in overall survival.

37. Sauer R, Becker H, Hohenberger W, et al. Preoperative versus postoperative chemoradiotherapy for rectal cancer. N Engl J Med 2004;351(17):1731–40.

38. Bujko K, Nowacki MP, Nasierowska-Guttmejer A, et al. Long-term results of a randomized trial comparing preoperative short-course radiotherapy with preoperative conventionally fractionated chemoradiation for rectal cancer. Br J Surg 2006;93(10):1215–23.

39. Ngan S, Fisher R, Goldstein D, et al. A randomised trial comparing local recurrence rates between short course and long course preoperative radiotherapy for clinical T3 rectal cancer: an intergroup trial (TROG, AGITG, CSSANZ). J Clin Oncol 2010;28(15s)Abstract 3509.

40. Radu C, Berglund A, Pahlman L, et al. Short-course preoperative radiotherapy with delayed surgery in rectal cancer – a retrospective study. Radiother Oncol 2008;87(3):343–9.

41. Hatfield P, Hingorani M, Radhakrishna G, et al. Short-course radiotherapy, with elective delay prior to surgery, in patients with unresectable rectal cancer who have poor performance status or significant comorbidity. Radiother Oncol 2009;92(2):210–4.

42. Pettersson D, Cedermark B, Holm T, et al. Interim analysis of the Stockholm III trial of preoperative

radiotherapy regimens for rectal cancer. Br J Surg 2010;97(4):580–7.

43. Stephens RJ, Thompson LC, Quirke P, et al. Impact of short-course preoperative radiotherapy for rectal cancer on patients' quality of life: data from the Medical Research Council CR07/National Cancer Institute of Canada Clinical Trials Group C016 randomized clinical trial. J Clin Oncol 2010;28(27):4233–9.

44. Peeters KC, van de Velde CJ, Leer JW, et al. Late side effects of short-course preoperative radiotherapy combined with total mesorectal excision for rectal cancer: increased bowel dysfunction in irradiated patients – a Dutch Colorectal Cancer Group study. J Clin Oncol 2005;23(25):6199–206.

45. Marijnen CA, van de Velde CJ, Putter H, et al. Impact of short-term preoperative radiotherapy on health-related quality of life and sexual functioning in primary rectal cancer: report of a multicenter randomized trial. J Clin Oncol 2005;23(9):1847–58.

46. Birgisson H, Pahlman L, Gunnarsson U, et al. Occurrence of second cancers in patients treated with radiotherapy for rectal cancer. J Clin Oncol 2005;23(25):6126–31.

47. Tiv M, Puyraveau M, Mineur L, et al. Long-term quality of life in patients with rectal cancer treated with preoperative (chemo)-radiotherapy within a randomized trial. Cancer Radiother 2010;14(6–7):530–4.

48. MERCURY Study Group. Extramural depth of tumor invasion at thin-section MR in patients with rectal cancer: results of the MERCURY study. Radiology 2007;243(1):132–9.

49. Taylor FG, Quirke P, Heald RJ, et al. Preoperative high-resolution magnetic resonance imaging can identify good prognosis stage I, II, and III rectal cancer best managed by surgery alone: a prospective, multicenter, European study. Ann Surg 2011;253(4):711–9.

50. Taylor FG, Quirke P, Heald RJ, et al. One millimetre is the safe cut-off for magnetic resonance imaging prediction of surgical margin status in rectal cancer. Br J Surg 2011;98(6):872–9.

51. Sebag-Montefiore D, Glynne-Jones R. When should pre-operative short course or long course chemoradiotherapy be used. 2012.

52. Rullier E, Sebag-Montefiore D. Sphincter saving is the primary objective for local treatment of cancer of the lower rectum. Lancet Oncol 2006;7(9):775–7.

53. Habr-Gama A, Perez RO. Non-operative management of rectal cancer after neoadjuvant chemoradiation. Br J Surg 2009;96(2):125–7.

54. Habr-Gama A, Perez RO, Proscurshim I, et al. Patterns of failure and survival for nonoperative treatment of stage c0 distal rectal cancer following neoadjuvant chemoradiation therapy. J Gastrointest Surg 2006;10(10):1319–29.

55. Habr-Gama A, Perez RO, Sao Juliao GP, et al. Nonoperative approaches to rectal cancer: a critical evaluation. Semin Radiat Oncol 2011;21(3):234–9.

56. Maas M, Beets-Tan RG, Lambregts DM, et al. Wait-and-see policy for clinical complete responders after chemoradiation for rectal cancer. J Clin Oncol 2011;29(35):4633–40.

57. Bach SP, Hill J, Monson JR, et al. A predictive model for local recurrence after transanal endoscopic microsurgery for rectal cancer. Br J Surg 2009;96(3):280–90.

7

Anal cancer

John H. Scholefield

Introduction

Anal cancer is rare, accounting for approximately 4% of large bowel malignancies; however, there is some evidence that its incidence is increasing. Most anal cancers arise from the squamous epithelium of the anal margin or anal canal, although a few arise from anal glands and ducts.

Traditionally, the anal region is divided into the anal canal and the anal margin or verge. The natural history, demography and surgical management of anal cancer differ between these areas. There is controversy regarding the exact definition of the anal canal. Anatomists see it as lying between the dentate line and the anal verge, whereas surgically it is defined as lying between the anorectal ring and the anal verge. For pathologists, the canal has been defined as corresponding to the longitudinal extent of the internal anal sphincter. The canal above the dentate line is lined by rectal mucosa, except for a small zone immediately above the dentate line called the transitional or junctional zone. Inferiorly, the canal is covered by stratified squamous epithelium. Further confusion relates to the definition of the anal canal and anal margin as sites for cancer. The anal margin is variously described as the visible area external to the anal verge, or as the area below the dentate line. This argument has become less important as surgery plays a lesser role in treatment, but reports of surgical results from past decades are confused by this variation in definition.

Over 80% of anal cancers are of squamous origin, arising from the squamous epithelium of the anal canal and perianal area; 10% are adenocarcinomas arising from the glandular mucosa of the upper anal canal, the anal glands and ducts. A very rare and particularly malignant tumour is anal melanoma. Lymphomas and sarcomas of the anus are even less common but have increased in incidence in recent years, particularly among patients with human immunodeficiency virus (HIV) infection. There has also been a rise in the incidence of other anal epidermoid tumours among patients with HIV.

Epidermoid tumours

Aetiology and pathogenesis

Anal squamous carcinomas are relatively uncommon tumours; there are between 300 and 400 new cases per year in England and Wales. Based on these figures, each consultant colorectal surgeon might expect to see one anal carcinoma every year or so. However, anal cancers are probably under-reported, since some anal canal tumours are misclassified as rectal tumours and some perianal tumours as squamous carcinomas of skin.

The SEER data (2005) quote an incidence of 1.5 per 100 000 population in the USA; similar incidence rates probably apply for the UK. The average age at presentation was 57 years for both sexes.

There is wide geographical variation in the incidence of anal cancers around the world. Areas with a high incidence of anal cancer usually also have a high incidence of cervical, vulval and penile tumours (reflecting the common aetiological agent – papillomaviruses).

The increasing incidence of HIV infection has resulted in a rise in the incidence of anal cancer; this has been seen particularly in areas such as San Francisco, with a large gay population, reportedly seeing a dramatic increase, but this is also seen in parts of the UK where there are large gay communities. Interestingly, there is also an increase in anal cancer seen in women in the last 10 years; a study from Denmark reported a doubling in the incidence of anal cancer in women over the last 10 years.[1]

✔✔ There is a disproportionately high incidence of anal cancer among male homosexual communities reported from San Francisco and Los Angeles. Daling et al.[2] identified risk factors for the development of squamous cell carcinoma of the anus: a history of receptive anal intercourse in males increased the relative risk of developing anal cancer by 33 times compared with controls with colon cancer, and a history of genital warts also increased the relative risk of developing anal cancer (27-fold in men and 22-fold in women). This reflects the likely aetiological link to human papillomaviruses in anal squamous cell carcinoma.

Epidemiological and molecular biological data have shown an association with human papillomavirus (HPV) type 16 DNA, and less commonly types 18, 31 and 33, and their DNA was consistently found to be integrated into the genome in cervical, vulval and penile squamous cell carcinomas. The same HPV DNA types have also been identified in a similar proportion of anal squamous cell carcinomas.[3] There are more than 60 types of HPV (a DNA virus), capable of causing a wide variety of lesions in squamous epithelium. Common warts can be found on the hands and feet of children and young adults, and are caused by the relatively infectious but otherwise innocuous HPV types 1 and 2. Anogenital papillomaviruses are less infective than HPV types 1 and 2 and are exclusively sexually transmitted. The epidemiology of genital papillomavirus infection is poorly understood, largely due to the social and moral taboos surrounding sexually transmissible infections. Anogenital papillomavirus-associated lesions range from condylomas through intraepithelial neoplasias to invasive carcinomas. The most common HPV types causing genital warts are types

6 and 11, which may also be isolated from genital warts and low-grade intraepithelial neoplasia. HPV types 16, 18, 31 and 33 are much less commonly associated with genital condylomata but are more commonly found in high-grade intraepithelial neoplasias and invasive carcinomas. Once one area of the anogenital epithelium is infected, spread of papillomavirus infection throughout the rest of the anogenital area probably follows, but remains occult in the majority of individuals. Although there is a commonly held belief that anal cancer occurs only in individuals who practise anal intercourse, this is unfounded.

Premalignant lesions

✔ Anal and genital papillomavirus-associated lesions may be identified clinically either by naked eye inspection or with an operating microscope (colposcope) and the application of acetic acid to the epithelium, resulting in an 'aceto-white' lesion. Colposcopic examination may suggest the degree of dysplasia and permits targeted biopsy of a lesion, but histological examination remains the diagnostic standard. The natural history of anal papillomavirus infection and intraepithelial neoplasia is in large part dependent on the infecting viral type and on the host immune state. In immunocompetent individuals the risk of malignant conversion from AIN III to invasive cancer is around 12% over 10 years, but in HIV patients the risk is nearer 30% in 10 years.

Anogenital intraepithelial neoplasia of the cervix (CIN), vulva (VIN), vagina (VAIN) and anus (AIN) is graded from I to III, according to the number of thirds of epithelial depth that appear dysplastic on histological section. Thus, in grade III the cells of the whole thickness of the epithelium appear dysplastic, being synonymous with carcinoma in situ.

High-grade anal intraepithelial lesions may be characterised by hyperkeratosis or changes in the pigmentation of the epithelium. Thus, carcinoma in situ may appear white, red or brown, the pigmentation commonly being irregular. The lesions may be flat or raised, but ulceration is suggestive of invasive disease. It is important that any suspicious area is biopsied and examined histologically. The terms 'Bowen's disease of the anus' and 'leucoplakia' are best avoided as they are confusing and convey no specific information, the malignant potential of leucoplakia being very uncertain.

At present, multifocal genital intraepithelial neoplasia represents a difficult clinical problem, which may be further complicated by the occurrence of synchronous or metachronous AIN.[4] The management of these lesions is largely one of regular observation with a low index of suspicion for biopsy. Ablation of the lesions has been popular in some centres – but in the author's opinion should be resisted as it destroys the histology and risks early recurrence of the disease from hair shafts and pilosebaceous units.

Histological types

Included within the category of epidermoid tumours are squamous cell, basaloid (or cloacogenic) carcinomas and muco-epidermoid cancers. The different morphological types of anal cancer do not appear to have different prognoses. Tumours arising at the anal margin tend to be well differentiated and keratinising, whereas those arising in the canal are more commonly poorly differentiated. Basaloid tumours arise in the transitional zone around the dentate line and form 30–50% of all anal canal tumours.

Patterns of spread

Anal canal cancer spreads locally, mainly in a cephalad direction, so that the tumour may appear to have arisen in the rectum. The tumour also spreads outwards into the anal sphincters and into the rectovaginal septum, perineal body, scrotum or vagina in more advanced cases (**Fig. 7.1**). Lymph node metastases occur frequently, especially in tumours of the anal canal. Spread occurs initially to the perirectal group of nodes and thereafter to inguinal, haemorrhoidal and lateral pelvic lymph nodes. The frequency of nodal involvement is related to the size of the primary tumour together with its depth of penetration. Approximately 14% of patients will present with inguinal lymph node involvement, but this rises to approximately 30% when the primary tumour is greater than 5 cm in diameter. Only 50% of patients with enlarged nodes at presentation will subsequently be shown to contain tumour. Synchronously involved nodes carry a particularly poor prognosis, whereas when metachronous spread develops the salvage rate is much higher.

Haematogenous spread tends to occur late and is usually associated with advanced local disease. The principal sites of metastases are the liver, lung and bones. However, metastases have been described in the kidneys, adrenals and brain.

Clinical presentation

The predominant symptoms of epidermoid anal cancer are pain and bleeding, which are present in about 50% of cases. The presence of a mass is noted by a minority of patients, around 25%. Pruritus and discharge occur in a similar proportion. Advanced tumours may involve the sphincter mechanism, causing faecal incontinence. Invasion of the posterior vaginal wall may cause a fistula.

Cancer of the anal margin usually has the appearance of a malignant ulcer, with a raised, everted, indurated edge. Lesions within the canal may not be visible, though extensive lesions spread to the anal verge, or can extend via the ischiorectal fossa to the

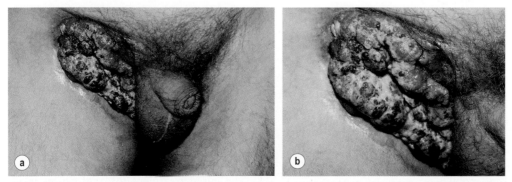

Figure 7.1 • Locally advanced anal cancer involving the anal canal, perianal skin, perineal skin and base of scrotum. Treatment with chemo-irradiation failed to control the disease and the patient underwent a salvage abdominoperineal excision.

skin of the buttock. Digital examination of the anal canal is usually painful, and may reveal the distortion produced by the tumour. Since anal cancer tends to spread upwards, there may be involvement of the distal rectum, giving the impression that the lesion has arisen there. Involvement of the perirectal lymph nodes may be palpable on digital examination. If the tumour has extended into the sphincter muscles, the characteristic induration of a spreading malignancy may be felt around the anal canal.

> ✓✓ Although up to one-third of patients will have inguinal lymph nodes that are enlarged, biopsy will confirm metastatic spread in only 50% of these; the rest are due to secondary infection. Biopsy or fine-needle aspiration is recommended by many to confirm involvement of the groin nodes if radical block dissection is contemplated. Distant spread is unusual in anal cancer, so hepatomegaly, though it must be looked for, is very uncommon. Frequently, other benign perianal conditions will exist in association with anal cancer, such as fistulas, condylomas or leucoplakia.

Investigation

> ✓ The most important investigation in the management of anal cancer is examination under anaesthetic. Examination under anaesthesia permits optimum assessment of the tumour in terms of size, involvement of adjacent structures and nodal involvement, and also provides the best opportunity to obtain a biopsy for histological confirmation. Magnetic resonance imaging (MRI) and computed tomography (CT) scanning are also essential in staging the disease. Routine positron emission tomography (PET) scanning remains controversial.

Clinical staging

No one system of staging for anal tumours has been adopted universally. However, that of the UICC is the most widely used. For anal canal lesions this system has been criticised as it has required assessment of involvement of the external sphincter. To overcome this a system has been suggested by Papillon et al.[5] as follows:

T1 <2 cm;

T2 2–4 cm;

T3 >4 cm, mobile;

T4a invading vaginal mucosa;

T4b extension into structures other than skin, rectal or vaginal mucosa.

MRI has taken over from endoanal ultrasound in staging these lesions. MRI is better than endoanal ultrasound, providing information on spread beyond the anal canal.

Serum tumour markers are unhelpful as they do not provide reliable information.

Treatment

Historical

Traditionally, anal cancer was treated as a 'surgical' disease. Anal canal tumours were treated by radical abdominoperineal excision and colostomy, whereas anal margin lesions were treated by local excision. Over the past 20 years, non-surgical radical treatments, i.e. radiotherapy with or without chemotherapy, have taken over as primary treatments of choice in most cases.

Overall, the results of surgery for anal cancer are disappointing for what is essentially a locoregional disease. For decades radical abdominoperineal excision of the rectum and anus was the preferred method of treatment at most centres around the world. Abdominoperineal excision for anal canal cancer differs little from the procedure used for rectal cancer, but particular care is taken to clear the space below the pelvic floor. Around 20% of cases are incurable surgically at presentation. Results published since the mid-1980s, reporting series collected over the previous several decades, have varied widely in their survival outcome, but on average the 5-year survival has been around 55–60%.

Around 75% of cancers at the anal margin have been treated in the past by local excision. The rationale for this was based on the perception that margin lesions rarely metastasise, though this has not always been confirmed by prolonged follow-up.

Current

> ✓✓ Radiotherapists have been treating anal tumours for many years, achieving equivalent survival rates but with the advantage of stoma avoidance in the majority of cases, which might otherwise have required radical surgery.

Radiation-alone therapy

The initial treatment for anal cancer was radiotherapy because the mortality and morbidity of surgical treatment of anal carcinoma were unacceptable. By the 1930s, however, it was recognised that the low-voltage radiotherapy used frequently produced severe radionecrosis. As surgery became safer, abdominoperineal excision for invading lesions, and local excision for small growths, became the standard treatment for the next four decades.

The development in the 1950s of equipment that could deliver high-energy irradiation by the cobalt source generator or, more recently, by linear accelerators, enabled radiotherapists to deliver higher penetrating doses to deeper placed structures with less superficial scatter of energy. Radiation damage to surrounding tissues was consequently reduced while simultaneously delivering an enhanced tumouricidal effect. Interstitial irradiation alone may produce local tumour control rates of 47%. Improved results have been described using a technique of external beam irradiation, combined with interstitial therapy: two-thirds survived for 5 years, the majority maintaining adequate sphincter function. In the UK high-dose external beam radiotherapy is most commonly used, for which 5-year survival rates of 75% at 3 years have been described.

Chemo-irradiation therapy (combined modality therapy)

✓✓ Combined modality therapy for anal cancer was championed by Norman Nigro. Nigro chose to use 5-fluorouracil (5-FU) and mitomycin C empirically as a preoperative regimen aimed at improving the results of radical surgery.[6] The radiotherapy then consisted of 30 Gy of external beam irradiation over a period of 3 weeks. A bolus of mitomycin C was given on the first day of treatment, and 5-FU was delivered in a synchronous continuous 4-day infusion during the first week of radiotherapy. After completion of radiotherapy, a further infusion of 5-FU was administered and patients later proceeded to abdominoperineal excision. It was evident to Nigro that the majority had quite dramatic tumour shrinkage: in his 1974 publication the tumour was reported to have disappeared completely in all three patients. No tumour was found in the surgical specimen in either of the patients who underwent abdominoperineal excision; the third refused surgery. Nigro's experience over the ensuing 10 years bore out his early enthusiasm. As he became more confident, he no longer routinely pressed his patients to undergo radical surgery, initially confining himself to excising the site of the primary tumour after combined modality therapy. Later, he dropped even this relatively minor surgical step if the primary site looked and felt normal after treatment.[7]

A variety of similar techniques have subsequently been described. With wider experience, it became clear that higher doses of radiotherapy (45–60 Gy) could be applied, usually split into two courses to minimise morbidity. Chemotherapy comprised intravenous infusion of 5-FU at the beginning and end of the first radiotherapy course, and a single bolus of mitomycin C given on the first day of treatment.[8] Modifications of chemotherapy dosage and prophylactic antibiotic therapy were necessary in elderly or frail patients, and those with extensive ulcerated tumours.

All the reported series describe excellent results, but there was a debate about whether chemotherapy added any advantage over radiotherapy alone.

The UK Coordinating Committee on Cancer Research compared chemo-irradiation with radiotherapy alone in a randomised multicentre study.[9] This study randomised 585 patients, making it the largest single trial in anal cancer. The trial showed that combined modality therapy gave superior local control of disease compared with radiotherapy alone. Only 36% of patients receiving combined therapy had 'local failure' compared with 59% of those receiving radiotherapy alone. Although there was no significant overall survival advantage for either treatment regimen, the risk of death from anal cancer was significantly less in the group receiving combined modality therapy (**Fig. 7.2**). As a result of this trial it seems that the standard treatment for anal squamous carcinoma should be a combination of radiotherapy and intravenous 5-FU with mitomycin, which remains the gold standard.

Mitomycin causes much of the toxicity of chemoradiation (a problem particularly in elderly patients) and thus trials of the use of cisplatin as an alternative to mitomycin have been performed (RTOG, 2006).[10] This trial randomised 652 patients but showed that cisplatin had no advantage over mitomycin and may be inferior. The search for the optimal regimen goes on.

Complications of chemoradiation for anal carcinoma include diarrhoea, mucositis, myelosuppression, skin erythema and desquamation. Late complications include anal stenosis and fistula formation. Many oncologists prefer to defunction anterior tumours in women as there is a high incidence of rectovaginal fistula formation in this group during radiotherapy treatment.

HIV patients with anal epidermoid cancers are probably best treated with chemoradiation, but have increased toxicity.[10]

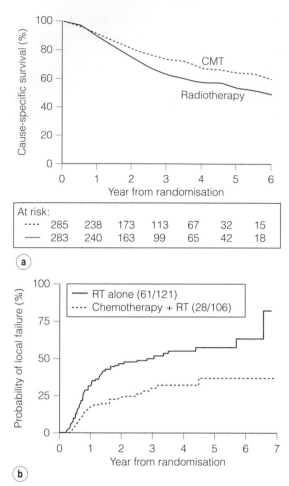

(a)

(b)

Figure 7.2 • (a) Deaths from anal cancer. Number of events: radiotherapy 105, combined modality therapy (CMT) 77 (RR = 0.71, 95% CI 0.53–0.95, P = 0.02). Number at risk = number alive. **(b)** UKCCCR Anal Cancer trial: risk of local failure (T1–2 and N0). Part **(a)**: UKCCCR Anal Cancer Trial Working Party. Lancet 1996; 348:1055, Figure 5. With permission from Elsevier. Part **(b)**: Northover J, Meadows A, Ryan C et al., on behalf of UKCCCR Anal Cancer Trial Working Party. Lancet 1996; 349:206. With permission from Elsevier.

Role of surgery today

Although surgeons no longer play the central therapeutic role, they nevertheless have important contributions to make.

Initial diagnosis

Most patients present to surgeons, who are best suited to perform examination under anaesthesia to confirm diagnosis and assess local extent.

Lesions at the anal margin

✅ Small lesions at the anal margin may still be treated by local excision alone, obviating the need for protracted courses of chemoradiation. There is some evidence that the risk of regional lymph node metastasis is not related to primary tumour size, which may explain the disappointing results sometimes reported after local excision; this conflicts with the view that tumour size is related to stage, which explains the excellent results of local excision in small tumours.

Treatment complications and disease relapse

Surgeons retain an important role in the treatment of anal cancer after failure of primary non-surgical therapy, either early or late. Four situations may require surgery after chemoradiation for anal cancer treatment: residual tumour, complications of treatment, incontinence or fistula after tumour resolution, and subsequent tumour recurrence.

1. The appearance of the primary site is often misleading after radiotherapy. In most patients complete remission is indicated by the tumour disappearing completely. In some, however, an ulcer remains, occasionally looking like an unchanged primary tumour. Only generous biopsy will reveal whether the residual ulcer contains tumour or consists merely of inflammatory tissue. Histological proof of residual disease is essential before radical surgery is recommended to the patient. For patients with proven residual disease, a salvage abdominoperineal resection may be the only option. In fit patients with extensive pelvic disease extending around the vagina or bladder, pelvic exenteration may need to be considered. This type of surgery carries a high morbidity with impaired wound healing due to the radiotherapy. A primary reconstruction of the perineal area using a myocutaneous flap is strongly recommended in salvage AP resections for anal cancer.

2. Complications of non-surgical treatment for anal cancer do occur in a proportion of patients, including radionecrosis, fistula and incontinence. Severe anal pain due to radionecrosis of the anal lining may necessitate either a colostomy, in the hope that the lesion may heal after faecal diversion, or radical anorectal excision with a flap used to reconstruct the perineum.

3. Occasionally, a tumour is so locally extensive that the patient will be rendered incontinent as a consequence of primary tumour shrinkage. Although rectovaginal fistula may be amenable to repair, sphincter damage is unlikely to improve with local surgery, necessitating abdominoperineal excision of the anorectum. Abdominoperineal excision of the rectum under these circumstances is usually best undertaken in conjunction with a rectus abdominis myocutaneous flap to aid perineal wound healing.

4. When there is recurrent disease developing after initial resolution, biopsy is mandatory before surgical intervention. These biopsies need to be of reasonable size, number and depth as the histological appearances following radiotherapy can make histopathological interpretation difficult. If high-dose radiotherapy was used for primary treatment, further non-surgical therapy for recurrence is usually contraindicated, making radical surgical removal necessary.

Inguinal metastases

There is a concern that irradiation of the groins as part of the radiotherapy protocol for anal squamous tumours may overtreat some patients. CT and MRI are not sensitive enough to discriminate between involved and uninvolved nodes. Inguinal sentinel node biopsy may provide an alternative to imaging-based staging for these nodes. As yet the data available are from small series only and the results are inconsistent.[11,12]

☑☑ Inguinal lymph nodes are enlarged in 10–25% of patients with anal cancers. Although inguinal lymph node involvement may be treated by radiotherapy, some argue in favour of surgery; however, histological or cytological confirmation is mandatory before radical groin dissection, as up to 50% of cases of inguinal lymphadenopathy may be due to inflammation alone. Enlargement of groin nodes some time after primary therapy is most likely to be due to recurrent tumour; radical groin dissection is indicated in this situation, with up to 50% 5-year survival.

Treatment of intraepithelial neoplasia

HPV infection of the anogenital area is very common; it is reported that over 70% of sexually active adults have at some time had occult or overt genital HPV infection. In most individuals the infection remains occult, but in a minority the infection manifests itself as either condylomas or intraepithelial neoplasia. As with other viral infections, it is impossible to eradicate HPV infection by surgical excision; for this reason, surgical excision of condylomas is effectively performed more for relief of symptoms and cosmesis.

Similarly, the natural history of low-grade AIN (I and II) is relatively benign and therefore a policy of observation alone is adequate. This is likely to be particularly advisable when large areas of the anogenital epithelium are affected. However, for high-grade AIN (III) the advice is more circumspect as we do not know the natural history of this condition. If the area of AIN III is small, it is probably prudent to excise it locally and then to observe the patient at regular intervals for a number of years. If the area of AIN III is too large for local excision without risk of anal stenosis, then a careful observational policy with 6-monthly review may be an option.

Aggressive surgical excision of the whole perianal skin and anal canal and resurfacing with split skin with a defunctioning colostomy has been used to treat wide areas of AIN III. This sort of surgery necessitates multiple procedures and carries significant morbidity, which for a condition of uncertain malignant potential may make the treatment worse than the disease.

The use of immunomodulators in AIN has been investigated as a potential therapeutic option. While some authors report encouraging results, these are all small studies of short duration. Photodynamic therapy using topical photosensitisers may be useful, but experience is currently very limited. All these treatments are painful and this often limits their use.

Rarer tumours

Adenocarcinoma

Adenocarcinoma in the anal canal is usually a very low rectal cancer that has spread downwards to involve the canal; however, true adenocarcinoma of the anal canal does occur, probably arising from the anal glands, which arise around the dentate line and pass radially outwards into the sphincter muscles. This is a very rare tumour, quite radiosensitive, and is increasingly being treated by chemoradiation.

Malignant melanoma

Another very rare tumour, this accounts for just 1% of anal canal malignant tumours. The lesion may mimic a thrombosed external pile due to its colour, although amelanotic tumours also occur. Anal melanomas have a dismal prognosis; the literature suggests a median survival of around 18 months after diagnosis and only 10–20% 5-year survival. All treatment options appear to be equally unsuccessful. Liver and lung metastases are common. As the chances of cure are minimal, radical surgery as primary treatment should be avoided, but local excision may provide useful palliation.[13]

Key points

- HPV is an aetiological factor in anal squamous cell carcinomas. Women with previous gynaecological lesions on the cervix and vulva and the immunosuppressed (transplant recipients and HIV patients) are at risk for AIN. These premalignant lesions may be rapidly progressive in immunocompromised patients.
- The management of anal squamous carcinoma has changed dramatically in the last few years. Chemo-irradiation is the treatment of first choice for most lesions.
- Surgery may be the primary treatment modality for small perianal lesions that can be locally excised.
- Melanoma of the anus is very rare and has a dismal prognosis. Radical surgery, chemotherapy and radiotherapy are of little benefit. Local excision may provide some useful palliation.

References

1. Frische M, Melbye M. Trends in the incidence of anal carcinoma in Denmark. Br Med J 1993;306:419–22.
2. Daling J, Weiss N, Hislop T, et al. Sexual practices, sexually transmitted diseases and the incidence of anal cancer. N Engl J Med 1987;317:973–7.
   Excellent epidemiological paper on anal squamous cell carcinoma.
3. Palmer JG, Scholefield JH, Shepherd N, et al. Anal cancer and human papillomaviruses. Dis Colon Rectum 1989;32:1016–22.
4. Scholefield J, Hickson W, Smith J, et al. Anal intraepithelial neoplasia: part of a multifocal disease process. Lancet 1992;340:1271–3.
5. Papillon J, Mayer M, Mountberon J, et al. A new approach to the management of epidermoid carcinoma of the anal canal. Cancer 1987;51:1830–7.
6. Nigro N, Vaitkevicius V, Considine Jr. B, et al. Combined therapy for cancer of the anal canal. A preliminary report. Dis Colon Rectum 1974;27:354–6.
   A classic paper – the first experience of using chemoradiation in anal cancer.
7. Nigro N. An evaluation of combined therapy for squamous cell cancer in the anal canal. Dis Colon Rectum 1984;27:763–6.
8. Cummings B, Keane T, O'Sullivan B, et al. Mitomycin in anal canal carcinoma. Oncology 1993;50(Suppl. 1):63–9.
9. UKCCCR Anal Cancer Trial Working Party. Epidermoid anal cancer: results from the UKCCCR randomised trial of radiotherapy alone versus radiotherapy, 5-fluorouracil, and mitomycin. Lancet 1996;348:1049–54.
   A large well-run randomised trial that changed the management of this cancer in the UK.
10. Uronis HE, Bendell JC. Anal cancer – an overview. Oncologist 2007;12:524–34.
11. Gretschel S, Warnick P, Bembenek A, et al. Lymphatic mapping and sentinel lymph node biopsy in epidermoid carcinoma of the anal canal. Eur J Surg Oncol 2008;34:890–4.
12. Hirche C, Dresel S, Krempien R, et al. Sentinel node biopsy by indocyanine green retention fluorescence detection for inguinal lymph node staging of anal cancer: preliminary experience. Ann Surg Oncol 2010;17:2357–62.
13. Ross M, Pezzi C, Pezzi T, et al. Patterns of failure in anorectal melanoma. A guide to surgical therapy. Arch Surg 1990;125:313–6.

8

Diverticular disease

Des Winter

Historical perspectives

Colonic diverticulosis is a common anatomical disorder characterised by acquired or false diverticula (mucosal protrusion through the muscle wall) with an age-dependent prevalence of over 50% by the seventh decade and beyond.[1] The term 'diverticulum' ('*divertikel*' in German) was used to describe what was an anatomical curiosity in the early 1800s until the recognition of 'perisigmoiditis' and related colovesical fistulas by the latter half of the 19th century.[2] Lord Berkeley Moynihan (1865–1936, Leeds) propagated the term 'diverticulitis' at the turn of the 20th century,[3] while diverticulosis was proposed as an umbrella term for asymptomatic individuals as well as attending patients.[4] For decades much of what was written about diverticular problems was based on erroneous assumptions. A lack of evidence and scientific endeavour in the field created a knowledge vacuum that was filled with the dogma of the era. We are left with a multiplicity of management protocols around the world based on local influence.

Anatomical and physiological perspectives

Colonic diverticulosis (the presence of a single diverticulum or multiple diverticula) and related disorders (diverticular disease) is traditionally thought to be a western-world, industrialised-country, mature-age-group phenomenon with clearly defined origins in meat-rich, fibre-poor diets. Some of the earliest descriptions date to the early 20th century[5] and the scientific basis for our current understanding is still limited. Parks described his findings on diverticula based on 300 cadaveric dissections in 1968.[1] He noted that diverticula tended to form rows in the lateral intertaenial (rather than antimesenteric) areas, that they were mainly in the sigmoid but could be scattered throughout the colon, and that frequently a blood vessel pierced the wall at the neck of the diverticulum. Much of what was determined about the incidence of diverticulosis was from this and other mid-twentieth century post-mortem studies.[6–8] Now confirmed in population-based data, diverticula are rare before 30, more common after 40, found in one-third after 60 and over 50% of those older than 70 years of age. The age-related phenomenon gives clues to the aetiology and points to general ageing processes including declining collagen strength or repair.

Incidence and geographical differences

Race and geography

Geographic disparities in the incidence of diverticulosis imply that it is predominantly a disease of westernised society associated with an ageing population and western diet. Diverticular disease is extremely rare in Asia and Africa compared to Europe and the USA,[9] with a reported prevalence of 0.5–1.7% in China and Korea.[10,11] As these countries become more industrialised, the incidence of diverticular disease increases.[12,13] This has been best described in Japanese immigrants to Hawaii, where necropsy studies demonstrate a dramatic increase in diverticulosis compared to age-matched mainland Japanese controls (52% vs. 0.5–1%).[13] However, the increasing incidence of diverticular disease is not solely due to adoption of a westernised lifestyle, and genetic factors may play a role. There are distinct differences in diverticulosis prevalence within ethnic groups living in the same region. For example, studies of ethnic groups living in Israel demonstrate differences in Ashkenazi Jews (16.2%), Sephardic Jews (3.8%) and Arabs (0.7%).[14,15]

Aside from differences in the geographic prevalence of diverticulosis, anatomical variations also exist, with a reported prevalence of right-sided diverticulosis of 20% in patients <40 years increasing to 40% in patients >60 years old in Asian populations.[16,17] As these countries become more westernised, the incidence of diverticular disease increases; however, the anatomical location (right colon) remains constant.[18,19]

Age and gender

Recent studies point towards age- and gender-related differences in patients presenting with diverticulitis. Males are more likely to develop diverticulitis at a younger age whereas there is a female predominance in older patients. In western populations, approximately one-fifth of patients with diverticulitis are under the age of 50 (reported incidence 18–34%[20–23]). There was a trend towards a more aggressive surgical approach in younger patients based on the hypothesis that the disease was more virulent in this subgroup.[24–26] Emerging evidence would suggest that younger age is a risk factor for recurrent disease rather than an indication for early intervention in the acute setting, as these patients are just as likely to settle with conservative management.[27,28]

Diet

Painter and Burkitt[2] described diverticular disease as a deficiency of dietary fibre, proposing that consumption of a refined western diet led to longer colonic transit times, decreased stool volume and increased intraluminal pressures.[29] Although a role for dietary fibre in the pathogenesis of diverticular

disease is plausible, there is little evidence to support this hypothesis. Conclusions are drawn from several randomised controlled trials with small patient numbers that produced conflicting results[30,31] and do not demonstrate an improvement in symptoms or diverticulitis recurrence overall. In addition to a high-fibre diet, controversy exists as to whether low-residue diets may improve symptoms. Residue refers to any indigestible food substance that remains in the intestinal tract and contributes to stool bulk.[32] Historically, low-residue diets were recommended for a number of gastrointestinal complaints.[33] Specifically, there was a concern that indigestible nuts and seeds could block a diverticulum, leading to diverticulitis or perforation. These concerns, however, have been dismissed following conclusive evidence from the healthcare professionals' follow-up study.[34]

> ✅ Low-fibre diet has an epidemiological association with the development of diverticular disease. However, recommending fibre as a treatment for diverticulosis is largely based on outdated, poorly controlled studies.
> Young patients (<50 years) may be more likely to suffer from recurrent diverticulitis. At present there is no evidence to support aggressive surgical intervention in cases of uncomplicated diverticular disease.

Aetiology and pathogenesis

There are several theories as to the pathogenesis of diverticular disease. Aside from luminal trauma, potential aetiological factors include elevated colonic pressures, compromised colon wall integrity and altered bacterial flora.[35–42]

Colonic wall abnormalities (specifically colonic wall thickening, increased collagen cross-linking,[43] muscle atrophy[44] and shortening of taeniae coli[45]) are thought to produce a 'stiffer', less compliant colon predisposing to diverticular herniation. In addition, abnormalities in cholinergic smooth muscle excitation and neuro-humoral signalling (serotonin, nitric oxide, vasoactive intestinal polypeptide) may contribute to disordered contractions and increased intraluminal pressures.[46–49]

Lifestyle

Large population studies have produced interesting information on the incidence of diverticular disease. Both the health professionals' follow-up study (47 228 men) and the Swedish mammography cohort study demonstrate a positive correlation between obesity and diverticular-associated complications.[50,51] Indeed, according to the American taskforce, obesity is recognised as a risk factor for diverticular disease.[52] This may be due to obesity-associated inflammation (cytokine secretion from metabolically active visceral fat[53]).

Smoking

Evidence for a potential association between diverticular disease and smoking is contradictory. Pathological examination of resected specimens demonstrates a higher incidence of strictures and perforation in smokers compared to non-smokers.[54] However, there appears to be a gender difference, with a higher likelihood of abscess or perforation in female smokers[51] compared to males.[55]

Non-steroidal anti-inflammatory drugs (NSAIDs)

It is hypothesised that NSAIDs may cause colonic injury via direct topical injury and/or impaired prostaglandin synthesis, compromising mucosal integrity, increasing permeability and enabling the influx of bacteria and other toxins.[41] Data from the health professional follow-up study showed an increased incidence of uncomplicated diverticular disease in patients who used NSAIDs compared with their asymptomatic counterparts.[56] In addition, NSAID use is associated with diverticular complications, including bleeding and perforation.[57] Other studies support these findings.[58,59]

Diverticulitis

The extent of the problem

It was misquoted for many years that about 25% of patients with diverticulosis will develop an acute inflammatory condition characterised by left iliac fossa pain, malaise and fever (diverticulitis), a figure that was rarely challenged although the basis for it is unclear. The origin of this overestimate may have been the misquoting of the proportion *re-presenting* following an episode of diverticular symptoms,[1] rather than the actual *prevalence* of

diverticulitis. A modern (1986–2004) population-based study found 1.7% of male healthcare professionals aged 40–75 developed diverticulitis, giving a crude annual incidence of 1 per 1000 (801 events in 47 228 persons over 18 years).[34] This figure has been confirmed as an accurate representation of the USA population, in whom there was an age-adjusted hospitalisation rate of 75 per 100 000 in 2005,[60] or 1 per 1000 in the present decade at the projected trajectory. The population trends seen in this national inpatient sample (1998–2005) reflect the worldwide finding of male predominance aged under 45 but female predominance in those older, as well as an increasing incidence in the under 45 age group. Fascinatingly, there was a large difference in the rates of diverticulitis admissions between the west (50.4 per 100 000) versus the other sectors of the USA (>70 per 100 000). The west of the USA also has a higher fibre intake and relatively lower colorectal cancer incidence than the rest of the country.[61]

Classification

It is now widely accepted that diverticulitis encompasses a wide spectrum of pathologies, ranging from acute uncomplicated diverticulitis to perforation with peritonitis. Although the underlying pathophysiology may be similar in all cases, the clinical manifestation of the disease differs greatly between individuals. In this regard it is helpful to further classify patients according to those who have 'mild diverticulitis' and those with 'severe diverticulitis' (see Table 8.1).[62] The adult prevalence of perforated diverticulitis is approximately 3.5 per 100 000 and the incidence has more than doubled in the last two

Table 8.1 • CT classification of acute diverticulitis

Moderate diverticulitis	Severe diverticulitis
Localised sigmoid colon wall thickening (>5 mm) Inflammation localised to pericolic fat	Moderate diverticulitis plus any of: Abdominopelvic abscess Free extraluminal gas Extraluminal contrast extravasation

From Ambrosetti P, Grossholz M, Becker C et al. Computed tomography in acute left colonic diverticulitis. Br J Surg 1997; 84(4):532–4.

decades.[63–66] Reasons why this may be are speculative, including NSAIDs, opioids, corticosteroids and smoking.[54,58,67] While this supports the historical assumption that high dietary fibre protects against the development of both disorders, the association is speculative until cofactors (hereditary, ethnic, socioeconomic, dietary, smoking, alcohol, etc.) are excluded.

Table 8.2 compares different classification systems for diverticulitis.

Segmental colitis associated with diverticulosis

Segmental colitis associated with diverticulosis (SCAD) is found in less than 1% of colonoscopy procedures.[72,73] The majority of these patients simply have bleeding per rectum rather than any significant change in bowel habit or constitutional symptoms. Many resolve without therapy such that medical treatment should be reserved for those with troublesome symptoms.[74,75]

Diagnosis and imaging

The diagnosis of diverticulitis is largely based on clinical impression.[76] Confirmatory imaging is helpful in determining the extent, degree and local consequences of the inflammatory process, as well as excluding other disorders.[77,78] Ultrasound is adequate, with reasonable sensitivity and specificity using graded compression and other tricks of waveform distortion that may not be readily available in every emergency room environment.[79,80] Although a relatively inexpensive, easily reproducible and safe modality, sonographic imaging displays reduced acoustic acuity in gas-distended or obese patients. Historically, a water-soluble (rather than barium-based) contrast enema with fluoroscopic images was used to confirm diverticulitis but the test was an unpleasant, messy, time-consuming endurance for patients and radiologists.[62] Not surprisingly, computed tomography (CT) in rapid, multiple slice scanners capable of variable plane reconstruction became the gold standard in determining the diagnosis and staging of diverticulitis[62,80]

Table 8.2 • Classification systems for diverticulitis

	Hinchey classification[68]	Köhler modification[69]	Modified Hinchey[70]	Hansen/Stock[71]
			0 Mild clinical diverticulitis	0 Diverticulosis
Stage I	Pericolic abscess confined by the mesocolon	Pericolic abscess	I Pericolic abscess or phlegmon Ia Colonic wall thickening/Confined pericolic inflammation Ib Confined small (<5 cm) pericolic abscess	Acute uncomplicated diverticulitis
Stage II	Pelvic abscess, distant from area of inflammation	IIa Distant abscess amenable to percutaneous drainage IIb Complex abscess with/without associated fistula	II Pelvic, distant intra-abdominal, or retroperitoneal abscess	Acute complicated diverticulitis IIa Phlegmon, peridiverticulitis IIb Abscess, sealed perforation IIc Free perforation
Stage III	Generalised peritonitis resulting from pericolic/pelvic abscess rupture into peritoneal cavity	Generalised purulent peritonitis	III Generalised purulent peritonitis	Recurrent diverticulitis
Stage IV	Faecal peritonitis resulting from free perforation of colonic diverticulum	Faecal peritonitis	IV Generalised faecal peritonitis	N/A

(**Figures 8.1** and **8.2**). Downsides include the allergic and nephrotoxic risks of intravenous contrast, so assessment of relevant history and biochemistry is essential. Widespread and repeated CT exposure to radiation is estimated to potentially harm individuals,[81] so patient age and exposure history is a factor. A pragmatic approach might be to use ultrasound initially, reserving CT for unclear cases or those in whom crisp anatomical definition is required (e.g. abscess needing drainage, suspicion of malignancy, unexpected or atypical sonographic findings, etc.; **Figures 8.3** and **8.4**).

Colonic imaging (either optical colonoscopy or CT colonography) is still performed routinely following an episode of diverticulitis to rule out neoplasia (either coexistent or mimicking an inflammatory

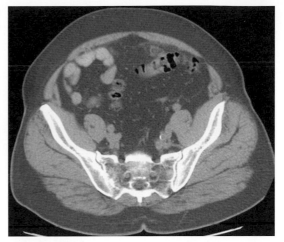

Figure 8.1 • CT image of moderate sigmoid diverticulitis.

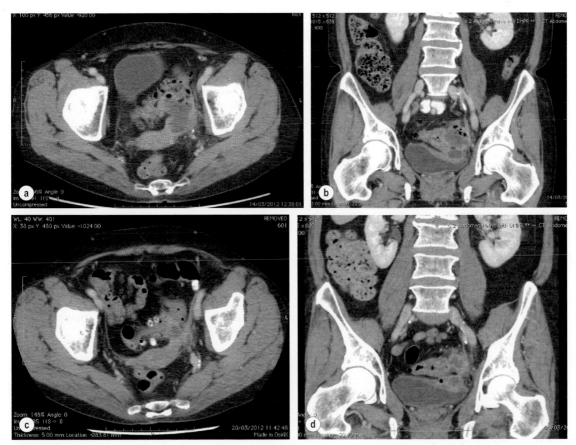

Figure 8.2 • Conservative management of diverticular abscess treated with IV antibiotics. **(a, b)** CT abdomen on presentation demonstrates a perisigmoid abscess (Hinchey II diverticulitis). **(c, d)** CT abdomen on day 7 following treatment with i.v. cefuroxime, ciprofloxacin and metronidazole demonstrates resolution of abscess.

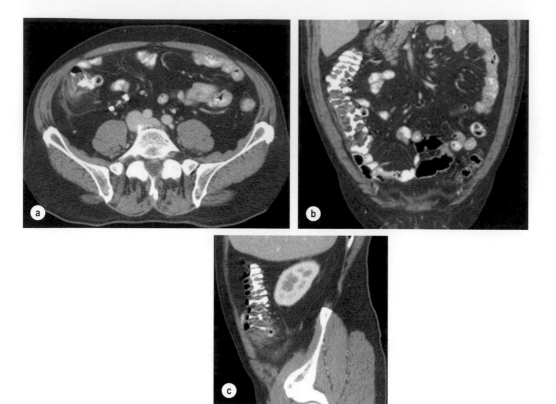

Figure 8.3 • Right-sided diverticulitis. CT may be useful in patients with atypical clinical findings. The above images demonstrate caecal diverticulitis as a cause for right iliac fossa pain in a 60-year-old male.

process). The utility of these procedures has been debated by authors from the Antipodes.[82,83] Where there has been good-quality cross-sectional imaging of relatively mild diverticulitis in an otherwise asymptomatic young patient with no premorbid reasons to screen, then diverticulitis is a soft indication for colonoscopy. Conversely, where there are atypical imaging features (i.e. localised lymphadenopathy, relative absence of diverticula, focal mass effect, more than one site of 'fat stranding') or complicated diverticulitis then early colonoscopy is very much indicated. While tradition considered that endoscopic insufflation would be too dangerous within 6 weeks of assumed diverticulitis,[84] there is little substance to this dogma and careful colonoscopy can be performed after an interval of 1–2 weeks where there is clinical suspicion of neoplasia (e.g. unresolved or progressive symptoms).

Magnetic resonance imaging (MRI) is of immense value in intestinal disorders because soft tissue delineation exceeds ultrasound or CT and additional benefits include fistulography, multiphase component separation and an absence of ionising radiation.[85–87] MRI is expensive, requires expert interpretation and scan platforms are claustrophobic, noisy places that patients must endure for prolonged periods. Open scanners have gone a long way to address the problem but they are few in number as yet.

> ✓✓ CT is the gold standard in diagnosing and staging the severity of diverticulitis.[88]
>
> Recent evidence suggests that routine follow-up colonoscopy may not be warranted and should be determined on a case-by-case basis depending on the level of clinical concern.[82,83]

Treatment

Conservative and medical options

Asymptomatic patients with diverticulosis do not require treatment. There was a historical vogue (until very recently) for advising patients to avoid nuts and seeds based on the misguided assumption that they precipitated symptomatic events by

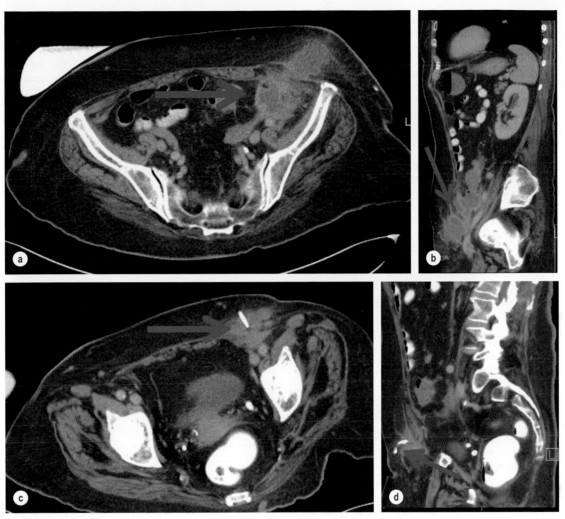

Figure 8.4 • (a, b) CT abdomen demonstrating a diverticular abscess involving the abdominal wall (red arrow; history of right hemicolectomy and end ileostomy). **(c, d)** The abscess was drained percutaneously with resolution of symptoms. Red arrow demonstrates placement of drain.

local trauma or obstruction. In keeping with the folklore of diverticular management in the 20th century, this was without scientific basis or fact.[34] Furthermore, although it seems unlikely to harm and may help prevent development of diverticula, there is scant proof that changing to a higher fibre intake can change the course of symptomatic diverticular problems.[31] Even when combined with non-absorbable antibiotics (rifaximin), any perceived benefit is small and not much better than placebo.[89] Lifestyle optimisation (i.e. high freshly sourced fibre intake, low animal fat/processed diet, smoking cessation, exercise, minimal anti-inflammatory drug intake, etc.) is central

to primary disease prevention and is sensible in all populations regardless of the presence of diverticula.

There are limited medical options for patients with recurrent or persistent symptoms deemed attributable to diverticulitis (or 'diverticular disease'). There is modest benefit to a prolonged course of 5-aminosalicylates or probiotics in short-term, small trials.[90,91] There is a relatively small side-effect profile to these agents due to their relatively specific intestinal drug delivery mechanism. However, the numbers needed to treat are probably high, the compliance poor and the overall applicability of the approach is low.

☑☑ Antibiotics for uncomplicated diverticulitis? According to present guidelines, bowel rest or intake of oral fluids and a 7- to 10-day regimen of broad-spectrum antibiotics is recommended in patients with uncomplicated diverticulitis.[92] As the aetiology is unknown, diverticulitis may be an inflammatory condition rather than an infective/bacterial problem. Current recommendations are based on expert opinion and it is yet to be established whether antibiotics are necessary in the primary treatment of acute mild diverticulitis.

The AVOD trial (open, multicentre trial) randomised patients (669 patients) to no antibiotics versus antibiotics for uncomplicated diverticulitis and found no significant difference in complication rate ($P = 0.3$), length of stay or recurrent diverticulitis ($P = 0.88$).[93]

The DIABOLO trial is a multicentre randomised clinical trial investigating the cost-effectiveness of treatment strategies with or without antibiotics for uncomplicated acute diverticulitis. This study is currently recruiting patients.[94]

There is no consensus on the most appropriate antibiotic regimen or route (oral/intravenous) for diverticulitis; however, broad-spectrum agents targeting Gram-negative organisms (*Escherichia coli*) are advised.

Emergency surgery

Historical perspectives

Henri Albert Hartmann (1860–1952, Paris, France) first described an alternative to abdominoperineal excision of the sigmoid and rectum for carcinoma at the French Surgical Association in 1921.[95,96] The dissection extended below the peritoneal reflection with transaction of the lower rectum, closure of the remaining short rectal stump and peritoneum, with formation of an end colostomy. Of course, this is not what was performed for acute diverticulitis in the 20th century but, amazingly, the eponymous term has endured regardless of the historical inaccuracy. This was due to the absence of a suitable alternative to describe what was, in essence, a non-restorative subtotal sigmoid colectomy with a long, intraperitoneal, closed rectosigmoid stump and end colostomy. This operation triumphed over previously performed three-stage procedures whereby an initial defunctioning loop colostomy was performed with subsequent resection and anastomosis (if and when the patient recovered), and eventually, colostomy closure. The mortality of this latter approach was unacceptably high and, while that of a 'Hartmann procedure' is still 10–15% in the present era, a one-stage non-restorative operation was thought safer. Short-term complications include persistent sepsis (often in the residual sigmoid stump due to persistent diverticulitis or opening of the staple line), stoma problems (necrosis, retraction, stenosis, etc.) and wound complications (including dehiscence). In the longer term, as many as half of patients are left with a permanent stoma due to the reluctance of the surgeon (or indeed the patient) to submit to the perils of another operation for anastomosis.

Does perforated diverticulitis require resection in all cases? Carl Eggers (1879–1956, New York, USA), a German-American surgeon and one of the founding members of the American College of Surgeons, described a series of patients with diverticulitis of whom he had managed a small number showing peritonitis with drainage alone.[97] Two randomised clinical trials (Denmark and France) in the 1980s and 1990s dealt with this question. Although both were underpowered, the data do support an organ-preserving approach. Patients in whom a drainage procedure (with or without a defunctioning stoma) alone was performed for purulent peritonitis had a lower mortality than those resected.[98,99] There may have been more short-term septic issues with an organ-preserving operation but this was in an age with fewer broad-spectrum antibiotics and less widespread availability of interventional radiology drainage of abscesses than now.

Laparoscopic peritoneal lavage for generalised purulent peritonitis

Alas, the trials were not enough to change practice at the time. They did give food for thought to another pioneering surgeon, Gerry O'Sullivan (1946–2012, Cork, Ireland), who considered it feasible to laparoscope a patient in whom there was generalised peritonitis and pneumoperitoneum on CT or plain radiography (erect chest or abdominal X-ray) due to perforated diverticulitis. By simply performing laparoscopic peritoneal lavage, his initial results were startling, with minimal morbidity, no stoma and low mortality[100] (see **Figure 8.5**). The utility and low mortality (<5%) of the approach to generalised peritonitis due to perforated, purulent diverticulitis has been confirmed in several small series, one multicentre experience and a systematic review.[101–105]

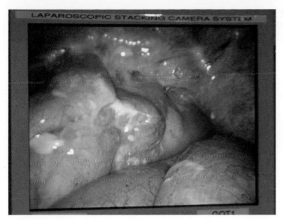

Figure 8.5 • Laparoscopic image of Hinchey III purulent diverticulitis.

Faecal peritonitis or the identification of a visible colonic wall breach are indications to resect the offending sigmoid colon, where many cases show features of stercoral rather than diverticular perforation (i.e. history of prolonged constipation, minimal or absent diverticula, large hole with focal necrosis not inflammation). A number of randomised clinical trials are under way across Europe (laparoscopic lavage versus resection; see Table 8.3).

Resection with primary anastomosis

Primary resection and anastomosis (PRA) with or without a defunctioning ileostomy has emerged as a worthy alternative to Hartmann's procedure (HP) in the setting of peritonitis secondary to diverticular perforation.[105] Indeed, some studies demonstrate superior outcomes compared to Hartmann's procedure, quoting mortality rates of 5% for PRA vs. 15% for HP.[106] Furthermore, PRA compares favourably in terms of postoperative morbidity, including wound and stoma complications and sepsis. In the most recent systematic review, anastomotic leak rates were of the order of 6%,[107] notably lower than the reported anastomotic leak rate in Hartmann's reversal (8%).

A treatment algorithm is shown in **Figure 8.6**.

Elective resection: facts, fiction and functional outcome

Elective resection for recurrent diverticulitis was once practised commonly after the second or third episode. However, the practice is risky, with reports of 1%

Table 8.3 • Randomised trials comparing laparoscopic lavage with resection

Name	Study	Objective	Inclusion criteria	Study number	Results
LADIES The Netherlands	Multicentre two-armed randomised trial LOLA arm; laparoscopic lavage, Hartmann's or resection and anastomosis (2:1:1) DIVA arm: for faeculent peritonitis Hartmann's or resection/anastomosis (1:1)	Patients with generalised peritonitis caused by perforated diverticulitis are randomised to undergo either laparoscopic lavage and drainage or resectional surgery by laparotomy	Free gas on CT, or upon the finding of peritonitis with diffuse fluid or gas on CT	LOLA arm: 264 DIVA arm: 212	Recruitment commenced 2009
LapLAND Ireland	Multicentre randomised trial	Laparoscopic lavage for perforated non-faeculent diverticulitis vs. Hartmann's or resection and anastomosis	Patients with generalised peritonitis and radiological evidence of free air on CT	300	Recruitment commenced 2010

LADIES: Swank HA, Vermeulen J, Lange JF et al. Dutch Diverticular Disease (3D) Collaborative Study Group. The LADIES trial: laparoscopic peritoneal lavage or resection for purulent peritonitis and Hartmann's procedure or resection with primary anastomosis for purulent or faecal peritonitis in perforated diverticulitis (NTR2037). BMC Surg 2010; 10:29.
LapLAND: http://clinicaltrialsfeeds.org/clinical-trials/show/NCT01019239

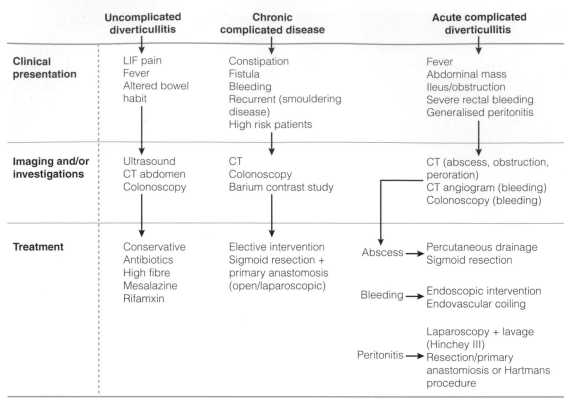

	Uncomplicated diverticulitis	Chronic complicated disease	Acute complicated diverticulitis
Clinical presentation	LIF pain Fever Altered bowel habit	Constipation Fistula Bleeding Recurrent (smouldering disease) High risk patients	Fever Abdominal mass Ileus/obstruction Severe rectal bleeding Generalised peritonitis
Imaging and/or investigations	Ultrasound CT abdomen Colonoscopy	CT Colonoscopy Barium contrast study	CT (abscess, obstruction, peroration) CT angiogram (bleeding) Colonoscopy (bleeding)
Treatment	Conservative Antibiotics High fibre Mesalazine Rifamxin	Elective intervention Sigmoid resection + primary anastomosis (open/laparoscopic)	Abscess → Percutaneous drainage Sigmoid resection Bleeding → Endoscopic intervention Endovascular coiling Peritonitis → Laparoscopy + lavage (Hinchey III) Resection/primary anastomiosis or Hartmans procedure

Figure 8.6 • Treatment algorithm. Based on: Klarenbeek BR, de Korte N, van der Peet DL et al. Review of current classifications for diverticular disease and a translation into clinical practice. Int J Colorectal Dis 2012; 27(2):207–14. With permission from Springer Science and Business Media.

mortality, 30–50% morbidity and as many as 10% receiving a stoma (at least in the short term) around the world.[108–110] The natural history of diverticulitis is such that one in six patients undergoes surgery at presentation while approximately 20–25% re-present, with a similar proportion requiring surgery such that less than 5% have more than two episodes.[111] In that series, six of the 78 patients readmitted with diverticulitis a second time died, a proportion commented to be twice that of those presenting for the first time. Parks did not suggest elective resection to improve this statistic, although many have used his data to support the premise of a 'prophylactic' operation. Indeed, he pointed out that several patients died in their first admission from suspected diverticulitis in whom radiology or necropsy tests were not performed so that they could not be classed as diverticular deaths in the paper. Had they been, the mortality was likely much higher for the first episode than reported for the second. The principles on which this outdated and flawed concept were founded predate modern cross-sectional imaging such that the diagnosis was clinical and inferred from subsequent barium enema.[112–114] Some patients had ongoing symptoms and others came to surgery for diverticulitis emergently so it was extrapolated that elective surgery was indicated to prevent a life-threatening event. We now know that diverticulitis follows a predictable course in the majority such that recurrence runs at 2% per year while the risk of requiring emergency surgery following diverticulitis is calculated to be only 1 in 2000 patient-years.[63] Furthermore, Mayo Clinic data suggest that diverticulitis is not a progressive disease in terms of severity or mortality risk.[115] Indeed, as it has been throughout the last century, the highest risk of extreme sepsis and death is with the first episode. The overwhelming majority of these patients have no history of diverticulitis and had no premorbid diagnosis of diverticulosis.[115–123]

There are certain diverticular-associated phenomena that are relative or absolute indications for elective surgery. These include fistula (e.g. colovesical, colovaginal, colocutaneous), obstruction from a stricture, and persisting diverticulitis ('smouldering diverticulitis') unresponsive to medical therapy. The latter is an uncommon event characterised by symptoms matched with a persistent subtle, tender mass in the left iliac fossa, persistently elevated markers of inflammation (e.g. C reactive protein), and no other abnormality on colonoscopy and cross-sectional imaging. Are there circumstances where a patient should consider elective resection for recurring episodes of diverticulitis, each of which resolve fully? After four defined episodes the risk of further episodes requiring admission and surgery is particularly high in the younger (<50 years of age) population.[124] Therefore, in young patients eager to avoid further morbidity and time off work in whom an elective operation can be performed with a mortality risk of <1%,[23] elective sigmoid resection is reasonable. However, the preoperative discussion should include the fact that recurrent diverticulitis may arise, that a stoma may be required (at least in the short term), that coexisting functional symptoms will persist, and that over 20% complain of urgency and even incontinence episodes.[125] The laparoscopic approach is attractive to patient and surgeon, as there are short-term advantages with smaller wounds, less morbidity and less time dependent on supportive care.[126]

✔ Indications for elective resection include fistula, diverticular stricture and disease refractory to conservative management.

Sigmoid resection may be considered in patients who have undergone abscess drainage or laparoscopic lavage; however, there is no evidence to support surgical intervention in these cases.

Diverticular haemorrhage

The proportion of patients with diverticulosis presenting with bleeding was originally thought to be as high as 3–5%.[127] However, this was based on a somewhat oversimplified quotient (number bleeding divided by number presenting to hospital with a diagnosis of diverticulosis) that would have hugely overestimated the prevalence. Modern population-based data would suggest fewer than 1 in 2000 person-years events (383 bleeds with only 70 requiring transfusion or intervention in 730 446 person-years of follow-up).[34] One group found no inflammation but non-uniform intimal thickening in the vasa recta of bleeding diverticula.[128,129] The majority of diverticular haemorrhages cease spontaneously. A requirement of more than 4 units of red cell concentrate may indicate patients at risk of ongoing bleeding.[130] Visceral angiography with embolisation[131–134] is preferable to blind colectomy, with which morbidity and mortality risks are high. One of the challenges to the surgeon faced with operating on an (all too often) elderly patient with lower gastrointestinal bleeding is what to remove. Many a young surgeon was caught out doing a left colectomy on the assumption that the sigmoid was the culprit, only to find ongoing bleeding –'diverticular' haemorrhage is right sided in over 50% and a proportion are due to angiodysplasia.

Key points

- The spectrum of diverticular disease encompasses asymptomatic diverticulosis, mild diverticulitis, complicated diverticular disease (abscess, perforation, stricture), diverticular bleeding and SCAD (segmental colitis with associated diverticulosis).
- The incidence of diverticulitis is approaching 1 per 1000 in western populations.
- There is a male predominance in younger patients while females are more likely to develop diverticulitis at an older age.
- The aetiology remains unknown but genetics, geographical location, ethnicity and lifestyle factors (smoking and obesity) play a role.
- There is a tenuous link between lack of dietary fibre and the development of diverticulosis; however, low-residue diets do not increase the likelihood of developing diverticulitis.
- Computed tomography is the gold standard for investigating diverticular disease. Follow-up colonoscopy may not be necessary if CT findings are consistent with diverticulitis and there is a low clinical concern for other pathologies (i.e. cancer).
- Antibiotics may not be necessary in the treatment of mild attacks.

- Complicated diverticular disease may be managed by a minimally invasive approach with percutaneous abscess drainage, laparoscopic washout or laparoscopic resection and primary anastomosis, with comparable results to open surgery (Hartmann's procedure).
- Elective sigmoid resection after two attacks of diverticulitis is unwarranted and the decision to undergo resection should be made on a case-by-case basis.

References

1. Parks TG. Post-mortem studies on the colon with special reference to diverticular disease. Proc R Soc Med 1968;61(9):932–4.

2. Painter NS, Burkitt D. Diverticular disease of the colon: a deficiency disease of the western civilisation. Br Med J 1971;2(5759):450–4.

3. Moynihan BG. An address on the pathology of the living: delivered before the Ashton-under-Lyne Division of the British Medical Association at the Opening of the Winter Session on October 18th, 1907. Br Med J 1907;2(2446):1381–5.

4. Spriggs EI, Marxer OA. An address on intestinal diverticula. Br Med J 1926;1(3395):130–4.

5. DeQuervain F. Diverticulitis and diverticulosis of the large intestine. Practioner 1927;18:352.

6. Welch CE, Allen AW, Donaldson GA. An appraisal of resection of the colon for diverticulitis of the sigmoid. Ann Surg 1953;138(3):332–43.

7. Horner JL. Natural history of diverticulosis of the colon. Am J Dig Dis 1958;3(5):343–50.

8. Hughes LE. Postmortem survey of diverticular disease of the colon: II. The muscular abnormality of the sigmoid colon. Gut 1969;10(5):344–51.

9. Kyle J, Adesola AO, Tinckler LF, et al. Incidence of diverticulitis. Scand J Gastroenterol 1967;2:77–80.

10. Guo-Zong P, Tong-Hua L, Min-Zhang C, et al. Diverticular disease of the colon in China: a 60-year retrospective study. Chin Med J 1984;97:391–4.

11. Kim EH. Hiatus hernia and diverticulum of the colon. N Engl J Med 1964;271:764–8.

12. Ogunbiyi OA. Diverticular disease of the colon in Idaban, Nigeria. Afr J Med Med Sci 1989;18:241–4.

13. Stemmerman GN, Yatani R. Diverticulosis and polyps of the large intestine. A necropsy study of Hawaii Japanese. Cancer 1973;31:1260–70.

14. Levy N, Luboshitzki R, Shiratzki Y, et al. Diverticulosis of the colon in Israel. Dis Colon Rectum 1977;20:477–81.

15. Levy N, Stermer E, Simon J. The changing epidemiology of diverticular disease in Israel. Dis Colon Rectum 1985;28:416–8.

16. Lee YS. Diverticular disease of the large bowel in Singapore. An autopsy survey. Dis Colon Rectum 1986;29:330–5.

17. Yap I, Hoe J. A radiological survey of diverticulosis in Singapore. Singapore Med J 1991;32:218–20.

18. Fong SS, Tan EY, Foo A, et al. The changing trend of diverticular disease in a developing nation. Colorectal Dis 2011;13(3):312–6.

19. Mimura T, Emanuel A, Kamm MA. Pathophysiology of diverticular disease. Best Pract Res Clin Gastroenterol 2002;16:563–76.

20. Guzzo J, Hyman N. Diverticulitis in young patients: is resection after a single attack always warranted? Dis Colon Rectum 2004;47:1187–90.

21. West SD, Robinson EK, Delu AN, et al. Diverticulitis in the younger patient. Am J Surg 2003;186:743–6.

22. Schweitzer J, Casillas RA, Collins JC. Acute diverticulitis in the young adult is not "virulent". Am Surg 2002;68(12):1044–7.

23. Masoomi H, Buchberg BS, Magno C, et al. Trends in diverticulitis management in the United States from 2002 to 2007. Arch Surg 2011;146(4):400–6.

24. Lahat A, Menachem Y, Avidan B, et al. Diverticulitis in the young patient – is it different? World J Gastroenterol 2006;12(18):2932–5.

25. Pautrat K, Bretagnol F, Huten N, et al. Acute diverticulitis in very young patients: a frequent surgical management. Dis Colon Rectum 2007;50:472–7.

26. Anderson DN, Driver CP, Davidson AI, et al. Diverticular disease in patients under 50 years of age. J R Coll Surg Edinb 1997;42:102–4.

27. Ritz JP, Lehmann KS, Stroux A, et al. Sigmoid diverticulitis in young patients: a more aggressive disease than in older patients? J Gastrointest Surg 2011;15:667–74.

28. Hjern F, Josephson T, Altman D, et al. Outcome of younger patients with acute diverticulitis. Br J Surg 2008;95:758–64.

29. Burkitt D, Painter NS. Effect of dietary fibre on stools and transit-times and its role in the causation of disease. Lancet 1979;2:1408–11.

30. Smith J, Humes DJ, Spiller RC. Should we treat uncomplicated symptomatic diverticular disease with fibre? Br Med J 2011;342:d2951. doi:10.1136/bmj.d2951.

31. Unlü C, Daniels L, Vrouenraets BC, et al. A systematic review of high-fibre dietary therapy in diverticular disease. Int J Colorectal Dis 2012;27(4):419–27.

32. Tarleton S, DiBaise JK. Low-residue diet in diverticular disease: putting an end to a myth. Nutr Clin Pract 2011;26(2):137–42.

33. Hosoi K, Alvarez WC, Mann FC. Intestinal absorption: a search for a low residue diet. Arch Intern Med 1928;41:112.

34. Strate LL, Liu YL, Syngal S, et al. Nut, corn, and popcorn consumption and the incidence of diverticular disease. JAMA 2008;300(8):907–14.

35. Almy TP, Howell DA. Medical progress: diverticular disease of the colon. N Engl J Med 1980;302(6):324–31.

36. Floch MH, Bina I. The natural history of diverticulitis: fact and theory. J Clin Gastroenterol 2004;38(Suppl. 5):S2–7.

37. Korzenik JR. Case closed? Diverticulitis: epidemiology and fiber. J Clin Gastroenterol 2006;40(Suppl. 3, 7):S112–6.

38. Laine L, Connors LG, Reicin A, et al. Serious lower gastrointestinal clinical events with non-selective NSAID or coxib use. Gastroenterology 2003;124(2):288–92.

39. Morris CR, Harvey IM, Stebbings WS, et al. Epidemiology of perforated colonic diverticular disease. Postgrad Med J 2002;78(925):654–8.

40. Morris CR, Harvey IM, Stebbings WS, et al. Do calcium channel blockers and antimuscarinics protect against perforated colonic diverticular disease? A case control study. Gut 2003;52(12):1734–7.

41. Lanas A, Sopena F. Nonsteroidal anti-inflammatory drugs and lower gastrointestinal complications. Gastroenterol Clin North Am 2009;38:333–52.

42. Whiteway J, Morson BC. Elastosis in diverticular disease of the sigmoid colon. Gut 1985;26(3):258–66.

43. Stumpf M, Cao W, Klinge U, et al. Increased distribution of collagen type III and reduced expression of matrix metalloproteinase 1 in patients with diverticular disease. Int J Colorectal Dis 2001;16:271–5.

44. Mimura T, Bateman AC, Lee RI, et al. Up-regulation of collagen and tissue inhibitors of matrix metalloproteinase in colonic diverticular disease. Dis Colon Rectum 2004;47:371–8.

45. Hughes LE. Postmortem survey of diverticular disease of the colon. I. Diverticulosis and diverticulitis. Gut 1969;10:336–44.

46. Yun AJ, Bazar KA, Lee PY. A new mechanism for diverticular diseases: aging-related vagal withdrawal. Med Hypotheses 2005;64:252–5.

47. Golder M, Burleigh DE, Belai A, et al. Smooth muscle cholinergic denervation hypersensitivity in diverticular disease. Lancet 2003;361:1945–51.

48. Jeyarajah S, Papagrigoriadis S. Review article: the pathogenesis of diverticular disease – current perspectives on motility and neurotransmitters. Aliment Pharmacol Ther 2011;33(7):789–800.

49. Huizinga JD, Waterfall WE, Stern HS. Abnormal response to cholinergic stimulation in the circular muscle layer of the human colon in diverticular disease. Scand J Gastroenterol 1999;34:683–8.

50. Strate LL, Liu YL, Aldoori WH, et al. Obesity increases the risks of diverticulitis and diverticular bleeding. Gastroenterology 2009;136(1):115–122.e1.

51. Hjern F, Wolk A, Håkansson N. Obesity, physical inactivity, and colonic diverticular disease requiring hospitalization in women: a prospective cohort study. Am J Gastroenterol 2012;107(2):296–302.

52. National Task Force on the Prevention and Treatment of Obesity. Overweight, obesity, and health risk. Arch Intern Med 2000;160(7):898–904.

53. Shoelson SE, Herrero L, Naaz A. Obesity, inflammation, and insulin resistance. Gastroenterology 2007;132:2169–80.

54. Turunen P, Wikström H, Carpelan-Holmström M, et al. Smoking increases the incidence of complicated diverticular disease of the sigmoid colon. Scand J Surg 2010;99(1):14–7.

55. Aldoori WH, Giovannucci EL, Rimm EB, et al. A prospective study of alcohol, smoking, caffeine and the risk of symptomatic diverticular disease in men. Ann Epidemiol 1995;5:221–8.

56. Aldoori WH, Giovannucci EL, Rockett HRH, et al. A prospective study of dietary fiber types and symptomatic diverticular disease in men. J Nutr 1998;128:714–9.

57. Strate LL, Liu YL, Huang ES, et al. Use of aspirin or nonsteroidal anti-inflammatory drugs increases risk for diverticulitis and diverticular bleeding. Gastroenterology 2011;140(5):1427–33.

58. Morris CR, Harvey IM, Stebbings WS, et al. Anti-inflammatory drugs, analgesics and the risk of perforated colonic diverticular disease. Br J Surg 2003;90:1267–72.

59. Goh H, Bourne R. Non-steroidal anti-inflammatory drugs and perforated diverticular disease: a case–control study. Ann R Coll Surg Engl 2002;84:93–6.

60. Nguyen GC, Sam J, Anand N. Epidemiological trends and geographic variation in hospital admissions for diverticulitis in the United States. World J Gastroenterol 2011;17(12):1600–5.

61. Lanza E, Jones DY, Block G, et al. Dietary fibre intake in the US population. Am J Clin Nutr 1987;46:790–7.

62. Ambrosetti P, Jenny A, Becker C, et al. Acute left colonic diverticulitis – compared performance of computed tomography and water-soluble contrast enema: prospective evaluation of 420 patients. Dis Colon Rectum 2000;43:1363–7.

63. Janes S, Meagher A, Frizelle FA. Elective surgery after acute diverticulitis. Br J Surg 2005;92:133–42.

64. Makela J, Kiviniemi H, Laitinen S. Prevalence of perforated sigmoid diverticulitis is increasing. Dis Colon Rectum 2002;45:955–61.

65. Morris CR, Harvey IM, Stebbings WS, et al. Incidence of perforated diverticulitis and risk factors for death in a UK population. Br J Surg 2008;95(7):876–81.

66. Humes DJ, Solaymani-Dodaran M, Fleming KM, et al. A population-based study of perforated diverticular disease incidence and associated mortality. Gastroenterology 2009;136(4):1198–205.

67. Piekarek K, Israelsson LA. Perforated colonic diverticular disease: the importance of NSAIDs, opioids, corticosteroids, and calcium channel blockers. Int J Colorectal Dis 2008;23(12):1193–7.

68. Hinchey EJ, Schaal PG, Richards GK. Treatment of perforated diverticular disease of the colon. Adv Surg 1978;12:85–109.

69. Köhler L, Sauerland S, Neugebauer E. Diagnosis and treatment of diverticular disease: results of a consensus development conference. The Scientific Committee of the European Association for Endoscopic Surgery. Surg Endosc 1999;13(4):430–6.

70. Wasvary H, Turfah F, Kadro O, et al. Same hospitalization resection for acute diverticulitis. Am Surg 1999;65(7):632–6.

71. Hansen O, Graupe F, Stock W. Prognostic factors in perforating diverticulitis of the large intestine. Chirurg 1998;69:443–9.

72. Makapugay LM, Dean PJ. Diverticular disease-associated chronic colitis. Am J Surg Pathol 1996;20(1):94–102.

73. Imperiali G, Meucci G, Alvisi C, et al. Segmental colitis associated with diverticula: a prospective study. Gruppo di Studio per le Malattie Infiammatorie Intestinali (GSMII). Am J Gastroenterol 2000;95(4):1014–6.

74. Imperiali G, Terpin MM, Meucci G, et al. Segmental colitis associated with diverticula: a 7-year follow-up study. Endoscopy 2006;38(6):610–2.

75. Freeman HJ. Natural history and long-term clinical behavior of segmental colitis associated with diverticulosis (SCAD syndrome). Dig Dis Sci 2008;53(9):2452–7.

76. Toorenvliet BR, Bakker RFR, Breslau PJ, et al. Colonic diverticulitis: a prospective analysis of diagnostic accuracy and clinical decision making. Colorectal Dis 2010;12:179–86.

77. Sarma D, Longo WE. Diagnostic imaging for diverticulitis. J Clin Gastroenterol 2008;42:1139–41.

78. Stoker J, van Randen A, Laméris W, et al. Imaging patients with acute abdominal pain. Radiology 2009;253:31–46.

79. Wilson SR, Toi A. The value of sonography in the diagnosis of acute diverticulitis of the colon. AJR Am J Roentgenol 1990;154:1199–202.

80. Lameris W, van Randen A, Bipat S, et al. Graded compression ultrasonography and computed tomography in acute colonic diverticulitis: meta-analysis of test accuracy. Eur Radiol 2008;18:2498–511.

81. Brenner DJ. Extrapolating radiation-induced cancer risks from low doses to very low doses. Health Phys 2009;97:505–9.

82. Westwood DA, Eglinton TW, Frizelle FA. Routine colonoscopy following acute uncomplicated diverticulitis. Br J Surg 2011;98(11):1630–4.
This was a retrospective longitudinal study of patients with an initial presentation of acute uncomplicated diverticulitis on the basis of CT criteria, at a single institution. Of 292 patients with acute diverticulitis, 205 underwent colonoscopy. The yield of advanced colonic neoplasia in this cohort was equivalent to, or less than, that detected on screening asymptomatic average-risk individuals. The authors conclude that in the absence of other indications, subsequent evaluation of the colon may not be required to confirm the diagnosis of diverticulitis.

83. Lau KC, Spilsbury K, Farooque Y, et al. Is colonoscopy still mandatory after a CT diagnosis of left-sided diverticulitis: can colorectal cancer be confidently excluded? Dis Colon Rectum 2011;54(10):1265–70.
This was a retrospective cohort study of 1088 patients with diverticultis on CT scanning. Colonoscopy was performed in 319 patients. The authors correlated CT findings with colorectal cancer diagnosis from the Western Australian Cancer Registry. They found a negative predictive value of diverticulitis diagnosed by CT for colorectal cancer of 97.9% (1065/1088) with a 95% confidence interval of 96.8–98.7%. Interestingly, in this study a significantly higher proportion of cancer cases were found in patients with abscess, local perforation or fistula.

84. Hale WB. Colonoscopy in the diagnosis and management of diverticular disease. J Clin Gastroenterol 2008;42:1142–4.

85. Schreyer AG, Furst A, Agha A, et al. Magnetic resonance imaging based colonography for diagnosis and assessment of diverticulosis and diverticulitis. Int J Colorectal Dis 2004;19:474–80.

86. Heverhagen JT, Sitter H, Zielke A, et al. Prospective evaluation of the value of magnetic resonance imaging in suspected acute sigmoid diverticulitis. Dis Colon Rectum 2008;51:1810–5.

87. Ravichandran S, Ahmed HU, Matanhelia SS, et al. Is there a role for magnetic resonance imaging in diagnosing colovesical fistulas? Urology 2008;72:832–7.

88. Rafferty J, Shellito P, Hyman NH, et al. Practice parameters for sigmoid diverticulitis. Standards Committee of American Society of Colon and Rectal Surgeons. Dis Colon Rectum 2006;49(7):939–44.
Practice parameters for sigmoid diverticulitis.

89. Maconi G, Barbara G, Bosetti C, et al. Treatment of diverticular disease of the colon and prevention of acute diverticulitis: a systematic review. Dis Colon Rectum 2011;54(10):1326–38.

90. Tursi A, Brandimarte G, Giorgetti GM, et al. Mesalazine and/or *Lactobacillus casei* in preventing recurrence of symptomatic uncomplicated diverticular disease of the colon: a prospective, randomized, open-label study. J Clin Gastroenterol 2006;40(4):312–6.

91. Tursi A, Joseph RE, Streck P. Expanding applications: the potential usage of 5-aminosalicylic acid in diverticular disease. Dig Dis Sci 2011;56(11):3112–21.

92. Rafferty J. Diverticulitis. American Society of Colon and Rectal Surgeons. Online. Available at http://www.fascrs.org/physicians/education/core_subjects/2005/diverticulitis; [accessed 28.06.12].
    See also Ref. 88. This is one of the most recent publications for the general management of diverticulitis; however, it is slightly outdated given more recent studies. The ASCRS recommend antibiotics (amoxicillin or ciprofloxacin/metronidazole) for the management of mild diverticulitis (Level III evidence, grade B).

93. Chabok A, Påhlman L, Hjern F, et al., for the AVOD Study Group. Randomized clinical trial of antibiotics in acute uncomplicated diverticulitis. Br J Surg 2012;99(4):532–9.
    This multicentre randomised trial involving 10 surgical departments in Sweden and one in Iceland recruited 623 patients with CT-verified acute uncomplicated left-sided diverticulitis. Patients were randomised to treatment with (314 patients) or without (309 patients) antibiotics for 7 days. Complications such as perforation or abscess formation were found in 1.9% who received no antibiotics and in 1.0% who were treated with antibiotics (P=0.3). The median hospital stay was 3 days in both groups. There was no difference in recurrent diverticulitis necessitating readmission to hospital at the 1-year follow-up.

94. Unlü C, de Korte N, Daniels L, et al., Dutch Diverticular Disease 3D Collaborative Study Group. A multicenter randomized clinical trial investigating the cost-effectiveness of treatment strategies with or without antibiotics for uncomplicated acute diverticulitis (DIABOLO trial). BMC Surg 2010;10:23.
    The results of the DIABOLO trial are awaited. This randomised trial aims to establish whether antibiotics are necessary in the primary treatment of acute mild diverticulitis. Inclusion criteria include patients admitted to hospital with left-sided diverticulitis diagnosed by CT or ultrasound. Treatment will comprise 48 hours of intravenous antibiotics (co-amoxiclav or ciprofloxacin/metronidazole). The primary end-point is time to full recovery at 6-month follow-up. Secondary end-points include: the proportion of patients who develop complicated diverticulitis; direct and indirect medical costs at 6 months; mortality; readmission rate within 6 months; and acute diverticulitis recurrence rates at 12 and 24 months follow-up.

95. Myers E, Winter DC. Adieu to Henri Hartmann? Colorectal Dis 2010;12(9):849–50.

96. Corman ML. Classic articles in colonic and rectal surgery. Henri Hartmann. Dis Colon Rectum 1984;27(4):273.

97. Eggers C. Diverticulitis and sigmoiditis. Ann Surg 1931;94(4):648–69.

98. Kronborg O. Treatment of perforated sigmoid diverticulitis: a prospective randomized trial. Br J Surg 1993;80(4):505–7.

99. Zeitoun G, Laurent A, Rouffet F, et al. Multicentre, randomized clinical trial of primary versus secondary sigmoid resection in generalized peritonitis complicating sigmoid diverticulitis. Br J Surg 2000;87(10):1366–74.

100. O'Sullivan GC, Murphy D, O'Brien MG, et al. Laparoscopic management of generalized peritonitis due to perforated colonic diverticula. Am J Surg 1996;171(4):432–4.

101. White SI, Frenkiel B, Martin PJ. A ten-year audit of perforated sigmoid diverticulitis: highlighting the outcomes of laparoscopic lavage. Dis Colon Rectum 2010;53(11):1537–41.

102. Taylor CJ, Layani L, Ghusn MA, et al. Perforated diverticulitis managed by laparoscopic lavage. Aust N Z J Surg 2006;76(11):962–5.

103. Myers E, Hurley M, O'Sullivan GC, et al. Laparoscopic peritoneal lavage for generalized peritonitis due to perforated diverticulitis. Br J Surg 2008;95(1):97–101.

104. Toorenvliet BR, Swank H, Schoones JW, et al. Laparoscopic peritoneal lavage for perforated colonic diverticulitis: a systematic review. Colorectal Dis 2010;12(9):862–7.

105. Constantinides VA, Tekkis PP, Athanasiou T, et al. Primary resection with anastomosis vs. Hartmann's procedure in nonelective surgery for acute colonic diverticulitis: a systematic review. Dis Colon Rectum 2006;49(7):966–81.

106. Salem L, Flum DR. Primary anastomosis or Hartmann's procedure for patients with diverticular peritonitis? A systematic review. Dis Colon Rectum 2004;47(11):1953–64.

107. Abbas S. Resection and primary anastomosis in acute complicated diverticulitis, a systematic review of the literature. Int J Colorectal Dis 2007;22(4):351–7.

108. Pessaux P, Muscari F, Ouellet JF, et al. Risk factors for mortality and morbidity after elective sigmoid resection for diverticulitis: prospective multicenter multivariate analysis of 582 patients. World J Surg 2004;28:92–6.

109. Killingback M, Barron PE, Dent OF. Elective surgery for diverticular disease: an audit of surgical pathology and treatment. Aust N Z J Surg 2004;74:530–6.

110. Oomen JL, Engel AF, Cuesta MA. Outcome of elective primary surgery for diverticular disease of the sigmoid colon: a risk analysis based on the POSSUM scoring system. Colorectal Dis 2006;8:91–7.

111. Parks TG. Natural history of diverticular disease of the colon. A review of 521 cases. Br Med J 1969;4:639–45.

112. Parks TG. Natural history of diverticular disease of the colon. Clin Gastroenterol 1975;4:3–21.

113. Manousos ON, Truelove SC, Lumsden K. Prevalence of colonic diverticulosis in general population of Oxford area. Br Med J 1967;3:762.

114. Sandler RS, Everhart JE, Donowitz M, et al. The burden of selected digestive diseases in the United States. Gastroenterology 2002;122:1500–11.

115. Chapman JR, Dozois EJ, Wolff BG, et al. Diverticulitis: a progressive disease? Do multiple recurrences predict less favourable outcomes? Ann Surg 2006;243:876–83.

116. Broderick-Villa G, Burchette RJ, Collins C, et al. Hospitalisation for acute diverticulitis does not mandate routine elective colectomy. Arch Surg 2005;140:576–81.

117. Salem TA, Molloy RG, O'Dwyer PJ. Prospective, five-year follow-up study of patients with symptomatic uncomplicated diverticular disease. Dis Colon Rectum 2007;50:1460–4.

118. Hart AR, Kennedy HJ, Stebbings WS, et al. How frequently do large bowel diverticula perforate? An incidence and cross-sectional study. Eur J Gastroenterol Hepatol 2000;12:661–5.

119. Makela J, Kiviniemi H, Laitinen S. Prevalence of perforated sigmoid diverticulitis is increasing. Dis Colon Rectum 2002;45:955–61.

120. Nylamo E. Diverticulitis of the colon: role of surgery in preventing complications. Ann Chir Gynaecol 1990;79:139–42.

121. Lorimer JW. Is prophylactic resection valid as an indication for elective surgery in diverticular disease? Can J Surg 1997;40:445–8.

122. Somasekar K, Foster ME, Haray PN. The natural history of diverticular disease: is there a role for elective colectomy? J R Coll Surg Edinb 2002;47:481–2.

123. Mueller MH, Glatzle J, Kasparek MS, et al. Long-term outcome of conservative treatment in patients with diverticulitis of the sigmoid colon. Eur J Gastroenterol Hepatol 2005;17:649–54.

124. Anaya DA, Flum DR. Risk of emergency colectomy and colostomy in patients with diverticular disease. Arch Surg 2005;140(7):681–5.

125. Levack MM, Savitt LR, Berger DL, et al. Sigmoidectomy syndrome? Patients' perspectives on the functional outcomes following surgery for diverticulitis. Dis Colon Rectum 2012;55(1):10–7.

126. Klarenbeek BR, Veenhof AA, Bergamaschi R, et al. Laparoscopic sigmoid resection for diverticulitis decreases major morbidity rates: a randomized control trial: short-term results of the Sigma Trial. Ann Surg 2009;249(1):39–44.

127. McGuire Jr HH, Haynes Jr BW. Massive hemorrhage for diverticulosis of the colon: guidelines for therapy based on bleeding patterns observed in fifty cases. Ann Surg 1972;175(6):847–55.

128. Meyers MA, Alonso DR, Baer JW. Pathogenesis of massively bleeding colonic diverticulosis: new observations. AJR Am J Roentgenol 1976;127(6):901–8.

129. Meyers MA, Alonso DR, Gray GF, et al. Pathogenesis of bleeding colonic diverticulosis. Gastroenterology 1976;71(4):577–83.

130. McGuire Jr. HH. Bleeding colonic diverticula. A reappraisal of natural history and management. Ann Surg 1994;220(5):653–6.

131. Khanna A, Ognibene SJ, Koniaris LG. Embolization as first-line therapy for diverticulosis-related massive lower gastrointestinal bleeding: evidence from a meta-analysis. J Gastrointest Surg 2005;9(3):343–52.

132. Millward SF. ACR appropriateness criteria on treatment of acute nonvariceal gastrointestinal tract bleeding. J Am Coll Radiol 2008;5(4):550–4.

133. Maleux G, Roeflaer F, Heye S, et al. Long-term outcome of transcatheter embolotherapy for acute lower gastrointestinal hemorrhage. Am J Gastroenterol 2009;104(8):2042–6.

134. Tan KK, Nallathamby V, Wong D, et al. Can superselective embolization be definitive for colonic diverticular hemorrhage? An institution's experience over 9 years. J Gastrointest Surg 2010;14(1):112–8.

9

Ulcerative colitis

Scott R. Kelley
Eric J. Dozois

Introduction

Ulcerative colitis (UC) is an idiopathic relapsing inflammatory bowel disease (IBD) involving the mucosa and lamina propria of the rectum and variable segments of the proximal colon. Characterised by remissions and exacerbations, the clinical spectrum of disease can range from inactive to fulminant. Medical management is generally effective in controlling ulcerative colitis, but ultimately 30–40% of patients will require surgical intervention. Criteria for the management of acute and chronic disease are well established, with surgery playing a fundamental role, as removal of the colon and rectum is essentially curative.

Epidemiology

Ulcerative colitis is an uncommon disease with varying incidence rates (0.5–$24.5/10^5$) and discernible differences are seen between different geographic and ethnic regions of the world.[1] Less common in Asia, Africa, South America and Southeastern Europe, UC has a varied incidence of between 2 and 15 cases per 100 000 persons per year in developed and industrialised western countries of North America, Northwestern Europe, and the UK. A significant trend of increasing incidence and prevalence rates has been reported in underdeveloped parts of the world as they become more industrialised, thus supporting the importance of environmental factors in the development of ulcerative colitis.

The onset of symptoms typically plateaus around the fourth decade of life, remaining fairly constant thereafter. A second peak of onset around the sixth to seventh decade has been described, though there is uncertainty as to whether this is truly a subsequent peak or merely difficulty in differentiating it from other colitides.[2]

Ulcerative colitis is seen with near equal frequency between males and females.[1] Caucasians and African Americans have a nearly equivalent incidence, while the Jewish populace experiences the highest documented rates. Hispanic, Native American, African, and Asian populations have the lowest incidence.[2]

Aetiopathogenesis

The pathogenesis of UC remains enigmatic, though multiple factors have been described as potential causative or protective agents in its occurrence and include: diet, alcohol and tobacco consumption, socioeconomic status, hygiene, urban living conditions, antibiotic usage, gut flora dysbiosis, probiotic use, non-steroidal anti-inflammatory agents, appendicectomy rates, breastfeeding, oral contraceptive use, stress, and familial and genetic causes.

Though a significant number of dietary factors have been evaluated as a causative agent for ulcerative colitis, no consensus has emerged.[2,3] A decreased risk has been associated with alcohol consumption, and the risk declined as daily alcohol consumption increased.[4]

Evidence demonstrates that smoking is protective against disease activity, and it has been shown that those who quit smoking are more likely to have a relapse. Ex-smokers are 70% more likely to develop ulcerative colitis when compared to those who have never smoked, though the causation remains unclear. Supplemental nicotine therapy has not consistently been shown to be more effective than placebo or conventional therapy (steroids/5-aminosalicylic acid), and has a significant side-effect profile.[2,3]

The hygiene hypothesis contends that cleaner living environments reduce the amount of organisms one is exposed to early in life, thus reducing the ability of the immune system to become tolerant, and subsequently causing an aberrant response when thus exposed.[5] Ulcerative colitis is more common among urban populations, indoor living, smaller families, and individuals of middle and upper socioeconomic status, who primarily reside in more sanitary surroundings.[6]

Antibiotic usage and the resulting gut flora dysbiosis are commonplace in developed countries, and hypothetically a potential cause of UC when taking into consideration that higher rates of utilisation are seen in industrialised and developed nations, though this is yet to be proven.[3] A correlation has been demonstrated in children with UC, who are more likely to have received antibiotics during their first year of life.[7]

A predisposition for UC has been reported to be as high as 29% in those with a positive family history, and between 10% and 20% of affected individuals have a first-degree relative with IBD. Twin studies have consistently shown a higher concordant disease rate in monozygotic compared to dizygotic pairs (approximately 50% versus nearly 0%), where the concordance among ordinary siblings was found to be around 5%.[8]

Clinical presentation

Colonic involvement at presentation can vary widely between different geographic regions, though proctosigmoiditis is the most common. In the USA 46% presented with proctosigmoiditis, 37% pancolitis and 17% with left-sided colitis.

Common symptoms associated with UC include urgency, diarrhoea, tenesmus and haematochezia. Constipation, a complaint in 15–20% of patients, is related to incomplete evacuation of the rectum.

Symptoms correlate with severity of disease, and increasing severity leads to worsening nausea, emesis, abdominal distension and weight loss. Protein-losing enteropathy may lead to loss of lean body mass and anaemia, and growth retardation in children. Haemodynamically significant haemorrhage is an uncommon complication, but is responsible for 10% of emergent colectomies. Severity can also have systemic manifestations, including tachycardia, pyrexia, leucocytosis, and increased fluid requirements, indicating toxicity.

Approximately 5–15% of patients with UC develop acute severe colitis, and up to 50% present initially with fulminant disease. Intense medical treatment has a high chance of inducing remission but when unsuccessful, emergent surgery will be necessary in up to 20% of patients. Perforation is a rare but serious occurrence with a mortality approaching 60%.

Extraintestinal manifestations

Upwards of 20% of patients with UC will develop extra-alimentary manifestations during the course of illness including, but not limited to, musculoskeletal (the most common), hepatopancreatobiliary, dermatological, thromboembolic and ophthalmological derangements.[9] Most extraintestinal manifestations present after an exacerbation of colonic inflammation, but they can also occur at the time of the acute flair. Colectomy is beneficial in inducing remission of peripheral arthropathy, erythema nodosum and iritis. Pyoderma gangrenosum does not universally respond, and axial arthropathy, primary sclerosing cholangitis, uveitis and episcleritis proceed independently of surgical intervention.

Musculoskeletal

Peripheral arthropathy asymmetrically involves numerous small and large joints (knees being the most common) affecting up to 20% of patients, with severity paralleling disease activity. The arthropathy is typically fleeting, rheumatoid factor negative (seronegative) and non-deforming. It disappears when medical treatment induces remission or after proctocolectomy, although it has been documented in patients with pouchitis after restorative proctocolectomy.[10]

Axial arthropathy (ankylosing spondylitis) involving the sacroiliac joints and one or more vertebrae occurs in up to 5% of patients. The majority of cases are HLA-B27 positive, unrelated to the activity of colitis and predominantly unresponsive to treatment. Asymptomatic sacroileitis is limited to the sacroiliac joint, HLA-B27 negative, largely unaffected by treatment and is radiographically detected in 24% of patients. Although both ankylosing spondylitis and asymptomatic sacroileitis have an overall poor response to treatment, anti-tumour necrosis factor (TNF)-α agents have recently shown promise.[10]

Hepatopancreatobiliary

Primary sclerosing cholangitis (PSC) is an idiopathic chronic and progressive disorder manifesting as stricturing, inflammation, and fibrosis of intra- and extrahepatic bile ducts. It is one of the most serious complications of UC. Patients with coexisting PSC and UC are at a markedly increased risk for colonic neoplasia (five times), necessitating close colonoscopic surveillance with extensive biopsy sampling. Around 5% of patients with UC will develop PSC, whereas upwards of 75% of patients with PSC are found to have concurrent UC.[11] The clinical course of PSC does not parallel underlying bowel disease and may present independently of colonic symptoms. An increased risk of development has been demonstrated in patients with human leucocyte antigen (HLA) B8, DR2, DR3 or DR6 haplotype positivity. Treatment of PSC with steroids, colectomy or antibiotics is ineffectual. Patients undergoing restorative proctocolectomy have a higher subsequent incidence of pouchitis and dysplasia in the ileal pouch mucosa.[12] Ultimately, the disease progresses to liver cirrhosis and eventual failure, which may prompt consideration for liver transplantation.

> ✅ The cumulative risk of pouchitis at 1, 2, 5 and 10 years after ileal pouch–anal anastomosis was 15.5%, 22.5%, 36% and 45.5% for the patients without PSC, and 22%, 43%, 61% and 79% for the patients with PSC.[12]

Cholangiocarcinoma is a rare association with UC, and PSC is the greatest risk factor for its development. The prognosis is dismal with a median survival of 9 months after diagnosis, and 12–15% of patients transplanted for PSC have cholangiocarcinoma.[13]

Dermatological

Erythema nodosum (EN) classically presents as tender, inflamed, red nodules mainly on the anterior surfaces of the lower extremities. The most common cutaneous lesion, it is seen in 10–20% of patients with UC. Exacerbations often parallel disease activity and frequently resolve after colonic disease subsides, although EN can precede bowel occurrence.[10]

Pyoderma gangrenosum (PG) occurs in 1–10% of patients with UC, and presents as plaques or pustules that break down and form painful ulcerations with undermined borders and necrotic centres. Legs are the most commonly affected area, though it can occur anywhere, including peristomally. Occurrences do not always parallel colonic disease activity.[10]

Thromboembolic

The incidence of deep venous thrombosis and pulmonary embolism in UC is threefold higher than the general population and associated with morbidity and mortality.[14] Though unproven, a hypercoagulable state in UC is hypothetically related to corticosteroid usage, activation of the coagulation cascade during a systemic inflammatory state, or up-regulation of acute phase reactants with flares.

Though rare, cerebral venous and dural sinus thrombosis can occur and results in a potentially devastating stroke. More commonly seen in patients with active disease, cases have been reported up to 10 years after a proctocolecotmy.

Ophthalmological

Manifestations of episcleritis, uveitis and scleritis can occur in up to 5% of patients. Ocular symptoms often present concurrently with peripheral arthritis and erythema nodosum. Episcleritis, the most common ophthalmopathy, presents with pain, burning and scleral injection. It usually occurs in parallel, as well as resolves with the treatment of colonic disease. Uveitis presents with pain, blurred vision, photophobia and headaches. Classically, the redness is most prominent centrally and dissipates radially. Uveitis does not typically coincide with flares, and prompt treatment is necessary to decrease the risk of visual impairment. Scleritis presents similarly to episcleritis, though is more severe and necessitates aggressive treatment in order to minimise retinal detachment and optic nerve impairment. In scleritis, unlike episcleritis, the sclera will appear pink or violet between the dilated surface vessels.[10]

Diagnosis and evaluation

With an extensive differential and no one exclusive pathognomonic test, a firm diagnosis of UC is dependent on several factors, including the clinical presentation, radiological work-up, endoscopic evaluation and histopathological determination of tissue biopsies. The differential diagnosis can include infectious (viral, bacterial, protozoal) as well as non-infectious causes (Crohn's disease, indeterminate colitis, collagenous colitis, ischaemic colitis, radiation colitis, diversion colitis, pharmacotherapy-induced colitis), and obtaining a detailed history and physical examination is imperative.

Microbiology

Colitides that can mimic UC include *Clostridium difficile*, *Escherichia coli* (serotype 0157:H7), *Salmonella*, *Shigella*, *Entamoeba* and *Campylobacter* infections. Stool studies for bacteria, ova and parasites should be obtained to confirm the true diagnosis and direct appropriate treatment. An increasing incidence of *Clostridium difficile* colitis in patients with IBD complicates their management and all patients with IBD hospitalised with an acute exacerbation should be assessed for synchronous infection.

Endoscopy

Endoscopy plays a pivotal role in the evaluation and diagnosis of UC, allowing for direct mucosal visualisation as well as providing an avenue for obtaining tissue biopsies. Other important indications include evaluating the proximal extent of colonic involvement, determining severity, differentiating from Crohn's disease, as well as monitoring responsiveness to medical management and surveillance.

During an acute attack, complete colonoscopy is generally avoided to decrease the risk of a potential perforation, while flexible or rigid proctoscopy is often utilised. Since inflammatory changes begin just above the anorectal junction and spread proximally, proctoscopy provides easy access to the lower rectum where biopsies can be obtained below the peritoneal reflection, minimising the risk of free perforation.

There is an overall lack of specific endoscopic features related to UC, though characteristic patterns of inflammation are appreciated. In the quiescent phase the mucosa will appear relatively normal, with the exception of neovascular changes. Oedema, erythema and an abnormal mucosal vascular pattern are endoscopically observed findings with mild inflammation. Loss of the vascular pattern (the submucosal vessels seen through the transparent mucosa) is a result of mucosal oedema, which makes it appear opaque. Oedema can also cause fine granularity in which there is a delicate regular stippled appearance of the mucosal surface. As the disease activity progresses to a moderate stage, superficial erosions, ulcerations and contact bleeding secondary to scope trauma are observed. Inflamed and regenerated mucosa surrounded by ulcerations lead to the development of pseudopolyps and a cobblestone appearance, which can also be appreciated during more severe conditions. Long-standing chronic inflammatory changes can give rise to a 'featureless microcolon' with mucosal atrophy, muscular hypertrophy, a decreased luminal diameter and loss of haustral folds.[15]

Histopathology

Inflammation in UC is confined to the rectum and colon. The mucosal columnar glandular epithelium extends into the anal canal to the level of the anal transitional zone. Segmental or skip areas do not occur, rather the inflammation in the colon and rectum is diffuse without intervening normal mucosa. The rectum is always involved, although the appearance of relative rectal sparing can occur in patients receiving transanally applied anti-inflammatory agents. A spared rectum not associated with local treatment should raise the suspicion of Crohn's disease. Backwash ileitis occurs only in cases with colonic extension to the ileocaecal junction.

Microscopic examination of a biopsy in early disease will demonstrate mucosal inflammation, goblet cell depletion, crypt of Lieberkuhn distortion, and vascular congestion. Mucin within goblet cells is expectorated, making them appear less evident or absent (goblet cell depletion). Branching of crypts may also be evident owing to regeneration following crypt epithelial damage. As severity progresses the lamina propria will exhibit infiltration by neutrophils, plasma cells, lymphocytes, eosinophils and mast cells. Neutrophils present within the epithelium of crypts (cryptitis) can aggregate in the crypt lumen, forming abscesses. Mucosal destruction, ulceration and subsequent atrophy are partly the result of rupturing of crypt abscesses. In advanced or late forms of UC, crypt destruction and loss occur as a result of damage to the crypt basal epithelium. Deeper submucosal or transmural inflammation with ulceration can also be observed, leaving large areas of exposed muscularis propria covered with granulation tissue giving the appearance of pseudopolyps. In the more chronic and quiescent phase a distorted architectural pattern with crypt distortion, branching and foreshortening can be identified.

Imaging

Although the reference standard for the diagnosis and follow-up of patients with UC is endoscopy, multiple traditional and emerging imaging modalities can also be utilised to assess patients with UC.

Conventional supine and upright abdominal X-rays are used to evaluate complications, including obstruction, dilatation or perforation. Dilatation of the transverse colon to greater than 6 cm is often seen in the face of toxic megacolon, and with imminent perforation is an indication for emergent surgical intervention.[16]

There has been a movement away from contrast roentography as endoscopic evaluation has become more commonplace. The earliest finding on double-contrast barium enema consists of a fine granular appearance in the rectosigmoid region as a result of mucosal oedema and hyperaemia. Advanced disease is characterised by the absence of haustral folds, narrowing and shortening of the colon, and diffuse ulceration. More chronic forms will present with colonic shortening, luminal narrowing, loss of haustral folds and widening of the presacral space.

In comparison to Crohn's disease, computed tomographic and magnetic resonance imaging studies for evaluating UC are less commonly obtained. Computed tomography (CT) is a relatively poor test for detecting the mucosal abnormalities of early disease, though more advanced UC often has a hallmark finding of diffuse colonic wall thickening. The benefit of CT lies in the ability to evaluate intraluminal and extraluminal disease, guide and monitor response to treatment, as well as detect complications.[16]

Colorectal cancer and surveillance

Prolonged duration, continuously active disease, severity of inflammation, PSC and diffuse involvement (pancolitis) are cumulative risk factors for the development of colorectal cancer in the setting of UC. Incidence rates for the development of cancer correspond to cumulative probabilities of 2% by 10 years, 8% by 20 years and 18% by 30 years.[17] As a general rule, beginning 10 years after the diagnosis of UC, the incidence of colorectal cancer increases by approximately 1% per year as long as the patient has their colon. The relative risk for cancer in relation to ulcerative proctitis has been estimated to be 1.7, left sided colitis 2.8 and pancolitis 14.8. In relation to the general population, there is an overall eightfold higher risk of colorectal cancer, with a 19-fold higher risk in patients with extensive colitis. It has been shown that roughly 17% of all deaths in UC are a result of colorectal cancer.

Dysplasia-associated lesion or mass (DALM) refers to a visibly raised dysplastic lesion within an area of inflammation, and confers a high risk of malignant potential. DALMs have been subdivided into adenoma-like (similar to sporadic adenomas) and non adenoma-like (sessile, irregular, ulcerated) lesions based solely on their endoscopic appearance. Some advocate treating adenoma-like DALMs with simple polypectomy and continued surveillance. The polyps must be discrete, completely removed and dysplasia must be absent elsewhere.[18] When dysplasia-associated lesions or masses are non-adenoma-like and cannot be entirely removed endoscopically, it is recommended to proceed with proctocolectomy because of the high probability of underlying neoplasia.

Flat low-grade dysplasia (LGD) detected during colonoscopic evaluation confers a reported ninefold increased risk of developing colorectal cancer and a 12-fold risk of developing an advanced lesion (high-grade dysplasia, or cancer).[19] Progression from colitis without dysplasia to colorectal cancer does not necessarily follow a sequence of low-grade dysplasia, high-grade dysplasia and ultimately carcinoma (inflammation–dysplasia–carcinoma sequence).

Rather, LGD can progress directly to colorectal cancer.[20] Low-grade dysplasia can present as unifocal or multifocal and treatment is to some extent controversial, with some advocating prophylactic colectomy, while others recommend intensive colonoscopic surveillance.[20] Flat low-grade dysplasia has been shown to be a strong predictor of progression to advanced neoplasia (53% at 5 years) in surveillance colonoscopy, and in patients who underwent a colectomy an unexpected advanced neoplasia (high-grade dysplasia or cancer) was found in nearly 24%.[21] Other studies have shown the presence of LGD is as likely as high-grade dysplasia (54% vs. 67%) to be associated with an already established cancer.[19] Repeated attempts to show low-grade dysplasia on endoscopic examinations should not be undertaken; rather, proctocolectomy is recommended to prevent progression to high-grade dysplasia or cancer.[22]

> ✓✓ A large meta-analysis of 20 surveillance studies showed the risk of developing cancer in patients with LGD is high. When LGD is detected on surveillance there is a ninefold risk of developing cancer and 12-fold risk of developing any advanced lesion.[19]

Flat high-grade dysplasia (HGD) has been shown to have a 42–45% rate of associated colorectal cancer at the time of colectomy, thus maintaining the recommendation that colectomy is mandatory in these patients, even if with incompletely resected HGD or with high-grade dysplasia found on random biopsies.[23]

Several studies have suggested that surveillance colonoscopy in patients with UC significantly reduces the risk of developing neoplasia. To date, no randomised controlled trials have documented a reduced risk of colorectal cancer development or death by utilising surveillance colonoscopy.[24] The American Gastroenterological Association and British Society of Gastroenterology share international guidelines recommending surveillance colonoscopy every 1–2 years starting 8–10 years after a diagnosis of pancolitis, or 15 years after left-sided colitis. Recommendations are also advocated for random non-targeted biopsies performed every 10 cm in all four quadrants, equating to 20–40 biopsies per colon. Colitis-associated cancers have been shown frequently to arise from flat mucosa, are multifocal, broadly infiltrating, anaplastic and

uniformly distributed throughout the colon. It is estimated that 33 non-targeted biopsies are required to detect dysplasia with 90% confidence, though studies show this is not often achieved.[25]

Patients with PSC and UC have an increased risk of colorectal cancer in comparison to those without PSC.[26] Cumulative colorectal cancer risk has been described as 33% at 20 years and 40% at 30 years after a diagnosis of UC. Surveillance colonoscopy is recommended at the time of diagnosis of PSC and yearly thereafter. In patients without a known diagnosis of UC, diagnostic colonoscopy with random biopsies is recommended to evaluate for subclinical evidence of disease.[23]

Flat and depressed colorectal lesions are often missed with conventional 'white light' colonoscopy and the utility of obtaining non-targeted random biopsies has been called into question.[27] Though highly specialised, time-consuming and not universally available, the use of high-magnification chromoscopic colonoscopy (dye spraying of the mucosal surface with indigo carmine or methylene blue) has been shown to have a significantly better correlation between endoscopic and histopathological findings than conventional colonoscopy, and also increased the number of neoplastic lesions identified. Chromoendoscopy (CE) has been repeatedly shown to increase the chance of detecting dysplasia compared to standard colonoscopic surveillance, allowing the endoscopist to take fewer, but rather higher yield, biopsies.[28]

Severity assessment

Disease severity is classified as mild, moderate or severe, and is based on the original descriptions provided by Truelove and Witts. Mild disease is characterised by less than four stools daily, with or without macroscopic blood, no signs of systemic toxicity (fever, tachycardia), mild to no anaemia, and a normal erythrocyte sedimentation rate (ESR). Severe disease results in six or more bloody bowel movements daily, signs of systemic toxicity, anaemia (less than 75% of normal value) and an increased ESR.

Unlike the Crohn's Disease Activity Index, no gold standard index exists for evaluating the severity of UC. Rather, multiple indices have been developed to measure disease severity and activity in clinical trials, many with overlapping measured variables. Some assess the clinical and biochemical aspects of disease (Truelove and Witts Severity Index, Lichtiger Index, Powel–Tuck Index, Activity

Index, Rachmilewitz Index, Physician Global Assessment, Ulcerative Colitis Clinical Score), others focus on endoscopy (Truelove and Witts Sigmoidoscopic Assessment, Baron Score, Powel–Tuck Sigmoidoscopic Assessment, Rachmilewitz Endoscopic Index), while further indices evaluate a combination of clinical and endoscopic criteria (Mayo Clinic Score, Sutherland Index). Common to all indices are numerical scoring systems. Scores at the elevated end of the spectrum indicate high disease activity, while lower scores signify milder or quiescent disease. Of the myriad scoring tools available to define disease activity, only two (Activity and Rachmilewitz Index) have been validated to date.[29]

Medical management

Inducing and maintaining clinical remission by promoting mucosal healing is the goal of medical treatment for UC. With several different medications to choose from (aminosalicylates, steroids, immunosuppresants, immunomodulators), therapy is modified in conjunction with the severity and extent of disease.

Clinical remission is characterised by symptom resolution of the inflammatory phase. This occurs with a decrease in diarrhoea, bleeding, urgency, tenesmus, the passage of mucopus and restoration of continence. Endoscopic remission will reveal regeneration of healthy mucosa, epithelial continuity, a return of a submucosal vascular pattern, and resolving ulceration, friability and granularity. Histological remission is achieved when an absence of neutrophils in the epithelial crypts is observed.

Just as there is no standard agreement amongst scoring systems measuring disease severity and activity, there are no universally validated means of defining disease remission. Prior to initiating maintenance therapy it is essential that clinical remission be achieved and verified. It has been demonstrated that high rates of relapse occur when endoscopic and histological remission has not been confirmed.[30]

✔✔ A prospective multicentre study revealed patients in clinical remission with less severe sigmoidoscopic scores (defined as normal-looking mucosa, with only mild redness and/or friability) after 6 weeks of acute treatment were less likely to relapse at 1 year than patients in clinical remission only (cumulative rate of relapse 23% vs. 80%, respectively; $P<0.0001$).[30]

Proctitis

Disease limited to the rectum is best treated with topical therapy, including foams, enemas and suppositories. Mesalamine suppositories (1–1.5 g/day) administered nightly, or in daily divided doses, have shown superiority in comparison to oral 5-aminosalicylic acid (5-ASA) compounds. Maximal response is noted within 4–6 weeks and, if unresponsive, combination therapy with topical corticosteroids has been shown to be more effective than either therapy alone. In patients unwilling to make use of, or failing to respond to, topical therapy, oral mesalamine may be given as an alternative, though higher doses are typically required. Systemic steroids are only administered in individuals refractory to topical and oral therapy, or in cases of severe disease.

Mild to moderate distal colitis

Mild to moderate distal colitis (30–40 cm) is primarily treated with a regimen of oral aminosalicylates, topical mesalamine or topical steroids. Mesalamine enemas are the treatment of choice and achieve higher rates of remission than oral 5-ASA compounds or topical steroids. Nightly administered mesalamine enemas (4 g/60 mL) have documented remission rates of between 60% and 70%, with rates increasing as the duration of therapy increases. If symptoms persist, and no response is seen within 2–4 weeks, an additional mesalamine or hydrocortisone enema can be administered each morning. Combination therapy has been shown to be superior to either therapy alone.[31] The systemic side-effects from corticosteroid enemas occur as a result of a low first-pass hepatic metabolism, and can be significant in some patients. Budesonide, a newer corticosteroid formulation that has a high first-pass hepatic metabolism, reduces the systemic side-effect profile, and has been shown to be as effective as conventional corticosteroid enemas. Oral mesalamine can be added in combination with topical therapy for patients showing a poor response, and is superior to oral or topical therapies alone. For patients not responding to or refusing topical therapy, oral mesalamine can be administered and has been shown to be a valuable alternative, though it is not as effective. Oral and intravenous corticosteroids are only administered in patients refractory to topical steroids and 5-ASA compounds (oral and topical), or in cases of severe disease.

Mild to moderate extensive colitis

Extensive colitis involves the colon beyond the reach of topical therapy and necessitates oral pharmacotherapy. Oral sulfasalazine (2–6 g/day) is the treatment of choice, showing remission rates of up to 80%, though with a significant systemic sulphonamide side-effect profile and high rates of intolerability (30–40%).[22] Newer non-sulphonamide 5-ASA formulations have been shown to be as effective as sulfasalazine, though better tolerated without dose-limiting systemic side-effects. Distal colonic and rectal disease topical therapy can also be concomitantly administered and this combination has been shown to be more successful in inducing remission at 8 weeks than oral therapy alone. Enteral steroids are implemented in cases not responding to oral mesalamine, or when the side-effects of the 5-ASA compounds cannot be tolerated. Prednisone is typically administered starting with doses of 40–60 mg/day until significant clinical improvement is observed. Once remission is achieved a taper of 5–10 mg/week is instituted until a daily dose of 20 mg is reached. A dose decrease of 2.5–5 mg/week is continued thereafter, while maintaining 5-ASA treatment, until completion.[22]

Thiopurines (6-mercaptopurine, azathioprine), with a primarily steroid-sparing benefit, are effective in patients who cannot be tapered off or tolerate corticosteroids. Their use is limited by a slow onset of action and prolonged duration is required to achieve optimal effectiveness (3–6 months).[22] Remicade (infliximab) has shown effectiveness in inducing remission in patients failing corticosteroid and/or thiopurine, as well as aminosalicylate therapy. Infliximab is intravenously administered over a 2-hour period at a dose of 5 mg/kg at weeks 0, 2 and 6, and then at 8-week intervals. Those who fail to respond after the initial two doses are unlikely to respond to a third dose. Shortening the interval between doses or increasing the dose to 10 mg/kg can treat those who eventually lose responsiveness after an initial response. For those not responding to an escalated dose and decreased interval, treatment discontinuation is recommended.[32]

☑☑ Two randomised, double-blind, placebo-controlled studies – the Active Ulcerative Colitis Trials 1 and 2 (ACT 1 and ACT 2, respectively) – showed patients with moderate-to-severe active ulcerative colitis treated with infliximab at weeks 0, 2 and 6 and every 8 weeks thereafter were more likely to have a clinical response at weeks 8, 30 and 54 than were those receiving placebo.[32]

Severe colitis

The mainstay of therapy for patients with severe/fulminant colitis is intravenous corticosteroids with a daily dose equivalent of 300 mg for hydrocortisone or 60 mg for methylprednisolone. Higher doses have not been proven to be beneficial, and 20–40% will fail to respond to therapy. Studies have been unable to confirm any incremental advantage in administering or continuing oral 5-ASA compounds and topical regimens. The utilisation of empiric broad-spectrum antibiotics, although routinely administered, has not shown benefit when treating patients with severe colitis. Intravenous ciclosporin (2–4 mg/kg/day continuous infusion) has been shown to be an effective adjuvant (82% response) in those lacking improvement while being treated with maximal medical therapy over a period of 3–5 days. Infliximab has shown short-term efficacy in limited small trials, with approximately half of treated patients requiring a colectomy at 5 years. Patients failing to respond to maximal medical therapy or showing signs of deterioration are candidates for surgery.[22] Though published data are somewhat conflicting, several studies have shown that higher rates of anastomotic and infectious complications are seen in patients following ileal pouch–anal anastomosis when infliximab has been given within an 8-week period prior to surgery. Given these findings, a discussion with a surgeon to review surgical options is prudent before beginning infliximab therapy.[33]

Surgical management

Surgery plays a pivotal role in the management of UC. Removal of the colon and rectum is essentially curative. Indications for removal include medical intolerability or unresponsiveness, intractability, life-threatening complications (perforation, bleeding, toxicity), dysplasia or malignancy, growth impediment in children, and for the attempted improvement of some extraintestinal manifestations refractory to medical treatment (pyoderma gangrenosum, erythema nodosum, peripheral arthritis, uveitis, iritis). The surgical approach depends on the presentation (emergent/urgent, elective) and can include: total abdominal colectomy with Brooke ileostomy, proctocolectomy with Brooke ileostomy, proctocolectomy with continent ileostomy, total abdominal colectomy with ileorectal anastomosis (IRA), and proctocolectomy with ileoanal reservoir/ileal pouch–anal anastomosis (IPAA). It is essential, when possible, to inform the patient, and have them site marked preoperatively by an enterostomal therapist.

Emergent/urgent

Toxic fulminant colitis, toxic megacolon, haemorrhage and perforation are life-threatening complications necessitating emergency colectomy. Urgent typically refers to hospitalised patients who are failing maximal medical therapy.

Historically, the Turnbull 'blow-hole' procedure was used in severely debilitated (septic, malnourished) patients with megacolon who could not withstand a major abdominal operation. A loop ileostomy, a transverse colostomy and, if needed, a sigmoid colostomy was created (**Fig. 9.1**). This allowed for faecal diversion, minimal handling of the bowel and patient convalesce for future colectomy, but did not eliminate the colitis nor the physiological impact of the inflammation on the patient. In rare circumstances (advanced pregnancy and toxic megacolon) the Turnbull approach could even now be considered.[34] Even so, recent experience in pregnant patients with fulminant disease suggests that total abdominal colectomy and Brooke ileostomy eliminates the systemic inflammatory consequences and can be done with low rates of maternal and foetal morbidity and mortality.[35]

> ✔ Subtotal colectomy and Brooke ileostomy for ulcerative colitis during pregnancy is safe. A multidisciplinary team that includes a gastroenterologist, high-risk obstetrician and experienced surgeon is necessary for an optimal outcome.[35]

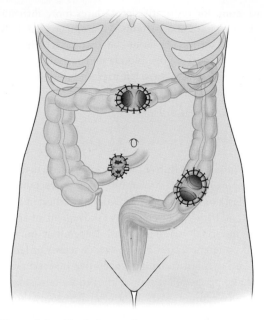

Figure 9.1 • Turnbull procedure.

For patients requiring urgent or emergent intervention, total abdominal colectomy with creation of a Brooke ileostomy and preservation of the rectum for a potential future restorative procedure is most commonly performed and recommended. It eliminates most of the disease and allows for restoration of health, as well as tapering of immunosuppressant medications.[36] When performing a total abdominal colectomy it is imperative to dissect as close to the ileocaecal valve as possible, thus preserving all of the ileocolonic branches for a possible restorative procedure. Deferring the proctectomy will simplify a restorative procedure by maintaining pelvic and presacral tissue planes. This not only reduces the potential complications (bleeding, infection, autonomic nerve damage) in an acutely ill patient, but also permits the opportunity pathologically to exclude Crohn's disease by examining the colonic specimen. Studies evaluating the outcome of a retained rectal stump have been conflicting. Some portend that leaving a diseased, thickened rectal stump is not associated with increased rates of postoperative pelvic sepsis or complications.[37] Others encourage exteriorisation (mucous fistula or subcutaneous placement) of long stumps, having found rates of pelvic sepsis as high as 12%, increased disease activity in the retained rectum and subsequent pelvic dissection for restorative procedures more difficult with a retained short stump.[38] If a mucous fistula is not done, the rectum should be irrigated with a rigid proctoscope to remove bloody mucous and a transanally placed rectal tube left in place for 48 hours to decrease pressure on the closed rectal stump.

Elective

Indications for elective surgery consist of medical unresponsiveness, intolerability or intractability, dysplasia or malignancy, growth retardation in children, and for the attempted improvement of some extraintestinal manifestations. Depending on patient preference, continence, age, concerns of fertility and dysplastic changes, operative inverventions include proctocolectomy with Brooke ileostomy, proctocolectomy with continent ileostomy, total abdominal colectomy with ileorectal anastamosis (IRA), and a restorative proctocolectomy with ileoanal reservoir/ileal pouch–anal anastamosis (IPAA).

Proctocolectomy with end ileostomy

A proctocolectomy with end Brooke ileostomy removes all disease and has a low rate of complications but leaves the patient with an incontinent stoma. Indications for this approach are patient preference, rectal cancer requiring pelvic radiation and poor sphincter function.

The patient is placed in stirrups in a modified lithotomy position. The colectomy portion of the procedure is carried out in a non-oncological approach unless neoplastic transformation has been identified. The rectal dissection and mobilisation may be done close to the perimuscular rectal wall in an attempt to minimise damage to the pelvic autonomic nerves. In the event of neoplastic changes both the colonic and rectal dissections are carried out in a standard oncological fashion. In the low anorectal region a perineal intersphincteric dissection is carried out, preserving the external sphincter and levator ani muscles, which significantly improves wound healing. The perineum is closed in layers and the greater omentum, if present, is mobilised and placed in the pelvis to prevent future bowel obstructions. After closure of the abdomen the ileostomy is matured in a standard evaginated Brooke fashion, with an attempted ideal projection of 2.5 cm (**Fig. 9.2**).

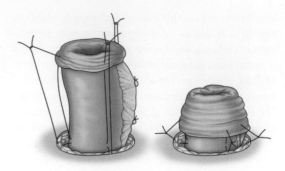

Figure 9.2 • Brooke ileostomy.

Stoma complications including retraction, peristomal skin excoriation, stenosis, prolapse and herniation can occur, with up to 30% of patients requiring operative revision. When delayed healing of the perineal wound occurs, evaluation for Crohn's disease and/or retained mucosa or foreign material (suture) should be carried out.

Proctocolectomy with continent ileostomy

Initially described by Nils Kock, the continent ileostomy still remains a viable alternative for motivated patients who are not candidates for an IPAA. Modifications and revisions to the original Kock continent ileostomy have been described and include the Barnett continent ileostomy reservoir (BCIR) and T-pouch, neither of which has supporting data to suggest they are better than the Kock pouch. Contraindications to construction of a continent ileostomy include Crohn's, obesity, marginal small bowel length, and anyone with a psychological or physical disability that would preclude understanding or being able to perform daily stomal intubation.

Surgical creation of a continent ileostomy is carried out by utilising 45–60 cm of terminal ileum and folding it into either a two-limb or S-pouch configuration. The pouch reservoir requires approximately 30 cm of ileum to construct, while a portion of the remaining distal outflow tract is intussuscepted to create a valve. As the pouch distends it causes an increase in pressure around the valve, thus occluding the outflow tract, preventing evacuation. The end of the ileum is brought out through the abdominal wall and matured flush with the skin. A wide-bore catheter is used to intubate the pouch by inserting it through the skin level stoma, which is placed to gravity drainage for approximately 10 days.

The pouch is slowly distended over time by intermittently clamping the catheter. When the catheter can be clamped for 8 hours without discomfort it is removed and intermittent intubation is carried out three to four times per day.

Postoperative pouch complications requiring reoperation are common and include skin-level or valve strictures, volvulus, herniation, fistulisation and valve slippage. Subluxation of the nipple valve is suggested by the onset of incontinence of the stoma and difficulty in inserting the catheter. Valve slippage is the most common complication, with reported rates of nearly 30%. Contrast studies may show partial or complete prolapse of the valve. Fistulas occur in approximately 10% of patients and typically originate from the base of the nipple valve or the pouch itself.[39,40] Despite the high morbidity and need for reoperative intervention with a continent ileostomy, patient satisfaction and quality of life are extremely high. It has been documented that over 90% would undergo the procedure again, as well as recommend it to friends and family.[41]

Ileorectal anastomosis

Colectomy with ileorectal anastomosis (IRA) should be considered only when the rectum is minimally inflamed, distensible and compliant, there is no rectal dysplasia, the patient has an intact sphincter mechanism and is willing to adhere to strict follow-up. Ileoproctostomy is an appealing alternative in younger patients of reproductive age in order to decrease the risk of impotence and reduced fecundity, as well as older patients with quiescent disease having colectomy for colonic dysplasia. Strict rectal surveillance must be adhered to due to the increased risk of future neoplastic changes. The risk of rectal carcinoma can reach up to 20% by 30 years.[42] Proctitis of the retained rectum can lead to bleeding, tenesmus, urgency, severe diarrhoea and pain. Topical, oral and systemic therapies can be utilised, but it has been documented that up to 45% of patients will not respond and eventually require a proctectomy.[43] In patients who require a completion proctectomy an end ileostomy, restorative IPAA or continent ileostomy are all options.

Restorative proctocolectomy/ileal pouch–anal anastomosis (IPAA)

Initially described in 1978 by Parks and Nicholls as an ileoanal ileal reservoir procedure, the restorative proctocolectomy has become the most common continence-preserving procedure performed for the management of UC in patients who are appropriate candidates. The restorative pouch can be fashioned in two-limb (J), three-limb (S), four-limb (W) or isoperistaltic (H) configurations (**Fig. 9.3**). The J-pouch, due to its ease of construction and excellent functional outcomes, has become the most common choice for most surgeons. The S-pouch provides additional length and can reduce anastomotic tension, though the 5-cm efferent limb of ileum projecting beyond the pouch can lead to evacuation difficulties and outlet obstruction. The isoperistaltic H-pouch, with its long outlet tract, can give rise to stasis, distension and pouchitis. The W-pouch has been shown to have similar functional results when compared to the J-pouch, but it is more time-consuming and technically difficult to construct.

The patient is placed in a modified lithotomy position to allow access to the anus and abdominopelvic cavity. A total colectomy is perfomed and the ileum is transected flush with the caecum (**Fig. 9.4**). In order to

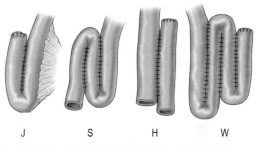
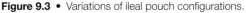

J   S   H   W

Figure 9.3 • Variations of ileal pouch configurations.

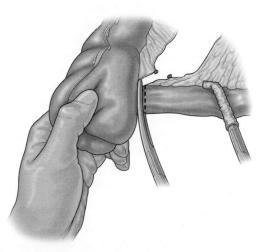

Figure 9.4 • Ileal transection adjacent to caecum.

provide adequate perfusion to the pouch it is imperative to preserve the ileal branches of the ileocolic and distal mesenteric arteries. At this point in the operation, if there is any doubt of the diagnosis, the colon should be removed and inspected with the pathologist. Once confident of the diagnosis of UC, evaluation for adequacy of reach of the small bowel to the deep pelvis should be undertaken. The proposed point of the pouch–anal anastomosis can be pulled down to the pubis, and if this point can be pulled 3–4 cm below the inferior edge of the pubis one can feel confident of successful reach for anastomosis. Strategies to decrease tension at the anastomosis include: complete mobilisation of the small-bowel mesentery to the root of the superior mesenteric artery cephalad to the head of the pancreas (**Fig. 9.5a**), proximal division of the ileocolic artery (**Fig. 9.5b**) and relaxing incisions of the mesentery over tension points along the superior mesenteric artery (**Fig. 9.5c**). Rectal dissection can be done in the total mesorectal excision (TME) plane or close to the rectal wall, depending on the concern for autonomic nerve damage and surgeon's experience with nerve-sparing proctectomy. Transection of the rectum should occur 2–3 cm above the dentate line in the anal transition zone, leaving a short rectal cuff (**Fig. 9.6**). After reach has been verified, a J configuration is fashioned, with each limb measuring between 12 and 15 cm in length. The limbs are paired in an antimesenteric fashion and are held in position with interrupted stay sutures (**Fig. 9.7**).

Double-stapled technique

For a stapled technique an enterotomy is made in the antimesenteric portion of the apex of the pouch and a linear cutting stapler is used to divide the walls of the two limbs, creating a common channel (**Fig. 9.8**). A purse-string suture is then fashioned around the enterotomy and the anvil from a circular stapler is placed inside the pouch, where it is held in place by tightening the purse-string (**Fig. 9.9**). The circular stapler is then placed transanally (**Fig. 9.10**). After appropriate orientation, the trocar is advanced either above or below the transverse staple line and attached to the anvil. The stapler is then closed, approximating the pouch and anus (**Fig. 9.11**).

Hand-sewn technique

For a hand-sewn pouch–anal anastomosis, an anal canal mucosectomy is performed, starting at the dentate line (**Fig. 9.12**). Raising the mucosa with a submucosal injection of dilute saline and epinephrine (1:200 000) facilitates the dissection of the mucosa away from the internal sphincter muscle (**Fig. 9.13a, b**). After the circumferential mucosa and proximal rectum have been removed, the pouch is gently brought down to the level of the dentate line. An enterotomy is made in the apex of the pouch, if not already created, and it is anchored in position by placing a suture in each of the four quadrants incorporating a full-thickness bite of the pouch, internal sphincter muscle and mucosa. Sutures are placed between the anchoring stitches, in a clockface orientation, to complete a mucosally intact anastomosis (**Fig. 9.14**). An air insufflation leak test is performed and a protective loop ileostomy fashioned (**Fig. 9.15**). The operation can be carried out without the creation of a diverting loop ileostomy in highly selected cases, with good results. However, in a meta-analysis of nearly 1500 patients the rate of anastomotic leakage was significantly higher in patients not given a defunctioning ileostomy.[44]

✔✔ A review of 17 studies comprising 1486 patients revealed restorative proctocolectomy without a diverting ileostomy resulted in functional outcomes similar to those of surgery with proximal diversion, but was associated with an increased risk of anastomotic leak. Diverting ileostomy should be omitted in carefully selected patients only.[44]

Outcomes in stapled versus hand-sewn anastomosis

Variations exist for the creation of a J-pouch, depending on the technique (hand-sewn versus double-stapled) chosen. A large meta-analysis demonstrated no significant differences between the two techniques. Nocturnal seepage and pad usage favoured the stapled anastomosis, in comparison to persisting symptoms due to inflammation or dysplasia in the cuff favouring the hand-sewn technique.[45] A single institution experience of over 3000 pouch procedures

---

✔✔ A large meta-analysis demonstrated no significant differences in postoperative complications between a mucosectomy and hand-sewn versus stapled anastomosis. Nocturnal seepage and pad usage favoured the stapled anastomosis, in comparison to persisting symptoms due to inflammation or dysplasia in the cuff favouring the hand-sewn technique.[45]

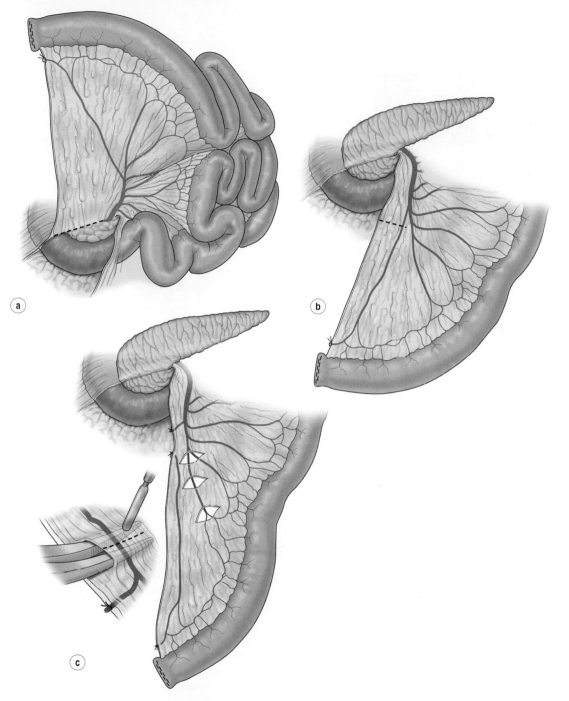

Figure 9.5 • **(a)** Mobilisation of the ileal mesentery around the duodenum. **(b)** Proximal division of the ileocolic artery. **(c)** Relaxing mesenteric incisions over the terminal portion of the superior mesenteric artery.

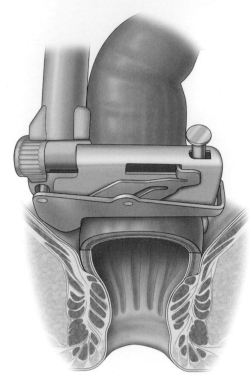

Figure 9.6 • Division of the rectum with stapler.

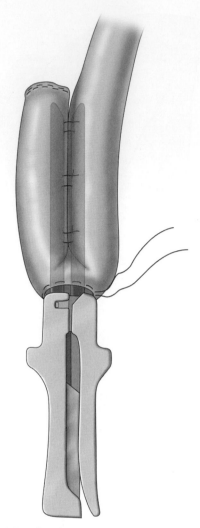

Figure 9.8 • Creation of reservoir with linear stapler.

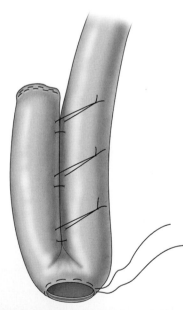

Figure 9.7 • J-pouch with orientation sutures.

(474 hand-sewn and 2635 stapled) revealed patients who underwent a stapled IPAA experienced better outcomes (incontinence, seepage, pad usage) and quality of life (dietary, social and work restrictions) in comparison to the hand-sewn group.[46]

Neoplastic changes observed in the retained anal transition zone in patients undergoing double-stapled technique are rare. The majority of reports have been associated with pathological findings of dysplasia or cancer in the initial operative specimen. A hand-sewn technique, including a completion mucosectomy, nearly eliminates the possibility of leaving columnar rectal mucosa behind, though not completely. Studies have been able to demonstrate 14–21% of excised pouches harbouring residual rectal mucosa.[47,48] A double-stapled technique, on the other hand, results in the retention of a small cuff of columnar mucosa. This can result in a 'cuffitis' or 'strip proctitis', and has been reported to occur in nearly 15% of stapled anastomoses, which can potentially progress to dysplasia.[49] Studies have

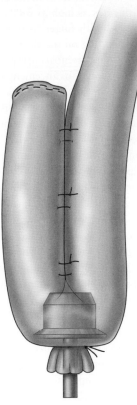

Figure 9.9 • Stapler anvil secured in J-pouch with purse-string suture.

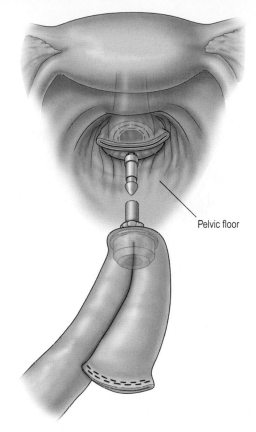

Figure 9.10 • Stapler placed transanally with spike posterior to transverse staple line.

Pelvic floor

demonstrated a 2.7–3.1% risk of developing low-grade dysplasia in the retained mucosa, although associated with a pre- or postoperative pathological diagnosis of concurrent dysplasia or cancer. In such patients a stapled technique may be less advisable and these authors recommend a mucosectomy and hand-sewn IPAA. For persistent or recurrent low-grade dysplasia, a completion mucosectomy, perineal pouch advancement and neo-ileal pouch–anal anastomosis is recommended.[50] Though studies recommending adequate pouch examination after an IPAA are lacking, long-term surveillance utilising annual endoscopy and biopsies is often recommended to monitor for dysplasia, although this is hard to achieve in practice.

Complications following pouch surgery

Major complications following pouch surgery include small-bowel obstruction, anastomotic stricture, pouch–vaginal fistula, pouchitis and pelvic sepsis. In several series, morbidity after IPAA is a significant problem, with documented rates of over 60%.[51]

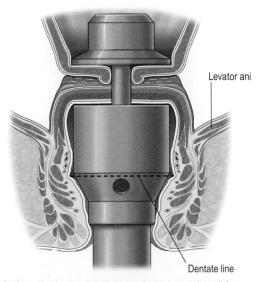

Levator ani

Dentate line

Figure 9.11 • Approximation of stapler and anvil for double-stapled anastomosis.

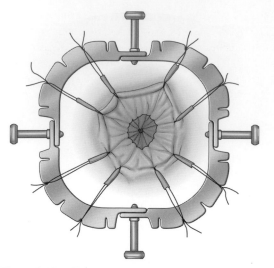

Figure 9.12 • Exposure for transanal mucosectomy using Lone Star retractor.

Small-bowel obstruction has been reported to occur in over 30% of patients, can present before or after loop ileostomy closure, and increases up to 10 years after operation. The cumulative risk has been shown to be 18% at 1 year, 27% at 5 years and 31% at 10 years. Adhesions are the most common cause of a small-bowel obstruction and surgical intervention is necessary in roughly 10% of patients by 10 years.[51,52]

Anastomotic strictures can cause pouch outlet obstruction with incomplete pouch evacuation and,

depending on how stricturing is defined, have been documented with rates as high as 38%. Stricturing can often be treated with finger or sequential dilator dilatation, depending on the degree of stenosis. If excessive fibrosis and stenosis are present, stricture excision and pouch advancement or removal may be necessary.[53]

Pouch–vaginal fistula is uncommon but is a devastating complication when it occurs. Obtaining a pouchogram prior to ileostomy closure, as well as a thorough vaginal and anal canal examination at the time of closure, can help exclude a fistula. Management depends on the level of the fistula (low versus high) and severity. Management includes placement of a seton, diversion, pharmacotherapy and transabdominal and perineal procedures.[54] A transanal or transvaginal approach for repairing low-lying fistulas has shown success in 50–70% of patients, though often requiring repeat procedures. Healing rates for higher fistulas after abdominal advancement of the pouch also show 50–70% documented success.[55] The presence of perianal abscess or fistula-in-ano preoperatively is associated with a 3.7- to 6-fold increase in the risk of developing pouch–vaginal fistula.[56]

The most common complication after IPAA is pouchitis, a non-specific inflammation of the pouch, which approaches 50% within 10 years. Symptoms include increased stool frequency, abdominal cramping, bleeding, urgency, tenesmus, incontinence

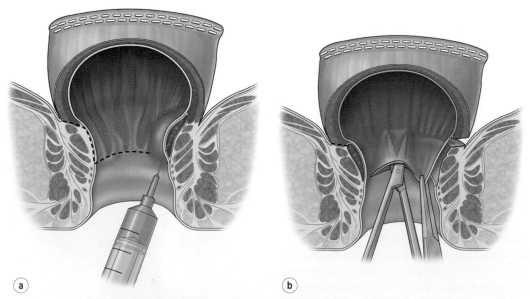

Figure 9.13 • (a) Submucosal injection. (b) Transanal mucosectomy.

and fevers. Diagnosis should be based on endoscopic and histological factors, rather than clinical symptoms alone. Hypothetically, pouchitis results from the overgrowth of anaerobic bacteria, local factors or ischaemia, though the exact aetiology is unknown. Extraintestinal manifestations, specifically primary sclerosing cholangitis, and high serological levels of perinuclear antineutrophil cytoplasmic antibody (p-ANCA) have been shown to correlate with higher levels of pouchitis and chronic pouchitis.[57,58] Smoking, on the other hand, has been shown to decrease rates of pouchitis and probiotics (VSL#3) have shown promise in reducing episodes of acute pouchitis as well as maintaining remission.[59,60] Treatment depends primarily on the administration of antibiotics (metronidazole and ciprofloxacin), with response rates documented in over 80% of patients, though topical steroid or 5-aminosalicylate therapy is occasionally required.[61] Recurrent and refractory pouchitis is difficult to manage. Diversion with a loop ileostomy does not always affect the degree of inflammation and excision with construction of a new reservoir can be followed by recurrent pouchitis. Crohn's disease should always be suspected in patients with chronic pouchitis. Pouch excision is rarely necessary.

Pelvic sepsis has been documented to occur in as many as 20% of patients, and has the most clinically significant implications. Sepsis occurring in the early postoperative period confers a fivefold increased risk of subsequent failure, necessitating aggressive treatment with major or minor procedures in order to attempt to preserve the pouch. Pelvic sepsis can often be managed with CT-guided percutaneous drainage, but extreme cases will require operative intervention. Pouch failure and loss can occur immediately or several years following septic complication, with estimated cumulative 3-, 5- and 10-year failure rates of 20%, 31% and 39%, respectively.[62] If pouch salvage occurs in the setting of pelvic sepsis, pelvic fibrosis leads to compromised function of the pouch.

> ✓✓ The frequencies of permanent defunctioning and excision of a pouch in 131 patients with septic complications were 24% and 6%, respectively. The 5-year pouch failure rate increased in a subgroup of patients with septic complications at the pouch–anal anastomosis when the anal sphincter was involved (50% vs. 29%). Surgery for septic complications is required in a high percentage of patients and repeated attempts are justified in order to decrease the risk of pouch loss.[62]

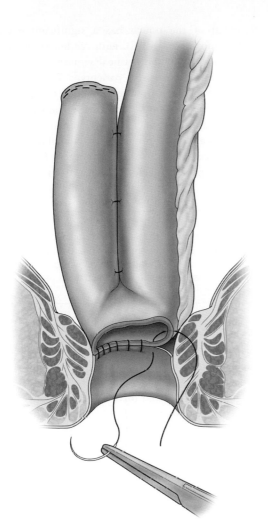

Figure 9.14 • Hand-sewn pouch–anal anastomosis.

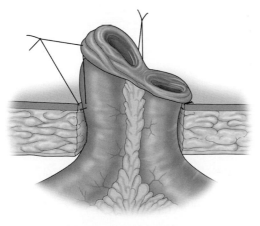

Figure 9.15 • Diverting loop ileostomy.

Female patients of reproductive age who undergo a proctocolectomy and creation of an IPAA have decreased postoperative fecundity, with reduced rates documented upwards of 50%.[63–66]

Studies have demonstrated no difference in fertility after a diagnosis of UC compared with before a diagnosis, but higher infertility rates (38%) in females who had pelvic pouch surgery in comparison to patients managed non-operatively (13%).[67] The decreased fertility is hypothetically related to tubal occlusion secondary to adhesions and a large percentage (67%) of patients have demonstrated abnormal hysterosalpingography when evaluated postoperatively.[68] The ability to carry a foetus to term and successfully deliver vaginally has not been shown to be affected by an ileal pouch–anal anastomosis. Pregnancy has also not been shown to decrease pouch function or increase complications when followed long term.[66,69] Men report statistically improved sexual quality and function in relation to sexual desire, intercourse satisfaction, erectile function and overall satisfaction after IPAA when compared with prior to surgery.[70]

✔✔ A meta-analysis of eight studies revealed that an IPAA can increase the risk of infertility, defined as achieving pregnancy within 12 months of attempting conception, in women with ulcerative colitis by approximately threefold. Counselling female patients regarding decreased rates of fecundity following an IPAA is imperative.[65]

Risk factors found to be independent predictors of pouch survival include: patient diagnosis, prior anal pathology, abnormal anal manometry, patient comorbidity, pouch–perineal or pouch–vaginal fistulas, pelvic sepsis, anastomotic stricture and separation.[56] Pouch failure, defined as pouch excision or permanent diversion, is reported in several large series to range from 7% to 10% at 10 years and in one study 8% at 20 years.[52,69,71]

Removal of the pouch has a significant early and late morbidity (62%), with readmissions and delayed healing of the perineal wound (persistent perineal sinus) in 40% of patients.[72] Thus, where failure is threatened by sepsis or poor function, it may be in the patient's interest to consider a salvage procedure that may be less traumatic and offers a chance of retaining satisfactory anal function. Recent success rates for salvage surgery following restorative proctocolectomy range from 75% to 94%.[73–75]

✔ The most common indications for pouch salvage are intra-abdominal sepsis, anastomotic stricture and retained rectal stump.[74] Surgical revision using a transanal or combined abdominoperineal approach has documented success rates of 74–94%.[73–75]

Functional outcomes

The frequency of bowel movements after an ileoanal–pouch anastomosis averages six in 24 hours, with minor incontinence of 11% during the day and 21% at night when followed for 20 years.[76] Nearly half will experience nocturnal leakage and minor spotting during the first 6 months, which improves over time with rates of 20% noted at 1 year.[77] Studies comparing quality of life before and after an IPAA procedure document greater freedom in role function, improved body image and reduced negative effects caused by colitis or life with an ileostomy. Over 90% of patients report overall satisfaction with good or excellent adjustment following IPAA. The long-term functional and clinical outcomes of a restorative proctocolectomy are excellent, and patient satisfaction and quality of life are extremely high.[78,79]

Key points

- Ulcerative colitis is an idiopathic relapsing inflammatory bowel disease involving the mucosa and lamina propria of the rectum and variable segments of the proximal colon.
- The incidence is between 2 and 15 cases per 100000 persons per year in more developed countries.
- The diagnosis is dependent on several factors, including the clinical presentation, radiological work-up, endoscopic evaluation and histopathological determination of tissue biopsies.
- Incidence rates for the development of cancer correspond to cumulative probabilities of 2% by 10 years, 8% by 20 years and 18% by 30 years.

- Toxic fulminant colitis, toxic megacolon, haemorrhage and perforation are life-threatening complications necessitating emergent surgical intervention, of which options are limited to the most expeditious and lowest risk procedures.
- Indications for elective surgery consist of medical unresponsiveness, intolerability or intractability, dysplasia or malignancy, growth retardation in children, and for the attempted improvement of some extraintestinal manifestations.
- Ileal pouch–anal anastomosis has become the most common continence-preserving procedure performed in patients who are appropriate candidates. Contraindications include incontinence, poor sphincter function and low rectal cancer.
- The foremost complication after completion of an IPAA is non-specific inflammation of the pouch (pouchitis), which approaches 50% within 10 years.
- Risk factors found to be independent predictors of pouch survival include: patient diagnosis, prior anal pathology, abnormal anal manometry, patient comorbidity, pouch–perineal or pouch–vaginal fistulas, pelvic sepsis, anastomotic stricture and separation.
- Pouch failure, defined as pouch excision or permanent diversion, is reported in several large series to range from 7% to 10% at 10 years and in one study 8% at 20 years.
- Success rates for salvage surgery following IPAA range from 75% to 94%.

References

1. Lakatos PL. Recent trends in the epidemiology of inflammatory bowel diseases: up or down? World J Gastroenterol 2006;12(38):6102–8.
2. Loftus Jr. EV. Clinical epidemiology of inflammatory bowel disease: incidence, prevalence, and environmental influences. Gastroenterology 2004;126(6):1504–17.
3. Bernstein CN. New insights into IBD epidemiology: are there any lessons for treatment? Dig Dis 2010;28(3):406–10.
4. Boyko EJ, Oerera DR, Koepsell TD, et al. Coffee and alcohol use and the risk of ulcerative colitis. Am J Gastroenterol 1989;84(5):530–4.
5. Bach JF. The effect of infections on susceptibility to autoimmune and allergic diseases. N Engl J Med 2002;347(12):911–20.
6. Blanchard JF, Bernstein CN, Wajda A, et al. Small-area variations and sociodemographic correlates for the incidence of Crohn's disease and ulcerative colitis. Am J Epidemiol 2001;154(4):328–35.
7. Shaw SY, Blanchard JF, Bernstein CN. Association between the use of antibiotics in the first year of life and pediatric inflammatory bowel disease. Am J Gastroenterol 2010;105(12):2687–92. Epub 2010 Oct 12.
8. Bengston MD, Aamodt G, Vatn MH, et al. Concordance for IBD among twins compared to ordinary siblings – a Norwegian population-based study. J Crohn's Colitis 2010;4(3):312–8.
9. Bernstein CN, Blanchard JF, Rawsthorne P, et al. The prevalence of extraintestinal diseases in inflammatory bowel disease: a population-based study. Am J Gastroenterol 2001;96(4):1116–22.
10. Levine JS, Burakoff R. Extraintestinal manifestations of inflammatory bowel disease. Gastroenterol Hepatol 2011;7(4):235–41.
11. Poritz LS, Koltun WA. Surgical management of ulcerative colitis in the presence of primary sclerosing cholangitis. Dis Colon Rectum 2003;46(2):173–8.
12. Penna C, Dozois R, Tremaine W, et al. Pouchitis after ileal pouch–anal anastomosis for ulcerative colitis occurs with increased frequency in patients with associated primary sclerosing cholangitis. Gut 1996;38(2):234–9.
13. Fevery J, Verslype C, Lai G, et al. Incidence, diagnosis, and therapy of cholangiocarcinoma in patients with primary sclerosing cholangitis. Dig Dis Sci 2007;52(11):3123–35.
14. Solem CA, Loftus EV, Tremaine WJ, et al. Venous thromboembolism in inflammatory bowel disease. Am J Gastroenterol 2004;99(1):97–101.
15. Fefferman DS, Farrell RJ. Endoscopy in inflammatory bowel disease: indications, surveillance, and use in clinical practice. Clin Gastroenterol Hepatol 2005;3(1):11–24.
16. Carucci LR, Levine MS. Radiographic imaging of inflammatory bowel disease. Gastroenterol Clin North Am 2002;31(1):93–117.

17. Eaden JA, Abrams KR, Mayberry JF. The risk of colorectal cancer in ulcerative colitis: a meta-analysis. Gut 2001;48(4):526–35.

18. Vieth M, Behrens H, Stolte M. Sporadic adenoma in ulcerative colitis: endoscopic resection is an adequate treatment. Gut 2006;55:1151–5.

19. Thomas T, Abrams KA, Robinson RJ, et al. Meta-analysis: cancer risk of low-grade dysplasia in chronic ulcerative colitis. Aliment Pharmacol Ther 2007;25(6):657–68.

    A large meta-analysis of 20 surveillance studies showed the risk of developing cancer in patients with LGD is high. When LGD is detected on surveillance there is a ninefold risk of developing cancer and 12-fold risk of developing any advanced lesion.

20. Ullman TA, Loftus Jr. EV, Kakar S, et al. The fate of low grade dysplasia in ulcerative colitis. Am J Gastroenterol 2002;97(4):922–7.

21. Ullman T, Croog V, Harpaz N, et al. Progression of flat low-grade dysplasia to advanced neoplasia in patients with ulcerative colitis. Gastroenterology 2003;125(5):1311–9.

22. Kornbluth A, Sachar DB. Ulcerative colitis practice guidelines in adults: American College of Gastroenterology, Practice Parameters Committee. Am J Gastroenterol 2010;105(3):501–23.

23. Ullman T, Odze R, Farraye FA. Diagnosis and management of dysplasia in patients with ulcerative colitis and Crohn's disease of the colon. Inflamm Bowel Dis 2009;15(4):630–8.

24. Rutter MD, Saunders BP, Wilkinson KH, et al. Thirty-year analysis of a colonoscopic surveillance program for neoplasia in ulcerative colitis. Gastroenterology 2006;130(4):1030–8.

25. Rodriguez SA, Eisen GM. Surveillance and management of dysplasia in ulcerative colitis by U.S. gastroenterologists: in truth, a good performance. Gastrointest Endosc 2007;1070.

26. Loftus Jr. EV, Harewood GC, Loftus CG, et al. PSC-IBD: a unique form of inflammatory bowel disease associated with primary sclerosing cholangitis. Gut 2005;54(1):91–6.

27. Rembacken BJ, Fujii T, Cairns A, et al. Flat and depressed colonic neoplasms: a prospective study of 1000 colonoscopies in the UK. Lancet 2000;355:1211–4.

28. Marion JF, Waye JD, Present DH, et al. Methylene blue spray targeted biopsies are superior to standard colonoscopic surveillance for detecting dysplasia in inflammatory bowel disease patients: a prospective endoscopic trial. Am J Gastroenterol 2008;103:2342–9.

29. D'Haens G, Sandborn WJ, Feagan BG, et al. A review of activity indices and efficacy end points for clinical trials of medical therapy in adults with ulcerative colitis. Gastroenterology 2007;132(2):763–86.

30. Meucci G, Fasoli R, Saibeni S, et al. Prognostic significance of endoscopic remission in patients with active ulcerative colitis treated with oral and topical mesalazine: a prospective, multicenter study. Inflamm Bowel Dis 2012;18(6):1006–10.

    A prospective multicentre study revealed patients in clinical remission with less severe sigmoidoscopic scores (defined as normal-looking mucosa, with only mild redness and/or friability) after 6 weeks of acute treatment were less likely to relapse at 1 year than patients in clinical remission only (cumulative rate of relapse 23% vs. 80%, respectively; $P < 0.0001$).

31. Banerjee S, Peppercorn MA. Inflammatory bowel disease. Medical therapy of specific clinical presentations. Gastroenterol Clin North Am 2002;31(1):185–202.

32. Rutgeerts P, Sandborn WJ, Feagan BG, et al. Infliximab for induction and maintenance therapy for ulcerative colitis. N Engl J Med 2005;353(23):2462–76.

    Two randomised, double-blind, placebo-controlled studies – the Active Ulcerative Colitis Trials 1 and 2 (ACT 1 and ACT 2 respectively) – showed patients with moderate-to-severe active ulcerative colitis treated with infliximab at weeks 0, 2, and 6 and every 8 weeks thereafter were more likely to have a clinical response at weeks 8, 30 and 54 than were those receiving placebo.

33. Selvasekar CR, Cima RR, Lawson DW, et al. Effect of infliximab on short-term complications in patients undergoing operation for chronic ulcerative colitis. J Am Coll Surg 2007;204(5):956–62.

34. Ooi BS, Remzi FH, Fazio VW. Turnbull-Blowhole colostomy for toxic ulcerative colitis in pregnancy: report of two cases. Dis Colon Rectum 2003;46(1):111–5.

35. Dozois EJ, Wolff BG, Tremaine WJ, et al. Maternal and fetal outcome after colectomy for fulminant ulcerative colitis during pregnancy: case series and literature review. Dis Colon Rectum 2006;49(1):64–73.

36. Alves A, Panis Y, Bouhnik Y, et al. Subtotal colectomy for severe acute colitis: a 20-year experience of a tertiary care center with an aggressive and early surgical policy. J Am Coll Surg 2003;197(3):379–85.

37. Brady RR, Collie MH, Ho GT, et al. Outcomes of the rectal remnant following colectomy for ulcerative colitis. Colorectal Dis 2008;10(2):144–50.

38. Carter FM, McLeod RS, Cohen Z. Subtotal colectomy for ulcerative colitis: complications related to the rectal remnant. Dis Colon Rectum 1991;34(11):1005–9.

39. Fazio VW, Church JM. Complications and function of the continent ileostomy at the Cleveland Clinic. World J Surg 1988;12(2):148–54.

40. Castillo E, Thomassie LM, Whitlow CB, et al. Continent ileostomy: current experience. Dis Colon Rectum 2005;48(6):1263–8.

41. Nessar G, Fazio VW, Tekkis P, et al. Long-term outcome and quality of life after continent ileostomy. Dis Colon Rectum 2006;49(3):336–44.

42. Juviler A, Hyman N. Ulcerative colitis: the fate of the retained rectum. Clin Colon Rectal Surg 2004;17(1):29–34.

43. Leijonmarck CE, Löfberg R, Ost A, et al. Long-term results of ileorectal anastomosis in ulcerative colitis in Stockholm County. Dis Colon Rectum 1990;33(3):195–200.

44. Weston-Petrides GK, Lovegrove RE, Tilney HS, et al. Comparison of outcomes after restorative proctocolectomy with or without defunctioning ileostomy. Arch Surg 2008;143:406–12.
A review of 17 studies comprising 1486 patients revealed that restorative proctocolectomy without a diverting ileostomy resulted in functional outcomes similar to those of surgery with proximal diversion but was associated with an increased risk of anastomotic leak. Diverting ileostomy should be omitted in carefully selected patients only.

45. Lovegrove RE, Constantinides VA, Heriot AG, et al. A comparison of hand-sewn versus stapled ileal pouch anal anastomosis (IPAA) following proctocolectomy: a meta-analysis of 4183 patients. Ann Surg 2006;244(1):18–26.
A large meta-analysis demonstrated no significant differences between a mucosectomy and hand-sewn versus a stapled anastomosis. Nocturnal seepage and pad usage favoured the stapled anastomosis in comparison to persisting symptoms due to inflammation or dysplasia favouring the hand-sewn technique.

46. Kirat HT, Remzi FH, Kiran RP, et al. Comparison of outcomes after hand-sewn versus stapled ileal pouch–anal anastomosis in 3,109 patients. Surgery 2009;146(4):723–9.

47. Heppell J, Weiland LH, Perrault J, et al. Fate of the rectal mucosa after rectal mucosectomy and ileoanal anastomosis. Dis Colon Rectum 1983;26:768–71.

48. O'Connell PR, Pemberton JH, Weiland LH, et al. Does rectal mucosa regenerate after ileoanal anastomosis? Dis Colon Rectum 1987;30:1–5.

49. Thompson-Fawcett MW, Mortensen NJ, Warren BF. "Cuffitis" and inflammatory changes in the columnar cuff, anal transitional zone, and ileal reservoir after stapled pouch–anal anastomosis. Dis Colon Rectum 1999;42(3):348–55.

50. Remzi FH, Fazio VW, Delaney CP, et al. Dysplasia of the anal transitional zone after ileal pouch–anal anastomosis: results of prospective evaluation after a minimum of ten years. Dis Colon Rectum 2003;46(1):6–13.

51. Fazio VW, Ziv Y, Church JM, et al. Ileal pouch–anal anastomoses complications and function in 1005 patients. Ann Surg 1995;222(2):120–7.

52. Meagher AP, Farouk R, Dozois RR, et al. J ileal pouch–anal anastomosis for chronic ulcerative colitis: complications and long-term outcome in 1310 patients. Br J Surg 1998;85(6):800–3.

53. Prudhomme M, Dozois RR, Godlewski G, et al. Anal canal strictures after ileal pouch–anal anastomosis. Dis Colon Rectum 2003;46(1):20–3.

54. Lolohea S, Lynch AC, Robertson GB, et al. Ileal pouch–anal anastomosis–vaginal fistula: a review. Dis Colon Rectum 2005;48(9):1802–10.

55. Heriot AG, Tekkis PP, Smith JJ, et al. Management and outcome of pouch–vaginal fistulas following restorative proctocolectomy. Dis Colon Rectum 2005;48(3):451–8.

56. Fazio VW, Tekkis PP, Remzi F, et al. Quantification of risk for pouch failure after ileal pouch anal anastomosis surgery. Ann Surg 2003;238(4):605–14.

57. Penna C, Dozois R, Tremaine W, et al. Pouchitis after ileal pouch–anal anastomosis for ulcerative colitis occurs with increased frequency in patients with associated primary sclerosing cholangitis. Gut 1996;38(2):234–9.

58. Fleshner PR, Vasiliauskas EA, Kam LY, et al. High level perinuclear antineutrophil cytoplasmic antibody (pANCA) in ulcerative colitis patients before colectomy predicts the development of chronic pouchitis after ileal pouch–anal anastomosis. Gut 2001;49(5):671–7.

59. Merrett MN, Mortensen N, Kettlewell M, et al. Smoking may prevent pouchitis in patients with restorative proctocolectomy for ulcerative colitis. Gut 1996;38(3):362–4.

60. Mimura T, Rizzello F, Helwig U, et al. Once daily high dose probiotic therapy (VSL#3) for maintaining remission in recurrent or refractory pouchitis. Gut 2004;53(1):108–14.

61. Shen B, Achkar JP, Lashner BA, et al. A randomized clinical trial of ciprofloxacin and metronidazole to treat acute pouchitis. Inflamm Bowel Dis 2001;7(4):301–5.

62. Heuschen UA, Allemeyer EH, Hinz U, et al. Outcome after septic complications in J pouch procedures. Br J Surg 2002;89(2):194–200.
The frequencies of permanent defunctioning and excision of a pouch in 131 patients with septic complications were 24% and 6%, respectively. The 5-year pouch failure rate increased in a subgroup of patients with septic complications at the pouch–anal anastomosis when the anal sphincter was involved (50% vs. 29%). Surgery for septic complications is required in a high percentage of patients and repeated attempts are justified in order to decrease the risk of pouch loss.

63. Olsen KO, Juul S, Berndtsson I, et al. Ulcerative colitis: female fecundity before diagnosis, during disease, and after surgery compared with a population sample. Gastroenterology 2002;122(1):15–9.

64. Gorgun E, Remzi FH, Goldberg JM, et al. Fertility is reduced after restorative proctocolectomy with ileal pouch anal anastomosis: a study of 300 patients. Surgery 2004;136(4):795–803.

65. Waljee A, Waljee J, Morris AM, et al. Threefold increased risk of infertility: a meta-analysis of infertility after ileal pouch anal anastomosis in ulcerative colitis. Gut 2006;55(11):1575–80.
A meta-analysis of eight studies revealed that an IPAA can increase the risk of infertility, defined as achieving pregnancy in 12 months of attempting conception, in women with ulcerative colitis by approximately threefold. Counselling female patients regarding decreased rates of fecundity following an IPAA is imperative.

66. Cornish JA, Tan E, Teare J, et al. The effect of restorative proctocolectomy on sexual function, urinary function, fertility, pregnancy and delivery: a systematic review. Dis Colon Rectum 2007;50(8):1128–38.

67. Johnson P, Richard C, Ravid A, et al. Female infertility after ileal pouch–anal anastomosis for ulcerative colitis. Dis Colon Rectum 2004;47(7):1119–26.

68. Oresland T, Palmblad S, Ellström M, et al. Gynaecological and sexual function related to anatomical changes in the female pelvis after restorative proctocolectomy. Int J Colorectal Dis 1994;9(2):77–81.

69. Hahnloser D, Pemberton JH, Wolff BG, et al. Pregnancy and delivery before and after ileal pouch–anal anastomosis for inflammatory bowel disease: immediate and long-term consequences and outcomes. Dis Colon Rectum 2004;47(7):1127–35.

70. Gorgun E, Remzi FH, Montague DK, et al. Male sexual function improves after ileal pouch anal anastomosis. Colorectal Dis 2005;7(6):545–50.

71. Tulchinsky H, Hawley PR, Nicholls J. Long-term failure after restorative proctocolectomy for ulcerative colitis. Ann Surg 2003;238(2):229–34.

72. Karoui M, Cohen R, Nicholls J. Results of surgical removal of the pouch after failed restorative proctocolectomy. Dis Colon Rectum 2004;47(6):869–75.

73. Dehni N, Remacle G, Dozois RR, et al. Salvage reoperation for complications after ileal pouch–anal anastomosis. Br J Surg 2005;92(6):748–53.

74. Tekkis PP, Heriot AG, Smith JJ, et al. Long-term results of abdominal salvage surgery following restorative proctocolectomy. Br J Surg 2006;93(2):231–7.

75. Shawki S, Belizon A, Person B, et al. What are the outcomes of reoperative restorative proctocolectomy and ileal pouch–anal anastomosis surgery? Dis Colon Rectum 2009;52(5):884–90.

76. Hahnloser D, Pemberton JH, Wolff BG, et al. Results at up to 20 years after ileal pouch–anal anastomosis for chronic ulcerative colitis. Br J Surg 2007;94(3):333–40.

77. Pemberton JH, Kelly KA, Beart Jr RW, et al. Ileal pouch–anal anastomosis for chronic ulcerative colitis. Long-term results. Ann Surg 1987;206(4):504–13.

78. Michelassi F, Lee J, Rubin M, et al. Long-term functional results after ileal pouch anal restorative proctocolectomy for ulcerative colitis: a prospective observational study. Ann Surg 2003;238(3):433–41.

79. Hahnloser D, Pemberton JH, Wolff BG, et al. The effect of ageing on function and quality of life in ileal pouch patients: a single cohort experience of 409 patients with chronic ulcerative colitis. Ann Surg 2004;240(4):615–21.

10

Crohn's disease

Mark W. Thompson-Fawcett
Neil J.McC. Mortensen

Introduction

Crohn's disease is a chronic transmural inflammatory process that can affect the gastrointestinal tract anywhere from mouth to anus and which may be associated with extraintestinal manifestations. The disease is commonly confined to a region of the gut. Frequent disease patterns observed include ileal, ileocolic and colonic. Perianal disease may coexist with any of these. Often there are discontinuous segments of disease with areas of normal mucosa intervening. Inflammation may cause ulceration, fissures, fistulas and fibrosis with stricturing. Histology reveals a chronic inflammatory infiltrate that is typically patchy and transmural, and may include classic granulomas with giant cell formation. Clinically, patients have abdominal pain and diarrhoea, and they may develop bowel obstruction or intestinal fistulas. A combination of the clinical, macroscopic, radiological and pathological features is required to make the diagnosis. It is a chronic disease with varying lengths of remission interspersed with acute episodes.

Epidemiology

Crohn's disease has an incidence of 6–15/100 000 and a prevalence of 50–200/100 000 in the West, but much lower in other, particularly warmer regions. Peak age of onset is 20–30 years, with a higher incidence in females in many higher incidence areas.

There is no association with socio-economic status or occupation, but an urban environment, cooler climate and higher standards of domestic hygiene may increase the risk. Incidence of Crohn's disease had steadily increased over recent decades but has now plateaued. Rates are lower but increasing in southern and eastern Europe, and Asia. Evidence of environmental effects is seen from studies of migrant populations. Current thinking is that environmental factors, rather than ethnicity, are a more important explanation for regional variation in incidence.[1]

Aetiology

Crohn's disease involves interplay between environmental and genetic factors. The specific cause of the exaggerated inflammatory response at the mucosal level remains unclear.

Smoking and oral contraception

Smoking increases the relative risk of Crohn's disease by a factor of 2, in contrast with ulcerative colitis where smoking provides a protective effect. Oral contraception may be associated with a small increase in risk, but whether this is causal or by association is not clear. Evidence suggests that oral contraceptive use has no effect on disease activity.[1]

Infection

Mycobacterium paratuberculosis causes a granulomatous inflammatory disorder in the intestine of cattle (Johne's disease) and it has been hypothesised that Crohn's is the human form of this disease. Many remain sceptical as the evidence is conflicting; the issue requires resolution.[1,2]

It has been controversially proposed that measles virus infection or vaccination may cause the granulomatous vasculitis observed in Crohn's disease, but this has now been dismissed.[1]

Genetic

Most inflammatory bowel disease (IBD) results from a genetic predisposition to an abnormal interaction between the immune system and environmental factors, especially the gut microbiota. Epidemiological studies have demonstrated familial aggregation: 2–22% of patients with Crohn's disease have a first-degree relative with IBD. There is greater concordance for IBD in monozygotic (20–50%) than dizygotic twins (0–7%). Early-onset disease has a higher familial prevalence rate, suggesting a greater genetic contribution compared with late-onset disease. Clinical patterns of IBD in affected parent–child and sibling pairs are concordant for each of disease type, extent and extraintestinal manifestations in the majority of cases. The relatives of patients with Crohn's disease also have an increased risk of developing ulcerative colitis. Crohn's disease and ulcerative colitis seem to be polygenic disorders with some shared susceptibility genes.[3]

These familial patterns have led to genome-wide scanning that has now identified 71 loci implicated in susceptibility to Crohn's disease.[4] Of these, all variants of IBD1 or the caspase recruitment domain family member 15 (CARD15) gene have generated most interest. CARD15 encodes the protein nucleotide-binding oligomerisation domain 2 (NOD2). It is associated with ileal disease, younger age at onset, ileocaecal resections and re-operation, and displays ethnic variation (less common in northern Europe and Asia).[5] Most evidence suggests CARD15 variants impair the innate immune system at mucosal level, limiting the ability of the intestinal epithelium to deal with pathogens or their components in the gut microbiota. It is hoped that further advances in genetics will improve phenotyping, help predict response to particular therapies and lead to the development of new targeted therapies.

Pathogenesis

Normally, the gut exists in a state of tolerance to the stream of microbial, dietary and other antigens in contact with the mucosa, but this tolerance and the ability to suppress an immune-mediated inflammatory response is lost in IBD. In Crohn's disease defects in immunoregulation are coupled with an increased mucosal permeability due to leaky paracellular pathways.

Defects in immunoregulation may include disturbed innate immune mechanisms at the epithelial barrier, problems with antigen recognition and processing by dendritic cells, and effects of psychosocial stress via a neuroimmunological interaction. In Crohn's disease the cell-mediated response is predominant, with excessive activation of effector T cells (Th1) that predominate over the regulatory T cells (Th3, Tr) that turn off the process. Proinflammatory cytokines released by effector T cells stimulate macrophages to release tumour necrosis factor (TNF)-α, interleukin (IL)-1 and IL-6. In addition, abnormal dendritic cell function may further drive the inflammatory response. Leucocytes then enter from the local circulation releasing further chemokines, amplifying the inflammatory process. The result is a local and systemic response, including fever, an acute-phase response, hypoalbuminaemia, weight loss, increased mucosal epithelial permeability, endothelial damage and increased collagen synthesis. Due to immune dysregulation the inflammatory response in the intestinal mucosa proceeds unchecked, producing a chronic inflammatory state.[6]

Pathology

Distribution

The macroscopic appearance and distribution are the first important considerations that provide key information towards differentiating Crohn's disease from other forms of IBD, particularly ulcerative colitis. Frequencies of regions involved are:

1. small bowel alone, 30–35%;
2. colon alone, 25–35%;
3. small bowel and colon, 30–50% (usually ileocolic);

4. perianal lesions, over 50%;
5. stomach and duodenum, 5% (minor subclinical mucosal abnormalities in 50%).

Skip lesions (areas of disease separated by normal bowel) strongly suggest Crohn's disease, although occasionally a periappendiceal or caecal patch of overt colitis may be observed with distal ulcerative colitis.

Macroscopic appearance

The unmistakable appearance of Crohn's disease is of a stiff, thick-walled segment of bowel with fat wrapping. There is creeping extension of mesenteric fat around the serosal surface of the bowel wall towards the antimesenteric border. This is part of the connective tissue changes that affect all layers of the bowel wall. As inflammation is full thickness, there can be fibrinous exudate and adhesions on the serosal surface. Narrow linear ulcers with intervening islands of oedematous mucosa give the mucosal surface its classic cobblestone appearance. Ulceration is discrete, and serpiginous linear ulcers usually run along the mesenteric aspect of the lumen. Deep fissuring from linear ulceration may lead to formation of fistulas through the bowel wall. Closer inspection may reveal multiple aphthous ulcers that usually develop on the surface of submucosal lymphoid nodules. Aphthous ulcers are the earliest macroscopic lesions in Crohn's disease and are seen before the classic appearances of more established disease. Inflammatory polyps are often found in the involved colon but are unusual in the small bowel. Enlarged lymph nodes may be present in the resected mesentery but are not caseated or matted together. Strictures can vary from 1 to 30 cm in length. These may be stiff like a hosepipe with turgid oedema, or tight fibrotic strictures from burnt-out inflammation. The narrowing of the lumen may be sufficient to produce obstruction and proximal dilatation, and there may be multiple dilated segments between multiple tight strictures. Fistulas, sinuses and abscesses are often present in the ileocaecal region but may arise from any segment of active disease and can communicate with other loops of bowel, stomach, bladder, vagina, skin or intra-abdominal abscess cavities.

Microscopy

Inflammation involves the full thickness of the bowel wall. Early mucosal changes show neutrophils attacking the base of crypts, causing injury and focal crypt abscesses. The formation of mucosal lymphoid aggregates followed by overlying ulceration produces aphthous ulcers. There is relative preservation of goblet cell mucin by comparison with ulcerative colitis, where there is usually mucin depletion. As the disease progresses, connective tissue changes occur in all layers of the bowel wall giving the stiff, thick-walled, macroscopic appearance. There is submucosal fibrosis and muscularisation. The muscularis mucosa and muscularis propria are thickened from increased amounts of connective tissue. Typically, the chronic inflammatory infiltrate and the architectural changes in the mucosa are patchy. Transmural inflammation is in the form of lymphoid aggregates seen throughout the bowel wall, leading to the formation of a Crohn's 'rosary' on the serosal surface. The following three features are diagnostic hallmarks of Crohn's disease:

1. deep non-caseating granulomas (excluding those that are mucosal or related to crypt rupture) are present in 60–70% of patients and are commonly located in the bowel wall but may be in the mesentery, regional lymph nodes, peritoneum, liver or contiguously involved tissue;
2. intralymphatic granulomas;
3. granulomatous vasculitis.

Pitfalls in differentiating Crohn's colitis from ulcerative colitis

Sometimes it is difficult even for an experienced gastrointestinal pathologist to differentiate between Crohn's colitis and ulcerative colitis on histology, and considerable interobserver variation is reported among pathologists. There can be overlap between the diseases and this can lead to the diagnosis of indeterminate colitis in 5–10% of patients with colonic involvement alone. During the course of the disease subsequent disease behaviour may change, leading to a change in diagnosis, usually towards Crohn's disease. For difficult cases, consideration of the macroscopic, microscopic, radiological and endoscopic features and the history and clinical picture is essential, for it is often the cumulative evidence that makes the diagnosis. A definitive diagnosis is more likely if the resected colon is available for assessment as opposed to mucosal biopsies. If only endoscopic biopsies are available, the endoscopic findings are important and must be discussed with the pathologist.

Rectal sparing may be seen in ulcerative colitis, especially if topical preparations have been used. Patchy inflammation is a feature of Crohn's disease, but treated ulcerative colitis can itself show patchy mucosal inflammation. Perianal disease is very suggestive of Crohn's, although patients with ulcerative colitis can develop cryptoglandular fistulas and abscesses. Lymphoid follicles may be seen in the base of the mucosa in severe ulcerative colitis, but they are a prominent feature of Crohn's disease, where they are transmural. In Crohn's disease there is relative preservation of goblet cell mucin, whereas mucin depletion is a feature of ulcerative colitis (with the exception of fulminant ulcerative colitis, where there may be surprisingly little mucin depletion). In established diversion proctitis or pouchitis it is difficult to exclude Crohn's disease as both these conditions may mimic Crohn's disease.

Clinical

Gastrointestinal symptoms

The clinical presentation varies depending on the site of disease. Acute first presentations of disease are uncommon, but ileal disease can mimic acute appendicitis and colonic disease may present as a fulminating colitis.

The majority of patients complain of diarrhoea (70–90%), abdominal pain (45–65%), rectal bleeding (30%) and perianal disease (10%). The symptom profile will reflect the disease location. Diarrhoea may result from mucosal inflammation, fistulation between loops of bowel, a short bowel from previous resections, bacterial overgrowth from obstructed segments, or bile salt malabsorption from terminal ileal disease. These latter two also produce steatorrhoea. Distal colitis and proctitis, and decreased rectal compliance, produce tenesmus and frequent bowel motions. Abdominal pain may be colicky from obstructing lesions or more continual from peritoneal irritation caused by acute inflammation. Terminal ileal disease is the most common site for obstructive lesions. Rectal bleeding is uncommon from terminal ileal disease, but does occur in 50% of patients with colonic disease. Massive bleeding occurs in 1–2%, though the site is often difficult to identify. When perianal disease is present, patients often complain of purulent discharge and minor leakage of faecal material with local discomfort. Fissures may be large,

indolent and painless. Significant perianal pain suggests undrained sepsis. Fistulas extending to the bladder can produce pneumaturia and recurrent urinary tract infection, while those extending to the vagina may cause wind or faeces vaginally.

Systemic symptoms

Weight loss is reported by 65–75% of patients. This is usually of the order of 10–20% of body weight and is the result of anorexia, food fear, diarrhoea and, less often, malabsorption. The latter may be caused by inflammatory disease but more commonly is due to bacterial overgrowth as a result of coloenteric fistulas, blind loops or stasis from chronic obstruction. If there is extensive small-bowel disease, there may be poor absorption of fat-soluble vitamins leading to symptoms and signs of osteomalacia (vitamin D) or a bleeding tendency (vitamin K). Other deficiencies are uncommon, usually resulting from inadequate intake rather than increased losses, but may include deficiencies of magnesium, zinc, ascorbic acid and the B vitamins. Symptoms of anaemia are common and usually result from iron deficiency due to intestinal blood loss and, less commonly, from vitamin B_{12} or folate deficiency. After resection of more than 50 cm of terminal ileum, vitamin B_{12} absorption falls below normal. Malabsorption of bile salts and fats, which can cause diarrhoea, usually only follows an ileal resection of greater than 100 cm. The inflammatory process produces a low-grade fever in 30–49% of patients; where high and spiking, or the patient reports rigors, it is likely that there is a suppurative intra-abdominal complication.[1]

Extraintestinal manifestations

These are outlined in Box 10.1 and are more common in association with Crohn's colitis than isolated small-bowel disease. They are similar to those that occur in ulcerative colitis, and may precede, be independent of or accompany active IBD, and can cause significant morbidity. They may be experienced by up to 50% of patients and be present for life in 25–30%. Gallstones are said to be common due to malabsorption of bile salts in the terminal ileum. However, symptomatic problems are not

Related to disease activity
- Aphthous ulceration (10%)
- Erythema nodosum (5–10%)
- Pyoderma gangrenosum (0.5%)
- Acute arthropathy (6–12%)
- Eye complications (conjunctivitis, etc.) (3–10%)
- Amyloidosis (1%)

Unrelated to disease activity
- Sacroiliitis (often minimal symptoms) (10–15%)
- Ankylosing spondylitis (1–2%)
- Primary sclerosing cholangitis (rare)
- Chronic active hepatitis (2–3%)
- Cirrhosis (2–3%)
- Gallstones (15–30%)
- Renal calculi (5–10%)

increased compared with the general population. Steatorrhoea promotes increased absorption of oxalate, thereby increasing the incidence of oxalate renal stones. Patients may have a fatty liver as a result of malnutrition or from receiving total parenteral nutrition. Mild abnormalities of liver function are common with active disease, and these do not imply significant liver disease.

Thromboembolic complications occur with IBD and are usually associated with severe active colonic disease. Common sites are the lower extremities and pelvic veins, but cerebrovascular accidents have also been reported. Metastatic Crohn's disease is an unusual complication in which nodular ulcerating skin lesions occur at distant sites including the vulva, submammary areas and extremities. Biopsies of these show non-caseating granulomas. Clubbing is seen in some cases of extensive small-bowel disease.

Amyloidosis is reported in 25% of patients with Crohn's disease at post-mortem but only 1% have clinical manifestations. It can occur in the bowel or within other organs, including the liver, spleen and kidneys. If renal function is affected, resection of the diseased bowel will result in regression of amyloid and improvement of renal function.[7]

Physical signs

Patients may appear well and have a normal physical examination. With more severe disease there may be evidence of weight loss, anaemia, iron deficiency,

clubbing, cachexia, proximal myopathy, easy bruising, elevated temperature, tachycardia and peripheral oedema. Signs of extraintestinal manifestations may be present.

Abdominal examination can be normal but tenderness in the right iliac fossa is common. Thickened loops of bowel may be palpable and if matted together can produce an abdominal mass. A psoas or intra-abdominal abscess produces signs and occasionally there is free peritonitis. Enterocutaneous fistulas are most common when there has been previous surgery and usually present through a scar. Acute or chronic strictures or carcinoma may produce signs of obstruction. Compared to the general population the relative risk of adenocarcinoma of the colon complicating Crohn's colitis is 1.4–1.9 and the relative risk of small-bowel carcinoma 21–27.[8] Perianal disease varies from an asymptomatic fissure or inflamed skin tag to severe disease that may look like a 'forest fire', with erythema, large fleshy skin tags, deep chronic fissures with bridges of skin and multiple fistulas creating the so-called 'watering-can perineum'. Fibrosis from chronic inflammation may have produced a woody, stiff anal canal or an anal or rectal stenosis.

Paediatric age group

In children and adolescents the gastrointestinal manifestations are similar but extraintestinal and systemic manifestations of disease become more important. About 15% have arthralgia and arthritis that often precedes bowel symptoms by months or years. Diagnosis may be delayed by a non-specific presentation with systemic symptoms of weight loss, growth failure and unexplained anaemia and fever. If active disease is dealt with promptly by medical or surgical treatment and adequate nutrition is maintained, retardation of growth and sexual development can usually be reversed.[7,8]

Pregnancy

This issue is often of concern as the disease frequently affects young adults. For the majority of patients with IBD fertility is normal but in some subgroups fertility rates are slightly reduced. Overall, patients with IBD do experience more adverse outcomes in pregnancy. In the absence of active disease, the outcome of pregnancy equals that of matched controls. With active disease at conception, there is an increase in spontaneous abortion and premature delivery, and a greater than 50% chance of relapsing disease during pregnancy. The risk of relapse is only 20–25% if disease is inactive at conception. It is therefore advisable to avoid conception during an acute phase of disease. Pregnancy probably does not affect the long-term course of the disease. Aminosalicylates, steroids and azathioprine are relatively safe in pregnancy. Azathioprine may be associated with a small increase in major congenital defects but this needs to be balanced against the importance of maintaining disease control. Methotrexate is contraindicated.[7,9]

Investigations

Laboratory

Anti-*Saccharomyces cervisiae* antibodies (ASCAs) and perinuclear antineutrophil cytoplasmic antibody (p-ANCA) can be useful to discriminate ulcerative colitis from Crohn's. ASCAs are positive in 35–50% of patients with Crohn's compared to less than 1% in ulcerative colitis. The specificity is around 90%. On the other hand, p-ANCA is often raised in ulcerative colitis, with a sensitivity of 55% and specificity of about 90%. If p-ANCA is elevated in Crohn's, it is only with colitis. Faecal calprotectin and lactoferrin can play a role in diagnosis, monitoring disease activity and predicting relapse.[10,11]

In more severe or established disease, magnesium, zinc and selenium levels should be checked. Serum albumin is often low in active disease due to downregulation of albumin synthesis by cytokines (IL-1, IL-2, TNF). Mild episodic elevations of liver function tests are common but persistent abnormalities require further investigation. Evidence of anaemia should be sought, and if present investigated. A neutrophil leucocytosis usually indicates active disease or septic complications. Of the serum protein markers for inflammation, C-reactive protein and orosomucoid most closely match clinical disease activity. Erythrocyte sedimentation rate is useful in Crohn's colitis but not in small-bowel disease. Faecal fat excretion may be increased if malabsorption is present. Severe ileocaecal involvement can cause right hydronephrosis or sterile pyuria, and an enterovesical fistula will lead to bacteria in the urine.

Radiology

Small-bowel imaging is usually carried out as part of the diagnostic work-up or soon after diagnosis to determine the extent of the disease. A small-bowel barium study has traditionally been the key to confirming the presence of small-bowel disease but this is being replaced by magnetic resonance enterography (MRE; or enteroclysis, the choice largely depending on local preference or radiologist). Good results are also achieved with computed tomography (CT) enterography and high-resolution ultrasound. The clinical question, local expertise, desire to minimise radiation, availability and cost are factors taken into account when choosing a modality.

A small-bowel barium follow-through provides the best resolution, but only assesses the lumen and carries a radiation burden similar to CT. It is debated whether a barium study is best done by barium meal and follow-through techniques (better tolerated) or by a small-bowel enema with a nasoduodenal tube (enteroclysis); probably most important is a radiologist committed to producing good-quality images. More subtle features of small-bowel Crohn's include thickening of the valvulae coniventes, a granular mucosal pattern and aphthous ulcers. As disease progresses features include wall thickening, cobblestoning and fissure-like ulcers, sinus tracts and fistulas. There may be stenosis causing obstructive symptoms, commonly in the terminal ileum (**Fig. 10.1**). Multiple tight stenoses with intervening dilated segments produce a 'chain of lakes' appearance (**Fig. 10.2**).

While CT enterography and MRE provide less luminal detail they provide information on wall thickening (>3 mm), oedema in the bowel wall and mesenteric fat, any increase in fat adjacent to bowel, lymph node involvement, increase in vascularity, fibrotic strictures, and sinuses and fistulas.

CT is frequently used to investigate acute abdominal pain. The diagnosis of Crohn's may be suggested in this context by seeing thickened small-bowel loops, especially in the terminal ileum (**Fig. 10.3**). CT is effective at detecting intra-abdominal abscesses and dilated segments of small bowel, and remains the most used modality for suspected acute complications including intra-abdominal sepsis and obstruction.

In addition to identifying stenosis (**Fig. 10.4**), magnetic resonance imaging (MRI) has the benefit of being able to demonstrate bowel wall oedema to assist in discriminating areas of inflammation from

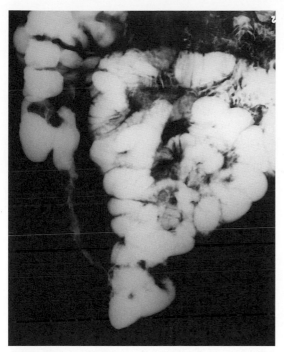

Figure 10.1 • Small-bowel enema with classic terminal ileal disease showing narrowing, cobblestone mucosa and fissures.

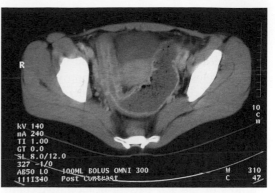

Figure 10.3 • CT scan showing thick-walled terminal ileum with proximal dilatation.

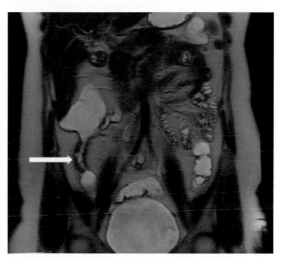

Figure 10.4 • MRI scan demonstrating strictured terminal ileum with thickened bowel wall.

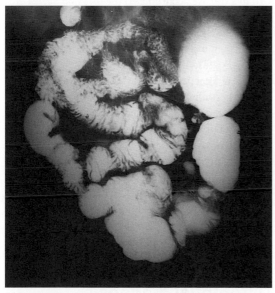

Figure 10.2 • Small-bowel barium enema showing multiple stenoses with intervening dilatation.

fibrosis. MRI is free of ionising radiation and not limited by poor renal function. Dynamic imaging also allows multiple sequences so contractions can be delineated from true strictures more easily. However, respiratory movement and claustrophobia may be a problem and it is more costly. Its advantages, mainly less radiation, mean MRI has become preferred over CT for routine imaging. If CT enterography is used a low-dose protocol should be considered. MRI is also the investigation of choice for complicated perianal sepsis. High-resolution ultrasound is popular in Europe and effective at detecting inflamed bowel, although operator dependent.

A double-contrast barium enema of the colon is now rarely done and has been replaced by colonoscopy. In severe acute presentations of Crohn's disease, plain abdominal films should be done initially to look for evidence of obstruction, mucosal oedema or dilatation. Plain films can also be useful to identify constipation proximal to a segment of colonic disease.

Endoscopy

Colonoscopy provides a macroscopic view that can be recorded, allows biopsies to aid in the differential diagnosis, can assess and biopsy strictures, and can clarify the situation where significant symptoms are not backed up by clinical evidence of disease. Intubation of the ileocaecal valve allows examination and biopsy of the terminal ileum. Small aphthous ulcers are the early features of Crohn's disease, in contrast with the erythema and loss of vascular pattern in ulcerative colitis. In more severe disease the oedematous mucosa is penetrated by deep fissuring ulceration to give a cobblestone appearance. Multiple biopsies should be taken even if the mucosa appears normal, as granulomas may be present that can confirm the diagnosis. There is not usually a role for routine follow-up endoscopy and endoscopic findings correlate poorly with clinical remission. There is a cancer risk in long-standing Crohn's colitis and most apply the same colonoscopic surveillance as they do in cases of extensive ulcerative colitis.

Endoscopy of the oesophagus, stomach and duodenum is necessary if there are appropriate symptoms, or abnormalities on a barium meal. Findings may include rugal hypertrophy, deep longitudinal ulcers and a cobblestone mucosa, the latter being the main differentiating feature from peptic ulcer disease. Biopsies should be taken but granulomas are often absent.

The diagnosis of Crohn's disease may be made by capsule endoscopy, and this may be in the context of investigating obscure chronic gastrointestinal bleeding when other investigations have been negative. Capsule endoscopy is more sensitive than MRE but only provides information from viewing the lumen. One of the technical problems is that the capsule may be held up by strictures and cause small-bowel obstruction. If there is any significant concern that this may happen, a dummy dissolvable capsule can be used first. Capsule endoscopy is considered second-line investigation by most.

Disease activity assessment and quality of life

For clinical purposes, disease activity is best assessed by clinical features and the investigations outlined above. It is usually categorised as mild, moderate or severe. If patients are asymptomatic (and off steroids) and/or have no obvious residual disease they are considered in remission. A number of indices of disease activity have been developed for Crohn's disease, including the Crohn's Disease Activity Index and the Harvey–Bradshaw index. Their role has largely been confined to clinical trials for standardisation and comparison of patient groups. However, with the widespread use of expensive biological agents, in publicly funded health services, a severity score over a certain threshold is often required to access these medications.

Health-related quality of life (HRQOL) is a quantitative measurement of the subjective perception a person has of their health state, including emotional and social aspects. If treatments are being compared, use of HRQOL instruments is essential for providing a valid and objective measure of a real change in health state.

Phenotyping

Different phenotypes of Crohn's disease are recognised and the clinical picture varies with the site and behaviour of the disease (i.e. stricturing or fistulating). To date it seems that the location of disease tends to be stable over time. However, the behaviour of Crohn's disease according to the location varies dramatically over the course of the disease. At 10 years, 46% of patients exhibit different disease behaviour than at diagnosis. Phenotype is important for genetic studies as differing phenotypes may correlate with particular genetic variations. Phenotype is also relevant for studying the outcome of therapy, medical or surgical. The Vienna classification was developed in 1998. This was modified to the current Montreal classification in 2005. At the time of diagnosis the following are recorded: age <16 years (A1), between 17 and 40 years (A2) or ≥40 years (A3), location of disease (ileal (L1), colonic (L2), ileocolonic (L3); isolated upper gastrointestinal disease (L4) if present is added to the others), behaviour (non-stricturing/non-penetrating (B1), stricturing (B2), penetrating (B3); perianal disease (p) is added if present).

Differential diagnosis

Small-bowel Crohn's disease

In most cases, after an appropriate work-up involving history and clinical, laboratory, radiological, endoscopic and pathological findings, the diagnosis will be fairly clear-cut. Table 10.1 shows

Table 10.1 • Differential diagnosis of small-bowel Crohn's disease

Differential diagnosis	Useful discriminating features
Appendicitis	History, CT scan
Appendix abscess	History, ultrasound/CT scan
Caecal diverticulitis	Older age, barium enema
Pelvic inflammatory disease	History
Ovarian cyst or tumour	Ultrasound
Caecal carcinoma	Barium enema/colonoscopy
Ileal carcinoid	Small-bowel enema
Behçet's disease	Painful ulceration of the mouth and genitalia
Systemic vasculitis affecting the small bowel	Underlying systemic connective tissue disorder
Radiation enteritis	History of radiotherapy
Ileocaecal tuberculosis	History of tuberculosis, circulating antibodies to *Mycobacterium*, stool cultures
Yersinia enterocolitica ileitis	Self-limiting, stool cultures, serology
Eosinophilic gastroenteritis	Gastric involvement, peripheral eosinophilia
Amyloidosis	Biopsy
Small-bowel lymphoma	Radiological appearance
Small-bowel lymphoma	Microscopy of fine-needle aspirate
Actinomycosis	Clinical picture and histology
Chronic non-granulomatous jejunoileitis	

the differential diagnoses of small-bowel Crohn's disease. Traditionally, perhaps the two that cause most difficulty are *Yersinia* and tuberculosis. With increased use of CT scanning for acute abdominal pain, thickened terminal ileum is a more common indication for a careful work-up.

Large-bowel Crohn's disease

When there is no small-bowel or perineal involvement, there are two areas where the diagnosis may be difficult. An isolated segment of disease, especially if it is a short segment, has to be differentiated from carcinoma, ischaemia, tuberculosis and lymphoma; occasionally, severe diverticular disease can appear as or disguise a segment of Crohn's disease. Inflamed diverticular disease can mimic Crohn's disease, with the presence of granulomas, transmural inflammation and fissuring ulceration. Isolated involvement of the sigmoid colon is not common in Crohn's disease, so care should be taken before making this diagnosis in the presence of diverticular disease. Differentiating Crohn's disease from ulcerative colitis has been discussed earlier.

Medical treatment

A summary of first-line medical treatment options for Crohn's disease is given in Box 10.2. The concept of treating Crohn's disease is to induce remission and then to maintain it. The most effective agent for inducing remission is a corticosteroid, and the second-line agents are the TNF inhibitors, infliximab or adalimumab. Budesonide has a role in ileocolic disease or right-sided colitis. It is not as effective for induction of remission as prednisolone or methyl-prednisone but has fewer side-effects. For moderate to severe disease, steroids are commenced and

Box 10.2 • Summary of medical treatment options for Crohn's disease

Induction of remission

Mild to moderate disease
- Prednisone 20–40 mg daily for 2–3 weeks then tapering
- Ileal and/or right colon: budesonide 9 mg per day
- Crohn's colitis: appropriate salicylate compound (oral and/or enema)
- Perianal disease: metronidazole 400 mg t.d.s. or ciprofloxacin 500 mg b.d.

Severe disease
- Intravenous prednisone 60–80 mg per day
- Infliximab, adalimumab or other biological

Maintenance of remission
- Azathioprine, 6-mercaptopurine, methotrexate, budesonide 6 mg per day (ileal and/or right colon)

at the same time immunosuppression, usually with azathioprine, is commenced. After some weeks or months, when the therapeutic benefit of immunosuppression commences, steroids can be removed. Aminosalicylates have modest efficacy for mild to moderate Crohn's colitis. For a more detailed discussion of medical therapy readers are referred to the British Society of Gastroenterolgy guidelines[12] and the United Kingdom National Health Service, National Institute for Health and Clinical Excellence (NICE) guidelines (http://guidance.nice.org.uk/TA187).

Multidisciplinary care

✅ For the safe and effective care of patients with IBD multidisciplinary care is essential. With the introduction of expensive biological drugs, with at times limited efficacy, and more powerful immunosuppressive regimes the surgeon must be involved in the complex decision-making for patients with moderate to severe Crohn's disease. Frequently patients do require surgery to achieve remission. Surgical input is needed to provide balanced decision-making, mindful that if the patient comes to surgery too late, the morbidity in a malnourished immmosuppressed patient is high. To contribute effectively to good decision-making the surgeon needs knowledge of the likely efficacy and outcome for the medical therapy options.

Aminosalicylates

Sulfasalazine and 5-aminosalicylic acid (5-ASA; also known as mesalazine or mesalamine) are used to treat disease of mild to moderate severity in the colon. Sulfasalazine consists of a sulfapyridine carrier linked to the active 5-ASA. In the colon bacteria cleave off the active 5-ASA, of which about 20% is absorbed. If 5-ASA is taken orally by itself, it is completely absorbed in the proximal small bowel. Although 5-ASA is the main active drug, the sulfapyridine produces most of the adverse effects, including nausea, vomiting, heartburn, headache, oligospermia and low-level haemolysis. These adverse effects are dose related. There are also a number of hypersensitivity reactions unrelated to drug levels, including worsening colitis. Adverse effects occur in 30% of people taking 4g daily of sulfasalazine. Other 5-ASA preparations use different carriers, or use pH- or time-dependent protective coatings that allow release to start in the jejunum, ileum or colon, thereby giving a much lower adverse effect profile.

Aminosalicylates have historically had a significant place in the management of Crohn's disease, but their indications are now limited. They can be used to treat colonic disease and to prevent recurrence after surgery, but their therapeutic benefit is limited. Mesalazine can be used for preventing recurrence after surgery with a number needed to treat (NNT) of 13.[13] Alternative treatments if indicated, such as azathioprine, are more effective, but mesalazine could be considered if other regimes are not desired. Aminosalicylates may have a limited role for mild to moderate colonic disease but have marginal efficacy over placebo.[12]

Steroids

Systemically absorbed corticosteroids are the most effective and commonly used drugs for moderate to severe Crohn's disease and will induce remission in 70–80% of cases. They are less effective if only the colon is involved. Doses of prednisone range from 20–40 mg/day orally for moderate disease to 60–80 mg/day intravenously for severe disease. Steroids should be used in short courses and must be tapered when a clinical response is achieved. They can be useful in resolving the obstructive symptoms in early disease caused by narrowing due to inflammatory oedema. Steroids will not help with obstructive symptoms caused by established fibrotic stenosis. Steroids are useful for maintaining a steroid-induced remission in the short term, which implies steroid-dependent disease, but they do not have a role in maintenance beyond this. There is no advantage in combining salicylate therapy with steroids.

Rectal administration of steroid is effective for left-sided colonic disease, but steroid is still absorbed systemically, and prolonged therapy can cause adrenal suppression. 5-ASA foam enemas are equally effective and can be used in combination with oral steroids in an exacerbation of disease.

To avoid systemic adverse effects, topically active corticosteroids have been developed. Budesonide, formulated as a slow-release oral preparation, acts in the small bowel and colon or can be given as an enema. The systemic bioavailability of budesonide is only 10–15% because of rapid first-pass metabolism in the liver, but it can still produce some suppression of plasma cortisol levels. The response rates are slightly less than prednisolone but with fewer side effects.

> ✔✔ In active Crohn's disease, budesonide produced remission in 51–60% of patients compared with 60–73% on systemic steroids, but with a halving of reported adverse effects from 60% to 30%. When budesonide 9 mg daily was compared with mesalamine 4 g daily for ileal and/or ascending colon disease, remission in the budesonide group at 16 weeks was 62% vs. 36% for mesalamine, and budesonide was better tolerated. Budesonide is not of value for maintenance therapy.[14,15] Budesonide was compared to placebo in a double-blind randomised controlled trial of endoscopic recurrence (at 3 and 12 months) after an ileal or ileocolic resection, with no overall benefit.[16]

Antibiotics

Metronidazole and ciprofloxacin are used to treat perianal disease. They both seem equally effective but ciprofloxacin may be better tolerated. They can reduce fistula discharge but probably have little impact on closure rates, and symptoms often return after cessation. Long-term use of metronidazole in doses >10 mg/kg/day is contraindicated because of the risk of peripheral neuropathy. There is evidence that metronidazole and ciprofloxacin have efficacy for ileal and colonic disease but are rarely used as alternative therapies are more effective.

Nutrition for therapy

The rationale for nutritional therapy is that intraluminal dietary antigens may drive the inflammatory response and that removal of these and bowel rest will bring remission.

> ✔✔ Total parenteral nutrition is effective in inducing remission in 60–80% of patients, which matches the effect of steroids, but combining both these therapies gives no added benefit over using only one. Relapse rates are high after cessation. Total enteral nutrition is equally as effective and has a similar relapse rate after cessation. Polymeric diets seem as effective as elemental and peptide-based diets, but polymeric diets are cheaper and more palatable and are therefore preferred.[12]

Polymeric or elemental intake as a proportion of the diet is also effective at maintaining remission.[17] Enteral nutrition is frequently chosen as the first-line therapy for children with Crohn's disease.[18]

Immunomodulatory therapy

This is used to reduce and eliminate steroid requirements, particularly after a remission has been achieved, and in refractory disease. Azathioprine and 6-mercaptopurine are purine analogues, azathioprine being quickly metabolised to 6-mercaptopurine. They inhibit cell proliferation and suppress cell-mediated events by inhibiting the activity of cytotoxic T cells and natural killer cells. The onset of a therapeutic effect takes 3–6 months. Toxicity occurs in 20–30%, including 3–15% of patients who will develop pancreatitis. A significant proportion of toxicity, and possibly lack of efficacy, can be due to genetic variability in the metabolism of azathioprine, that can be tested for and managed.[19]

> ✔✔ Fever, rash, arthralgias and hepatitis may occur and marrow suppression is dose related. In trials to improve disease or to decrease steroid requirements, there is a success rate of about 70–80%, and this applies equally to all disease sites, including perianal disease. In Cochrane reviews the odds ratio for inducing remission compared to placebo is 2.43 and for maintaining remission 2.32. If disease recurs after stopping therapy it seems it can be successfully reintroduced (Prefontaine E, Macdonald JK, Sutherland LR. Azathioprine or 6-mercaptopurine for induction of remission in Crohn's disease. Cochrane Database Syst Rev. 2010(6):CD000545). Methotrexate is used occasionally for treating Crohn's disease. Limited data suggest it is as effective as azathioprine or 6-mercaptopurine and it is prescribed for patients who do not tolerate or respond to the latter two drugs.[12,20]

'Biological agents'

'Biological agents' is the term used to refer to monoclonal antibodies targeted at mediators of the inflammatory response. The two agents in common clinical use are infliximab, introduced in the late 1990s, followed several years later by adalimumab. A number of other agents are under evaluation. Infliximab is a mouse–human chimeric monoclonal antibody to TNF-α delivered by intravenous infusion. Adalimumab is a fully human monoclonal antibody also directed at TNF-α, but has the added convenience of being able to be delivered by subcutaneous injection. The randomised controlled trials (RCTs) evaluating these drugs are funded by the manufacturers, are complex in design with frequent crossovers, and require careful study to determine the real clinical efficacy. Occasional severe adverse reactions are reported and infectious diseases, especially tuberculosis, need to be excluded before treatment. There may be the possibility of an increase in the risk of malignancy long term. Unfortunately, because of crossovers in RCTs there are few patients who remain purely in placebo arms to generate reliable long-term data on adverse outcomes. Perhaps the biggest drawback of these agents is their high cost.

✔✔ The initial placebo-controlled trial with infliximab addressed induction of remission after a single dose. At 4 weeks after a single dose, an initial treatment response was seen in 65% (54 of 83) who received infliximab and 17% (4 of 24) in the placebo group; at 12 weeks this was 41% and 12%, respectively.[21] The ACCENT I study followed and addressed the maintenance of remission with a year of treatment with infliximab; 573 patients were recruited. After an initial infusion, 58% responded. The responders were then randomised to placebo or infliximab at 2 and 6 weeks and then 8-weekly up to 54 weeks. At week 54, of initial responders, about 15% in the placebo group and 35% in the treatment group were in clinical remission.[22]

Similar results with initial moderate efficacy have been demonstrated using infliximab to treat fistulas. The ACCENT II study recruited patients with perianal (90%) and enterocutaneous draining fistulas. The primary end-point of the study was a reduction in the number of fistulas by 50% or more. After three infusions at 0, 2 and 6 weeks, the study randomised responders at week 14 to placebo or infliximab infusions 8-weekly to week 54. The primary end-point was loss of response, with fistulas reactivating or reappearing. Of 306 patients enrolled, 195 (64%) responders were randomised at week 14. At week 54, 23 of 98 patients receiving placebo maintained a response compared with 42 of 91 receiving infliximab. This means that of all 306 patients entered into the study, about 30% of patients treated with infliximab will maintain a response at 1 year, 22% having a complete response. In the placebo group after initial infliximab response, 19% (19 of 98) had a complete response.[23] The efficacy at 1 year judged by complete response is therefore modest.

Adalimumab (a human anti-TNF monoclonal antibody) has been evaluated in the CLASSIC I and II[24,25] and CHARM studies,[26] and has similar efficacy to infliximab. Adalimumab may be beneficial if infliximab therapy has not been successful and vice versa.

The CHARM study looked at maintenance therapy with adalimumab for 12 months using hospitalisation as an end-point. After induction all patients were randomised to adalimumab or placebo. The Crohn's-related hospitalisation rate at 12 months was 8.4% on adalimumab and 15.5% on placebo. This means 14 patients are treated to prevent one admission. The study also looked at surgery rates. Three of 517 patients who had adalimumab and 10 of 261 who had placebo required major Crohn's-related surgery in the 12 months. Rates of surgery were higher but the follow-up is short.

✔ In clinical practice biological agents are best used short term as an agent to induce remission when conventional modalities have been ineffective, with a view to following on with conventional immunosuppression.

Large national datasets have not shown any drop in surgical intervention rates for Crohn's since the introduction of biologicals. Similarly, no alterations in surgical intervention rates were observed in the 1990s when the use of azathioprine and methotrexate became widespread.[27,28]

✔ In the modest proportion of patients who remain in remission on these agents (perhaps 1 in 5), continuing length of treatment is unknown. NICE recommends stopping therapy after 1 year and restarting if disease reactivates. A recent systematic review suggested infliximab may be cost-effective for induction but not maintenance, compared to standard therapy.[29]

Surgery and immunosuppression

With increasing use of immunosuppressive therapies there is concern about the impact of these treatments on perioperative morbidity. Azathioprine does not cause problems in the perioperative period. However, there are now a number of reports that there is an increase in septic complications if surgery is carried out within several months of receiving biological therapy. Rates may be about double that of matched controls.[30] One recent paper however suggests no difference.[31] Use of greater than 20 mg prednisone for more than 6 weeks probably has an impact and steroids should be reduced before surgery if possible.

Prophylaxis against recurrent disease after surgery

After surgery medical treatment can be used to prevent recurrence. Patients often prefer to be medication free when these treatments have limited efficacy. For smokers it remains very important to stop, to halve their rate of recurrence. There was a phase of excitement for using mesalazine a decade ago. With more data the efficacy of this was questioned.

> ✓✓ However, after a series of updated meta-analyses there is probably a 15% difference in clinical recurrence. If used Therapy recommended after small-bowel resection is at a dose of >2 g/day should continue for 2 years starting 2 weeks after surgery.[32]

Many clinicians use azathioprine for what they perceive as 'higher-risk patients' but the data are not strong and the benefit at best modest; in addition, it is hard to define high risk for recurrence except for smoking.[33] The European (ECCO) guidelines have an algorithm for using azathioprine for postoperative prophylaxis, but the UK British Society of Gastroenterology guidelines do not, citing a lack of evidence to support its use in this context.

Other drugs

Antidiarrhoeal medication and anticholinergic agents to relieve colicky pain are useful in mild to moderate disease but should be avoided in severe exacerbations. Non-steroidal anti-inflammatory drugs should also be avoided as they may make the disease worse, and opioids can increase bowel spasm. Cholestyramine is useful for treating bile salt diarrhoea.

Surgery

Development of surgery

Crohn and colleagues initially described radical resection of involved segments of bowel, but high recurrence rates led to a vogue for bypassing affected segments. Frequent complications with the bypassed segments caused a return to resectional surgery.

> ✓ Modern surgery for Crohn's disease involves resecting the least amount of bowel to re-establish satisfactory intestinal function. This is based on the concept that Crohn's is a gut-wide disease and that microscopic disease at the resection margin does not influence recurrence of disease.[34,35]

Furthermore, one small study has shown that asymptomatic endoscopic small-bowel lesions remaining after ileocolic resection did not correlate with clinical recurrence.[36] Although the term 'recurrence of disease' is widely used, a better term is 'recrudescence', implying a new outbreak of already present disease.

It is important to avoid any unnecessary sacrifice of gut as these patients may need resections of further segments for future disease recrudescence. In the move to conservatism, however, it is important not to procrastinate when there is an indication for surgery. When patients were questioned on the timing of their surgery, most would have preferred to have had the procedure 12 months earlier because of the benefits it gave.[37] Low quality-of-life scores with active disease improve to normal when remission is obtained, whether by surgery or medical treatment.[38] When medical treatment does not induce remission or the adverse effects of therapy are unacceptable, in most cases the best course of action for the patient is to proceed to surgery.

Laparoscopic surgery is often feasible. Most surgeons would favour an extracorporeal anastomosis and, where possible, extracorporeal ligation of the mesentery. For ileocolic resections this can usually be accomplished with relative ease, giving the patient a small 3–5 cm midline incision through the umbilicus. Sometimes the incison will need to be lengthened to accommodate a large inflammatory mass. A meta-analysis has shown quicker short-term recovery after laparoscopic ileocolic resection.[39] However, equivalent early discharge can be achieved with enhanced recovery after open surgery.[40] As for laparoscopic colorectal surgery in general, patients usually prefer a laparoscopic approach, with its cosmetic advantage. Perioperative care, as for open surgery, should incorporate the principles of enhanced recovery pathways to optimise the benefits of smaller wounds.

Risk of operation and re-operation

Accurate population figures about patterns of disease and complications are not easy to obtain.

Many of the data presented in this chapter are from specialist centres and these figures may not always apply to the Crohn's population at large. In perhaps the largest population-based cohort reported of 1936 patients from Sweden, the cumulative rate of intestinal resection was 44%, 61% and 71% at 1, 5 and 10 years, respectively, after diagnosis; the subsequent risk of recurrence was 33% and 44% at 5 and 10 years, respectively.[41] In another population-based study involving 210 patients with Crohn's disease at a mean of 11 years from disease onset, 56% required surgery; by life-table analysis the re-operation rate was 25% at 10 years and 56% at 20 years.[42]

In a tertiary referral centre experience of 592 patients with Crohn's disease, 74% required surgery at a median of 13 years, follow-up. The chance of surgery varied with the site of disease and was 65% in those with small-bowel involvement, 58% in those with colonic or anorectal disease, and 91% in those with ileocolic disease.[43] Half of the patients in a tertiary referral centre who have had one operation will require re-operation for further disease with follow-up of more than 10 years.[44,45] Most studies report the annual rate of symptomatic recurrence to be 5–15% and the annual re-operation rate to be 2–10%. Recurrence is at the site of previous disease in the majority, but may be at a new site.[46] For patients presenting to a surgical service, the cumulative chance of a permanent stoma at 20 years is 14% and of a temporary stoma 40%.[47]

Risk factors for recurrence

Many studies have looked at risk factors for recurrence. Recurrence (or recrudescence) can be defined by radiological findings, endoscopic findings, the return of symptoms or the need for further surgery. Most studies have been retrospective, and although some claim to identify risk factors, others report no association for the same risk factor. There is no consistently robust evidence that age of onset of disease, gender, site of disease, number of resections, length of small-bowel resection, proximal margin length, microscopic disease at the resection margin, fistulising vs. obstructive disease, number of sites of disease, presence of granulomas or blood transfusion have an important impact on recurrence.[48,49]

Although a recurrence frequently occurs immediately proximal to the previous anastomosis, there is no consistent or high-quality evidence to date that anastomotic technique (side-to-side, end-to-end, end-to-side, hand-sewn or stapled) affects recurrence.

> ✓✓ In an RCT it has been shown that there is no difference between a stapled side-to-side and a hand-sewn end-to-end anastomosis.[50]
>
> However, it is now clear that continuing to smoke after a surgical resection doubles the risk of recurrence and patients must be urged to stop smoking.[51–53] As above, prophylactic use of 5-ASA has a modest effect to reduce recurrence (as discussed above) by 15%, giving an NNT of 8.

The use of azathioprine is also discussed above.

Principles of surgery for Crohn's disease

Perioperative considerations

Excellent perioperative care is essential for a good outcome in patients with Crohn's disease. As there is always potential for colonic or rectal involvement with small-bowel disease, this should be borne in mind when planning surgery. Deep vein thrombosis prophylaxis using higher prophylactic doses of low-molecular-weight heparin, compression stockings plus or minus intermittent calf compression devices is important as patients with IBD are at higher risk of thrombotic complications.[54] Full postoperative anticoagulation may need to be considered if there is a history of thrombosis. Patients will often be at risk of adrenal suppression and the need for intravenous steroid cover should be considered every time. Before elective surgery, significant malnutrition should be restored by either enteral or parenteral nutrition, all potential electrolyte problems corrected and sepsis controlled. If these goals cannot be achieved, consideration should be given to a temporary stoma rather than an anastomosis. Joint management with a gastroenterologist is an essential principle in the decision-making and hospital care, and psychological well-being needs to be addressed.

Technique

Patients with Crohn's disease can be among the most technically difficult cases a surgeon will face. Compromise of good technique can be unforgiving. Any part of the bowel can be affected or involved with Crohn's disease, so if there is any doubt the patient should be placed in a modified lithotomy or Lloyd–Davies position. For open surgery a midline infraumbilical incision gives good access, is more easily reopened in the future and will not interfere with stomas that may be needed on either side of the abdomen. At each operation a full examination of the bowel should be carried out to stage the disease and the length of remaining and resected bowel measured. In the event of recurrence it is helpful to have marked anastomotic sites with a metal clip. At the first abdominal operation for Crohn's disease, consideration should be given to removing the appendix to prevent future diagnostic problems and confusion.

> ✅ Thick oedematous vascular mesenteric pedicles require special mention. A standard clamp and tie technique may allow a vessel to retract into the mesentery, resulting in a mesenteric haematoma with potential to compromise the blood supply to large segments of bowel. Thick pedicles should be dealt with very carefully and some recommend double-suture ligation. Spillage of gastrointestinal contents must be minimised and controlled, and meticulous haemostasis is important as there may be inevitable loss from oozing, inflamed, raw surfaces. Great care should be taken not to damage or perforate other loops of bowel or other organs in the presence of difficult adhesions and inflammation.

One of the benefits of laparoscopic surgery may be a decrease in adhesion formation, facilitating easier re-operation.

Surgery for small-bowel and ileocolic Crohn's disease

Indications

Surgery for small-bowel Crohn's disease is aimed at treating complications not amenable to medical therapy. Surgical interventions are required for:

1. stenosis causing obstructive symptoms;
2. enterocutaneous or intra-abdominal fistulas to other organs;
3. draining intra-abdominal or retroperitoneal abscesses;

4. controlling acute or chronic bleeding;
5. free perforation.

Of these, obstruction is the most frequent indication.

Gastroduodenal disease

Symptomatic gastroduodenal disease is present in 0.5–4% of patients and is usually associated with disease in other sites. The first and second parts of the duodenum are most commonly involved and the disease often extends into the gastric antrum. Most patients who require surgery require it for problems of stenosis or occasionally bleeding. Often it is difficult at endoscopy to differentiate Crohn's from peptic ulcer disease but a trial of medical ulcer therapy may help. Gastrojejunostomy is the standard procedure for duodenal or pyloric stenosis. Historically, vagotomy was often added to reduce stomal ulceration. Proton-pump inhibitors can now be effective in this role and the potential side-effects of vagotomy avoided.

In selected cases pyloric or duodenal strictureplasty may be considered, and produce better function. Results of a duodenal strictureplasty are variable and complications can be significant.[55,56] Massive acute upper gastrointestinal bleeding is rare, but if endoscopic methods are unsuccessful, bleeding should be controlled by under-running the bleeding vessel with a suture. Balloon dilatation of benign upper gastrointestinal tract strictures is safe, but the limited experience in Crohn's disease suggests dilatation has little long-term benefit. Fistulas involving the duodenum occur in 0.5% of patients with Crohn's disease and generally arise from other diseased segments fistulating into the duodenum. Surgical therapy for these is usually successful and prognosis relates to the severity of disease in the primary segment. Closure of secondary duodenal defects with a jejunal serosal patch or Roux-en-Y limb may be preferable to primary suture.

Ileocolic disease

The cumulative operation rate for patients with distal ileal disease at 5 years from the time of diagnosis is up to 80%. Ileocaecal disease is treated with a limited ileocaecal resection, including a few centimetres of macroscopically normal bowel at each end, and either a side-to-side or end-to-end anastomosis is satisfactory.[50]

After a first operation the re-operation rate at 5 years is 20–25% and at 10 years 35–40%.

Re-operation rates after second and subsequent operations are the same. Further disease is usually on the ileal side of the anastomosis and it is important to stress that this is new disease and does not relate to an inadequate resection margin. Although recurrent disease rates are high and on average a patient will need an operation every 10 years, surgery is highly successful at relieving symptoms and restoring health when disease is refractory to medical treatment.

Balloon dilatation of selected symptomatic ileocolic strictures, usually short anastomotic strictures, is a treatment option with at least short-term benefit in 60–80% (with a risk of perforation of 2–11%) and with longer-term benefit in 40–60%.[57]

Ileal and jejunal multisite disease

If there is isolated small-bowel disease, it is most commonly in the terminal ileum and is usually suited to a limited resection. More extensive disease can produce obstructive strictures throughout the small bowel. In the past, these patients requiring surgery had multiple resections, with a risk of short-bowel syndrome. In an endeavour to maximise conservation of bowel length the concept of strictureplasty was introduced, and this technique is now preferred for all suitable lesions. It is ideally suited to short fibrotic strictures but it may be used for strictures up to 10–15 cm long. Long strictures with active inflammation are usually better managed with resection unless there is concern about bowel length because of previous resections. In most series half the patients having a strictureplasty will also have a segmental resection.

Strictureplasty is carried out using the same methods as used for pyloroplasty. The Heineke–Mikulicz technique is usually used. In a small number of cases with longer strictures where bowel conservation is required, a Finney or a Jaboulay strictureplasty may be used. For even longer narrowed segments a side-to-side isoperistaltic technique described by Michelassi et al. may be used.[58] The diseased bowel is divided at its midpoint, the diseased portion opened on the antimesenteric border, the ends spatulated, and the proximal and distal ends advanced so that the diseased segments lie side by side, where they are anastomosed to each other, trying to ensure stenotic segments are complemented with dilated segments. Despite often long suture lines, results are similar to other strictureplasty techniques. Most candidates for strictureplasty have three or four strictureplasties but in some cases there may be 10–15. To ensure no significant strictures have been missed a Foley catheter can be passed along the small bowel through an enterotomy. The balloon is then inflated to a diameter of 25 mm and pulled back through the bowel, and strictures not easily seen externally will be identified. Alternatively, a marble, steel or wooden ball with a diameter of 25 mm can be traced through the bowel to identify strictures.

Results of strictureplasty have proved it to be a safe and effective technique. Overall morbidity is 10–20%. Postoperative abdominal septic complications occur in 5–10%, and overall 98–99% have symptomatic relief. Postoperative bleeding from a strictureplasty site occurs in about 3% of patients, but this usually resolves with conservative measures. Recurrence requiring re-operation is about 30% at 5 years. Re-operation rates after a strictureplasty are similar whether or not a limited resection is included in the operation. The re-operation rates are similar after first, second and third recurrences requiring surgery. Less than 10% of the strictureplasties themselves restricture, so most of the recurrent disease occurs at new sites.[59–63]

Fistulas and abscesses

Enteric fistulas may affect up to 30% of patients with Crohn's disease and in a referral centre about 40% are internal, 40% external and 20% mixed. Internal fistulas are usually spontaneous and external ones postoperative. Fistula tracts have an associated abscess, at least initially, in most cases. In expert hands surgical repair is successful in closing the fistula in more than 95% of cases, but failure after an attempt at definitive surgery can result in life-threatening morbidity.

Enterocutaneous fistulas and intra-abdominal abscess

Enterocutaneous fistulas in Crohn's disease are a common cause of intestinal failure and patients who develop intestinal failure are best managed in a specialised unit with a multidisciplinary team. Intra-abdominal abscesses that are drained externally will often result in a fistula. When abscesses complicate existing fistulas it is necessary to convert these fistula/abscess complexes into a well-draining fistula. Fistulas, whether postoperative or spontaneous, will drain along the line of least resistance, which is often previous scar tissue from incisions or drain sites.

Management principles

Although spontaneous and postoperative fistulas behave differently, the same management principles apply. The steps are outlined below.

1. Resuscitate the patient, correcting electrolytes and restoring haemoglobin levels. Control sepsis by open or percutaneous drainage and antibiotics; occasionally, exteriorisation of the bowel ends will be required. Attempts at repair and anastomosis should never be made in a patient with significant nutritional compromise or sepsis. Protect the skin from the fistula output by expert application of stoma appliances.

> ✔✔ There has been a vogue for using somatostatin analogues to decrease fistula output but it has shown no benefit.[64] Some may still argue to use it for very high volume proximal fistulas that were not part of this trial.

2. Establish nutrition by either enteral feeding or total parenteral nutrition.
3. Support morale as these patients are often emotionally very fragile. They are upset and angry about what has happened to them and often demoralised and frightened as well. The surgeon should at all times recognise this and be prepared directly to address these issues with the patient.
4. Mobilise the patient. If it is reasonable to anticipate closure with conservative measures, or the fistula is postoperative, wait for at least 6 weeks. If a fistula has not closed by 12 weeks, it probably never will. However, a fistula will generally close spontaneously by 6 weeks unless it:
   (a) originates from a diseased segment of bowel;
   (b) arises from an anastomotic breakdown greater than 50% of the circumference of the bowel;
   (c) has a very short tract or communication between skin and mucosa;
   (d) has bowel obstruction distal to it.
5. Plan a definitive operation with:
   (a) complete enterolysis;
   (b) en bloc resection of the diseased or damaged bowel and the fistula tract with primary anastomosis.

The work-up includes radiological imaging to (i) define the extent of intestinal disease, (ii) exclude any obstructing lesions and (iii) delineate the fistula tracts. Avoid the temptation to carry out earlier and repetitive imaging unless the results will alter management. There are reports of vacuum-assisted dressings and gelfoam embolisation of the fistula tract achieving closure; whether the closure is simply accelerated or whether surgery can be avoided is unknown.

Spontaneous enterocutaneous fistulas

In Crohn's disease this implies that there is a segment of diseased bowel that will require resection. This group generally benefits from earlier surgery for the following reasons:

1. The fistula will not heal spontaneously.
2. There is no concern about a more recent laparotomy making surgery difficult.
3. The bowel perforation occurs slowly and abdominal sepsis is usually localised, lessening the initial systemic insult.
4. Although the aim is to optimise the patient's general and nutritional state before surgery, active Crohn's disease will limit what is achievable.

Postoperative fistulas

In contrast to spontaneous fistulas, these will usually close with conservative measures if there is no downstream obstruction because the previously diseased bowel has been removed. However, the patient is often very ill and can have extensive abdominal contamination, which will usually drain by the incision or a drain site but may require added open or percutaneous drainage. On occasions the abdominal wound may be better left open initially and managed with a vacuum-assisted dressing, although there are some concerns that enterocutaneous fistulas can be induced in this way.

Intra-abdominal fistulas

These fistulas are usually spontaneous. The origin of the fistula, or primary defect, may arise from any segment of diseased bowel but is most commonly from the ileocaecal region. Similar management principles apply to these fistulas as to those described above, but the patients are generally in better health and less symptomatic. About half of the fistulas are diagnosed clinically, the remainder being asymptomatic and discovered at surgery. A fistula should always be suspected between two loops of adherent bowel. The secondary defect can occur in the stomach, duodenum, vagina, fallopian tube, ureter or urethra, but the sigmoid colon, small bowel and bladder are the most common sites. Most high vaginal fistulas are from the rectum but some are from the ileum.

Surgery involves en bloc resection of the primary defect and fistula with primary anastomosis and often only simple closure of the secondary defect, but with the exception of the duodenum.

Spontaneous free perforation in the small bowel or colon

Free perforation occurs in about 1% of patients with Crohn's disease and involves the small bowel and colon with similar frequency. Best results are from operation within 24 hours, with resection of the diseased segment and exteriorisation of the bowel ends.

Surgery for colonic and rectal Crohn's disease

Indications

The most common indication for colonic surgery is intractable disease that is not well controlled with medical therapy. The need for surgery and the choice of operation will depend on the extent of the disease. About one-third will have segmental disease, a third left-sided disease and a third total colitis. Overall a third will have associated perianal disease. After 10 years about half will have had surgery and a quarter will have an ileostomy.[65] Many of those with severe colitis will settle with medical treatment. However, half of these patients will require colectomy within 1–2 years.[66]

Emergency colectomy and colectomy and ileostomy

Acute colectomy for Crohn's disease constitutes a small portion of operations for acute Crohn's disease. The indications for this include toxic dilatation, haemorrhage, perforation and severe colitis not responding to medical therapy. If medical treatment brings a response in 48–72 hours and urgent surgery is avoided, early elective colectomy should

be considered as the chance of recurrent toxic colitis in the following years is significant and symptomatic control is often poor. Severe haemorrhage and perforation both occur in about 1% of patients with colitis. Urgent surgery is usually a total colectomy and ileostomy.

Completion proctectomy, if possible, is usually left until the patient is in good health, but severe haemorrhage can be a problem. The rectal stump, if left initially, will usually need to be removed to control residual symptoms. If the rectum is retained long term there is a risk of cancer and surveillance is required. In selected cases a loop ileostomy can be used to defunction moderately severe colitis. This will allow clinical improvement in over 80%. Half will be able to have the stoma closed initially, but only 20% continue without relapse after medium-term follow-up.[67]

Other than an urgent colectomy or a high-risk patient, colectomy and ileostomy may be used in the presence of substantial anorectal disease when there is concern about perineal wound healing. After colectomy with a period of maximal medical therapy the perianal disease may settle, facilitating better results with proctectomy, but doubt remains as to whether this is effective.

Segmental colectomy

Segmental colectomy is appropriate for a symptomatic stricture. In some cases it may be required to exclude cancer. The pattern of recurrence is similar to that seen with segmental small-bowel disease (Table 10.2). A meta-analysis of case series has compared segmental colectomy to colectomy and ileorectal anastomosis. If there were multiple colonic segments involved recurrence was earlier with segmental resections, but there was no difference in permanent stoma rates. Treatment choices should be guided by the extent of colonic disease.[68]

Total colectomy and ileorectal anastomosis

In patients needing a colectomy for Crohn's colitis, 25% have rectal sparing, with a normally functioning rectum and sphincter mechanism. These patients are suitable for an ileorectal anastomosis. Some patients with a mild proctitis and/or mild perianal disease may even achieve reasonable function. With more severe disease colectomy and ileorectal anastomosis may be done in two stages.

Table 10.2 • Long-term outcome of patients with segmental colonic Crohn's disease who have a segmental resection

Reference	n	Mean follow-up (years)	Clinical recurrence (%)	Re-operation rate at 10 years (%)	Permanent stoma avoided (%)
Allan et al.[91]	36	–	–	66	–
Makowiec et al.[92]	142	12	60	32	88
Prabhakar et al.[93]	48	14	77	33	86
Polle et al.[94]	91	8.3	–	33 (at mean 8.3 years)	56*

The series by Prabhakar et al. includes 10 patients who had the majority of their colon removed.
*Some patients had a stoma formed after segmental resection.

Clinical recurrence is reported in 50% at 10 years. Of those who lose their ileorectal anastomosis, many will still have obtained 4–5 years of useful function, and this can be particularly important if a stoma is deferred for teenage and young adult years. At 10 years over half will retain their rectum. The development of perianal disease usually leads to proctectomy.

Panproctocolectomy

This operation is the gold standard for treating colorectal disease and is associated with the lowest recurrence rate, albeit at the price of a stoma. Recurrence usually involves small-bowel disease, but it can be from perineal Crohn's after removal of the anorectum. Recurrence rates after panproctocolectomy are of the order of 15–25% at 10 years. Patients report a good quality of life after colectomy and ileostomy for disease confined to the colon.[44] In addition, a portion will need revisional surgery for ileostomy complications.[47]

Removal of the rectum requires particular care not to damage the pelvic nerves, and a technique of intersphincteric and perimuscular dissection (close to the rectal wall) of the rectum has been used. As there is no natural anatomical plane, perimuscular dissection is more vascular and time-consuming than dissection in the mesorectal plane. It is probably safe for the specialist to carry out most of the dissection in the mesorectal plane, perhaps coming inside the mesorectal plane at the critical points, anteriorly and laterally in relation to the parasympathetic nerves. Whichever technique is preferred, the surgeon has to be prepared to modify this to take account of severe perineal or perirectal disease that can make the dissection very difficult. The perineal wound is best treated with primary closure and suction drainage (if desired) from above. Delayed wound healing is frequently a problem, although 60–80% will have uncomplicated healing. Up to 30% will take 4–6 months to heal completely, but vacuum-assisted closure systems can now reduce this in many cases. About 10% will have longer-term problems with perineal sinuses, most of which settle with further surgical procedures. These may include several attempts at scraping the sinus tract to remove necrotic tissue and freshen the walls, and excluding an enteroperineal fistula (**Fig. 10.5**) and cutaneous Crohn's disease. In troublesome cases of active perineal disease after proctectomy, there is a role for wide excision and a vertical rectus abdominis transpelvic musculocutaneous flap reconstruction.

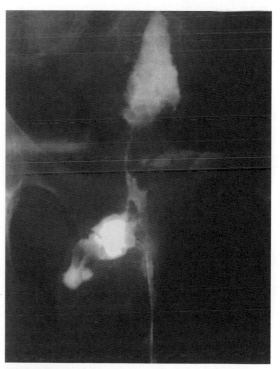

Figure 10.5 • Sinogram examination demonstrating an enteroperineal fistula.

Disappointingly, in a small number the flap of normal skin can also develop granulomatous cutaneous Crohn's disease.

Restorative proctocolectomy

Crohn's disease has traditionally been regarded as a contraindication for an ileal pouch because of the risk of developing small-bowel or perianal disease that will lead to pouch excision. Now some surgeons are prepared to offer an ileal pouch to a well-informed patient who has isolated colonic Crohn's and requires a proctocolectomy. Other surgeons still regard Crohn's as an absolute contraindication.[32] The risk of pouch failure (and excision) is in the range of 10–45%, and is higher than for ulcerative colitis. However, for Crohn's disease at other sites re-operation rates of 50% at 10 years are acceptable, and small-bowel recurrence probably involves a similar sacrifice of bowel to that of excising a pouch.[69,70] The group in Paris who controversially promoted pouches in selected patients with colorectal Crohn's disease have reported 10-year follow-up documenting Crohn's-related events in 35%, with 10% requiring pouch excision.[71]

Crohn's colitis and cancer

With extensive Crohn's colitis it is now accepted that there is an increased risk of colorectal cancer similar to ulcerative colitis.[72–74] Field change in the colonic mucosa with areas of dysplasia is observed as in ulcerative colitis.[75] Surveillance colonoscopy should be offered to patients with Crohn's colitis and this is probably best done with dye spray and targeted biopsies. Particular care is needed in the presence of colonic strictures, which should always be regarded as malignant until proven otherwise; this may entail a resection to make the diagnosis.

Perianal disease

Perianal disease should be considered as a separate entity or phenotype of Crohn's disease. It is associated with more severe luminal disease and earlier age of onset. Some 30–70% of patients with Crohn's disease will have a degree of involvement of the anal canal, ranging from minor skin tags to severe disease. However, only a much smaller proportion will need surgical intervention for anal disease.[76] In different cohorts perianal disease has been reported either as more frequent in association with colonic disease or rectal disease or ileal disease.[77,78] A small percentage of patients have their initial presentation with anal disease, but over time half of these will develop disease at other intestinal sites. The activity of anal disease is unrelated to more proximal disease activity.

Generally, the prognosis is good, with only 5–10% of patients with perianal Crohn's requiring a proctectomy. If rectal disease is also present, proctectomy will be needed in up to twice this number. Fissures or fistulas may be asymptomatic, and after some years about half will have healed spontaneously and a further 20–30% will heal after a surgical procedure. Carcinoma is a rare but recognised complication, and hidradenitis suppurativa may coexist. The benign course of most perianal lesions caused by an incurable disease has led many (but not all) surgeons to a general policy of conservative treatment. Carefully selected cases without active disease can benefit from active surgical management. Preserving a functioning sphincter must remain a paramount concern in these patients. Box 10.3 outlines a classification of lesions described by Hughes and Taylor.[79] This classification is useful to help understand the aetiology and development of anal lesions. In practice lesions are usually described as

---

Box 10.3 • Hughes' classification of perianal lesions in Crohn's disease

Primary lesions
- Anal fissure
- Ulcerated oedematous pile
- Cavitating ulcer
- Aggressive ulceration

Secondary lesions
- Skin tags
- Anal/rectal stricture
- Perianal abscess/fistula
- Anovaginal/rectovaginal fistula
- Carcinoma

Incidental lesions
- Piles
- Perianal abscess or fistula
- Skin tags
- Cryptitis
- Hidradenitis suppurativa

From Hughes LE, Taylor BA. Perianal lesions in Crohn's disease. In: Allan R, Keighley M, Alexander-Williams J et al. (eds) Inflammatory bowel disease, 2nd edn. Edinburgh: Churchill Livingstone, 1990; pp. 351–61. With permission from Churchill Livingstone.

they are observed. Surgery is most frequently indicated for secondary and incidental lesions.

Investigation

Careful examination, often under anaesthesia, is the most useful investigation and often an essential part of the work-up. In complicated cases, MRI and/or endoanal ultrasound in combination with examination under anaesthesia allow accurate identification of obscure tracts and collections.[80]

Medical treatment

Ciprofloxacin, metronidazole, azathioprine, infliximab and adalimumab are probably effective at controlling or improving perianal disease (see above), but most of the claims in the literature are anecdotal and the impact of medical therapy on reducing complications or the need for surgery is not known. Case series suggest that while the initial response rate is reasonable, the long-term closure rate is little improved by adding infliximab to established medical and surgical treatment.[81] In those with active disease, however, it seems reasonable to employ any measure that is likely to help the symptomatic patient and avert proctectomy. Ciprofloxacin or metronidazole are often used for septic problems and should be the first-line medical treatment. Ciprofloxacin is better tolerated but more expensive.

Anal fissure

Most fissures are in the midline posteriorly, one-third are multiple and two-thirds are asymptomatic. Anal canal pressures are similar to those in controls and 50–70% heal with conservative or concurrent medical therapy.[82] Initially a conservative approach should be adopted for chronic fissures. Treatment options include topical glyceryl trinitrate and diltiazem, and botulinum toxin injection. All efforts should be made to conserve the internal anal sphincter in Crohn's disease. However, if all else fails and the patient has significant symptoms, the fissure will usually heal after a lateral anal sphincterotomy without compromising continence. This should probably not be done in the presence of active proctitis. Healing the fissure may prevent future abscesses and fistulas arising from its base.[83]

Abscesses

Abscesses may arise from deep cavitating ulcers or distorted anal glands (**Fig. 10.6**). The first sign of an abscess is often increasing perianal pain. An MRI can confirm clinical suspicion if little is obvious on initial

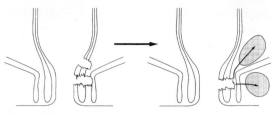

Figure 10.6 • Pathogenesis of anal suppurative disease. Deep cavitating ulcers give rise to extrasphincteric and supralevator abscesses.

examination. Occasionally, abscesses may be above the levator muscles. Examination under anaesthesia will identify the problem, in combination with MRI for difficult cases. Collections should be drained by removing a small area of overlying skin. In larger cavities it may be useful to insert a mushroom catheter to facilitate drainage and irrigation. It is usually inadvisable to lay open a primary tract at this stage.

Anal fistulas

Fistulous disease may range from an incidental fistula to a 'watering-can' perineum. If a fistula has been judged incidental or there is no active inflammation in the perianal region or rectum it is reasonable to progress to a standard surgical procedure. If there is active disease no more than drainage and seton insertion should be considered until the disease is in remission, as healing is likely to be poor and medical therapy should be implemented. Once acute inflammatory disease is controlled or absent, options to eliminate the fistula may be considered. Sphincter preservation is particularly important. A lay open or fistulotomy may be done if the tract is superficial. If the fistula is higher and transphincteric a rectal advancement flap or ligation of intersphincteric tract (LIFT) procedure are options, giving a success rate as high as 50–70% at 2–3 years.[76,84] Later recurrence after initial success is not uncommon. Bovine collagen fistula plugs are likely to be more successful with single tracts than complex fistulas and seem to work in about 50% of cases where applied.[85] A covering stoma is probably not of benefit for the majority of cases. In complicated fistulas or in the presence of active inflammation, the aim is to establish adequate drainage and this is best done with a loose seton, which may be left long term with a good functional result. Supralevator fistulas are a difficult problem and usually involve perforating disease from the rectum or even more proximal bowel. Again, the primary aim is drainage and identification of the internal origin, but these cases are more likely to need a proctectomy. Fistulas arising from deep cavitating ulcers are difficult to manage and proctectomy is often unavoidable in the long term.

Rectovaginal fistulas

The distressing problem of passing faeces or wind per vaginam means that these fistulas usually require surgical therapy. They occur in 10% of women presenting to specialist centres with Crohn's disease. In one series 37% had a proctectomy, but only one-third of these were primarily for the rectovaginal fistula.[86] They are more frequently associated with colon rather than small-bowel disease. The fistula, if low, will usually be identified on examination that may need to be done under anaesthesia with initial insertion of a seton to control sepsis. An MRI will give information about surrounding sepsis and may identify the fistula. For difficult high fistulas a vaginogram may be used.

Medical therapy should be optimised. It is doubtful whether biologicals are helpful to close the fistula. If the disease is quiescent a variety of surgical approaches can be employed. Depending on the condition of local tissues, options include a rectal advancement flap, anocutaneous advancement flaps, vaginal flaps, a Martius graft, a gracilis interposition or sphincteroplasty.[87,88] With persistence and possibly more than one procedure, closure rates of over 50% may be a reasonable expectation. A temporary stoma may be considered for complex repairs.

Defunctioning ileostomy for perianal disease

A temporary ileostomy has a role in providing symptomatic relief to the desperate patient while more definitive treatment options are discussed or tried. In this situation, the majority will experience symptomatic improvement but with longer follow-up only a small number have intestinal continuity restored and following this an even smaller number remain in clinical remission.[67]

Long-term complications of perianal disease

Longer-term complications of perianal Crohn's disease may include rectal or anal strictures and incontinence due to fibrosis and sphincter damage. Symptomatic strictures should be gently dilated to not more than 20 mm, remembering that with an impaired sphincter there is a risk of precipitating or worsening incontinence. About half the patients who develop an anal or rectal stricture will require proctectomy.[89]

Prognosis

Standardised mortality rates are higher for patients with Crohn's disease, with a ratio of 1.4. This particularly relates to patients who have the onset of their disease before the age of 20 years, and the risk is particularly high early in the course of the disease, although the absolute numbers dying remain small. Causes of death include sepsis, perioperative complications, electrolyte disturbances and gastrointestinal tract cancers.[8]

Quality-of-life issues are important to these patients and they express concerns over energy levels, fear of surgery and body image. Often, loss of energy and malaise contribute more to functional disability than specific gastrointestinal symptoms. In terms of academic success and advancement, patients are not hampered by the disease, and employment rates are the same as for matched healthy controls. However, patients frequently express impairment of employment, recreation, and interpersonal and sexual relationships. Most patients continue to function optimistically and adapt successfully. However, Crohn's patients are twice as likely to suffer anxiety and depression disorders and are more likely to require treatment with psychotropic drugs. Disease relapses produce considerable stress, and psychological support from counsellors, psychiatrists, non-medical and patient support groups should be utilised.[90]

Key points

- Patients with Crohn's disease usually enjoy reasonable health punctuated by periods of increased disease activity, initially managed medically.
- Many patients will require surgery at some stage.
- Multidisciplinary management has taken on increased importance now that biological treatments are well established. Sensible, safe and cost-effective management is essential. Surgical input into medical treatment decisions is paramount.

- Surgery is restricted to dealing with troublesome segments that cannot be managed medically.
- Surgery for small-bowel disease is usually necessary because of complications of disease such as strictures and fistulas.
- Surgery for large-bowel disease is usually necessary because of inability of medical treatment to control symptoms.
- Severe disease in young people can be life threatening and expert surgical care is required.

References

1. Carbonnel F, Jantchou P, Monnet E, et al. Environmental risk factors in Crohn's disease and ulcerative colitis: an update. Gastroentérol Clin Biol 2009;33(Suppl. 3(0)):S145–57.

2. Sartor RB. Does Mycobacterium avium subspecies paratuberculosis cause Crohn's disease? Gut 2005;54(7):896–8.

3. Nunes T, Fiorino G, Danese S, et al. Familial aggregation in inflammatory bowel disease: is it genes or environment? World J Gastroenterol 2011;17(22):2715–22.

4. Franke A, McGovern DPB, Barrett JC, et al. Genome-wide meta-analysis increases to 71 the number of confirmed Crohn's disease susceptibility loci. Nat Genet 2010;42(12):1118–25.

5. Büning C, Genschel J, Bühner S, et al. Mutations in the NOD2/CARD15 gene in Crohn's disease are associated with ileocecal resection and are a risk factor for reoperation. Aliment Pharmacol Ther 2004;19(10):1073–8.

6. Baumgart DC, Carding SR. Inflammatory bowel disease: cause and immunobiology. Lancet 2007;369(9573):1627–40.

7. Satsangi J, Sutherland LR, editors. Inflammatory bowel diseases. Elsivier; 2003.

8. Peyrin-Biroulet L, Loftus Jr EV, Colombel J-F, et al. Long-term complications, extraintestinal manifestations, and mortality in adult Crohn's disease in population-based cohorts. Inflamm Bowel Dis 2011;17(1):471–8.

9. Orchard T, Goldin R, Tekkis P, et al. Part II: Complications and comorbidities – Chapter 8: Fertility and inflammatory bowel disease. Oxford: Clinical Publishing, an imprint of Atlas Medical Publishing Ltd; 2011. p. 73–7.

10. Nikolaus S, Schreiber S. Diagnostics of inflammatory bowel disease. Gastroenterology 2007;133(5):1670–89.

11. Lewis JD. The utility of biomarkers in the diagnosis and therapy of inflammatory bowel disease. Gastroenterology 2011;140(6):1817–26.e2.

12. Mowat C, Cole A, Windsor A, et al. Guidelines for the management of inflammatory bowel disease in adults. Gut 2011;60(5):571–607.
   IBD section of the British Society of Gastroenterology UK guidelines.

13. Ford AC, Khan KJ, Talley NJ, et al. 5-Aminosalicylates prevent relapse of Crohn's disease after surgically induced remission: systematic review and meta-analysis. Am J Gastroenterol 2011;106(3):413–20.
   Most recent meta-analysis of 5-ASA to prevent recurrence after surgery showing an NNT of 10

14. Benchimol EI, Seow CH, Otley AR, et al. Budesonide for maintenance of remission in Crohn's disease. Cochrane Database Syst Rev 2009;(1):CD002913.

15. Thomsen O, Cortot A, Jewell D, et al. A comparison of budesonide and mesalamine for active Crohn's disease. N Engl J Med 1998;339:370–4.
   Budesonide is twice as effective as mesalamine in treating active Crohn's, with the benefit of fewer side-effects than systemic steroids.

16. Hellers G, Cortot A, Jewell D, et al. Oral budesonide for prevention of postsurgical recurrence in Crohn's disease. Gastroenterology 1999;116:294–300.
   Budesonide does not have a role in prophylaxis after surgery.

17. Akobeng AK, Thomas AG. Enteral nutrition for maintenance of remission in Crohn's disease. Cochrane Database Syst Rev 2007;(3):CD005984.

18. El-Matary W. Enteral nutrition as a primary therapy of Crohn's disease: the pediatric perspective. Nutr Clin Pract 2009;24(1):91–7.

19. Zabala-Fernandez W, Barreiro-de Acosta M, Echarri A, et al. A pharmacogenetics study of TPMT and ITPA genes detects a relationship with side effects and clinical response in patients with inflammatory bowel disease receiving azathioprine. J Gastrointestin Liver Dis 2011;20(3):247–53.

20. Elton EHS. Review article: the medical management of Crohn's disease. Aliment Pharmacol Ther 1996;10:1–22.
   A review article that includes data on the effect of parenteral and enteral nutrition that are as effective as steroids at inducing remission, but the effect ends as soon as normal diet is reintroduced.

21. Targan SR, Hanauer SB, van Deventer SJ, et al. A short-term study of chimeric monoclonal antibody cA2 to tumor necrosis factor alpha for Crohn's disease. Crohn's Disease cA2 Study Group. N Engl J Med 1997;337:1029–35.
   The first RCT of biological agents in Crohn's disease demonstrating moderate efficacy in inducing remisson.

22. Hanauer SB, Feagan BG, Lichtenstein GR, et al. Maintenance infliximab for Crohn's disease: the ACCENT I randomised trial. Lancet 2002;359(9317):1541–9.
Many centres took part with small numbers each. There is drug company representation on the writing committee. Infliximab is moderately effective at inducing remission but at 12 months is only a little better than placebo. The data need to be interpreted carefully; infliximab is very expensive, has a poor cost–benefit ratio, and there are concerns about serious long-term side-effects. On the other hand, there are many anecdotes of dramatic clinical responses when other measures have failed. It has a role to induce remission in refractory cases.

23. Sands BE, Anderson FH, Bernstein CN, et al. Infliximab maintenance therapy for fistulizing Crohn's disease. N Engl J Med 2004;350(9):876–85.
This study looks at the role of infliximab for fistulating Crohn's disease and is a similar design to ACCENT I. Similar comments apply as for ACCENT I above.

24. Hanauer SB, Sandborn WJ, Rutgeerts P, et al. Human anti-tumor necrosis factor monoclonal antibody (adalimumab) in Crohn's disease: the CLASSIC-I trial. Gastroenterology 2006;130(2):323–33.
The first RCT to establish the efficacy of induction therapy with adalimumab.

25. Sandborn WJ, Hanauer SB, Rutgeerts P, et al. Adalimumab for maintenance treatment of Crohn's disease: results of the CLASSIC II trial. Gut 2007;56(9):1232–9.
The first RCT to demonstrate the efficacy of adalimumab for maintenance of remission out to 56 weeks after successful induction therapy with adalimumab in CLASSIC I.

26. Colombel JF, Sandborn WJ, Rutgeerts P, et al. Adalimumab for maintenance of clinical response and remission in patients with Crohn's disease: the CHARM trial. Gastroenterology 2007;132(1):52–65.
This RCT looked at the frequency of dosing for maintenance of remission, every other week (40%) versus every week (47%) versus placebo (17%) at 56 weeks.

27. Jones DW, Finlayson SRG. Trends in surgery for Crohn's disease in the era of infliximab. Ann Surg 2010;252(2):307–12.

28. Cosnes J, Nion-Larmurier I, Beaugerie L, et al. Impact of the increasing use of immunosuppressants in Crohn's disease on the need for intestinal surgery. Gut 2005;54(2):237–41.

29. Dretzke J, Edlin R, Round J, et al. A systematic review and economic evaluation of the use of tumour necrosis factor-alpha (TNF-alpha) inhibitors, adalimumab and infliximab, for Crohn's disease. Health Technol Assess 2011;15(6):1–244.

30. Appau K, Fazio V, Shen B, et al. Use of infliximab within 3 months of ileocolonic resection is associated with adverse postoperative outcomes in Crohn's patients. J Gastrointest Surg 2008;12(10):1738–44.

31. Waterman M, Xu W, Dinani A, Steinhart AH, Croitoru K, Nguyen GC, et al. Preoperative biological therapy and short-term outcomes of abdominal surgery in patients with inflammatory bowel disease. Gut 2013;62(3):387–94.

32. Travis SP, Stange EF, Lemann M, et al. European evidence based consensus on the diagnosis and management of Crohn's disease: current management. Gut 2006;55(Suppl. 1):i16–35.
European Crohn's and Colitis Organisation Consensus Development Conference series. Evidence-based consensus statement that includes opinions of experts both for and against the various recommendations.

33. Peyrin-Biroulet L, Deltenre P, Ardizzone S, et al. Azathioprine and 6-mercaptopurine for the prevention of postoperative recurrence in Crohn's disease: a meta-analysis. Am J Gastroenterol 2009;104(8):2089–96.
Meta-analysis that outlines the modest efficacy of these drugs to prevent postoperative recurrence.

34. Fazio VW, Marchetti F, Church M, et al. Effect of resection margins on the recurrence of Crohn's disease in the small bowel. A randomized controlled trial. Ann Surg 1996;224:563–71.
From restrospective reviews and now a small randomised trial it seems highly likely microscopic involvement of resection margin does not increase recurrence rates.

35. McLeod RS. Resection margins and recurrent Crohn's disease. Hepatogastroenterology 1990;37(1):63–6.

36. Klein O, Colombel JF, Lescut D, et al. Remaining small bowel endoscopic lesions at surgery have no influence on early anastomotic recurrences in Crohn's disease. Am J Gastroenterol 1995;90(11): 1949–52.

37. Scott NA, Hughes LE. Timing of ileocolonic resection for symptomatic Crohn's disease – the patient's view. Gut 1994;35(5):656–7.

38. Thirlby RC, Land JC, Fenster LF, et al. Effect of surgery on health related quality of life in patients with inflammatory bowel disease: a prospective study. Arch Surg 1998;133:826–32.

39. Tilney HS, Constantinides VA, Heriot AG, et al. Comparison of laparoscopic and open ileocecal resection for Crohn's disease: a metaanalysis. Surg Endosc 2006;20(7):1036–44.

40. Andersen J, Kehlet H. Fast track open ileo-colic resections for Crohn's disease. Colorectal Dis 2005;7(4):394–7.

41. Bernell O, Lapidus A, Hellers G. Risk factors for surgery and postoperative recurrence in Crohn's disease. Ann Surg 2000;231:38–45.

42. Shivananda S, Hordijk ML, Pena AS, et al. Crohn's disease: risk of recurrence and reoperation in a defined population. Gut 1989;30(7):990–5.

43. Farmer RG, Whelan G, Fazio VW. Long-term follow-up of patients with Crohn's disease. Relationship between the clinical pattern and prognosis. Gastroenterology 1985;88(6):1818–25.

44. Halme LE. Results of surgical treatment of patients with Crohn's disease. Ann Chir Gynaecol 1992;81(3):277–83.

45. Nordgren SR, Fasth SB, Oresland TO, et al. Long-term follow-up in Crohn's disease. Mortality, morbidity, and functional status. Scand J Gastroenterol 1994;29(12):1122–8.

46. Fichera A, Lovadina S, Rubin M, et al. Patterns and operative treatment of recurrent Crohn's disease: a prospective longitudinal study. Surgery 2006;140(4):649–54.

47. Post S, Herfarth CH, Schumacher H, et al. Experience with ileostomy and colostomy in Crohn's disease. Br J Surg 1995;82(12):1629–33.

48. Borley NR, Mortensen NJ, Jewell DP. Preventing postoperative recurrence of Crohn's disease. Br J Surg 1997;84:1493–502.

49. Yamamoto T. Factors affecting recurrence after surgery for Crohn's disease. World J Gastroenterol 2005;11(26):3971–9.

50. McLeod RS, Wolff BG, Ross S, et al., Investigators of the CT. Recurrence of Crohn's disease after ileocolic resection is not affected by anastomotic type: results of a multicenter, randomized, controlled trial. Dis Colon Rectum 2009;52(5):919–27.
Good-quality RCT to finally address the question about technique for ileocolic anastomosis.

51. Cottone M, Rosselli M, Orlando A, et al. Smoking habits and recurrence in Crohn's disease. Gastroenterology 1994;106:643–8.
A study of 182 patients looking for risk factors for recurrence of Crohn's after surgical resection. The study found that smoking doubles your risk of recurrence of Crohn's disease.

52. Moskovitz D, McLeod RS, Greenberg GR, et al. Operative and environmental risk factors for recurrence of Crohn's disease. Int J Colorectal Dis 1999;14:224–6.
A retrospective study of 92 patients that confirms the findings of other studies that show a doubling of recurrence rate for those who continue to smoke after surgical resection.

53. Sutherland LR, Ramcharan S, Bryant H, et al. Effect of cigarette smoking on recurrence of Crohn's disease. Gastroenterology 1990;98:1123–8.
The first of a number of papers that have shown the powerful effect of smoking on recurrence. Evidence is probably level 3 but the strength of the effect is such that there is little doubt.

54. Hudson M, Chitolie A, Hutton RA, et al. Thrombotic vascular risk factors in inflammatory bowel disease. Gut 1996;38:733–7.

55. Worsey MJ, Hull T, Ryland L, et al. Stricturoplasty is an effective operation in the operative management of duodenal Crohn's. Dis Colon Rectum 1999;42:596–600.

56. Yamamoto T, Bain IM, Connolly AB, et al. Outcome of stricturoplasty for duodenal Crohn's disease. Br J Surg 1999;86:259–62.

57. Sabate JM, Villarejo J, Bouhnik Y, et al. Hydrostatic balloon dilatation of Crohn's strictures. Aliment Pharmacol Ther 2003;18(4):409–13.

58. Michelassi F, Taschieri A, Tonelli F, et al. An international, multicenter, prospective, observational study of the side-to-side isoperistaltic strictureplasty in Crohn's disease. Dis Colon Rectum 2007;50(3):277–84.
A large multicentre collection of cases of this advanced strictureplasty technique demonstrating safety and efficacy.

59. Fearnhead NS, Chowdhury R, Box B, et al. Long-term follow-up of strictureplasty for Crohn's disease. Br J Surg 2006;93(4):475–82.

60. Ozuner G, Fazio VW, Lavery IC, et al. How safe is strictureplasty in the management of Crohn's disease? Am J Surg 1996;171(1):57–60.

61. Serra J, Cohen Z, McLeod RS. Natural history of strictureplasty in Crohn's disease: 9-year experience. Can J Surg 1995;38(6):481–5.

62. Yamamoto T, Bain IM, Allan RN, et al. An audit of strictureplasty for small-bowel Crohn's disease. Dis Colon Rectum 1999;42:797–803.

63. Yamamoto T, Fazio VW, Tekkis PP. Safety and efficacy of strictureplasty for Crohn's disease: a systematic review and meta-analysis. Dis Colon Rectum 2007;50(11):1968–86.

64. Scott NA, Finnegan S, Irving MH. Octreotide and postoperative enterocutaneous fistulae: a controlled prospective study. Acta Gastroenterol Belg 1993;56(3–4):266–70.
Octreotide is not helpful in closing enterocutaneous fistula. There still may be a role, though, to help manage high output fistulas. This subgroup is not specifically addressed by the study.

65. Lapidus A, Bernell O, Hellers G, et al. Clinical course of colorectal Crohn's disease, a 35 year follow-up study of 507 patients. Gastroenterology 1998;114:1151–60.

66. Kornbluth A, Marion JF, Salomon P, et al. How effective is current medical therapy for severe ulcerative and Crohn's colitis? An analytic review of selected trials. J Clin Gastroenterol 1995;20(4):280–4.

67. Edwards CM, George BD, Jewell DP, et al. Role of a defunctioning stoma in the management of large bowel Crohn's disease. Br J Surg 2000;87(8):1063–6.

68. Tekkis PP, Purkayastha S, Lanitis S, et al. A comparison of segmental vs subtotal/total colectomy for colonic Crohn's disease: a meta-analysis. Colorectal Dis 2006;8(2):82–90.

69. Panis P, Poupard B, Neneth J, et al. Ileal pouch–anal anastomosis for Crohn's disease. Lancet 1996;347:854–7.

70. Phillips RKS. Ileal pouch–anal anastomosis for Crohn's disease. Gut 1998;43:303–8.

71. Regimbeau JM, Panis Y, Pocard M, et al. Long-term results of ileal pouch–anal anastomosis for colorectal Crohn's disease. Dis Colon Rectum 2001;44(6):769–78.

72. Gillen CD, Walmsley RS, Prior P, et al. Ulcerative colitis and Crohn's disease: a comparison of the colorectal cancer risk in extensive colitis. Gut 1994;35(11):1590–2.

73. Maykel JA, Hagerman G, Mellgren AF, et al. Crohn's colitis: the incidence of dysplasia and adenocarcinoma in surgical patients. Dis Colon Rectum 2006;49(7):950–7.

74. Collins PD, Mpofu C, Watson AJ, et al. Strategies for detecting colon cancer and/or dysplasia in patients with inflammatory bowel disease. Cochrane Database Syst Rev 2006;(2):CD000279.

75. Sigel JE, Petras RE, Lashner BA, et al. Intestinal adenocarcinoma in Crohn's disease: a report of 30 cases with a focus on coexisting dysplasia. Am J Surg Pathol 1999;23:651–5.

76. Sangwan YP, Schoetz Jr DJ, Murray JJ, et al. Perianal Crohn's disease. Results of local surgical treatment. Dis Colon Rectum 1996;39(5):529–35.

77. Halme LA, Sainio P. Factors related to frequency, type and outcome of anal fistulas in Crohn's disease. Dis Colon Rectum 1995;38(1):55–9.

78. Eglinton T, Reilly M, Chang C, et al. Ileal disease is associated with surgery for perianal disease in a population-based Crohn's disease cohort. Br J Surg 2010;97(7):1103–9.

79. Hughes LE, Taylor BA. Perianal lesions in Crohn's disease. In: Allan R, Keighley M, Alexander-Williams J, Hawkins C, editors. Inflammatory bowel disease. 2nd ed. Edinburgh: Churchill Livingstone; 1990. p. 351–61.

80. Schwartz DA, Wiersema MJ, Dudiak KM, et al. A comparison of endoscopic ultrasound, magnetic resonance imaging, and exam under anesthesia for evaluation of Crohn's perianal fistulas. Gastroenterology 2001;121(5):1064–72.

81. Hyder SA, Travis SP, Jewell DP, et al. Fistulating anal Crohn's disease: results of combined surgical and infliximab treatment. Dis Colon Rectum 2006;49(12):1837–41.

82. Sweeney JL, Ritchie JK, Nicholls RJ. Anal fissure in Crohn's disease. Br J Surg 1988;75(1):56–7.

83. Fleshner PR, Schoetz Jr DJ, Roberts PL, et al. Anal fissure in Crohn's disease: a plea for aggressive management. Dis Colon Rectum 1995;38(11):1137–43.

84. Sonoda T, Hull T, Piedmonte MR, et al. Outcomes of primary repair of anorectal and rectovaginal fistulas using the endorectal advancement flap. Dis Colon Rectum 2002;45(12):1622–8.

85. O'Riordan JM, Datta I, Johnston C, et al. A systematic review of the anal fistula plug for patients with Crohn's and non-Crohn's related fistula-in-ano. Dis Colon Rectum 2012;55(3):351–8.

86. Radcliffe AG, Ritchie JK, Hawley PR, et al. Anovaginal and rectovaginal fistulas in Crohn's disease. Dis Colon Rectum 1988;31(2):94–9.

87. Andreani SM, Dang HH, Grondona P, et al. Rectovaginal fistula in Crohn's disease. Dis Colon Rectum 2007;50(12):2215–22.

88. Songne K, Scotte M, Lubrano J, et al. Treatment of anovaginal or rectovaginal fistulas with modified Martius graft. Colorectal Dis 2007;9(7):653–6.

89. Linares L, Moreira LF, Andrews H, et al. Natural history and treatment of anorectal strictures complicating Crohn's disease. Br J Surg 1988;75(7):653–5.

90. Loftus Jr EV, Guerin A, Yu AP, et al. Increased risks of developing anxiety and depression in young patients with Crohn's disease. Am J Gastroenterol 2011;106(9):1670–7.

91. Allan A, Andrews H, Hilton CJ, et al. Segmental colonic resection is an appropriate operation for short skip lesions due to Crohn's disease in the colon. World J Surg 1989;13(5):611–4.

92. Makowiec F, Paczulla D, Schmidtke C, et al. Crohn's colitis: segmental resection or colectomy. Gastroenterology 1996;110:A1402.

93. Prabhakar LP, Laramee C, Nelson H, et al. Avoiding a stoma: the role of segmental colectomy in Crohn's colitis. Dis Colon Rectum 1997;40:71–8.

94. Polle SW, Slors JF, Weverling GJ, et al. Recurrence after segmental resection for colonic Crohn's disease. Br J Surg 2005;92(9):1143–9.

11

Incontinence

Paul-Antoine Lehur
Mark T.C. Wong

Introduction

Faecal incontinence (FI), the involuntary loss of solid or liquid stool, is a debilitating condition with potentially devastating consequences on both the physical and psychosocial well-being of afflicted individuals. Although surveys of the general adult population have estimated the prevalence of FI to be between 1% and 18%,[1,2] the majority of sufferers do not seek medical help due to embarrassment and social stigmatisation.[3,4] As a result, the condition remains largely undiagnosed.

It is estimated that FI affects over half a million adults in the UK. This symptom/functional disorder has very profound negative consequences for the patient. Fear of embarrassment, even at worst public humiliation, can impose major restrictions on individuals and their families.[3]

> ✅ FI occurs when a person loses the ability to control their anal sphincter and bowel movements, resulting in leakage of faeces.

Aetiology

The ability to maintain continence to stool relies on a coordinated interplay of several factors, including stool consistency, rectal capacity and compliance, intact neural pathways, normal anal sphincter and pelvic floor function, and normal anorectal sensation. Deficiencies or failures in any component can lead to incontinence. In many cases, the aetiology of FI is multifactorial and it is impossible to ascertain the relative contribution of each factor, further adding to the complexity of managing this condition.[5]

FI is more commonly an acquired disorder, so finding a cause is the first step to manage the disorder adequately (**Fig. 11.1**).

Faecal loading or impaction is a major contributor for FI in an elderly, frail population. A rectum impacted with faeces can result in 'overflow incontinence'. It is easily diagnosed on digital examination. A rectally administered treatment is required to clear the bowel, followed by regular checks to avoid recurrence.[3] When 'empty' on digital examination or when there is no relief from incontinence after evacuation of the rectum, the three main mechanisms (sometimes acting in combination) are: diarrhoea or loose stool, a rectal volume/compliance reduction, and anatomical and/or functional injuries to the anal sphincter complex (Fig. 11.1).

Sphincter injury

In adult females, the most common cause of sphincter injury is obstetric trauma. After vaginal delivery, up to 10% of primiparous women have a clinically recognised sphincter disruption (**Fig. 11.2a**), and the incidence of occult injuries diagnosed sonographically can be as high as 30% after normal delivery.[6,7] More complicated deliveries, such as those involving instrumental delivery (forceps/vacuum-assisted), a

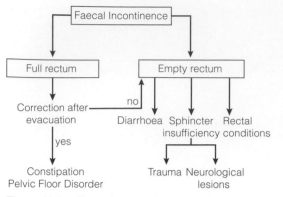

Figure 11.1 • The various mechanisms responsible for faecal incontinence: a guide to identifying a cause.

large birth weight and a prolonged second stage of labour have been shown to increase the risk of FI, and an episiotomy has not been shown consistently to protect against sphincter injury.[6–10]

Anorectal surgical procedures responsible for direct trauma to the anal sphincters with resultant incontinence include haemorrhoidectomy and fistulotomy.[11] With the former, some patients can occasionally report minor degrees of incontinence to flatus and/or faecal soiling due to loss of the normal anal cushions allied to sensory impairment in the anal canal. Risk factors for incontinence following fistula-in-ano surgery include high or complex fistulas or repeated procedures for recurrence or

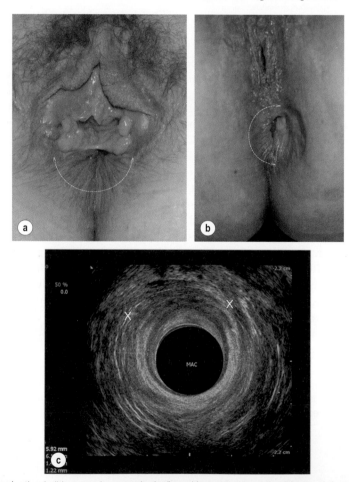

Figure 11.2 • **(a)** Examination in lithotomy (gynaecological) position: anterior anal sphincter defect, a sequela of fourth degree tear following vaginal delivery. (Obstetric injury) of the perineum is classified as a first-degree tear if confined to vaginal mucosa and perineal skin, second degree if the perineal muscles are torn, third degree if the anal sphincter is torn, and fourth degree if both sphincter and anorectal mucosa is torn. In the illustrated situation, the anal sphincter muscles and perineal body have separated, leaving a large anterior hemi-circumferential defect splaying open the anal sphincters in a horseshoe-type configuration (arrows). Here the defect was such that the anal and vaginal mucosa have healed to form a cloacal defect. **(b)** Examination in lithotomy (gynaecological) position: left lateral anal sphincter defect, sequela of an extensive fistulotomy for complex anal fistula, resulting in a gaping anus (arrows). **(c)** Endoanal ultrasonography (EAUS). Anterior defect of internal and external sphincters (marks) visualised on two-dimensional image of the anal canal.

persistence (**Fig. 11.2b**). Manual anal dilatation for anal fissures has been associated in the past with incontinence rates of up to 20% (by contrast, the current use of lateral internal sphincterotomy has resulted in much lower rates). Incontinence can also arise following major colorectal resections, such as low anterior resection with coloanal anastomosis, due to the reduction in or loss of the rectal reservoir capacity, and also to the disruption of intramural nerve pathways. Function can be further adversely affected by chemotherapy and/or radiation.

Trauma to the perineum or pelvis, such as pelvic fractures after road traffic accidents or impalement injuries, can be associated with significant soft tissue damage to both the anal sphincter and its nerve supply,[1,8] along with collateral damage to other pelvic floor structures, such as the bladder and urethra. Occasionally, injuries associated with a sexual assault may result in faecal incontinence.

Neurological diseases, such as multiple sclerosis, muscular dystrophies or congenital myelomeningocoele (spina bifida), can cause incontinence frequently coupled with constipation and evacuation problems.[3]

The sequelae from congenital abnormalities, like anal agenesis or Hirschsprung's disease treated in childhood, can also be responsible for later faecal incontinence, with their own specific management.

Rectal compliance

The rectum can become stiff and uncompliant so that it will not adapt to filling due to conditions such as inflammatory bowel disease (Crohn's disease, ulcerative colitis), radiation proctitis and irritable bowel syndrome.[12]

'Idiopathic' faecal incontinence

Often, the precise aetiology is unclear and the incontinence is termed 'idiopathic'. Pudendal neuropathy, conceptually demonstrated by delayed pudendal nerve terminal motor latency and an increase in mean nerve fibre density (which can be hard to show in practice), is considered to be present in the majority of these patients.[13] Low squeeze pressures and decreased anal canal sensation are usually found. Idiopathic faecal incontinence may result from chronic straining during defecation

and perineal descent, as first described by Parks et al.[14] Perineal descent also appears to be related to the number of vaginal deliveries, thereby leading to another way in which the pudendal nerves can be damaged. Indeed, a majority of cases of faecal incontinence secondary to obstetric damage is due to a combination of traumatic injury to the anal sphincters and the associated trauma to the pelvic floor nerve supply, the latter only becoming evident many years later at the onset of menopause. To make matters worse, these patients present frequently with associated urinary incontinence (double incontinence), which has to be identified and managed accordingly.

This multifactorial aetiology results in a wide variation in clinical presentation and much overlap between the above groups.[3] Clinically, patients may present with either a pattern of 'urge incontinence', where they are unable to actively defer a bowel movement, 'passive incontinence', with the patient unaware of stool leakage, or a 'mixed pattern'. While a patient presenting with urge incontinence may suggest external anal sphincter pathology, this may also be a feature of rectal pathology, such as proctitis or carcinoma. Conversely, passive soiling is more suggestive of a deficient internal anal sphincter or an anatomical deformity from a fistula-in-ano or post-surgical scarring.

Added to the complexity is the frequent coexistence of other pelvic floor pathologies, such as rectal intussusception, which can itself result in patients presenting with varying combinations and severity of urge and passive incontinence or post-defecatory leakage. Indeed, up to 75% of patients with rectal intussusception have incontinence, with some presenting only with this symptom.[15] Although the exact mechanism remains unclear, it is postulated that rectal intussusception stretches the internal anal sphincter and inappropriately triggers the rectoanal inhibitory reflex, leading to temporary reversal of the pressure gradient in the anal canal and soiling. The accompanying incomplete rectal emptying of this defecatory disorder can also contribute to post-defecatory leakage.

> ✔ Faecal incontinence is a symptom, not a diagnosis. This symptom should not be ignored as something can be done.[3] It is important to identify the underlying causes for each individual and this is often multifactorial.

Presentation

History

Clinical assessment starts with a detailed history. The frequency and severity of incontinence episodes are best quantified on a 3-week stool diary filled out by the patient. It is an essential and simple tool to ascertain a baseline of incontinence episodes. It will serve as a useful comparator when referred back to during treatment. Standardised scoring systems are a useful complement and provide an objective assessment tool (Table 11.1).[16] It is also important to assess stool consistency using the Bristol stool chart, which rates it on a seven-point scale from hard to liquid. Finally, a quality of life assessment is provided by the Faecal Incontinence Quality of Life (FIQoL) instrument that attempts to measure any impairment in quality of life 'due to accidental bowel leakage' in four different domains: lifestyle, coping and behaviour, depression, and embarrassment.[17]

The history offers clues to the possible aetiology of incontinence. In women, clearly an obstetric history is mandatory, including number of pregnancies, mode of delivery, birth weight and type of presentation.[10] The hormonal status is recorded, as well as the presence of any concomitant urinary incontinence, which could suggest a more global pelvic floor deficiency. A history of anal surgery is important, particularly in men, because up to 25% of male patients with faecal incontinence have an iatrogenic sphincter injury.

It is too simplistic to attribute all patients with urge incontinence and all patients with passive in-continence as having external and internal sphincter weakness, respectively. The scenario is often more complex, with patients presenting with an overlap of symptoms. Some may even present with mixed symptoms of faecal incontinence and obstructed defecation, which should make the clinician consider a possible posterior compartment prolapse syndrome.[18]

Examination

A general examination (abdomen and neurological examination of the back and lower limbs) should be performed. Next, the perianal skin should be inspected for any scars of trauma or surgery (Fig. 11.2), as well as skin excoriation that could suggest long-term seepage of stool. The pelvic floor should be examined for evidence of a descended perineum. A gaping anal orifice when pulling apart the buttocks suggests decreased resting tone, an absent or weak voluntary contraction, and pudendal neuropathy. The patient should be asked to strain to accentuate a descending perineum or exteriorise any rectal prolapse or rectocele. In addition, when examining the patient in the gynaecological position any mid- or anterior compartment deficiencies might be visible, including utero-vaginal prolapse and cystocoele respectively.

Sensory perception at the anal margin must be checked and a digital rectal examination performed to assess resting and squeeze anal pressures and contractions of the puborectalis muscle, as well as to confirm the presence of a rectocele. With an educated finger, defects in the sphincter muscles can be felt, and straining can also reveal subtle cases of rectal

Table 11.1 • St Mark's Incontinence Score[16]

	Never	Rarely	Sometimes	Weekly	Daily
Incontinence for solid stool	0	1	2	3	4
Incontinence for liquid stool	0	1	2	3	4
Incontinence for gas	0	1	2	3	4
Alteration in lifestyle	0	1	2	3	4
			No	Yes	
Need to wear a pad or plug			0	2	
Taking constipating medicines			0	2	
Lack of ability to defer defecation for 15 minutes			0	4	

Definitions
Never: no episodes in the past four weeks. Rarely: one episode in the past 4 weeks. Sometimes: more than one episode in the past 4 weeks but less than one a week. Weekly: one or more episodes a week but less than one per day. Daily: one or more episodes a day. Add one score from each row: minimum score= 0 (perfect continence); maximum score= 24 (totally incontinent).

intussusception and enterocele. Finding impacted stool suggests overflow as a possible mechanism for incontinence.

Investigations

The indications and extent for a diagnostic work-up should be guided by the duration and severity of symptoms, the response to initial conservative management, and ultimately the fitness for surgery (see Box 11.1). It is also imperative to exclude any coexisting organic pathology that could lead to symptoms of faecal incontinence and warrant urgent attention.

Anorectal physiology studies are essential in providing an objective assessment of anal sphincter pressures, rectal sensation, rectoanal reflexes and rectal compliance, all of which guide management.[8] Manometry is a simple method for measuring internal (resting) and external anal sphincter (squeeze) tone, which are usually low in patients with faecal incontinence. Although the findings of anorectal physiology studies do not consistently correlate with symptom severity, they may influence the treatment options under consideration and guide biofeedback training modalities.[3,5]

Endoanal ultrasonography (EAUS) provides a dynamic assessment of the thickness and structural integrity of the external and internal sphincter muscle using an intra-anal probe. It is the procedure of choice to diagnose sphincter defects in patients with suspected sphincter injury. When performed by an experienced clinician, EAUS approaches 100% sensitivity and specificity in identifying internal and external sphincter defects.[19] However, the presence of a sphincter defect does not necessarily correlate with incontinence. In a study of 335 patients with incontinence, 115 patients who were continent and 18 asymptomatic female volunteers, EAUS detected sphincter defects in 65%, 43% and 22%, respectively.[20]

Dynamic standard or magnetic resonance imaging (MRI) defaecography is not a routine test in incontinent patients as it relies on the patient's ability to retain paste. However, it is useful in selected cases when there are mixed symptoms, including obstructed defecation, where an occult prolapse may be responsible for the incontinence, particularly when other tests have failed to identify a clear cause (e.g. normal or near-normal anal pressures and intact anal sphincters).

At first glance, pelvic floor electrophysiological assessment, including pudendal nerve terminal motor latency, might be considered useful, but lack of a direct impact on treatment strategy, the operator-dependent nature of the test and patient discomfort have significantly limited its use in many centres.

> ✅ Baseline assessment in faecal incontinence relies on a structured evaluation, including patient reporting of symptoms, careful and sensible clinical examination, and investigations that arise from this focused history taking and examination.

Management of faecal incontinence in adults

The treatment of faecal incontinence is mainly guided by the severity of symptoms, the aetiology and the structural integrity of the sphincter muscles. Despite a number of publications on the topic, it has to be borne in mind that current recommendations are based more on expert opinion than high-quality

---

Box 11.1 • Work-up for faecal incontinence: a summary

A. Symptom assessment

- Careful history taking
- Three-week stool diary
- Faecal Incontinence score[16]
- Bristol stool chart
- Faecal Incontinence Quality of Life instrument[17]
- Urinary incontinence
- Constipation

B. Clinical assessment

- General examination (neurological)
- Anorectal examination
- Assessment of the anterior compartment
- Cognitive assessment (if needed)

C. Investigations

- Exclude organic pathology
  - Colonoscopy – or Flexible sigmoidoscopy
  - Mammogram – pelvic ultrasound – cervical smears
- Anorectal physiology tests
- Endoanal ultrasonography
- Standard or MRI dynamic defecography

In the modern, structured approach to management of faecal incontinence, start by addressing reversible factors and, only if this fails to restore continence, progress to specialised investigations and treatment options.[3]

evidence. Given this absence of truly objective evidence, the patient's own views are all the more important.[3]

> ✅ Management of faecal incontinence is often multidisciplinary, often involving several specialists working to provide holistic care to help the patient cope with the broad range of needs, including consideration of the psychological impact of this potentially stigmatising handicap.

Conservative measures

First-line treatment measures of faecal incontinence are conservative.[1,3] These can also be used as adjuncts to subsequent surgical procedures.

Dietary modification and medications

Faecal incontinence is exacerbated by liquid stools. An increase in dietary fibre may improve stool consistency. Stool bulking agents (e.g., psyllium) also improve stool consistency and decrease symptoms of incontinence. The recommended dose is 25–30 g/day. A gradual increase of fibre intake will reduce the associated abdominal bloating and discomfort. Dairy products should be avoided in patients with lactose intolerance. Antidiarrhoeal agents are also useful and the first drug of choice should be loperamide (0.5–16 mg/day as required). This should be started with low doses (less than 2 mg) to avoid constipation, and consider loperamide hydrochloride syrup if fractions of a conventional dose are required. People unable to tolerate loperamide hydrochloride should be offered codeine phosphate or co-phenotrope.[3] Cholestyramine chelates bile salts, the latter being occasionally responsible for diarrhoea, and may be worth a try.

Small retrograde enemas and suppositories can promote more complete bowel emptying and as a consequence reduce soiling. In more intractable cases such as spinal-cord injured patients with overflow incontinence from severe faecal impaction, a regular enema programme using specially designed apparatus has proved to be highly effective[21] (**Fig. 11.3**). This can also be useful in situations where the patients have cognitive impairment or in the elderly infirm in order to prevent skin excoriation and infections from frequent soiling.[1,3]

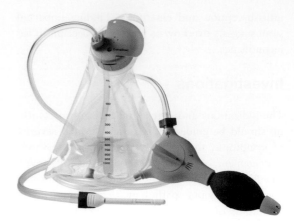

Figure 11.3 • Conservative management: dedicated material for transanal retrograde colonic enemas/irrigation.

Biofeedback, pelvic floor muscle training and electrostimulation

Biofeedback (BFB) – also known as 'behavioural therapy' – uses either visual, auditory or verbal feedback techniques, with three main goals: strength training, sensory training and coordination training.[3] The treatment protocol should be customised for each patient based upon the supposed underlying pathophysiological mechanism. A set of 10–15 sessions (two per week) is recommended to assess the efficacy of the biofeedback, with regular 'recall' sessions every 6 months for surveillance of progress. Supportive counselling and practical advice regarding diet and skin care play an important role in the success of biofeedback.

The benefit of BFB varies, with a wide range of improvement reported (64–89%).[8] Largely due to the different definitions of success and therapeutic regimens, the varied selection criteria, fluctuating individual motivations and therapist enthusiasm. Improved rectal sensation after biofeedback is one of the most consistent predictors for improved continence.

However, recent controlled trials have raised questions as to whether BFB provides a specific benefit relative to education and good clinical management, despite a large body of uncontrolled studies supporting its efficacy.[22] The current consensus is that BFB as a treatment for faecal incontinence is possibly effective and is recommended because it is painless and risk-free, after other behavioural and medical management has been tried and inadequate symptom relief has been obtained (level C).[3,23] Pelvic floor muscle exercises are recommended as an early intervention based upon low cost, no morbidity and some weak evidence suggesting efficacy. Based on the available data from a Cochrane review, there is a suggestion that electrical stimulation may have a therapeutic effect, but the current evidence... Current evidence does not support the use of faradic stimulation for faecal incontinence.[24]

Anal plug

Anal plugs are diposable devices that expand when soaked with faecal content and control continence by blocking the passage of stool. Although they are not well tolerated by all patients, they may be helpful in preventing faecal incontinence in selected groups, such as patients with neurological impairment (spina bifida) who have less anal sensation and thus a greater toleration.[25]

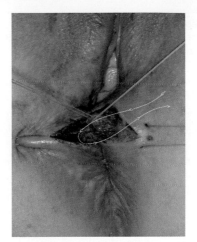

Figure 11.4 • Sphincteroplasty for anterior sphincter defect following obstetric injury. Overlapping anal sphincter repair: two edges of detached sphincter muscles dissected free and mobilised with the scar tissue; The U-shaped suturing (arrows) uses either non-absorbable or absorbable sutures to bring both muscle ends together.

✔ A patient is referred for surgical consideration after conservative treatment has failed. The surgeon should ensure that these measures of conservative management have been correctly and adequately administered before embarking on surgery.

Surgery

Surgical treatment for faecal incontinence is reserved for patients who have failed conservative therapy. The available techniques range from direct repair of damaged sphincters (e.g. sphincteroplasty) to techniques that augment the function (e.g. injectables, sacral nerve stimulation) or replace the native anal sphincter complex (e.g. artificial bowel sphincter, dynamic graciloplasty). A stoma should not be perceived as a failure of management and when appropriately chosen can significantly improve nursing care and provide a better quality of life for affected patients.

Sphincteroplasty

'Anal sphincteroplasty' describes a secondary (delayed) repair of the anal sphincter muscles. It is distinct from an 'anal sphincter repair', a term used to describe primary (immediate) repair of the anal sphincters following direct trauma (not discussed here). Anterior sphincteroplasty following an obstetric injury is the most common type of reconstruction performed.

Overlapping sphincteroplasty is the standard of care (**Fig. 11.4**). It is performed under general anaesthesia with the patient either in the prone jack-knife or lithotomy position. An incision is made transversely between the anus and the vaginal introitus. The scar tissue and muscle ends are dissected from the rectum posteriorly and the vagina anteriorly without separate identification and repair of the internal anal sphincter. Adequate mobilisation is necessary to ensure a tension-free wrap. The scar tissue is then divided transversely. The two ends are overlapped over the midline and stitched with 2/0 mattress sutures. A levatorplasty can be added, taking great care not to narrow the vagina excessively, which can cause dyspareunia. A T-closure with interrupted absorbable sutures is often feasible. A small opening in the centre of the wound is left or a Penrose drain is inserted.[26] It has recently been suggested that a biological implant to reinforce the anal muscles could be advantageous.[27]

> ✅ Preoperative counselling should highlight postoperative wound infection and delayed healing as the most common complication.[28]

Sphincteroplasty confers substantial benefits in patients with localised (from 90 to 180 degrees) sphincter defects. Predictors of worse outcome are older age (≥50 years), deep wound infection, and isolated external anal sphincter defects.[29] Short-term outcomes suggest good-to-excellent results in a majority of patients. There is, however, increasing evidence that continence deteriorates with long-term follow-up with studies having shown that, after 5–10 years, only 40–45% of patients were satisfied with the functional outcome.[30,31] Adjuvant biofeedback therapy after surgery may improve quality of life and help sustain symptomatic improvement with time. At present, no single preoperative manometric variable can predict outcome after a sphincter repair.[32]

Previous sphincter repair does not seem to affect the clinical outcome of a subsequent repair. In a comparative study, the outcome was similar between patients with or without a previous sphincter repair, with good results obtained in 50% and 58% of patients respectively.[33] Indeed, the long-term benefit of a repeat sphincter repair was similar to an initial repair.[34]

Pelvic floor repair (postanal, preanal or total)

Different types of pelvic floor repair have been described in the past.[35,36] The aim of postanal repair was to increase the length of the anal canal, restore the anorectal angle and recreate the flap valve mechanism, which at the time was thought essential for maintaining faecal continence. Despite initial improvement, the long-term results of postanal repair or total pelvic floor repair for neurogenic faecal incontinence have been disappointing.

Postanal repair or total pelvic floor repair now have no place in the treatment of neuropathic faecal incontinence, as better options are available.[28]

Sphincter reconstruction – muscle transposition

Non-stimulated and stimulated muscle transpositions have been devised to replace the anal sphincter (*neosphincter*) when local repair is not possible or has failed. Transposition of one or both gluteal muscles from the buttock (*gluteoplasty*) has been used as well as transposition of the gracilis muscle from the leg, being wrapped around the anus to form a new sphincter (*graciloplasty*). Variable success rates have been reported with non-stimulated muscle transplants. Due to limited efficacy and significant morbidity these procedures are no longer used.

The addition of an implanted electrical stimulator permits permanent contraction of the transposed muscle and thus a better closure of the anus. The so-called 'stimulated' or *dynamic gracioplasty*, first reported in 1988, has been the most developed procedure of this type.[37] Its principle is to induce the fast-twitch, fatiguable type II muscle fibres of the gracilis muscle to change into the slow-twitch, fatigue-resistant type I muscle fibres that resemble the internal anal sphincter. Dynamic gracioplasty is most appropriate for patients with extensive sphincter disruption precluding a direct surgical repair, severe neural damage or congenital disorders (anal atresia). It has also been used in total anorectal reconstuction after abdominoperineal resection for low rectal or recurrent anal cancers.[38] The results of dynamic gracioplasty have been variable, with satisfactory continence restoration being achieved only in specialised high-volume centres. Multicentre trials that included less experienced surgeons have shown a high morbidity and a poorer functional outcome.[39,40] Due to some reported mortality, high infection and other morbidities rates and a limited success rate, this technique has not gained wide acceptance.[28] With virtually no published reports over the last 5 years, dynamic gracioplasty appears to have been replaced nowadays by other less aggressive options.

Artificial sphincters

Artificial sphincters can be defined as any kind of implanted device intended to replace or reinforce the native sphincteric mechanism. They aim to be a substitute for normal sphincters.[28] As such, it is necessary that they are efficient for both terminal bowel functions, of continence and evacuation; their implantation is safe and reproducible, with a limited need for patient/medical intervention and follow-up after implantation; finally, they should be cost effective.

Artificial bowel sphincter

Artificial sphincters currently used in humans are silicone-made, pressure-regulated devices restoring continence through an inflatable cuff placed around the lower rectum or upper anal canal.

Three models have been on the market. Over the last 5 years, there have been no publications on two of them: the prosthetic bowel sphincter (PBS), developed in the UK, and the Agency for Medical Innovations (AMI) soft anal band system, once popular in Germany and Austria. The only recent available data concern the Acticon Neosphincter™ (American Medical Systems (AMS), Minnetonka, MN, USA) artificial bowel sphincter (ABS).

The ABS, a modified model of the AMS 800 artificial urinary sphincter, has been in use since 1996 for the management of severe faecal incontinence. In short, it comprises a fluid-filled cuff that encircles and compresses the anal canal. A pressure-regulating balloon is implanted in the retropubic space of Retzius. The system is controlled by a pump placed in the labia majora or scrotum, which is accessible to the patient (**Fig. 11.5**). The pressurisation fluid is an isotonic solution, as the artificial sphincter walls are semipermeable membranes and radio-opaque (except in the case of iodine allergy where normal saline is used; **Fig. 11.6**). To initiate defecation, squeezing the pump empties the cuff by transferring fluid into the balloon, permitting passage of stool. The cuff then refills automatically from pressure built up in the balloon.

The role of the ABS in treating faecal incontinence has been reaffirmed in several reports from different groups,[41-44] as well as being supported in the current recommendations of both the National Institute for Health and Clinical Excellence (NICE) and the American Society of Colon and Rectal Surgeons (ASCRS).[3,5] The ABS is especially indicated for patients with 'severe end-stage faecal incontinence'.

Careful patient selection and sound operative technique are critical components for success with artificial sphincter implantation. Exclusion criteria include morbid obesity, insulin-dependent diabetes mellitus, Crohn's disease, pelvic sepsis and radiation proctitis. Individuals who practice anoreceptive intercourse are also not candidates for the procedure. It is also vital to ensure that all patients are adequately motivated and have sufficient manual dexterity to operate the device independently.

The artificial bowel sphincter provides good restoration of continence for solid and liquid stool in patients who retain the device, with all studies reporting good restoration of continence and a positive impact

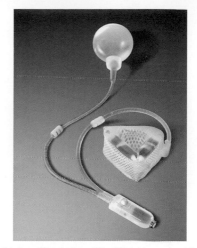

Figure 11.5 • The Acticon™ artificial bowel sphincter.

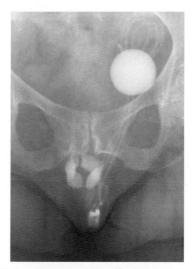

Figure 11.6 • The Acticon™ artificial bowel sphincter: device in place, inflated with isotonic radiopaque fluid, in a female patient (X-ray plain AP view).

on quality of life. The risk of constipation after implantation of an ABS is a concern as the cuff, even when widely open, can still narrow the anal canal enough to prevent complete and easy evacuation.[45]

Along with an evident beneficial effect in treating severe faecal incontinence, studies have also highlighted the associated risks of infection and mechanical failure. However, severe morbidity is rare and no mortality has ever been reported. Explantation of the device generally solves any problems without long-term sequelae.

The primary concern with ABS implantation is infection, with rates ranging from 20% to 45%.

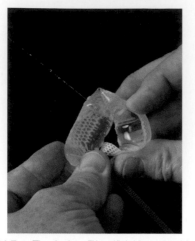

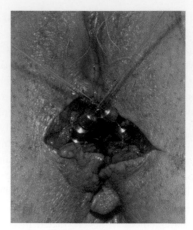

Figure 11.7 • The Acticon™ artificial bowel sphincter – microperforation on a leaking cuff responsible for a mechanical failure.

Figure 11.8 • The Fenix™ magnetic anal sphincter.

The time between ABS implantation and first bowel movement, as well as a history of perineal sepsis, were found to be independent risk factors for early-stage infection.[44] Mechanical failure is also a well-recognised complication after ABS implantation. The most common cause is microperforation at the folds of the cuff membrane, which leads to a loss of fluid and pressurisation of the system (**Fig. 11.7**). Cuff perforation is easily perceived by the patient as both a return to incontinence and a non-functioning flat control pump. Cuff perforation reflects intrinsic wear and tear of the device components over time and contributes to the need for revision procedures, especially in patients with satisfactory functional ABS results. As such, it has been shown that revision rate is directly proportional to the length of follow-up. These concerns suggest that an appropriate component upgrade by the manufacturer might lead to improved long-term results and a lower cost.[41]

Magnetic anal sphincter

Studied in small trials, the magnetic anal sphincter (MAS; FENIX™, Torax Medical Inc., Shoreview, MN, USA) is a novel device designed to augment the native anal sphincter. It consists of a series of titanium beads with magnetic cores hermetically sealed inside. The beads are interlinked with independent titanium wires to form a flexible ring that rests around the external anal sphincter in a circular fashion. The device is manufactured in different

lengths determined by the number of beads (14–20) necessary to accommodate the variation in anal canal circumference (**Fig. 11.8** and **11.9**).

One of the advantages of this still investigational device over the previous artificial sphincters is that it begins working immediately once implanted, without the need for subsequent manipulation by either the patient or surgeon. The procedure for implantation is also substantially simpler than the ABS because access to the perineum alone is required.

A recent multicentre feasibility study demonstrated good short-term restoration of continence with limited morbidity.[46] In a subsequent non-randomised comparative cohort study assessing results of the MAS and the ABS, it was shown that the two devices were similarly effective in restoring continence and quality of life, without any difference in morbidity.[47] A further comparative study with sacral nerve stimulation showed similar results.[48]

Based on these results, MAS was granted a CE mark on November 2011 and its commercial use has commenced in selected centres in Europe with further large scale reports expected.

Presently the place of the MAS in the treatment algorithm of faecal incontinence remains to be determined. It appears to be a promising innovation as it offers a less invasive and simpler alternative of anal reinforcement than the ABS. However, with only short-term follow-up available, it remains to be seen if the MAS can withstand the test of time.

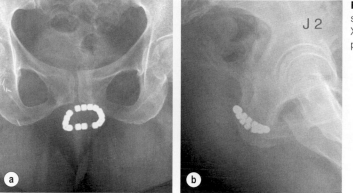

Figure 11.9 • The Fenix™ magnetic anal sphincter: implanted device visualised on X-ray AP **(a)** and lateral **(b)** views of the pelvis.

Sacral nerve stimulation

Sacral nerve stimulation (SNS) was first described for use in urological disorders. It was adapted for use in faecal incontinence in 1995.[49] Although not completely elucidated, it is believed that the premise behind SNS is the stimulation of the sacral nerves to recruit additional function from the anal sphincters and pelvic floor musculature, as well as having effects on colonic motility and the local spinal reflex arcs, which reduce the rectal sensory threshold and increase rectal blood flow.[50]

SNS consists of a *screening phase* of peripheral nerve evaluation (PNE), followed by a second *therapeutic phase* of permanent neurostimulator implantation (**Fig. 11.10**). In the initial diagnostic phase of PNE, which can be performed under local or general anaesthesia with the patient in the prone position, the S3 foramen is preferentially cannulated under fluoroscopic guidance with an electrode through which stimulation is performed, looking for an appropriate 'bellows response' of the pelvic floor and plantar flexion of the ipsilateral great toe. This is sometimes repeated on the contralateral side to select the best response, with some routinely screening the S2 and S4 positions as well. Once a location is decided upon, the electrode is secured in place and connected to a portable external stimulator. The patient then undergoes a 3-week trial of stimulation while filling out a bowel-habit diary. Only patients with significant clinical improvement, demonstrated by a reduction in frequency of episodes or days of faecal incontinence of at least 50%, are then selected for the *therapeutic phase*, of the permanent stimulator implantation (**Fig. 11.11a, b**). The permanent stimulator is placed subcutaneously in the gluteal area under local anaesthesia. The pulse generator is activated and stimulation parameters are set by telemetry. It can be deactivated by the patient with a small, hand-held device, the 'patient programmer'.[28]

> ✅ SNS is a minimally invasive technique with low morbidity. The decision to implant a permanent neurostimulator is made on the basis of clinical improvement during test stimulation.

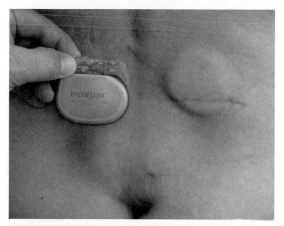

Figure 11.10 • Sacral nerve stimulation: Interstim™ pulse generator (left) and the implanted generator in a thin patient (right).

Sacral nerve stimulation is therefore an attractive treatment option for several reasons. It is minimally invasive, a trial phase allows one to decide on the suitability for permanent implantation, and it has minimal morbidity with no reported mortality.[51–54] Studies have shown that SNS is feasible, with sustainable long-term results. In a series of 52 patients with a follow-up lasting at least 5 years, it has been reported that 74% of patients experienced at least

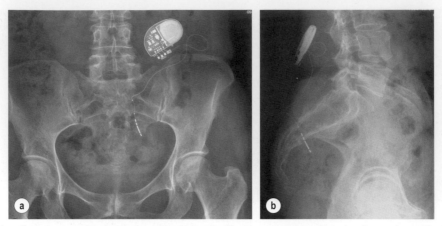

Figure 11.11 • Sacral nerve stimulation: implanted Interstim™ pulse generator with extension and quadripolar electrode on a plain X-ray AP **(a)** and lateral **(b)** views.

50% improvement in continence, with quality of life improved in all domains.[53] In a recent US report, at 3 years follow-up, 86% of patients had at least a 50% reduction in incontinent episodes per week compared to baseline, with significant improvements in quality of life.[54]

However, this technique is not free of complications, with reported morbidity including implant site pain (28%), paraesthesia (15%), change in sensation of stimulation (12%) and infection (10%), with less than 5% requiring device explantation. A recent meta-analysis (34 studies) reported an overall complication rate of 15% in permanently implanted patients with 3% requiring explantation.[55] The latter results were similarly echoed in a separate study from an expert centre, which reported that at a median follow-up of 33 months, 17.6% of patients required explantation of the device or discontinued treatment entirely.[56]

As encouraging as SNS outcomes may be, this modality is very expensive and furthermore not all patients respond favourably to PNE. In an attempt to improve patient selection and eventual outcomes, several studies have tried to identify negative predictive factors for PNE, such as old age, the need for repeat PNE procedures and the use of temporary electrodes, but to date no consensus has been reached and selection criteria remain subjective at best.[57,58] Current patient selection is therefore based upon a pragmatic 'trial-and-error' approach, using the PNE test. Test stimulation is indicated not by an underlying physiological condition, but by the existence of an anal sphincter with reduced or absent voluntary

squeeze function and intact reflex activity, and nerve–muscle connection.

Contraindications to SNS include pathological conditions of the sacrum preventing adequate electrode placement, skin disease at the area of implantation, severe anal sphincter damage, pregnancy, bleeding risk, psychological instability, low mental capacity and the presence of a cardiac pacemaker or implantable defibrillator.

The use of SNS in patients with a sphincter defect is presently fiercely debated.[29,59] Some series have shown that SNS was able to correct faecal incontinence in patients with associated sphincter defects. In light of the current available evidence, a pragmatic approach is required based on the patient's age and personal views, type of defect, and visible contraction of the remaining sphincter. Day-to-day decision-making is therefore relatively simple.

> ✅ SNS is an expensive therapy that requires a dedicated team for an optimal outcome. It can yield dramatic improvement in some, and yet provide no benefit in others.

Percutaneous and transcutaneous tibial nerve stimulation

Another form of neurostimulation, known as tibial nerve stimulation, either percutaneous (PTNS) or transcutaneous (TENS), has been investigated. This peripheral, temporary, ambulatory stimulation of the tibial nerve with surface or needle electrodes at the level of the malleolus relies on intact neuronal connections of this nerve with the sacral plexus. It aims to mimic the effect seen when direct stimulation

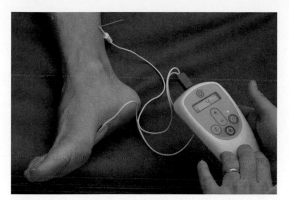

Figure 11.12 • Posterior tibial nerve stimulation (PTNS): needle placement at the ankle for therapy.

is used, as with SNS. Scattered preliminary data from short-term studies indicate a therapeutic effect in mild idiopathic faecal incontinence and incontinence due to partial spinal trauma. Larger patient studies are awaited (**Fig. 11.12**).[60–62]

Injection therapy

Injectable bulking agents were first described for use in faecal incontinence in 1993. The technique relies on the bulking effect of the injected materials with subsequent fibrosis/collagen deposition helping to enhance continence. These materials are usually injected into either the submucosa or the intersphincteric plane, with some reports suggesting the routine use of ultrasound guidance to improve outcomes.[63] A variety of materials have been used, including autologous fat, glutaraldehyde cross-linked collagen (Contigen™), pyrolytic carbon beads (Durasphere™) and silicone biomaterial or PTQ™. The most recent addition to this group has been the use of polyacrylonitrile (Gatekeeper™), a shape memory hydrophylic material that enlarges in diameter seven times its initial diameter of 1.2 mm once in contact with human tissue. An initial single-centre report showed a sustained improvement in incontinence and quality-of-life scores over a mean follow-up of 33 months. Larger studies with longer follow-up are required to confirm these early encouraging results.[64]

Despite the relative simplicity of the procedure, the available data suggest that the effects of bulking agents appear to be short-lived and of limited efficacy. As such, they could be recommended for use in only selected cases of mild passive faecal incontinence related to internal sphincter dysfunction and soiling.[63]

Currently there is little evidence for the effectiveness of injectable bulking agents in managing passive faecal incontinence.[65] The available injectable bulking agents appear to be safe, with only minor complications reported.[66] In a systematic review, variations in the practice of injection of bulking agents have been identified that appear to influence the likelihood of complications and outcomes after treatment.[67]

Stoma

Antegrade continence enema

This procedure was first described in 1990 for children.[68] The concept of irrigation is to ensure emptying of the colon and/or rectum to prevent seepage of stool. Various procedures have been described to provide an access to the right colon. Initially, the appendix was used to create a continent stoma, an 'appendicostomy', by invaginating the tip of the appendix into the caecum to create a one-way valve. The base of the appendix is then brought out to the abdominal wall and the patient can then introduce antegrade enemas.[68] Other options now include a caecal or ileal tube.[69,70] This procedure can also be performed percutaneously guided by a colonoscope during which a specially designed catheter (CHAIT Trapdoor™) is introduced into the caecum using the following method: (1) fixation of the caecum to the abdominal wall using anchors, (2) dilation of the caecostomy site and (3) placement of a CHAIT trapdoor catheter (**Fig. 11.13**).[70] This minimally invasive approach has been shown to be safe and useful for both paediatric patients and adults.

In a recent long-term review of 75 adult patients, with a median follow-up of 4 years, up to 91% of patients were still performing antegrade enemas, while maintaining a significant reduction in incontinence scores compared to preoperative values.[71] However, some morbidity has been reported with this procedure the most common being wound infection and leakage from the ministoma.

End stoma

A stoma is appropriate for patients with severe end-stage faecal incontinence in which all other available treatments have failed, are inappropriate because of comorbidities, or when preferred by the patient. While a stoma may be associated with significant psychosocial issues and stoma-related

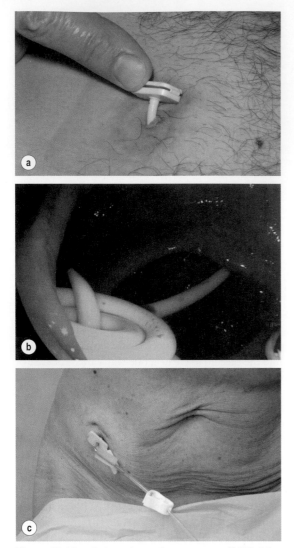

Figure 11.13 • Antegrade continence enema (ACE). **(a)** Malone opening on the abdomen right lower quadrant with a CHAIT Trapdoor™ in place for ACE. **(b)** View of the endoscopically placed pigtail CHAIT Trapdoor™ for access to the right colon for ACE. **(c)** Irrigation through the CHAIT Trapdoor™ for ACE in a faecally incontinent patient.

complications, it can conversely allow the patient to resume normal activities and improves quality of life.[72] In a survey of patients who had a colostomy created to manage their faecal incontinence, 83% reported a significant improvement in lifestyle and 84% would choose to have the stoma again.[73]

An end sigmoid colostomy without proctectomy is usually recommended as a procedure of choice for patients who elect to have a colostomy. A colostomy, however, can result in its own problems in some patients, such as diversion colitis of the rectal

stump and mucus leakage, unfrequently necessitating a secondary proctectomy.[74]

> ✅ A colostomy can be a good option for patients who suffer from severe faecal incontinence, offering symptom relief with improved quality of life.

Conclusion

Despite all the currently available treatment procedures presented and discussed above, each patient needs an individualised management approach, taking into account his own needs and preferences. Evidence is unfortunately not robust for most assessment and treatment methods described. Thus, decision-making often relies on expert opinion and personal experience which should in turn be in the context of a multidisciplinary team of specialists. This is essential for optimizing patient outcomes, with the colorectal surgeon being only a part of the support process.[3]

It has to be kept in mind that there is active research in this area and newer therapies will soon be with us (Secca, sling implantation, new nerve-stimulation techniques or stem cell injection).

Finally on the basis of current knowledge, it is recommended that a graduated treatment approach be adopted, tailored to the cause and severity of the patient's symptoms, beginning first with less invasive options and progressing in a stepwise manner to more advanced treatments. When surgery for faecal incontinence is considered, the anal sphincter assessment is essential to define whether a surgical procedure may be aimed at correcting an obvious anatomical defect, or augmenting a functionally deficient but structurally intact sphincter complex (**Fig. 11.14**).

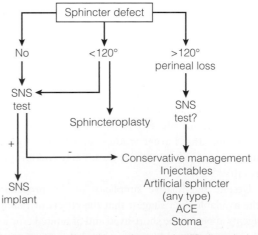

Figure 11.14 • Faecal incontinence: simplified surgical treatment algorithm.

Key points

- Faecal incontinence (FI) is defined as the involuntary loss of solid or liquid stool.
- The frequency and severity of incontinence episodes and urgency best assessed on stool diaries guide the treatment choice.
- FI is multifactorial: the identification of mechanism and cause of FI is key for subsequent management.
- Conservative management including dietary counselling, medication and pelvic floor retraining is first-line.
- Overlapping sphincteroplasty can be offered to patients with significant FI and a documented sphincter injury, frequently a sequelae of obstetrical trauma. Most patients improve after sphincteroplasty, but outcomes deteriorate over time.
- Lap ventral rectopexy for an associated rectal prolapse (overt or internal) may solve FI.
- Sacral nerve stimulation is an effective therapy for patients with significant FI who fail conservative management. The technique has the advantage of allowing a therapeutic trial prior to permanent stimulator implantation.
- Artificial anal sphincter has been shown to have reasonable success but is associated with significant morbidity. It remains a useful technique in carefully selected patients with end-stage FI.
- Colostomy provides restoration of a more normal lifestyle and improves quality of life. An end sigmoidostomy alone is recommended. Antegrade colonic enemas could also be an option in refractory FI.
- Newer therapies including stimulation techniques, slings, injectables of various types and magnetic sphincters are currently assessed, outlining how research is active in the field of FI.

References

1. Madoff RD, Parker SC, Varma MG, et al. Faecal incontinence in adults. Lancet 2004;364:621–32.

2. Sharma A, Marshall RJ, Macmillan AK, et al. Determining levels of faecal incontinence in the community: a New Zealand cross-sectional study. Dis Colon Rectum 2011;54:1381–7.

3. National Institute for Health and Clinical Excellence (NICE) Clinical Guideline 49. Faecal incontinence: the management of faecal incontinence in adults. http://www.nice.org.uk/nicemedia/pdf/CG49NICEGuidance; June2007[accessed January 2012].

4. Johanson JF, Mafferty J. Epidemiology of fecal incontinence; the silent affliction. Am J Gastroenterol 1996;91:33–6.

5. Tjandra JJ, Dykes SL, Kumar RR, et al., and the Standards Practice Task Force of the American Society of Colon and Rectal Surgeons. Practice parameters for the treatment of fecal incontinence. Dis Colon Rectum 2007;50:1497–507.

6. Sultan A, Kamm M, Hudson C, et al. Anal-sphincter disruption during vaginal delivery. N Engl J Med 1993;329:1905–11.

7. Sultan AH, Kamm MA, Bartram CI, et al. Third degree obstetric anal sphincter tears: risk factors and outcome of primary repair. Br Med J 1994;308:887–91.

8. Rao SS. Diagnosis and management of fecal incontinence. Am J Gastroenterol 2004;99:1585–604.

9. Mazouni C, Bretelle F, Battar S, et al. Frequency of persistent anal symptoms after first instrumental delivery. Dis Colon Rectum 2005;48:1432–6.

10. Eogan M, O'Brien C, Daly L, et al. The dual influence of age and obstetric history on faecal incontinence in parous women. Int J Obstet Gynaecol 2011;112:93–7.

11. Lindsey I, Jones OM, Smigin-Humphreys MM, et al. Patterns of fecal incontinence after anal surgery. Dis Colon Rectum 2004;47:1643–9.

12. Lundby L, Krogh K, Jensen VJ, et al. Long-term anorectal dysfunction after postoperative radiotherapy for rectal cancer. Dis Colon Rectum 2005;48:1343–9.

13. Kiff ES, Swash M. Slowed conduction in the pudendal nerves in idiopathic (neurogenic) faecal incontinence. Br J Surg 1984;71:614–6.

14. Parks AG, Porter NH, Hardcastle JD. The syndrome of the descending perineum. Proc R Soc Med 1966;59:477–82.

15. Collinson R, Wijffels N, Cunningham C, et al. Laparoscopic ventral rectopexy for internal rectal prolapse: short-term functional outcomes. Colorectal Dis 2010;12:97–104.

16. Vaizey CJ, Carapeti E, Cahill JA, et al. Prospective comparison of faecal incontinence grading systems. Gut 1999;44:77–80.

17. Rockwood TH, Church JM, Fleshman JW, et al. Fecal Incontinence Quality of Life scale: quality of life instrument for patients with fecal incontinence. Dis Colon Rectum 2000;43:9–16.

18. Jones OM, Cunningham C, Lindsey I. Paradigm shifts in the management of faecal incontinence. Aust N Z J Surg 2010;80:205–7.

19. Berger N, Tjandra JJ, Solomon M. Endoanal and endorectal ultrasound: applications in colorectal surgery. Aust N Z J Surg 2004;74:71–5.

20. Karoui S, Savoye-Collet C, Koning E, et al. Prevalence of anal sphincter defects revealed by sonography in 335 incontinent patients and 115 continent patients. AJR Am J Roentgenol 1999;173:389–92.

21. Christensen P, Bazzocchi G, Coggrave M, et al. A randomized, controlled trial of transanal irrigation versus conservative bowel management in spinal cord-injured patients. Gastroenterology 2006;131:738–47.

22. Norton C, Chelvanayagam S, Wilson-Barnett J, et al. Randomized controlled trial of biofeedback for fecal incontinence. Gastroenterology 2003;125:1320–9.

23. Norton C, Whitehead WE, Bliss DZ, et al. Management of fecal incontinence in adults. Neurourol Urodyn 2010;29:199–206.

24. Hosker G, Norton C, Brazzelli M. Electrical stimulation for faecal incontinence in adults. Cochrane Database Syst Rev 2002;2.

25. Kim J, Shim MC, Choi BY, et al. Clinical application of continent anal plug in bedridden patients with intractable diarrhea. Dis Colon Rectum 2001;44: 1162–7.

26. Goetz LH, Lowry AC. Overlapping sphincteroplasty: is it the standard of care? Clin Colon Rectal Surg 2005;18:22–31.

27. Zutshi M, Ferreira P, Hull T, et al. Biological implants in sphincter augmentation offer good short-term outcomes after a sphincter repair. Colorectal Dis 2012;14:866–71.

28. Abrams P, Andersson KE, Birder L, et al. Fourth International Consultation on Incontinence: Recommendations of the International Scientific Committee: Evaluation and treatment of urinary incontinence, pelvic organ prolapse, and fecal incontinence. Neurourol Urodyn 2010;29:213–40.

29. Oom DM, Gosselink MP, Schouten WR. Anterior sphincteroplasty for fecal incontinence: a single center experience in the era of sacral neuromodulation. Dis Colon Rectum 2009;52:1681–7.

30. Malouf AJ, Norton CS, Engel AF, et al. Long-term results of overlapping anterior anal sphincter repair for obstetric trauma. Lancet 2000;355:260–5.

31. Bravo Gutierrez A, Madoff RD, Lowry AC, et al. Long-term results of anterior sphincteroplasty. Dis Colon Rectum 2004;47:727–31.

32. Gearhart S, Hull T, Floruta C, et al. Anal manometric parameters: predictors of outcome following anal sphincter repair? J Gastrointest Surg 2005;9:115–20.

33. Giordano P, Renzi A, Efron J, et al. Previous sphincter repair does not affect the outcome of repeat repair. Dis Colon Rectum 2002;45:635–40.

34. Vaizey CJ, Norton C, Thornton MJ, et al. Long-term results of repeat anterior anal sphincter repair. Dis Colon Rectum 2004;47:858–63.

35. Setti Carraro P, Kamm MA, Nicholls RJ. Long-term results of postanal repair for neurogenic faecal incontinence. Br J Surg 1994;81:140–4.

36. Pinho M, Ortiz J, Oya M, et al. Total pelvic floor repair for treatment of neuropathic faecal incontinence. Am J Surg 1992;163:340–3.

37. Baeten C, Spaans F, Fluks A. An implanted neuromuscular stimulator for fecal continence following previously implanted gracilis muscle: report of a case. Dis Colon Rectum 1988;31:134–7.

38. Rosen HR, Urbarz C, Novi G, et al. Long-term results of modified graciloplasty for sphincter replacement after rectal excision. Colorectal Dis 2002; 4: 266–9.

39. Thornton MJ, Kennedy ML, Lubowski DZ, et al. Long-term follow-up of dynamic graciloplasty for faecal incontinence. Colorectal Dis 2004;6:470–6.

40. Chapman AE, Geerdes B, Hewett P, et al. Systematic review of dynamic graciloplasty in the treatment of faecal incontinence. Br J Surg 2002;89:138–53.

41. Wong MT, Meurette G, Wyart V, et al. The artificial bowel sphincter: a single institution experience over a decade. Ann Surg 2011;254:951–6.

42. Michot F, Lefebure B, Bridoux V, et al. Artificial anal sphincter for severe fecal incontinence implanted by a transvaginal approach: experience with 32 patients treated at one institution. Dis Colon Rectum 2010;53:1155–60.

43. Melenhorst J, Koch SM, van Gemert WG, et al. The artificial bowel sphincter for FI: a single centre study. Int J Colorectal Dis 2008;23:107–11.

44. Wexner SD, Jin HY, Weiss EG, et al. Factors associated with failure of the artificial bowel sphincter: a study of over 50 cases from Cleveland Clinic Florida. Dis Colon Rectum 2009;52:1550–7.

45. Gallas S, Leroi AM, Bridoux V, et al. Constipation in 44 patients implanted with an artificial bowel sphincter. Int J Colorectal Dis 2009;24:969–74.

46. Lehur PA, McNevin S, Buntzen S, et al. Magnetic anal sphincter augmentation for the treatment of fecal incontinence: a preliminary report from a feasibility study. Dis Colon Rectum 2010;53:1604–10.

47. Wong MT, Meurette G, Stangherlin P, et al. The magnetic anal sphincter versus the artificial bowel sphincter: a comparison of 2 treatments for fecal incontinence. Dis Colon Rectum 2011;54:773–9.

48. Wong MT, Meurette G, Wyart V, et al. Does the magnetic anal sphincter compare favourably with sacral nerve stimulation in the management of faecal incontinence? Colorectal Dis 2012;14:e323–9.

49. Matzel K, Stadelmaier M, Hohenfellner FP. Electrical stimulation of sacral spinal nerves for treatment of faecal incontinence. Lancet 1995;346:1124–7.

50. Kenefick NJ, Emmanuel A, Nicholls RJ, et al. Effect of sacral nerve stimulation on autonomic nerve function. Br J Surg 2003;90:1256–60.

51. Jarrett ME, Varma JS, Duthie GS, et al. Sacral nerve stimulation for faecal incontinence in the UK. Br J Surg 2004;91:755–61.

52. Leroi AM, Parc Y, Lehur PA, et al. Efficacy of sacral nerve stimulation for fecal incontinence: results of a multicentre double-blind crossover study. Ann Surg 2005;242:662–9.

53. Altomare DF, Ratto C, Ganio E, et al. Long-term outcome of sacral nerve stimulation for fecal incontinence. Dis Colon Rectum 2009;52:11–7.

54. Mellgren A, Wexner SD, Coller JA, et al. Long-term efficacy and safety of sacral nerve stimulation for fecal incontinence. Dis Colon Rectum 2011;54:1065–75.

55. Tan E, Ngo N-T, Darzi A, et al. Meta-analysis: sacral nerve stimulation versus conservative therapy in the treatment of faecal incontinence. Int J Colorectal Dis 2011;26:275–94.

56. Maeda Y, Lundby L, Buntzen S, et al. Suboptimal outcome following sacral nerve stimulation for faecal incontinence. Br J Surg 2011;98:140–7.

57. Altomare DF, Rinaldi M, Lobascio P, et al. Factors affecting the outcome of temporary sacral nerve stimulation for faecal incontinence. The value of the new tined electrode. Colorectal Dis 2010;13:198–202.

58. Govaert B, Melenhorst J, Nieman FH, et al. Factors associated with percutaneous nerve evaluation and permanent sacral nerve modulation outcome in patients with fecal incontinence. Dis Colon Rectum 2009;52:1688–94.

59. Nicholls J. Sphincter repair for incontinence. Colorectal Dis 2009;11:545–6.

60. Boyle DJ, Prosser K, Allison M, et al. A percutaneous tibial nerve stimulation for the treatment of urge fecal incontinence. Dis Colon Rectum 2010;53:432–7.

61. Govaert B, Pares D, Delgado-Aros S, et al. A prospective multicenter study to investigate percutaneous tibial nerve stimulation for the treatment of faecal incontinence. Colorectal Dis 2010;12:1236–41.

62. Queralto M, Portier G, Cabarrot PH, et al. Preliminary results of peripheral transcutaneous neuromodulation in the treatment of idiopathic faecal incontinence. Int J Colorectal Dis 2006;21:670–2.

63. Tjandra JJ, Lim JF, Hiscock R, et al. Injectable silicone biomaterial for fecal incontinence due to internal anal sphincter dysfunction is effective. Dis Colon Rectum 2004;47:2138–46.

64. Ratto C, Parello A, Donisi L, et al. Novel bulking agent for faecal incontinence. Br J Surg 2011;98:1644–52.

65. Maeda Y, Laurberg S, Norton CA. Perianal injectable bulking agents for treatment for faecal incontinence. Cochrane Database Syst Rev 2009;(3).

66. Luo C, Samaranayake CB, Plank LD, et al. Systematic review on the efficacy and safety of injectable bulking agents for passive faecal incontinence. Colorectal Dis 2010;12:296–303.

67. Hussain ZI, Lim M, Stojkovic SG. Systematic review of perianal implants in the treatment of faecal incontinence. Br J Surg 2011;98:1526–36.

68. Malone PS, Ransley PG, Kiely EM. Preliminary report: the antegrade continence enema. Lancet 1990;336:1217–8.

69. Worsøe J, Christensen P, Krogh K, et al. Long-term results of antegrade colonic enema in adult patients: assessment of functional results. Dis Colon Rectum 2008;51:1523–8.

70. Biyani D, Barrow E, Hodson P, et al. Endoscopically placed caecostomy buttons: a trial ACE procedure. Colorectal Dis 2007;9:373–6.

71. Chereau N, Lefevre JH, Shields C, et al. Antegrade colonic enema for FI in adults: long-term results of 75 patients. Colorectal Dis 2011;13:e238–42.

72. Saltzstein RJ, Romano J. The efficacy of colostomy as a bowel management alternative in selected spinal cord injury patients. J Am Paraplegia Soc 1990;13:9–13.

73. Norton C, Burch J, Kamm MA. Patients' views of a colostomy for fecal incontinence. Dis Colon Rectum 2005;48:1062–9.

74. Catena F, Wilkinson K, Phillips RK. Untreatable faecal incontinence: colostomy or colostomy and proctectomy? Colorectal Dis 2002;4:48–50.

12

Functional problems and their surgical management

Nicola S. Fearnhead

Introduction

Pelvic floor pathology tends to be complex and crosses several disciplines. Treatment of urogynaecological pathology in isolation is likely to have an adverse impact on defecatory function, and vice versa.[1] Ideal care of women with pelvic floor disorders involves specialist urologists, gynaecologists and colorectal surgeons, and allied specialities including radiology, physiotherapy, specialist nursing, physiology, gastroenterology, psychiatry and chronic pain clinics. Preoperative assessment may include questionnaires on obstetric and urogynaecological history, constipation and incontinence scoring, visual analogues for pain, quality-of-life questionnaires, careful clinical examination, proctoscopy with or without colonoscopy, defecography, transit studies, anorectal physiology and endoanal ultrasound. Increased understanding of the anatomical and functional aspects of pelvic floor problems has led to the establishment of multidisciplinary pelvic floor clinics and teams.[2,3]

Rectal prolapse

Rectal prolapse is protrusion of the rectum through the anus. Prolapse is either mucosal, where only the mucosal layer prolapses, or full thickness, with circumferential protrusion through the anus of all layers of the rectal wall. It occurs occasionally in young children but is most common in elderly women.

Risk factors include connective tissue disorders, for example Marfan's and Ehlers–Danlos syndromes,[4] and a history of anorexia nervosa.[5] The latter patients may present some years after resolution of the psychiatric disorder, the prolapse resulting from poor cross-linking of collagen fibres in the pelvic floor musculature during adolescence. Other risk factors for pelvic organ prolapse include high body mass index and high birth weight babies delivered vaginally.[6,7]

Mucosal prolapse

Mucosal prolapse may occur in isolation, but is commonly associated with obstructive defecation syndrome (ODS) and solitary rectal ulcer syndrome (SRUS). It may cause symptoms of perianal discomfort, passage of mucus or blood per rectum, constipation and straining at stool. The treatment of mucosal prolapse initially involves bulking agents and increased fibre intake. If surgical intervention is required, outpatient procedures such as suction banding or sclerotherapy or day case procedures such as surgical excision or plication of the prolapse or radiofrequency ablation[8–10] are commonly used. More recently some patients with mucosal prolapse and ODS have been treated with the procedure for prolapse and haemorrhoids (PPH) or stapled transanal rectal resection (STARR)[11,12] (see below).

Full-thickness rectal prolapse (see Table 12.1)

Although conservative treatment with increased fibre and bulking laxatives may improve symptoms to some extent, the definitive treatment for full-thickness rectal prolapse is almost exclusively surgical. Indeed, the Cochrane Library's review on prolapse surgery failed to identify any trials comparing surgery to non-operative management.[13] Surgical repair may be undertaken either from an abdominal or perineal approach. There is also the option of concurrent resection being undertaken either by abdominal (resection rectopexy) or perineal (Altemeier's procedure) approaches.

Choice of surgical approach

The choice of approach is largely influenced by surgeon preference as well as patient factors, including comorbidity, age, gender and sexual activity. Most surgeons prefer perineal procedures in elderly or frail patients and abdominal approaches in fit patients,[14] although there is increasing evidence that laparoscopic procedures are safe even in the very elderly.[15] The choice of procedure should also take into account the presence of concurrent genital prolapse, constipation, evacuatory difficulties, faecal incontinence and history of pelvic floor injury.[16] Resection rectopexy has traditionally been recommended for patients who have both constipation and rectal prolapse, although there is little evidence to support this practice (see below). Men tend to be offered perineal procedures in view of the potential for erectile dysfunction from rectal mobilisation during abdominal approaches.

✔✔ A revised meta-analysis of randomised controlled trials in prolapse surgery was undertaken by the Cochrane Library in 2008 but only identified 12 trials with 380 patients.[13] The reviewers had set out to address the issues of abdominal vs. perineal approaches, rectopexy methods, open vs. laparoscopic approaches, and no resection vs. resection. The paucity of data, small sample sizes and methodological problems resulted in a complete lack of useful conclusions being drawn from the analysis. In particular, there was no difference in recurrence rates between abdominal and perineal approaches.[13]

Perineal approaches

The principal perineal approaches are the Delorme and Altemeier procedures. Delorme's procedure involves resection of the sleeve of redundant rectal mucosa and plication of the prolapsed muscle wall without resection.[17] Altemeier's procedure (perineal rectosigmoidectomy) involves dissection into the peritoneal cavity via the prolapsed peritoneal lining of the pouch of Douglas, followed by excision of the rectosigmoid and a coloanal anastomosis[18] (**Figs 12.1 and 12.2**). The latter is usually done by hand but can be done with a circular stapler.[19] Pelvic floor repair or levatorplasty may be used in conjunction with perineal procedures to treat incontinence.[20]

Delorme's procedure for full-thickness rectal prolapse has remained in favour as it is well tolerated in the elderly, has low morbidity and mortality, and minimal impact on continence and bowel function. Recurrence rates are, however, high, varying between 5% and 26.5%, although the procedure may be repeated.[21,22]

Altemeier's procedure carries the potential complication of pelvic sepsis from anastomotic dehiscence, but nevertheless appears well tolerated, even in the elderly. The largest published series report complication rates of 12–14% with very low mortality and improved continence in around half of patients, but rates of recurrent prolapse are still high at 10–16%.[21,22]

✔✔ A small randomised trial (20 participants) compared Altemeier's procedure with abdominal resection rectopexy, both procedures being combined with pelvic floor repair.[23] One patient in the Altemeier's arm had recurrent full-thickness prolapse although two patients in each arm developed mucosal prolapse. Both groups experienced significant postoperative morbidity, but symptoms of incontinence were significantly improved only in the abdominal resection rectopexy group.[23]

Abdominal approaches

Abdominal surgery may be performed either open or laparoscopically. Abdominal rectopexy entails rectal mobilisation and fixation to the sacrum with non-absorbable sutures or mesh.

✔✔ A recent randomised trial of 252 patients has confirmed the traditional view that fixation of the rectum to the sacrum (rectopexy) is an integral part of the success of transabdominal prolapse repair.[24]

Table 12.1 • Randomised controlled trials in rectal prolapse surgery

Authors (reference)	Year	n	Length of follow-up	Trial procedures	Outcomes
Speakman et al.[29]	1991	26	Median 12 months	Open polypropylene mesh rectopexy with division vs. preservation of lateral ligaments	Lateral ligament preservation was associated with less postoperative constipation but an increased rate of recurrent prolapse
Luukkonen et al.[38]	1992	30	6 months	Open resection suture rectopexy vs. open polyglycolic acid mesh rectopexy	Resection rectopexy resulted in less postoperative constipation
McKee et al.[39]	1992	18	Mean 20 months	Open resection rectopexy vs. open suture rectopexy (with division of the lateral ligaments)	Resection rectopexy resulted in less postoperative constipation but less improvement in faecal incontinence
Selvaggi et al.[30]	1993	20	Mean 14 (range 6–24) months	Open Marlex®/Mersilene® rectopexy with division vs. preservation of lateral ligaments	Lateral ligament preservation was associated with less postoperative constipation
Winde et al.[35]	1993	49	Mean 50.5 months	Open abdominal rectopexy (with anterior mesh sling) comparing polyglycolic acid vs. polyglactin mesh	No significant differences in postoperative complications or recurrence rates
Novell et al.[34]	1994	63	Median 47 (range 44–50) months	Open abdominal Ivalon® sponge rectopexy vs. suture rectopexy	No significant difference in recurrence rates. Significantly higher incidence of postoperative constipation in Ivalon® sponge group
Deen et al.[23]	1994	20	Median 17 (8–22) months	Altemeier's procedure with pelvic floor repair vs. abdominal resection rectopexy with pelvic floor repair	Similar recurrent full thickness and mucosal prolapse rates. Significant postoperative morbidity in both groups. Incontinence significantly improved in resection rectopexy group only
Galili and Rabau[36]	1997	37	Mean 3.7 years	Open abdominal mesh rectopexy (with anterolateral rectal mesh fixation) comparing polyglycolic acid vs. polypropylene mesh	No significant differences in postoperative complications or recurrence rates
Boccasanta et al.[43]	1998	21	Mean 29.5 (range 8–45) months	Laparoscopic vs. open Marlex®/Mersileneeg® mesh rectopexy versus open suture mesh (with anterolateral rectal mesh fixation)	No significant difference in recurrence rates
Mollen et al.[31]	2000	18	Mean 3.5 years	Posterior mesh rectopexy with division vs. preservation of lateral ligaments	No statistical difference in functional outcome
Solomon et al.[42]	2002	40	Mean 24.2 (range 2–52) months	Laparoscopic vs. open abdominal mesh rectopexy	No significant difference in recurrence rate. Laparoscopic approach was associated with significantly less morbidity, shorter hospital stays and longer operating times

Table 12.1 • (*cont.*) Randomised controlled trials in rectal prolapse surgery

Authors (reference)	Year	n	Length of follow-up	Trial procedures	Outcomes
Boccasanta et al.[19]	2006	40	Mean 28 months	Altemeier's procedure with levatorplasty comparing monopolar electrocautery dissection and handsewn anastomosis vs. harmonic scalpel dissection and circular stapled anastomosis	No significant difference in functional outcomes or recurrence rates. Operating time, blood loss and hospital stay were significantly reduced in the stapled group
Karas et al.[24]	2011	252	5 years (10.6% patients lost to follow-up)	Transabdominal rectal mobilisation without rectopexy vs. with rectopexy (mesh or sutures)	Significantly higher 5-year recurrence rate in no rectopexy (8.6%) vs. rectopexy group (1.5%) ($P=0.003$)
PROSPER (Prolapse Surgery: Perineal or Rectopexy) trial, www.prosper. bham.ac.uk		292	Trial has closed and follow-up results awaited	First randomisation or surgeon preference to select abdominal vs. perineal approach. Second randomisation in abdominal approach of suture vs. resection rectopexy and in perineal approach of Delorme vs. Altemeier operations (see Fig. 12.1)	48 patients randomised to approach, 78 to abdominal methods and 212 to perineal methods. Primary end-point of recurrent prolapse abandoned in favour of secondary end-points of bowel function and quality of life when recruitment one-third of anticipated

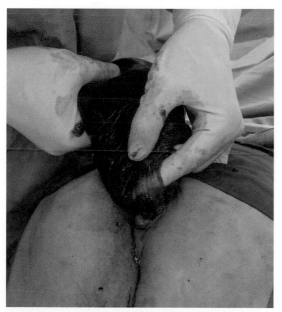

Figure 12.1 • Division of peritoneal reflection during Altemeier's procedure. Photograph printed with permission of Dr Tracy Hull, Cleveland Clinic, Cleveland, Ohio.

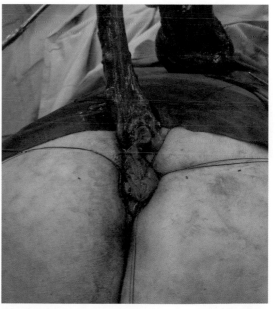

Figure 12.2 • Resection of rectosigmoid prior to coloanal anastomosis during Altemeier's procedure. Photograph printed with permission of Dr Tracy Hull, Cleveland Clinic, Cleveland, Ohio.

Rectopexy may be performed either posteriorly with Ivalon sponge (Wells's procedure), fascia lata (Orr–Loygue operation) or mesh, or anteriorly with an anterior mesh sling around the rectum to the sacrum (Ripstein's procedure) or ventral mesh rectopexy. Resection during an abdominal rectopexy (Frykman–Goldberg procedure) usually involves resection of the sigmoid colon with an anastomosis at the sacral promontory.[25]

✔✔ A multicentre pooled analysis of 643 patients who underwent abdominal procedures for rectal prolapse over a 22-year period found age, gender, surgical technique, approach (open or laparoscopic) and method of rectopexy had no impact on recurrence rates.[26] Nevertheless, this study was retrospective and probably not powered to show significant differences between the different surgical techniques of rectal mobilisation only, mobilisation with resection and rectopexy, or mobilisation and rectopexy.[26] Another retrospective meta-analysis using data from six studies on abdominal approaches to rectal prolapse repair again found no difference in recurrence rates with age, sex or surgical technique.[27]

Defecatory disorders are common after abdominal rectopexy and may present as novel or worsening constipation, evacuatory difficulties or faecal incontinence. Although many studies include analysis of these problems, their actual extent is difficult to quantify. In one small series, 23 patients undergoing abdominal rectopexy were evaluated prospectively for bowel function: symptoms of incontinence improved in 82%, 36% of patients with preoperative constipation improved with surgery, and 42% developed new-onset constipation.[28] Faecal incontinence was reportedly improved in most series of abdominal rectopexy.[22]

✔✔ Three trials have compared the effects of conservation versus division (with potential rectal denervation) of the lateral ligaments during posterior mesh rectopexy,[29–31] although all studies only involved small numbers of participants. Two of these trials found that preservation of the lateral ligaments was associated with less postoperative constipation,[29,30] although one also found an increased rate of recurrent prolapse with this technique.[29] A more recent, but still small, prospective randomised study found that division of the lateral ligaments during posterior Teflon® mesh rectopexy had no impact on postoperative constipation.[31]

A number of studies have examined different methods of rectal fixation during rectopexy. The principal concerns with mesh are infection and extrusion. Although the incidence of infection is low,[32,33] the consequences are serious when it occurs. Complete peritoneal closure over non-absorbable mesh may also reduce the incidence of postoperative small bowel obstruction.

✔✔ A randomised trial in 63 patients comparing Ivalon® sponge to suture rectopexy found no difference in recurrence rates, although there was a significantly higher incidence of postoperative constipation in the Ivalon® sponge arm.[34] The authors concluded that there was no need to use prosthetic materials to perform successful rectopexy.
Two trials looking at the relative benefits of different types of mesh in rectopexy surgery found no significant differences in either postoperative complications or recurrence rates with either absorbable or non-absorbable meshes.[35,36]

Resection is usually performed in combination with suture rectopexy in view of the excess risk of infection if non-absorbable mesh is used.[33] However, a small series of 35 cases of resection rectopexy with non-absorbable mesh in young patients reported good functional outcomes and no instances of mesh infection or anastomotic leakage.[37]

✔✔ Two trials with a combined total of 48 patients have examined the impact of concomitant sigmoid resection during open abdominal rectopexy.[38,39] One trial randomised patients between resection rectopexy and polyglycolic acid mesh rectopexy[38] and the other compared resection rectopexy with suture rectopexy.[39] If the results of these two small studies are combined, there is a statistically significant difference in rates of postoperative constipation, with a lower incidence in the resection arms of each trial.[40] However, one of the trials involved division of the lateral ligaments,[39] which may in itself have contributed to the high incidence of postoperative constipation. This trial also demonstrated that there was no improvement in incontinence symptoms in the resection group.[39]

Laparoscopic approaches

No prospective randomised trial has been conducted with a treatment arm including either laparoscopic suture rectopexy or laparoscopic resection rectopexy. A meta-analysis conducted to compare open and laparoscopic rectopexy in 688 patients[41] included

12 studies, only one of which was prospective and randomised.[42] The rectopexy techniques included resection, suture and mesh. The meta-analysis concluded that laparoscopic rectopexy was safe, took longer and had comparable recurrent prolapse rates to open surgery.[41]

✔✔ Two randomised trials have compared open and laparoscopic mesh rectopexy.[42,43] The first trial (21 patients) involved anterolateral rectal fixation of non-absorbable mesh (Marlex® or Mersilene®) to the sacral promontory and found no difference in recurrence rates between the different approaches at just over 2 years.[43] The second trial (40 patients) described full rectal mobilisation with posterior mesh rectopexy to the sacral promontory with a single spiked chromium staple and lateral fixation with hernia staples.[42] It too confirmed no difference in recurrence rates at 2 years (with one recurrence in the open group) but did show that the laparoscopic approach was associated with significantly less morbidity, a shorter hospital stay but a longer operating time.[42]

A feasibility study has examined the technique of robot-assisted laparoscopic rectopexy and concluded that it could be safely undertaken with similar functional outcomes but higher recurrence rates than open rectopexy.[44]

The surgical management of combined rectal and urogenital prolapse is probably best carried out from an abdominal approach, and laparoscopic repairs are particularly suited to repairing abnormalities of the rectum, vagina, bladder and pelvic floor,[45,46] allowing nerve-sparing surgery and minimally invasive techniques. A combined approach may also serve to lessen the impact of prolapse repair in one compartment on symptoms in another. If mesh is used, procedures that open the vagina should be avoided to reduce the chance of mesh erosion. Vaginal hysterectomy in the setting of combined rectal and urogynaecological prolapse surgery may be associated with higher morbidity.[47]

The PROSPER trial

Uncertainty over the best surgical procedure for rectal prolapse led to the PROSPER (Prolapse Surgery: Perineal or Rectopexy) trial being initiated in the UK in 2001. It had an unusual pragmatic design in that randomisation occurred at either one or two steps within the treatment pathway (**Fig. 12.3**). The first potential randomisation was based on the

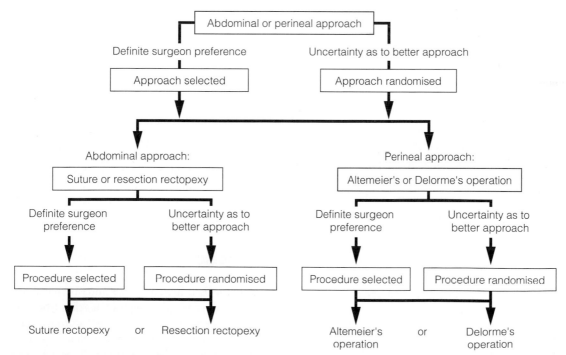

Figure 12.3 • Randomisation options within the PROSPER trial. Derived from trial design information (www.prosper.bham.ac.uk).

surgeon's uncertainty as to whether an abdominal or perineal approach was more appropriate. If the surgeon had a preference, this randomisation was avoided. The second potential point for randomisation occurred in the decision between suture or resection rectopexy for the abdominal approach, or between Delorme's and Altemeier's operation for the perineal approach.

The primary outcome for the first randomisation between abdominal and perineal approaches was recurrent rectal prolapse, but this was later relegated to a secondary outcome measure in favour of bowel function and quality-of-life scores when recruitment to the trial failed to meet anticipated levels. The primary outcome measures for the second randomisation between procedures were bowel function and quality of life. Substantially more patients were randomised in the perineal than the abdominal arm. The original recruitment target was 1000 and the trial was completed in 2007 after the target was revised to 300. The final results on the 292 patients recruited are awaited; 48 were randomised to the approach, 78 to the abdominal method (resection/suture rectopexy) and 212 to the perineal method (Delorme's/Altemeier's).

✔✔ An interim report on the first 153 patients in the PROSPER trial reported five (3.7%) serious adverse events, including three (2%) deaths. There were 23 (15%) recurrent (11 mucosal and 12 full-thickness) prolapses. Thirty-two patients (20.9%) experienced postoperative complications (www.prosper.bham.ac.uk/poster.pdf). Initial assessment of defecatory function using Kamm scores showed a dramatic improvement in continence and evacuation.

Recurrent rectal prolapse

Recurrence rates following rectal prolapse surgery vary widely. As all of the approaches carry a risk of recurrence, a number of patients will come to a second procedure. There is, however, little in the literature on management of recurrent rectal prolapse. Abdominal approaches are used more commonly than perineal approaches for recurrent full-thickness prolapse by some groups,[48] while others point out that perineal procedures can be safely repeated.[49] Recurrent prolapse in more than one compartment may be best treated via an abdominal approach.[50] Irrespective of approach, surgery for recurrent prolapse carries a significant risk of postoperative bowel dysfunction, either with obstructive or incontinent symptoms.[48,49]

Obstructive defecation, rectocele and rectal intussusception

The cardinal symptoms of obstructive defecation are straining at stool, a sense of incomplete evacuation, and the need for rectal, vaginal or perineal digitation in order to achieve evacuation. Paradoxical contraction of the puborectalis muscle during straining at stool is better termed pelvic floor dyssynergia. The latter is more commonly associated with urogynaecological, gastrointestinal and psychological problems than with slow-transit constipation. Many 'constipated' patients will have improvement in their symptoms with treatment of ODS. Treatment is predominantly medical with dietary manipulation, use of laxatives and biofeedback training.[51]

An anterior rectocele and/or rectal intussusception (internal rectal prolapse) are often found in association with ODS. The syndrome is very complex and the symptomatology variable. Symptoms of ODS may mask a number of occult disorders, including anxiety and depression, gynaecological prolapse, anismus, rectal hyposensitivity and slow-transit constipation. Many problems associated with obstructive defecation may not be immediately apparent.[52] Recognition and anticipation of occult pathology allow treatment to be tailored to the individual patient.

Objective assessment of the symptoms of ODS is particularly important when trying to assess the impact of new surgical interventions for the condition. The Cleveland Clinic Constipation Scoring System is already widely used but is not specific for obstructive defecation.[53] A new system using a structured questionnaire and giving a possible maximum score of 31 points has recently been suggested.[54] This gives weight to time spent at defecation, the number of attempts at defecation each day, use of digitation, use of laxatives and enemas, the presence of incomplete evacuation, straining at stool, and stool consistency.[54]

Rectocele

A rectocele is a hernia of the anterior rectal wall through the rectovaginal septum. It arises from muscular and nerve damage sustained during vaginal delivery, as a result of hormonal changes following the menopause, or due to paradoxical contraction of the puborectalis. Rectoceles occur due to a pressure gradient between the rectum and vagina during coughing and straining due to weakness in the puborectalis and bulbocavernosus muscles.[55] Suspensory surgery on the anterior vaginal wall, e.g. anterior colporrhaphy or Burch colposuspension, may predispose to development of a rectocele.[56] Posterior rectoceles are rare, and usually result from traumatic injury or surgical interventions breaching the anococcygeal ligament.

An anterior rectocele is a common finding in patients with ODS, but may also occur in asymptomatic patients. It is commonly seen on defecography[57] and magnetic resonance (MR) proctography.[58] Associated symptoms include difficulty in evacuation, constipation, the need for perineal or vaginal digitation during defecation and rectal discomfort. Anal digitation is not usually a symptom caused by a rectocele. Rectoceles vary in size, both in the extent of protrusion into the vagina and in the length of involvement of the rectovaginal septum, but size does not necessarily correlate with severity of symptoms.

The mainstays of treatment of symptomatic rectocele are dietary manipulation and biofeedback.[59–61] Rectocele repair can lead to improved defecatory symptoms in selected patients who have failed to respond to conservative treatment.[62] Surgical repair, by either gynaecologists or colorectal surgeons, gives highly variable results and may be performed via transvaginal, perineal, transanal or transabdominal routes. A variety of techniques employ suture plication, mesh reinforcement of the rectovaginal septum, resection of redundant tissue, fixation of the rectum, vagina or perineal body, or reinforcement of the pelvic floor musculature. There has been a recent vogue for repair of rectocele with laparoscopic ventral rectopexy,[63] or transanal excision using linear[64,65] and circular staplers (see section on stapled transanal rectal resection).

The Block procedure involves full-thickness suture plication of the rectocele with absorbable sutures via a transanal approach.[66] The Sarles procedure consists of an elliptical transanal mucocutaneous flap, plication of the anterior rectal muscle with non-absorbable sutures, resection of redundant mucosa and reapplication of the flap to the anal verge with absorbable sutures[67] (much like an anterior Delorme operation). Transanal approaches may compromise the integrity of the sphincter complex with consequent faecal

incontinence,[68,69] although other studies have shown no effect on continence or sexual function.[70]

Abdominal repair may be performed by open or laparoscopic approaches and involves dissection of the rectovaginal septum via the pouch of Douglas; repair of the rectocele can then be carried out with or without concomitant rectopexy or sacrocolpopexy.

Although a number of authors report series of varying sizes, there have been very few prospective randomised controlled trials (Table 12.2).

✓ A retrospective multicentre study examined the results of rectocele repair in 317 patients by transanal approaches (*n*=141), perineal levatorplasty (*n*=126) or combined transanal repair and perineal levatorplasty (*n*=50).[71] None of the procedures was functionally superior, but bleeding complications were more common in transanal procedures, and dyspareunia and delayed perineal wound healing were more frequent after perineal levatorplasty. About half of the patients who had preoperative faecal incontinence and underwent perineal levatorplasty had improved continence scores postoperatively.[71]

✓✓ Two small randomised trials (see Table 12.2) have compared transanal rectocele repair with posterior colporrhaphy in 57 and 30 patients, respectively.[72,73] A Cochrane Database Review pooled the results of these to perform a meta-analysis of posterior vaginal wall surgery in women.[74] Both approaches resulted in improved defecatory function, with a greater proportion of patients in the vaginal approach group achieving successful outcomes and a significantly higher rate of symptomatic recurrent posterior vaginal wall prolapse in the transanal group.[74] A recent trial in multiparous women with obstructed defecation randomised patients to three different types of rectocele repair: transperineal repair with or without levatorplasty and transanal repair. All three methods improved the anatomical appearances of rectocele on defecography but transperineal repair with levatorplasty was associated with the best functional outcome.[75]

Rectal intussusception

Rectal intussusception refers to the invagination of the rectal wall during defecation. The bowel wall will descend to varying degrees, which are classified to the leading edge of the intussusception. The

Table 12.2 • Randomised controlled trials in rectocele surgery

Authors	Year	n	Length of follow-up	Procedures	Outcomes
Kahn et al.[72]	1999	63	25 months	Posterior colporrhaphy (24) vs. transanal repair (33)	• Longer length of stay and higher narcotic usage in vaginal approach group • Successful repair higher in vaginal group (87.5%) vs. transanal group (69.7%)
Sand et al.[111]	2001	160	12 months	Anterior and posterior colporrhaphy without vs. with Vicryl™ mesh (Ethicon)	• No difference in rates of recurrent rectocele at 1 year: 10% vs. 8.2% ($P=0.71$) • Cystocele recurrence greater in group without mesh (43%) than with mesh (25%) ($P=0.02$)
Boccasanta et al.[112]	2004	50	23.4±5.1 months vs. 22.3±4.8 months	Stapled transanal prolapsectomy with perineal levatorplasty vs. STARR procedure	• STARR group had less postoperative pain ($P<0.0001$) and greater decrease in rectal sensitivity threshold volume ($P=0.012$) • No differences in functional outcomes or early and late complication rates • Significantly higher incidence of dyspareunia in prolapsectomy with levatorplasty group (20%) over STARR group (none) ($P=0.018$)
Nieminen et al.[73]	2004	30	12 months	Posterior colporrhaphy (15) vs. transanal repair (15)	• Improved defaecatory function 93% vs. 73% ($P=0.08$) • Recurrent symptomatic rectocele/ enterocele 7% vs. 40% ($P=0.04$)
Paraiso et al.[113]	2006	106	17.5±7 months	Posterior colporrhaphy (37) vs. site-specific rectocele repair (37) vs. site-specific rectocele repair with graft augmentation (32)	• No difference in symptom improvement among groups (15% functional failure rate overall) • Anatomical failure rate 46% in graft augmentation group compared to 14% and 22% in other groups ($P=0.02$) • No differences in improvement in sexual function or dyspareunia rates • Bowel symptoms at 12 months were improved significantly in all groups[62]
Farid et al.[75]	2010	48	6 months	Transperineal repair with levatorplasty (16) vs. transperineal repair without levatorplasty (16) vs. transanal repair (16)	• Significant reduction in rectocele size on defaecography in all groups • Best functional outcome in transperineal groups with levatorplasty giving best outcomes

intussusception may remain entirely within the rectum, reach the dentate line, protrude into the anus or (in the case of full-thickness prolapse) protrude through the anus. There is, however, little correlation between the degree of intussusception seen on evacuation defecography and the symptoms experienced by the patient. Rectal intussusception is also seen in asymptomatic individuals.

Rectal intussusception may be associated with symptoms of obstructive defecation. It may be diagnosed at rigid sigmoidoscopy by an experienced practitioner on asking the patient to strain during withdrawal of the sigmoidoscope. It is more commonly seen during contrast or MR defecography. Internal rectal intussusception is initially treated conservatively. Surgical procedures in the event of failure of conservative management include abdominal rectopexy,[76,77] an internal Delorme procedure,[78] laparoscopic ventral rectopexy[79,80] and the stapled transanal rectal resection (STARR) procedure.[81,82]

Laparoscopic ventral rectopexy

Working on the premise that rectal prolapse is initiated by anterior rectal wall intussusception, ventral rectosacropexy with no other rectal mobilisation was introduced. The operation can be performed open or laparoscopically. Laparoscopic ventral rectopexy involves peritoneal mobilisation over the pouch of Douglas to gain access via the rectovaginal septum to the pelvic floor, mesh fixation to the septum distally and, with either sutures or a ProTack™ stapling device, proximally to the sacrum, and extraperitonealisation of the mesh by full peritoneal closure.[46] A simultaneous colporrhaphy to treat an enterocele or vaginal prolapse may be performed by anchoring the posterior vagina to the mesh with sutures. A prospective series of 109 cases treated using this technique reported low morbidity (minor complications in 7%) and low recurrent prolapse rates (4%).[46] Another series of 80 patients reported complications in 21% but no recurrence at a median follow-up of 54 months; there was also marked improvement in symptoms of either faecal incontinence or ODS.[45] There was no mesh infection or erosion in either series.

Proponents of ventral rectopexy for full-thickness rectal prolapse propose that avoidance of posterior mobilisation reduces rectal denervation and may lessen postoperative symptoms of constipation.[83,84] Improvement of constipation symptoms after rectopexy in patients with external prolapse has led to the introduction of ventral rectopexy as a treatment for other disorders associated with obstructed defecation, including internal rectal intussusception and rectocele.[63,79,80,83,85]

✅ There are no randomised controlled trials to assess ventral rectopexy. A systematic review on ventral rectopexy for rectal prolapse and intussusception examined the outcomes of 728 patients in 12 case series. Recurrence rates appeared reasonable at 0–15.6%. Avoidance of posterior mobilisation appeared to reduce the postoperative incidence of new-onset constipation or faecal incontinence, but the review emphasised the heterogeneity of the studies included and the relatively short follow-up.[86]

Stapled transanal rectal resection (STARR)

STARR was first used in ODS following the introduction of the procedure for prolapse and haemorrhoids (PPH). The latter uses a circular stapling device (Proximate PPH-01™, Ethicon Endo-Surgery®). The STARR technique was described by Altomare et al. in 2002,[87] who combined dissection of the rectovaginal septum via a perineal incision with a single transanal firing of the PPH-01™ stapling gun. The PPH technique was modified for STARR by using a purse-string suture, which was full thickness anteriorly and only mucosal posteriorly. The initial study described the results in eight female patients, all of whom had symptoms of ODS associated with an anterior rectocele.[87] The PPH-03™ (Ethicon Endo-Surgery®) stapling device has been modified to reduce the risk of haemorrhagic complications.[88]

STARR is normally carried out in the Lloyd–Davies position, although some surgeons prefer the prone jack-knife or Kraske position. STARR consists of a full-thickness circumferential resection of the lower rectum using stapling devices. There are two principal methods. Using the PPH stapling device, purse-string sutures to encompass the full thickness of rectal wall are placed 4 cm above the dentate line and used to pull the rectal wall into the circular gun to resect the rectum, and the stapler is then closed with a finger in the vagina to protect the rectovaginal septum. The alternative is a circumferential technique involving four or five firings of a curved linear stapler (Contour Transtar™, Ethicon Endo-Surgery®), which allows more accurate placement of the purse strings and each firing of the stapler to be done under direct observation.[89] With either method the end result should be a circumferential row of staples. Any bleeding points are oversewn with an absorbable suture. A small study using dynamic magnetic resonance imaging (MRI) for pre- and early postoperative comparison has shown that STARR reduces the size of rectocele and eliminates rectal intussusception in patients with ODS.[90]

✅✅ Two randomised trials have compared use of the double-firing PPH stapling technique to Transtar.[91,92] Both studies showed an improvement in functional outcome at 12 months, but there was a higher rate of recurrent ODS in the PPH groups in both studies (see Table 12.3). One of the studies reported a significantly higher incidence of postoperative faecal urgency in the PPH group.[91]

Table 12.3 • Randomised controlled trials of stapled transanal rectal resection (STARR)

Authors	Year	n	Length of follow-up	Procedures	Outcomes
Boccasanta et al.[112]	2004	50	23.4±5.1 months vs. 22.3±4.8 months	Stapled transanal prolapsectomy with perineal levatorplasty vs. STARR procedure	• STARR group had less postoperative pain ($P<0.0001$) and greater decrease in rectal sensitivity threshold volume ($P=0.012$) • No differences in functional outcomes or early and late complication rates • Significantly higher incidence of dyspareunia in prolapsectomy with levatorplasty group (20%) over STARR group (none) ($P=0.018$)
Lehur et al.[114]	2008	119	12 months	STARR ($n=59$) vs. biofeedback therapy ($n=60$) for women with ODS, rectocele and rectal intussusception	• Only 54 STARR patients and 39 biofeedback patients completed the follow-up period • ODS and QoL scores improved significantly in both groups ($P=0.0001$) • Successful functional outcomes were observed in 44 (81.5%) STARR vs. 13 (33.3%) biofeedback patients ($P<0.0001$) • Complications occurred in 8 (15%) STARR patients (including 1 SAE – bleeding) and in 1 (2%) biofeedback patient who experienced anal pain
Boccasanta et al.[91]	2011	100	3 years	STARR with double firing PPH-01™ vs. CCS-30 Contour Transtar™	• Functional outcomes improved significantly in both groups ($P<0.001$) • Operating time was significantly shorter in STARR group ($P=0.008$) • Faecal urgency incidence was 34.0% in STARR group and 14.0% in TRANSTAR group ($P=0.035$) • Recurrence rates at 3 years were 12.0% in STARR group and none in TRANSTAR group ($P=0.035$)
Renzi et al.[92]	2011	63	2 years	STARR with double-firing PPH-01™ vs. CCS-30 Contour Transtar™	• Functional outcomes improved significantly in both groups at 12 months ($P<0.0001$) • Improvement in functional outcome was only maintained in Transtar group at 24 months • No significant differences in length of stay or complication rates

ODS, obstructed defaecation syndrome; SAE, serious adverse event; STARR, stapled transanal resection rectopexy.

Chapter 12

One of the major concerns about the STARR technique is the potential threat to structures anterior to the rectal wall in the pouch of Douglas. As an enterocele is fairly common in patients with pelvic floor disorders, it is important to establish the presence of an enterocele with defecography or MRI prior to performing a STARR procedure. A German group has advocated the use of laparoscopy during the procedure in patients known to have an enterocele[93] and another study has performed STARR with relative safety in patients with ODS and enterocele.[94] Early concern about the STARR procedure arose from a report of 29 patients of whom half had severe postoperative complications or recurrent symptoms.[95] Complications included severe intraoperative or early postoperative bleeding requiring re-operation or rectal tamponade, pelvic and retroperitoneal sepsis, persistent severe perianal pain, and new-onset faecal incontinence. Seven patients had recurrent symptoms of ODS and one underwent resection of recurrent rectal internal mucosal prolapse.[95] The authors discussed potential errors in technique, including the possibility of stapling too close to the dentate line, undetected co-pathology including pelvic floor dyssynergia, or poor patient selection. The study suggested that parity, pelvic floor dyssynergia and anxiety states were risk factors predisposing to failure of STARR.[95] Small rectal diameter, marked pelvic floor descent and low sphincter pressures are also poor prognostic indicators, whereas rectocele, enterocele and intussusception are positive predictors for a favourable outcome.[96]

✔️✔️ The Milan group reported a randomised trial between single stapled transanal prolapsectomy with perineal levatorplasty and the STARR procedure.[97] The STARR group had consistently lower postoperative pain scores but there were otherwise no differences in operative time, hospital stay or return to work. The stapled prolapsectomy group showed improvement in constipation symptoms in 76% compared to 88% in the STARR group. Both groups experienced similar complication rates, with a significant incidence of delayed perineal wound healing in the prolapsectomy group. Late complications were similar, with urgency of defecation, incontinence to flatus and anal stenosis occurring in both groups. Dyspareunia affected 20% of the prolapsectomy group but did not occur within the STARR group.[97]

STARR became widely used without good published evidence for its efficacy and safety, raising concerns about the need for evidence-based practice with this procedure.[98] International registries were established to address these concerns.

✔️✔️ In 2009, the European STARR registry reported the combined UK, Italian and German 1-year follow-up results of 2224 patients who had undergone a STARR procedure.[99] The mean age for undergoing a STARR procedure was 54.7 years and 83.3% were female. While significant improvements were seen in obstructed defecation and symptom severity scores, and in quality-of-life assessment, the complication rate was high at 36%. Complications included urgency (20%), persistent pain (7.1%), urinary retention (6.9%), postoperative bleeding (5%), sepsis (4.4%), staple line complications (3.5%) and incontinence (1.8%). Single cases each of rectal necrosis and rectovaginal fistula were reported, although there was no perioperative mortality. The conclusions urged better methods of patient selection and optimisation of technique to reduce postoperative defecatory urgency and pain.[99]

Reports of significant complication rates persist, which is of particular concern in surgery for benign disease. Rare but serious complications include rectovaginal fistula,[99,100] retroperitoneal sepsis,[97] rectal perforation requiring colostomy,[100] necrotising pelvic fasciitis requiring emergency laparotomy with Hartmann's procedure and hysterectomy and subsequent early death from multi-organ failure.[101]

The external pelvic rectal suspension (EXPRESS) procedure

The EXPRESS procedure was developed as an alternative surgical repair for patients with symptoms of ODS in conjunction with rectal intussusception with or without a rectocele. The procedure was first described using Gore-Tex® mesh[102] and then Permacol® (Tissue Science Laboratories).[103]

EXPRESS involves dissection of the rectovaginal septum via perineal incision, mobilisation of the lateral rectal wall, blind tunnelling through the retropubic space anterior to the bladder to allow suture fixation to the lower end of the recti muscles and fixation of a T-shaped piece of Permacol® in the rectovaginal septum. Any associated rectocele is repaired via the perineal wound by dissecting into the ischiorectal fossa on either side to expose the ischial tuberosities. The Tbar of the mesh is passed underneath the puborectalis muscle and is sutured to the ischial tuberosity on either side and anchored to the rectum.

There is one reported series of 17 patients treated with the EXPRESS procedure for ODS. Intraoperative complications included small vaginal perforations in two patients and anterior rectal wall perforations in three; all were recognised at the time of surgery and repaired. One patient developed sepsis in the rectovaginal plane and required subsequent surgical drainage and a diverting stoma. Two other patients also developed postoperative sepsis, one requiring surgical drainage. Three complained of neuralgic pain, but all resolved with time. There was significant improvement in symptom and quality of life, and no reported change in sexual function. Although the authors concluded that postoperative morbidity was lower than the STARR procedure and functional results similar,[102–104] EXPRESS is still only performed in a single centre.

Solitary rectal ulcer syndrome (SRUS)

SRUS may be caused by paradoxical contraction of the anal sphincter muscle during defecation, is frequently associated with anal digitation, and results in anterior mucosal trauma and ulceration. It is characterised by classical symptoms, endoscopic findings and histopathological changes.[105] Treatment involves dietary changes, bulking agents and biofeedback to reverse the underlying defecatory disorder.[106] Surgical intervention is rarely indicated and should only be used for patients with concomitant demonstrable prolapse or intractable symptoms refractory to conservative management. A number of surgical options have been described in SRUS management, including transanal excision of the ulcer, stapled mucosal resection, modified anterior Delorme procedure, abdominal rectopexy, and colostomy formation.[107] Simple resection without biofeedback does not resolve the symptoms.[108] Rectopexy has high failure rates of up to 50%,[107,109] although early results of the STARR procedure in refractory SRUS appear encouraging.[110]

Key points

- Patients being considered for surgical management of functional disorders of defecation are best managed within the setting of a multidisciplinary clinic or team.
- The management of full-thickness prolapse is almost exclusively surgical.
- There is no current evidence to support the superiority of abdominal or perineal approaches to rectal prolapse repair, although the results of the PROSPER trial are awaited.
- Fixation of the rectum to the sacrum is a key component of successful rectopexy. Mesh and suture techniques give equivalent results in abdominal rectopexy.
- Preservation of the lateral ligaments during rectal mobilisation is associated with fewer postoperative defecatory symptoms.
- Laparoscopic approaches to abdominal rectopexy are as effective as open approaches, and may have benefits in terms of recovery times and lower morbidity.
- Laparoscopic surgery may have particular benefits for management of combined genital and rectal prolapse.
- Rectocele repairs should only be offered to patients who remain symptomatic after conservative management of obstructed defecation with dietary manipulation, bulking agents and biofeedback, and who digitate vaginally or perineally (i.e. not anal digitators).
- There is limited evidence to suggest that transvaginal approaches to rectocele repair may be functionally superior to transanal approaches.
- The STARR procedure or ventral rectopexy may offer symptomatic relief in carefully selected patients with obstructive defecation syndrome.
- The Transtar technique of STARR may be associated with less postoperative faecal urgency and more sustained long-term results.
- The EXPRESS procedure provides an alternative surgical repair for patients with symptoms of obstructive defecation associated with rectal intussusception or rectocele but needs validation.

References

1. Davis K, Kumar D. Posterior pelvic floor compartment disorders. Best Pract Res Clin Obstet Gynaecol 2005;19(6):941–58.

2. Kapoor DS, Sultan AH, Thakar R, et al. Management of complex pelvic floor disorders in a multidisciplinary pelvic floor clinic. Colorectal Dis 2008;10(2):118–23.

3. Finco C, Luongo B, Savastano S, et al. Selection criteria for surgery in patients with obstructed defecation, rectocele and anorectal prolapse. Chir Ital 2007;59(4):513–20.

4. Carley ME, Schaffer J. Urinary incontinence and pelvic organ prolapse in women with Marfan or Ehlers Danlos syndrome. Am J Obstet Gynecol 2000;182(5):1021–3.

5. Dreznik Z, Vishne TH, Kristt D, et al. Rectal prolapse: a possibly underrecognized complication of anorexia nervosa amenable to surgical correction. Int J Psychiat Med 2001;31(3):347–52.

6. Karasick S, Spettell CM. The role of parity and hysterectomy on the development of pelvic floor abnormalities revealed by defecography. Am J Roentgenol 1997;169(6):1555–8.

7. Swift S, Woodman P, O'Boyle A, et al. Pelvic Organ Support Study (POSST): the distribution, clinical definition, and epidemiologic condition of pelvic organ support defects. Am J Obstet Gynecol 2005;192(3):795–806.

8. Chew SS, Marshall L, Kalish L, et al. Short-term and long-term results of combined sclerotherapy and rubber band ligation of hemorrhoids and mucosal prolapse. Dis Colon Rectum 2003;46(9):1232–7.

9. Gupta PJ. Randomized controlled study: radiofrequency coagulation and plication versus ligation and excision technique for rectal mucosal prolapse. Am J Surg 2006;192(2):155–60.

10. Kleinubing Jr H, Pinho MS, Ferreira LC. Longitudinal multiple rubber band ligation: an alternative method to treat mucosal prolapse of the anterior rectal wall. Dis Colon Rectum 2006;49(6):876–8.

11. Orrom W, Hayashi A, Rusnak C, et al. Initial experience with stapled anoplasty in the operative management of prolapsing hemorrhoids and mucosal rectal prolapse. Am J Surg 2002;183(5):519–24.

12. Corman ML, Carriero A, Hager T, et al. Consensus conference on the stapled transanal rectal resection (STARR) for disordered defaecation. Colorectal Dis 2006;8(2):98–101.

13. Tou S, Brown SR, Malik AI, et al. Surgery for complete rectal prolapse in adults. Cochrane Database Syst Rev 2008;(4):CD001758.
Cochrane meta-analysis of randomised controlled trials in prolapse surgery identified 12 trials with 380 patients. There was no difference in recurrence rates between abdominal and perineal approaches.

14. Brown AJ, Anderson JH, McKee RF, et al. Strategy for selection of type of operation for rectal prolapse based on clinical criteria. Dis Colon Rectum 2004;47(1):103–7.

15. Wijffels N, Cunningham C, Dixon A, et al. Laparoscopic ventral rectopexy for external rectal prolapse is safe and effective in the elderly. Does this make perineal procedures obsolete? Colorectal Dis 2011;13(5):561–6.

16. Farouk R, Duthie GS. The evaluation and treatment of patients with rectal prolapse. Ann Chir Gynaecol 1997;86(4):279–84.

17. Christiansen J, Kirkegaard P. Delorme's operation for complete rectal prolapse. Br J Surg 1981;68(8):537–8.

18. Altemeier WA, Culbertson WR, Schowengerdt C, et al. Nineteen years' experience with the one-stage perineal repair of rectal prolapse. Ann Surg 1971;173(6):993–1006.

19. Boccasanta P, Venturi M, Barbieri S, et al. Impact of new technologies on the clinical and functional outcome of Altemeier's procedure: a randomized, controlled trial. Dis Colon Rectum 2006;49(5):652–60.

20. Agachan F, Reissman P, Pfeifer J, et al. Comparison of three perineal procedures for the treatment of rectal prolapse. Southern Med J 1997;90(9):925–32.

21. Madiba TE, Baig MK, Wexner SD. Surgical management of rectal prolapse. Arch Surg 2005;140(1):63–73.

22. Marderstein EL, Delaney CP. Surgical management of rectal prolapse. Nat Clin Pract Gastroenterol Hepatol 2007;4(10):552–61.

23. Deen KI, Grant E, Billingham C, et al. Abdominal resection rectopexy with pelvic floor repair versus perineal rectosigmoidectomy and pelvic floor repair for full-thickness rectal prolapse. Br J Surg 1994;81(2):302–4.
A randomised controlled trial of Altemeier's procedure with pelvic floor repair compared to abdominal resection rectopexy with pelvic floor repair. Similar recurrent prolapse rates and significant postoperative morbidity were observed in both groups. Incontinence significantly improved in the resection rectopexy group only.

24. Karas JR, Uranues S, Altomare DF, et al. No rectopexy versus rectopexy following rectal mobilization for full-thickness rectal prolapse: a randomized controlled trial. Dis Colon Rectum 2011;54(1):29–34.
A randomised trial of 252 patients confirmed that fixation of the rectum to the sacrum (rectopexy) is an integral part of the success of prolapse repair.

25. Madoff RD, Williams JG, Wong WD, et al. Long-term functional results of colon resection and rectopexy for overt rectal prolapse. Am J Gastroenterol 1992;87(1):101–4.

26. Raftopoulos Y, Senagore AJ, Di Giuro G, et al. Recurrence rates after abdominal surgery for

complete rectal prolapse: a multicenter pooled analysis of 643 individual patient data. Dis Colon Rectum 2005;48(6):1200–6.

27. DiGiuro G, Ignjatovic D, Brogger J, et al. How accurate are published recurrence rates after rectal prolapse surgery? A meta-analysis of individual patient data. Am J Surg 2006;191(6):773–8.

28. Madden MV, Kamm MA, Nicholls RJ, et al. Abdominal rectopexy for complete prolapse: prospective study evaluating changes in symptoms and anorectal function. Dis Colon Rectum 1992;35(1):48–55.

29. Speakman CT, Madden MV, Nicholls RJ, et al. Lateral ligament division during rectopexy causes constipation but prevents recurrence: results of a prospective randomised study. Br J Surg 1991;78(12):1431–3.

30. Selvaggi F, Scotto di Carlo E, Silvestri L, et al. Surgical treatment of rectal prolapse: a randomised study (Abstract). Br J Surg 1993;80:89.

31. Mollen RM, Kuijpers JH, van Hoek F. Effects of rectal mobilization and lateral ligaments division on colonic and anorectal function. Dis Colon Rectum 2000;43(9):1283–7.

32. Keighley MR, Fielding JW, Alexander-Williams J. Results of Marlex mesh abdominal rectopexy for rectal prolapse in 100 consecutive patients. Br J Surg 1983;70(4):229–32.

33. Athanasiadis S, Weyand G, Heiligers J, et al. The risk of infection of three synthetic materials used in rectopexy with or without colonic resection for rectal prolapse. Int J Colorectal Dis 1996;11(1):42–4.

34. Novell JR, Osborne MJ, Winslet MC, et al. Prospective randomized trial of Ivalon sponge versus sutured rectopexy for full-thickness rectal prolapse. Br J Surg 1994;81(6):904–6.
A prospective randomised trial comparing Ivalon® sponge to suture rectopexy found no difference in recurrence rates, although there was a significantly higher incidence of postoperative constipation in the Ivalon® sponge arm.

35. Winde G, Reers B, Nottberg H, et al. Clinical and functional results of abdominal rectopexy with absorbable mesh-graft for treatment of complete rectal prolapse. Eur J Surg 1993;159(5):301–5.

36. Galili Y, Rabau M. Comparison of polyglycolic acid and polypropylene mesh for rectopexy in the treatment of rectal prolapse. Eur J Surg 1997;163(6):445–8.

37. Lechaux JP, Arienza P, Goasguen N, et al. Prosthetic rectopexy to the pelvic floor and sigmoidectomy for rectal prolapse. Am J Surg 2001;182(5):465–9.

38. Luukkonen P, Mikkonen U, Jarvinen H. Abdominal rectopexy with sigmoidectomy vs. rectopexy alone for rectal prolapse: a prospective, randomized study. Int J Colorectal Dis 1992;7(4):219–22.

39. McKee RF, Lauder JC, Poon FW, et al. A prospective randomized study of abdominal rectopexy with and without sigmoidectomy in rectal prolapse. Surg Gynecol Obstet 1992;174(2):145–8.

40. Bachoo P, Brazzelli M, Grant A. Surgery for complete rectal prolapse in adults. Cochrane Database Syst Rev 2000;2:CD001758.

41. Sajid MS, Siddiqui MR, Baig MK. Open vs laparoscopic repair of full-thickness rectal prolapse: a re-meta-analysis. Colorectal Dis 2010;12(6):515–25.

42. Solomon MJ, Young CJ, Eyers AA, et al. Randomized clinical trial of laparoscopic versus open abdominal rectopexy for rectal prolapse. Br J Surg 2002;89(1):35–9.
No significant difference was found in recurrence rates but the laparoscopic approach was associated with significantly less morbidity, shorter hospital stays and longer operating times.

43. Boccasanta P, Rosati R, Venturi M, et al. Comparison of laparoscopic rectopexy with open technique in the treatment of complete rectal prolapse: clinical and functional results. Surg Laparosc Endosc 1998;8(6):460–5.

44. de Hoog DENM, Heemskerk J, Nieman FHM, et al. Recurrence and functional results after open versus conventional laparoscopic versus robot-assisted laparoscopic rectopexy for rectal prolapse: a case–control study. Int J Colorectal Dis 2009;24(10):1201–6.

45. Slawik S, Soulsby R, Carter H, et al. Laparoscopic ventral rectopexy, posterior colporrhaphy and vaginal sacrocolpopexy for the treatment of rectogenital prolapse and mechanical outlet obstruction. Colorectal Dis 2008;10(2):138–43.

46. D'Hoore A, Penninckx F. Laparoscopic ventral recto(colpo)pexy for rectal prolapse: surgical technique and outcome for 109 patients. Surg Endosc 2006;20(12):1919–23.

47. Boccasanta P, Venturi M, Spennacchio M, et al. Prospective clinical and functional results of combined rectal and urogynecologic surgery in complex pelvic floor disorders. Am J Surg 2010;199(2):144–53.

48. Hool GR, Hull TL, Fazio VW. Surgical treatment of recurrent complete rectal prolapse: a thirty-year experience. Dis Colon Rectum 1997;40(3):270–2.

49. Fengler SA, Pearl RK, Prasad ML, et al. Management of recurrent rectal prolapse. Dis Colon Rectum 1997;40(7):832–4.

50. Gauruder-Burmester A, Koutouzidou P, Rohne J, et al. Follow-up after polypropylene mesh repair of anterior and posterior compartments in patients with recurrent prolapse. Int Urogynecol J Pelvic Floor Dysfunct 2007;18(9):1059–64.

51. Lau CW, Heymen S, Alabaz O, et al. Prognostic significance of rectocele, intussusception, and abnormal perineal descent in biofeedback treatment for constipated patients with paradoxical puborectalis contraction. Dis Colon Rectum 2000;43(4):478–82.

52. Pescatori M, Spyrou M, Pulvirenti d'Urso A. A prospective evaluation of occult disorders in obstructed defecation using the 'iceberg diagram'. Colorectal Dis 2006;8(9):785–9.

53. Agachan F, Chen T, Pfeifer J, et al. A constipation scoring system to simplify evaluation and management of constipated patients. Dis Colon Rectum 1996;39(6):681–5.

54. Altomare DF, Spazzafumo L, Rinaldi M, et al. Set-up and statistical validation of a new scoring system for obstructed defaecation syndrome. Colorectal Dis 2008;10(1):84–8.

55. Shafik A, El-Sibai O, Shafik AA, et al. On the pathogenesis of rectocele: the concept of the rectovaginal pressure gradient. Int Urogynecol J Pelvic Floor Dysfunct 2003;14(5):310–5.

56. Wiskind AK, Creighton SM, Stanton SL. The incidence of genital prolapse after the Burch colposuspension. Am J Obstet Gynecol 1992;167(2):399–405.

57. Agachan F, Pfeifer J, Wexner SD. Defecography and proctography. Results of 744 patients. Dis Colon Rectum 1996;39(8):899–905.

58. Kaufman HS, Buller JL, Thompson JR, et al. Dynamic pelvic magnetic resonance imaging and cystocolpoproctography alter surgical management of pelvic floor disorders. Dis Colon Rectum 2001;44(11):1575–84.

59. Mimura T, Roy AJ, Storrie JB, et al. Treatment of impaired defecation associated with rectocele by behavioral retraining (biofeedback). Dis Colon Rectum 2000;43(9):1267–72.

60. Heymen S, Scarlett Y, Jones K, et al. Randomized, controlled trial shows biofeedback to be superior to alternative treatments for patients with pelvic floor dyssynergia-type constipation. Dis Colon Rectum 2007;50(4):428–41.

61. Koh CE, Young CJ, Young JM, et al. Systematic review of randomized controlled trials of the effectiveness of biofeedback for pelvic floor dysfunction. Br J Surg 2008;95(9):1079–87.

62. Gustilo-Ashby AM, Paraiso MF, Jelovsek JE, et al. Bowel symptoms 1 year after surgery for prolapse: further analysis of a randomized trial of rectocele repair. Am J Obstet Gynecol 2007;197(1):76e1–5.

63. Wong M, Meurette G, Abet E, et al. Safety and efficacy of laparoscopic ventral mesh rectopexy for complex rectocele. Colorectal Dis 2011;13(9):1019–23.

64. Ayav A, Bresler L, Brunaud L, et al. Long-term results of transanal repair of rectocele using linear stapler. Dis Colon Rectum 2004;47(6):889–94.

65. D'Avolio M, Ferrara A, Chimenti C. Transanal rectocele repair using EndoGIA: short-term results of a prospective study. Tech Coloproctol 2005;9(2):108–14.

66. Block IR. Transrectal repair of rectocele using obliterative suture. Dis Colon Rectum 1986;29(11):707–11.

67. Sarles JC, Arnaud A, Selezneff I, et al. Endorectal repair of rectocele. Int J Colorectal Dis 1989;4(3):167–71.

68. Ho YH, Ang M, Nyam D, et al. Transanal approach to rectocele repair may compromise anal sphincter pressures. Dis Colon Rectum 1998;41(3):354–8.

69. Ayabaca SM, Zbar AP, Pescatori M. Anal continence after rectocele repair. Dis Colon Rectum 2002;45(1):63–9.

70. Heriot AG, Skull A, Kumar D. Functional and physiological outcome following transanal repair of rectocele. Br J Surg 2004;91(10):1340–4.

71. Boccasanta P, Venturi M, Calabro G, et al. Which surgical approach for rectocele? A multicentric report from Italian coloproctologists. Tech Coloproctol 2001;5(3):149–56.

72. Kahn MA, et al. Posterior colporrhaphy is superior to the transanal repair for treatment of posterior vaginal wall prolapse. Neurourol Urodyn 1999;18(4):329–30.

73. Nieminen K, Hiltunen KM, Laitinen J, et al. Transanal or vaginal approach to rectocele repair: a prospective, randomized pilot study. Dis Colon Rectum 2004;47(10):1636–42.

74. Maher CM, Feiner B, Baessler K, et al. Surgical management of pelvic organ prolapse in women: the updated summary version Cochrane review. Int Urogynecol J 2011;22(11):1445–57.
Cochrane review that analyses two trials comparing transanal rectocele repair with posterior colporrhaphy. Outcomes favour the transvaginal approach.

75. Farid M, Madbouly KM, Hussein A, et al. Randomized controlled trial between perineal and anal repairs of rectocele in obstructed defecation. World J Surg 2010;34(4):822–9.

76. Kruyt RH, Delemarre JB, Gooszen HG, et al. Selection of patients with internal intussusception of the rectum for posterior rectopexy. Br J Surg 1990;77(10):1183–4.

77. Christiansen J, Zhu BW, Rasmussen OO, et al. Internal rectal intussusception: results of surgical repair. Dis Colon Rectum 1992;35(11):1026–9.

78. Trompetto M, Clerico G, Realis Luc A, et al. Transanal Delorme procedure for treatment of rectocele associated with rectal intussusception. Tech Coloproctol 2006;10(4):389.

79. Collinson R, Wijffels N, Cunningham C, et al. Laparoscopic ventral rectopexy for internal rectal prolapse: short-term functional results. Colorectal Dis 2010;12(2):97–104.

80. Sileri P, Franceschilli L, de Luca E, et al. Laparoscopic ventral rectopexy for internal rectal prolapse using biological mesh: postoperative and

short-term functional results. J Gastrointest Surg 2012;16(3):622–8.

81. Ommer A, Albrecht K, Wenger F, et al. Stapled transanal rectal resection (STARR): a new option in the treatment of obstructive defecation syndrome. Langenbecks Arch Surg 2006;391(1):32–7.

82. Pechlivanides G, Tsiaoussis J, Athanasakis E, et al. Stapled transanal rectal resection (STARR) to reverse the anatomic disorders of pelvic floor dyssynergia. World J Surg 2007;31(6):1329–35.

83. Portier G, Kirzin S, Cabarrot P, et al. The effect of abdominal ventral rectopexy on faecal incontinence and constipation in patients with internal intra-anal rectal intussusception. Colorectal Dis 2011;13(8):914–7.

84. Boons P, Collinson R, Cunningham C, et al. Laparoscopic ventral rectopexy for external rectal prolapse improves constipation and avoids de novo constipation. Colorectal Dis 2010;12(6):526–32.

85. van den Esschert JW, van Geloven AAW, Vermulst N, et al. Laparoscopic ventral rectopexy for obstructed defecation syndrome. Surg Endosc 2008;22(12):2728–32.

86. Samaranayake CB, Luo C, Plank AW, et al. Systematic review on ventral rectopexy for rectal prolapse and intussusception. Colorectal Dis 2010;12(6):504–12.

87. Altomare DF, Rinaldi M, Veglia A, et al. Combined perineal and endorectal repair of rectocele by circular stapler: a novel surgical technique. Dis Colon Rectum 2002;45(11):1549–52.

88. Arroyo A, Perez-Vicente F, Serrano P, et al. Evaluation of the stapled transanal rectal resection technique with two staplers in the treatment of obstructive defecation syndrome. J Am Coll Surg 2007;204(1):56–63.

89. Lenisa L, Schwandner O, Stuto A, et al. STARR with Contour® Transtar™: prospective multicentre European study. Colorectal Dis 2009;11(8):821–7.

90. Schwandner T, Hecker A, Hirschburger M, et al. Does the STARR procedure change the pelvic floor: a preoperative and postoperative study with dynamic pelvic floor MRI. Dis Colon Rectum 2011;54(4):412–7.

91. Boccasanta P, Venturi M, Roviaro G. What is the benefit of a new stapler device in the surgical treatment of obstructed defecation? Three-year outcomes from a randomized controlled trial. Dis Colon Rectum 2011;54(1):77–84.

92. Renzi A, Brillantino A, Di Sarno G, et al. PPH-01 versus PPH-03 to perform STARR for the treatment of hemorrhoids associated with large internal rectal prolapse: a prospective multicenter randomized trial. Surg Innov 2011;18(3):241–7.

93. Petersen S, Hellmich G, Schuster A, et al. Stapled transanal rectal resection under laparoscopic surveillance for rectocele and concomitant enterocele. Dis Colon Rectum 2006;49(5):685–9.

94. Reibetanz J, Boenicke L, Kim M, et al. Enterocele is not a contraindication to stapled transanal surgery for outlet obstruction: an analysis of 170 patients. Colorectal Dis 2011;13(6):e131–6.

95. Dodi G, Pietroletti R, Milito G, et al. Bleeding, incontinence, pain and constipation after STARR transanal double stapling rectotomy for obstructed defecation. Tech Coloproctol 2003;7(3):148–53.

96. Boenicke L, Reibetanz J, Kim M, et al. Predictive factors for postoperative constipation and continence after stapled transanal rectal resection. Br J Surg 2012;99(3):416–22.

97. Boccasanta P, Venturi M, Salamina G, et al. New trends in the surgical treatment of outlet obstruction: clinical and functional results of two novel transanal stapled techniques from a randomised controlled trial. Int J Colorectal Dis 2004;19(4):359–69.

98. Jayne DG, Finan PJ. Stapled transanal rectal resection for obstructed defaecation and evidence-based practice. Br J Surg 2005;92(7):793–4.

99. Jayne DG, Schwandner O, Stuto A. Stapled transanal rectal resection for obstructed defecation syndrome: one-year results of the European STARR Registry. Dis Colon Rectum 2009;52(7):1205–14.
    The European STARR registry report on follow-up in 2224 patients undergoing the STARR procedure. Complications were reported in 36% of patients.

100. Martellucci J, Talento P, Carriero A. Early complications after stapled transanal rectal resection performed using the Contour® Transtar device. Colorectal Dis 2011;13(12):1428–31.

101. Gagliardi G, Pescatori M, Altomare DF, et al. Results, outcome predictors, and complications after stapled transanal rectal resection for obstructed defecation. Dis Colon Rectum 2008;51(2):186–95.

102. Williams NS, Giordano P, Dvorkin LS, et al. External pelvic rectal suspension (the Express procedure) for full-thickness rectal prolapse: evolution of a new technique. Dis Colon Rectum 2005;48(2):307–16.

103. Williams NS, Dvorkin LS, Giordano P, et al. EXternal Pelvic REctal SuSpension (Express procedure) for rectal intussusception, with and without rectocele repair. Br J Surg 2005;92(5):598–604.

104. Dench JE, Scott SM, Lunniss PJ, et al. Multimedia article. External pelvic rectal suspension (the Express procedure) for internal rectal prolapse, with or without concomitant rectocele repair: a video demonstration. Dis Colon Rectum 2006;49(12):1922–6.

105. Vaizey CJ, van den Bogaerde JB, Emmanuel AV, et al. Solitary rectal ulcer syndrome. Br J Surg 1998;85(12):1617–23.

106. Malouf AJ, Vaizey CJ, Kamm MA. Results of behavioral treatment (biofeedback) for solitary rectal ulcer syndrome. Dis Colon Rectum 2001;44(1):72–6.

107. Sitzler PJ, Kamm MA, Nicholls RJ, et al. Long-term clinical outcome of surgery for solitary rectal ulcer syndrome. Br J Surg 1998;85(9):1246–50.

108. Marchal F, Bresler L, Brunaud L, et al. Solitary rectal ulcer syndrome: a series of 13 patients operated with a mean follow-up of 4.5 years. Int J Colorectal Dis 2001;16(4):228–33.

109. Tweedie DJ, Varma JS. Long-term outcome of laparoscopic mesh rectopexy for solitary rectal ulcer syndrome. Colorectal Dis 2005;7(2):151–5.

110. Boccasanta P, Venturi M, Calabro G, et al. Stapled transanal rectal resection in solitary rectal ulcer associated with prolapse of the rectum: a prospective study. Dis Colon Rectum 2008;51(3):348–54.

111. Sand PK, Koduri S, Lobel RW, et al. Prospective randomized trial of polyglactin 910 mesh to prevent recurrence of cystoceles and rectoceles. Am J Obstet Gynecol 2001;184(7):1357–64.

112. Boccasanta P, Venturi M, Stuto A, et al. Stapled transanal rectal resection for outlet obstruction: a prospective, multicenter trial. Dis Colon Rectum 2004;47(8):1285–97.

113. Paraiso MF, Barber MD, Muir TW, et al. Rectocele repair: a randomized trial of three surgical techniques including graft augmentation. Am J Obstet Gynecol 2006;195(6):1762–71.

114. Lehur PA, Stuto A, Fantoli M, et al. Outcomes of stapled transanal rectal resection vs. biofeedback for the treatment of outlet obstruction associated with rectal intussusception and rectocele: a multicenter, randomized, controlled trial. Dis Colon Rectum 2008;51(11):1611–8.

13

Functional problems and their medical management

Anton V. Emmanuel

Introduction

Symptoms related to functional gastrointestinal disorders (FGIDs) are highly prevalent. In community-based studies, up to 22% of 'normal' UK subjects can be diagnosed as having irritable bowel syndrome (IBS) and up to 28% have functional constipation.[1] These disorders are constellations of symptoms – they are not diseases. As such, the emphasis of management of these patients is based on simple principles: the exclusion of organic disease, making a confident diagnosis, explaining why symptoms occur, alteration of lifestyle where appropriate and avoidance of surgery. Education about healthy lifestyle behaviours, reassurance that the symptoms are not due to a life-threatening disease such as cancer and establishment of a therapeutic relationship are essential, and patients have a greater expectation of benefit from lifestyle modification than drugs. This chapter will deal primarily with IBS and functional constipation, leaving the treatment of faecal incontinence to Chapter 11. Similarly, rectal prolapse, which is a frequent comorbidity of chronic constipation, is dealt with in Chapter 12.

The prevalence of functional disorders depends on the exact diagnostic criteria used; the current standards are the Rome III criteria.[2] The core diagnostic requirement for IBS is abdominal pain related to bowel function in association with altered stool form or frequency. The definition of functional constipation requires the presence of at least two of the following: less than three bowel actions a week, need

to strain or manually assist evacuation on >25% of occasions, passage of hard stools on >25% of occasions or a sensation of abnormal evacuation on >25% of occasions. These symptoms need to be chronic, and organic disease needs to have been excluded. Although these criteria can be criticised for being over-inclusive, what is clear is that FGIDs represent a major burden on secondary and tertiary outpatient clinics and IBS is the commonest diagnosis in gastrointestinal clinics.[3] An important confounding factor to be borne in mind when reviewing the literature on FGIDs is that the overwhelming majority of studies originate from tertiary centres. Patients attending such institutions are known to have disproportionately high scores on scales of depression, health-related anxiety and somatisation,[4] representing a potentially biased, self-selected group. One further compounding variable in assessing studies of FGIDs is that there is a notoriously high placebo response, ranging from 30% to 80%.[5]

Irritable bowel syndrome

The key to successful management of IBS is empathic reassurance. This will need to be individually directed according to the patient's symptoms, beliefs and anxieties.[6] Early and positive diagnosis is essential. Helpful factors in establishing a diagnosis are: (i) presence of symptoms for more than 6 months; (ii) frequent consultations for non-gastrointestinal symptoms; (iii) self-report that stress aggravates symptoms.

A key component of the reassurance is provision of a simple explanation of the benign nature and prognosis of the condition. Patients should be advised that no more than 2% of patients need their diagnosis of IBS to be revised at 30 years of follow-up.[1] Equally, it is important to remember that 88% of patients had recurring episodes of gastrointestinal symptoms, and so reassurance should be allied to advice about the need for long-term symptom control.[1]

Investigation

The presence of alarm features such as symptom onset after age 50, rectal bleeding, significant weight loss or abdominal mass mandates serological and luminal investigation to exclude organic disease. Investigations in these frequently young patients (the majority of patients at presentation are aged less than 35[1]) should otherwise be avoided since they may both exacerbate patients' anxieties and undermine their confidence in the clinician. The search for a simple diagnostic test of IBS remains, and faecalcalprotectin is emerging as a possible candidate to differentiate IBS from an organic cause of diarrhoea.[7]

> ✅✅ An important diagnosis to consider, especially in the presence of low-grade anaemia, is coeliac disease.

Approximately 5% of patients fulfilling IBS diagnostic criteria will have histological evidence of coeliac disease compared to 0.5% of controls without IBS symptoms.[8]

Treatment

Lifestyle modification
No strong, reproducible clinical trial evidence exists in favour of any particular dietary intervention in IBS.

> ✅ Behavioural training to encourage patients to alter patterns of phobic avoidance of public toilets is a central component of biofeedback, and is of undoubted value in some patients.[9]

True food allergies are much rarer than lay perception would predict,[10] and food fads and avoidances should be discouraged. One helpful dietary intervention worth considering in diarrhoea-predominant IBS patients (d-IBS) is reduction of excess caffeine and sorbitol (found in chewing gum and sweeteners).[11]

Studies have been carried out on the effect of dietary fibre augmentation in some constipation-predominant IBS (c-IBS) patients.[12,13] Early placebo-controlled crossover studies showed some acceleration of transit but no significant effect on symptoms.[12] Later studies have corroborated the absence of beneficial effect on symptoms and suggested that there is an increase in abdominal bloating, discomfort and flatulence during dietary fibre supplementation.[13] In summary, the effect of dietary fibre in IBS is not significantly beneficial, and the diet is frequently difficult to adhere to in the long term.[14] Current guidelines generally recommend avoiding fibre supplementation in IBS patients (www.nice.org/uk/CG061).

Pharmacological treatments
Most patients with FGIDs do not need drug therapy. The strongest evidence for a single agent in IBS patients is in d-IBS, where loperamide is a well-tolerated and effective treatment of diarrhoea and urgency.[15]

The popular aetiological theory that IBS symptoms relate to gut spasm has led to a huge number of uniformly low-quality studies of antispasmodics in IBS patients. These have been subject to meta-analysis.[16] In essence, what can be concluded is that, even allowing for publication bias in favour of positive studies, there is no evidence that anticholinergic (such as dicycloverine, hyoscine) or antispasmodic drugs (mebeverine, peppermint) have any advantage over placebo in treating the symptoms of IBS.

> ✅✅ In contrast, the data for the efficacy of tricyclic antidepressants show unequivocal benefit in favour of low-dose usage of these agents.[17] Doses of amitriptyline or nortriptyline of 10–50 mg act at both the central (anxiety and depression) and peripheral (neuromodulatory) mechanisms of IBS.

One putative mechanism of action of tricyclic agents is through an effect on gut serotonin receptors.

✔ Many drugs that agonise or antagonise serotonin receptors have been developed, and the effect of all these drugs amounts to about 20% advantage over placebo.[18]

None of these agents are licensed for use in the UK at the time of writing, with some having been withdrawn due to safety concerns. Serotonin agents are amongst a number of emerging agents targeting enteric neurotransmitter receptors, some of which may have a role in relieving the sensory symptoms of IBS.[19] In contrast to studies of low-dose tricyclics, standard doses of newer antidepressants (selective serotonin reuptake inhibitors) lead to a less impressive improvement in IBS, and at greater cost.[20] Finally, preliminary evidence suggests the possibility that some probiotic strains of bacteria may have a beneficial influence in patients with IBS, though this is very much emerging information.[21]

Psychological treatments

✔✔ A landmark study by Creed et al. showed that cognitive behavioural therapy directed towards bowel symptoms is effective in treating women with IBS, with a 'number needed to treat' of 3.[22]

The essence of such treatment is that it is gut focused, since general cognitive behavioural and relaxation therapies are no more effective than standard care. The Creed study also showed that such treatment is cost-effective and beneficial in the long term.[22]

✔✔ A number of studies in the literature show the value of hypnotherapy in IBS with benefit in the long-term setting, at up to 6 years following the cessation of therapy.[19]

In brief, three-quarters of patients report symptom alleviation after hypnotherapy, and over 80% of these responders remain well at a median follow-up of 5 years.[23]

Surgery

Patients with IBS are disproportionately more likely to undergo abdominal and pelvic surgery than age- and sex-matched controls.[24,25] IBS patients have a prevalence of cholecystectomy of 4.6% compared with 2.4% in controls, and a prevalence of hysterectomy of 18% versus 12% in controls. There is also evidence that IBS patients are more likely to undergo appendicectomy (35% prevalence compared to 8% in control patients with ulcerative colitis).[25] [Editor's comment: although patients with ulcerative colitis have a lower than normal prevalence of appendicectomy.] Furthermore, these examinations are more likely to yield normal findings macroscopically and histologically in IBS patients.[26]

Abdominal or pelvic surgery may predispose to the development of functional symptoms through mechanical, neural or hormonal impairments. Heaton et al. reported that 44% of subjects develop new symptoms of urgency after cholecystectomy and 27% report constipation symptoms beginning after hysterectomy.[27] In contrast, women undergoing gynaecological surgery for non-pain indications did not develop IBS more often than non-operated controls.[28] What these studies do highlight is the key importance of trying to minimise surgery in patients with FGIDs. In those patients who do undergo an operation it is implicit that there is complete explanation of the possibility of developing new symptoms postoperatively. The corollary of this is that patients in whom there is a high suspicion of FGID (based on symptoms and normal investigations) should be dissuaded from undergoing diagnostic laparoscopy, which is not usually revealing and which may result in new complaints.

Functional constipation

Estimates from the USA suggest that 1.2% of the population consult a physician every year with the complaint of constipation.[29] Since 85% of these consultations result in the prescription of a laxative, it should come as no surprise that the estimated annual expenditure on prescription laxatives in the UK is £48 million,[30] more than is spent on treating hypertension. This figure does not include the cost of over-the-counter laxatives nor the costs of specialist investigation and work absenteeism. What these figures reflect is the importance of the role of the hospital specialist in identifying appropriate patients to put through further investigation and specific treatments.

In terms of pathophysiology, functional constipation is considered to be due to either slow whole-gut transit ('colonic inertia'), rectal evacuatory dysfunction or a combination of both of these abnormalities. The commonest cause of slow transit in general practice is as a side-effect of drug therapy for other reasons. The commonest culprit drugs are opiates, anticholinergics, antihypertensives, iron supplements, antacids and non-steroidal anti-inflammatory drugs.[30]

Investigation

As in the case of patients with IBS, luminal investigation is reserved for patients with a short history or alarm symptoms, in whom there is the need to exclude colorectal cancer. In addition to the drug causes listed above, which can be identified from careful history-taking, the other common associations are with neurological disease (multiple sclerosis, Parkinson's disease and diabetic autonomic neuropathy). Causes of constipation that can be identified from simple serological testing include hypothyroidism, hypercalcaemia and hypokalaemia.

Whereas the diagnosis of IBS is one of exclusion, there are investigations available both to define the pathophysiological abnormality and confirm the presence of constipation. Colonic transit can be simply measured by use of radio-opaque markers followed by a plain abdominal X-ray. One well-described assessment comprises ingestion of three sets of radiologically distinct markers that are ingested at 24-hour intervals and an abdominal X-ray taken 120 hours after the first ingestion; retention of more than the normal range for any one of the three sets of markers reflects slow transit.[31] The test is cheap, sensitive and reproducible, and provides clinically helpful information in the management of patients with constipation.[30]

Defecating proctography (using barium or magnetic resonance contrast gel) and the balloon expulsion test are means of quantifying the anatomical and physiological disturbances of rectal evacuation in patients with functional constipation. Abnormalities such as paradoxical anal sphincter contraction, impaired pelvic floor relaxation, anal intussusception and rectal prolapse can be demonstrated by these techniques.[32] No firm evidence exists as to the value of these abnormalities in the management of patients with constipation.[32] The place of anorectal manometry in patients with chronic constipation is primarily in the exclusion of Hirschsprung's disease.[32]

Treatment

Dietary fibre supplementation

This is the traditional first line of therapy for chronic constipation, and by the time of specialist referral most patients would have already undertaken trials of such therapy. Fibre supplementation increases gut transit and stool bulk by a fraction of the starting value, and as such is only effective in patients with mild constipation.[33] In those small numbers of patients seen in hospital who have not tried fibre supplementation, advice needs to be offered about a gradual stepwise increase in fibre intake. Patients need to be counselled that the effect is not apparent until therapy has been established for several weeks.

> ✔ Patients need to continue with the diet in the long term,[34] and there is evidence that this can be difficult for a significant proportion. Increasing liquid intake and attempting to maintain regular meal-time patterns seem also to have a place in improving symptoms, although the evidence is strongest in the elderly.[33]

Laxatives, suppositories, enemas and novel prokinetics

There are widely held misconceptions of the danger of 'self-poisoning' without a daily bowel action. Given the limited evidence base for the use of laxatives, the first step in the management of constipation is to discourage laxative overuse.[30,35] The effect of laxatives in chronic constipation is modest at best. Only a very small number of trials have compared a laxative regimen with placebo, and meta-analysis would not be statistically or clinically meaningful.[35] Compared to the dearth of placebo-controlled studies, there are a number of open and blinded comparisons between different laxatives. These have been systematically reviewed recently[35] and as might be predicted the opinion of the reviewers is that methodological flaws and inconsistencies prevent meaningful conclusions being drawn. The conclusions that can be drawn are listed below. Overall there is an increase in stool frequency with bulking agents of 1.4 bowel movements per week, and with other laxative classes of 1.5 bowel movements per week.

Bulk laxatives have a limited role in chronic constipation. They should be reserved for patients who are unable to consume adequate dietary fibre. They have no role in either patients with severe constipation or those who need rapid relief of symptoms.

> ✅ **Osmotic agents** comprise either poorly absorbed ionic salts or non-absorbed sugars and alcohols. Dose titration is possible with osmotic laxatives, which have a particular place in the management of megacolon and megarectum once the patient has been disimpacted.

> ✅ **Stimulant laxatives** (anthranoid compounds such as senna, or polyphenolic compounds such as bisacodyl) usually have an effect on stool output within 24 hours of ingestion, and are most suitable for occasional, rather than regular, use.

The effect of these drugs is unpredictable and dose escalation is often required. Nevertheless, they appear to be harmless and are frequently used in chronic severe constipation. What is clear is that the previous fears that chronic use of anthranoid laxatives may result in enteric nerve damage is highly unlikely.[36] **Stool softeners** and **compound mixtures** of the above classes of laxative are also commonly used, although their efficacy has not been rigorously demonstrated.

Some **suppositories** induce a chemically induced reflex rectal contraction. **Enemas** act either by stimulating rectal contraction or by softening hard stool.

> ✅ Suppositories and enemas can be effective in alleviating the symptoms of evacuation difficulty if dietary modification and behavioural therapy have been unsuccessful. Used on an as-required basis, enemas have a particular place in managing rectal impaction.

Cisapride was the first **prokinetic** to be studied in chronic functional constipation, showing limited short-lived effect. Prucalopride and tegaserod are agonists at the serotonin-4 receptor and seem to accelerate both upper and lower gut transit.[37] Both drugs improve transit and pain/bloating symptoms, although the optimal duration of treatment remains uncertain. Further pharmacological options for chronic constipation have been developed, targeting intestinal chloride secretion (lubiprostone) and guanylate cyclase (linaclotide) and opioid receptors (methylnaltrexone).[38]

> ✅✅ In laxative refractory patients, novel prokinetic drugs offer a therapeutic alternative to behavioural therapy or surgery.

Behavioural therapy (biofeedback)

Gut-directed behavioural therapy, biofeedback, is now an established therapy for functional constipation, and in a number of specialist centres is first-line therapy for new referrals.[39,40] Biofeedback is a learning strategy based on operant conditioning. The main focus is on abdominal and pelvic coordination and it is undoubtedly beneficial in patients with dyssynergic evacuation,[39] but it also seems benificial in patients with slow transit.[40]

> ✅✅ Short- and long-term benefit is evident in over 60% of unselected patients in specialist centres.[9,40,41]

The effect of treatment is seen not only in symptoms (improved bowel frequency, reduced need to strain), but also in terms of reduced laxative use and improved quality-of-life scores.[9]

Biofeedback seems to have its effect through alteration of a variety of pathophysiological disturbances. There is evidence that successful outcome with biofeedback is associated with specifically improved autonomic innervation to the colon, and improved transit time for patients with slow and normal transit.[9]

> ✅ Additionally, treatment may improve pelvic floor coordination,[40] thereby allowing antegrade peristalsis and preventing retrograde movement of colonic content. What is important is that biofeedback is successful not just in patients with mild symptoms, but also in those with intractable symptoms who are being considered for surgery.[41]

Surgical treatment for constipation

Surgery for rectal evacuation symptoms in the context of structural anorectal disturbance is described elsewhere in this book. In those patients with proven slow transit who have failed to respond to dietary modification, biofeedback, long-term trials of laxatives and prokinetics, the traditional algorithm dictates consideration of a surgical approach. The standard surgical procedure has been total colectomy (performed to the level of the sacral promontory) and ileorectal anastomosis.[42] Ileorectostomy is reported as being more successful than ileosigmoidostomy in terms of successful relief of constipation and, providing greater than 7–10 cm of rectum is left intact, then bowel frequency and urgency are not unacceptably frequent.[42]

Almost every major colorectal institution and a huge number of other centres have published on their experience of subtotal colectomy for slow transit constipation. Results vary widely, with satisfaction rates varying from 39% to 100%.[40] Whilst median scores of bowel frequency tend to show statistically significant improvements, what these composite figures mask are the facts that, firstly, approximately one in three patients do not improve at all and, secondly, that some patients develop diarrhoea.

> ✅ The strongest argument against colectomy for slow transit constipation is that the disorder is a pan-enteric one, and so mere removal of the colon is unlikely to yield sustained benefit.[43,44]

There are two unequivocal conclusions that come out of the welter of small studies in the literature. Firstly, adverse effects occur in over half of all patients. Most common is episodic subacute small bowel obstruction (occurring in up to two-thirds of some series), need for further abdominal surgery (in up to one-third of patients), persisting constipation (in up to one-quarter), diarrhoea (in up to one-quarter) and faecal incontinence (in up to 10%).

> ✅ The second conclusion, related to the incidence of adverse events, is the importance of careful patient selection.

Thus, of the many patients complaining of constipation in the community, only a tiny proportion (approximately 1%) are referred to tertiary care, of whom only a small fraction (less than 5%) might benefit from surgical treatment.[45] Patient selection must initially be on clinical grounds (including careful consideration of potential psychiatric disorders) and the physiological demonstration of slow transit. Some authors have recommended extensive anorectal sensory and motor physiological testing, defecating proctography and upper gut motility studies to aid identification of subgroups in whom surgery may be more successful.[46] In contrast, Rantis et al.[47] identified only 23% of patients in whom such extensive testing altered clinical management; additionally, the cost of this testing was great (US $140 000 in 1997).

In view of the controversy about subtotal colectomy, a vogue for alternative surgical therapies arose. Two particular surgical approaches have received sustained study: stoma formation and segmental colonic resection. However, the data on efficacy and morbidity of these techniques are little different and no less controversial than those for subtotal colectomy.[48] There is unequivocally no place for division of the puborectalis in an attempt to treat rectal evacuatory dysfunction.[49]

A less invasive surgical approach to functional constipation has been the antegrade continence enema (the Malone procedure). Initially used in patients with constipation secondary to neurological disease, the technique has been widely reported in functional constipation.[50] Patients intubate their stoma (appendix or plastic conduit) and irrigate with either water, a stimulant or osmotic laxative. Although there are stomal complications in over 50% of patients (stenosis, mucus leak, pain), three-quarters of patients report 'high' or 'very high' satisfaction with the procedure.[50]

Current trials of medical therapy for FGIDs require quality-of-life data to complement conventional efficacy data. The surgical literature to date shows that although stool frequency may improve, gut-specific quality of life does not.[51]

Putative treatments for constipation

> ✅ Recent surgical developments have looked at modifications of subtotal colectomy. Small, short-term studies have shown that ileosigmoid or antiperistaltic caecorectal anastomoses may improve bowel frequency and quality of life.[52,53]

However, the major recent development with regard to surgical therapy for constipation has been sacral nerve stimulation.[54] In the single publication to date, two patients were studied in a double-blind crossover fashion with their sacral nerve stimulator either turned on or off.

> ✅ There was a clear improvement in both symptoms and quality of life with the stimulator turned on, potentially extending the role of sacral nerve stimulation from its existing licence for the treatment of faecal incontinence.

Idiopathic megarectum and megacolon

Megarectum and megacolon are uncommon clinical conditions of unknown aetiology that present typically, but not exclusively, with intractable constipation in the first two decades of life.[55] Other conditions presenting with constipation in the context of gut dilatation (e.g. Hirschsprung's disease, chronic intestinal pseudo-obstruction) are not included since the aetiology of these disorders is known. Patients with idiopathic megarectum tend to present with faecal incontinence in the context of recurrent faecal impaction frequently requiring surgical disimpaction. In contrast, patients with idiopathic megacolon more frequently present with abdominal pain and distension in the context of chronic constipation.[55]

✔ The majority of patients with idiopathic megarectum and megacolon can be successfully managed by disimpaction followed by the use of osmotic laxatives. The osmotic agent needs titration in order that the patient obtains a semiformed ('porridgey') stool that is passed three times a day. Occasionally, rectal evacuation techniques (such as suppository use or biofeedback therapy) are required actually to empty the rectum of the semiformed stool.[56]

When medical therapy fails (due to compliance failure or lack of success in avoiding recurrent impaction), surgical therapy is warranted. A number of surgical procedures have been performed, with variable reports of success. As with reports of surgery for idiopathic constipation, the longer the duration of follow-up, the worse the documented outcome. Anorectal physiology, whole-gut transit studies and evacuation proctography do not help identify patients who may benefit or help with choice of surgical procedure.[57] Anorectal physiology testing does have a role in identifying the presence of a rectoanal inhibitory reflex, which excludes the differential diagnosis of Hirschsprung's disease.

✔✔ With regard to resectional surgery, colectomy offers good results in the majority of patients (80%), with ileorectal anastomosis yielding the greatest levels of patient satisfaction.[57]

Outcomes with the Duhamel procedure, anal myomectomy and restorative proctocolectomy are also favourable in the majority of cases, approaching 70% in the majority of series. Restorative proctocolectomy is suitable in patients with dilatation of both the colon and rectum, whilst the recent procedure of vertical reduction rectoplasty has been proposed for those with dilatation confined to the rectum.[57]

✔ In situations where initial surgery has failed, formation of a stoma (colostomy or ileostomy) is associated with excellent results.[58]

Stoma formation as a primary procedure is also successful in the vast majority of cases.[58] The ultimate choice of surgical procedure will depend on available expertise, patient physical and psychological factors, and the patient's choice.

Key points

- Dietary manipulation is rarely helpful in managing symptoms in hospital-referred patients with functional disorders.
- Drug therapy is rarely needed in treating patients with IBS.
- Loperamide is unequivocally beneficial in patients with loose stools and urgency.
- Low-dose tricyclic antidepressants are effective in relieving functional abdominal pain.
- A comprehensive approach to therapy of functional disorders requires close liaison with psychological services. The effect of laxatives in chronic constipation is minimally superior to placebo.
- Biofeedback is effective in almost two-thirds of patients with constipation, whether due to slow transit or evacuatory dysfunction.
- Subtotal colectomy and ileorectal anastomosis is beneficial in a small number of highly selected patients, although surgical morbidity is frequently high.
- The majority of patients with idiopathic megarectum and megacolon can be managed by disimpaction and initiation of osmotic laxatives.

References

1. Jones R, Lydiard S. Irritable bowel syndrome in the general population. Br Med J 1991;304:87–90.
2. Longstreth GF, Thompson WG, Chey WD, et al. Functional bowel disorders. Gastroenterology 2006;130:1480–91.
3. Drossman DA, Sandler RS, McKee DC, et al. Bowel patterns among subjects not seeking health care: use of a questionnaire to identify a population with bowel dysfunction. Gastroenterology 1982;83:529–34.
4. Emmanuel AV, Mason HJ, Kamm MA. Relationship between psychological state and level of activity of extrinsic gut innervation in patients with a functional gastrointestinal disorder. Gut 2001;49:214–9.
5. Patel SM, Stason WB, Legezda A, et al. The placebo effect in irritable bowel syndrome trials: a meta-analysis. Neurogastroenterol Motil 2005;17:332–40.
6. Thompson WG. Review article: the treatment of the irritable bowel syndrome. Aliment Pharm Ther 2002;16:1395–406.
7. Keohane J, O'Mahony C, O'Mahony L. Irritable bowel syndrome type symptoms in patients with inflammatory bowel disease: a real association or reflection of occult inflammation? Am J Gastroenterol 2010;105:1789–94.
8. Sanders DS, Carter MJ, Hurlstone DP, et al. Association of adult coeliac disease with irritable bowel syndrome: a case control study in patients fulfilling the Rome II criteria referred to secondary care. Lancet 2001;358:1504–8.
9. Emmanuel AV, Mason HJ, Kamm MA. Response to a behavioural treatment, biofeedback, in constipated patients is associated with improved gut transit and autonomic innervation. Gut 2001;49:209–13.
10. Pearson DJ. Pseudo food allergy. Br Med J 1986;292:221–2.
11. Hyams JS. Sorbitol intolerance: an unappreciated cause of functional gastrointestinal complaints. Gastroenterology 1983;84:30–3.
12. Lucey MR, Clark ML, Lowndes J, et al. Is bran efficacious in irritable bowel syndrome? A double blind placebo-controlled crossover study. Gut 1987;28:221–5.
13. Snook J, Shepherd HA. Bran supplementation in the treatment of irritable bowel syndrome. Aliment Pharm Ther 1994;8:511–4.
Whilst some patients can expect improvement in stool output with bran, the majority of patients experience an increase in abdominal distension and discomfort.
14. Hillman LC, Stace NH, Pomare EW. Irritable bowel patients and their long-term response to a high fibre diet. Am J Gastroenterol 1984;79:1–7.
15. Cann PA, Read NW, Holdsworth CD, et al. Role of loperamide and placebo in management of irritable bowel syndrome. Dig Dis Sci 1984;29:239–47.
Loperamide is effective in slowing gut transit, reducing stool frequency and urgency in patients with IBS.
16. Poynard T, Regimgeau C, Benhamou Y. Meta-analysis of smooth muscle relaxants in the treatment of irritable bowel syndrome. Aliment Pharm Ther 2001;15:355–61.
17. Jackson AL, O'Malley PG, Tomkins G, et al. Treatment of functional gastrointestinal disorders with antidepressant medications. Am J Med 2000;108:65–72.
Meta-analysis of studies using a variety of tricyclic antidepressants in varying doses in patients with FGIDs showing clear benefit for low-dose tricyclics over placebo.
18. Spiller R, Aziz Q, Creed F, et al. Guidelines on the irritable bowel syndrome: mechanisms and practical management. Gut 2007;56:1770–98.
Practical and up-to-date review of management options available for IBS, encompassing minimum investigation, pharmacological, dietary and lifestyle treatment.
19. Maneerattanaporn M, Chang L, Chey WD. Emerging pharmacological therapies for the irritable bowel syndrome. Gastroenterol Clin N Am 2011;40(1):223–43.
20. Tack J, Broekaert D, Fischler B, et al. A controlled crossover study of the selective serotonin reuptake inhibitor citalopram in irritable bowel syndrome. Gut 2006;55:1095–103.
21. Whorwell PJ, Altringer L, Morel J, et al. Efficacy of an encapsulated probiotic Bifidobacterium infantis 35624 in women with irritable bowel syndrome. Am J Gastroenterol 2006;101:1581–90.
22. Creed F, Fernandes L, Guthrie E, et al. The cost-effectiveness of psychotherapy and paroxetine for severe irritable bowel syndrome. Gastroenterology 2003;124:303–17.
23. Gonsalkorale WM, Miller V, Afzal A, et al. Long term benefits of hypnotherapy for irritable bowel syndrome. Gut 2003;52:1623–9.
24. Kennedy TM, Jones RH. Epidemiology of cholecystectomy and irritable bowel syndrome in a UK population. Br J Surg 2000;87:1658–63.
25. Kennedy TM, Jones RH. The epidemiology of hysterectomy and irritable bowel syndrome in a UK population. Int J Clin Pract 2000;54:647–50.
26. Lu CL, Liu CC, Fuh JL, et al. Irritable bowel syndrome and negative appendectomy: a prospective multivariable investigation. Gut 2007;56:655–60.
27. Heaton KW, Parker D, Cripps H. Bowel function and irritable bowel symptoms after hysterectomy and cholecystectomy – a population based study. Gut 1993;34:1108–11.

28. Sperber AD, Morris CB, Greemberg L, et al. Development of abdominal pain and IBS following gynecological surgery: a prospective, controlled study. Gastroenterology 2008;134:75–84.

29. Sonnenberg A, Koch TR. Physician visits in the United States for constipation: 1958–1986. Dig Dis Sci 1989;34:606–11.

30. Emmanuel AV. The use and abuse of laxatives in the elderly. In: Potter J, Norton C, Cottenden AM, editors. Bowel care in frail older people. London: Royal College of Physicians; 2002[Chapter 6].

31. Evans RC, Kamm MA, Hinton JM, et al. The normal range and a simple diagram for recording whole gut transit. Int J Colorectal Dis 1992;7:15–7.

32. Diamant NE, Kamm MA, Wald A, et al. AGA technical review on anorectal testing techniques. Gastroenterology 1999;116:735–54.

33. Harari D, Gurwitz JH, Minaker KL. Constipation in the elderly. J Am Geriatr Soc 1993;41:1130–40.

34. Jones MP, Talley NJ, Nuyts G, et al. Lack of objective evidence of efficacy of laxatives in chronic constipation. Dig Dis Sci 2002;47:2222–30.

35. Tramonte SM, Brand MB, Mulrow CD, et al. The treatment of chronic constipation in adults. J Gen Intern Med 1997;12:15–24.
    Systematic review of the placebo-controlled laxative studies and those comparing different laxative classes. The limited benefit of these drugs over placebo is highlighted.

36. Kieman JA, Heinicke EA. Sennosides do not kill myenteric neurons in the colon of the rat or mouse. Neuroscience 1989;30:837–42.

37. Emmanuel AV, Roy AJ, Nicholls TJ. Prucalopride, a systemic enterokinetic, for the treatment of constipation. Aliment Pharm Ther 2002;16:1347–56.
    Large, single-centre study of the effect of a serotonin agonist on gut physiology and symptoms in patients with functional constipation.

38. Emmanuel AV, Tack J, Quigley EM, et al. Pharmacological management of constipation. Neurogastroenterol Motil 2009;21(Suppl. 2):41–54.

39. Heymen S, Scarlett Y, Jones K, et al. Randomized, controlled trial shows biofeedback to be superior to alternative treatments for patients with pelvic floor dyssynergia-type constipation. Dis Colon Rectum 2007;50:428–41.

40. Chiotakakou-Faliakou E, Kamm MA, Roy AJ, et al. Biofeedback provides long term benefit for patients with intractable slow and normal transit constipation. Gut 1998;42:517–21.
    Demonstration of long-term efficacy of biofeedback in patients who have an initially good response to treatment.

41. Brown SR, Donati D, Seow-Chen F, et al. Biofeedback avoids surgery in patients with slow transit constipation: report of four cases. Dis Colon Rectum 2001;44:737–9.

42. Vasilevsky CA, Nemer FD, Balcos EG, et al. Is subtotal colectomy a viable option in the management of chronic constipation? Dis Colon Rectum 1988;31:679–81.

43. Knowles CH, Scott M, Lunniss PJ. Outcome of colectomy for slow transit constipation. Ann Surg 1999;230:627–38.
    Systematic review of most of the small reports of subtotal colectomy showing that efficacy is inversely related to duration of follow-up. A rationale for patient selection is presented.

44. Altomare DF, Portincasa P, Rinaldi M, et al. Slow transit constipation: solitary symptom of a systemic gastrointestinal disease. Dis Colon Rectum 1999;42:231–40.

45. Rex DK, Lappas JC, Goulet RC, et al. Selection of constipated patients as subtotal colectomy candidates. J Clin Gastroenterol 1992;15:212–7.

46. Redmond JM, Smith GW, Barofsky I, et al. Physiologic tests to predict long-term outcome of total abdominal colectomy for intractable constipation. Am J Gastroenterol 1995;90:748–53.

47. Rantis PC, Vernava AM, Daniel GL, et al. Chronic constipation – is the work-up worth the cost? Dis Colon Rectum 1997;40:280–6.

48. Lundin E, Karlbom U, Pahlman L, et al. Outcome of segmental colonic resection for slow-transit constipation. Br J Surg 2002;89:1270–4.

49. Kamm MA, Hawley PR, Lennard-Jones JE. Lateral division of puborectalis in the management of severe constipation. Br J Surg 1988;75:661–3.

50. Marshall J, Hutson JM, Anticich N, et al. Antegrade continence enemas in the treatment of slow-transit constipation. J Pediatr Surg 2001;36:1227–30.

51. FitzHarris GP, Garcia-Aguilar J, Parker SC, et al. Quality of life after subtotal colectomy for slow-transit constipation: both quality and quantity count. Dis Colon Rectum 2003;46:433–40.

52. Feng Y, Jianjiang L. Functional outcomes of two types of subtotal colectomy for slow-transit constipation: ileosigmoidal anastomosis and cecorectal anastomosis. Am J Surg 2008;195:73–7.

53. Marchesi F, Sarli L, Percalli L, et al. Subtotal colectomy with antiperistaltic cecorectal anastomosis in the treatment of slow-transit constipation: long-term impact on quality of life. World J Surg 2007;31:1658–64.

54. Kenefick NJ, Vaizey CJ, Cohen CR, et al. Double-blind placebo-controlled crossover study of sacral nerve stimulation for idiopathic constipation. Br J Surg 2002;89:1570–1.

55. Gattuso JM, Kamm MA. Clinical features of idiopathic megarectum and idiopathic megacolon. Gut 1997;41:93–9.
    The only true prospective comparison of symptoms, pathophysiology and management between patients with idiopathic megarectum and megacolon.

56. Mimura T, Nicholls T, Storrie JB, et al. Treatment of constipation in adults associated with idiopathic megarectum by behavioural retraining including biofeedback. Colorectal Dis 2002;4:477–82.

57. Gladman MA, Scott SM, Lunniss PJ, et al. Systematic review of surgical options for idiopathic megarectum and megacolon. Ann Surg 2005;241:562–74.

A definitive systematic review of the published data on surgical procedures for idiopathic megacolon and megarectum in adults.

58. Stabile G, Kamm MA, Hawley PR, et al. Results of stoma formation for idiopathic megarectum and megacolon. Int J Colorectal Dis 1992; 7:82–4.

14

Anal fistula: evaluation and management

Peter J. Lunniss
Robin K.S. Phillips

Introduction

Anorectal sepsis is common, presenting as either an acute abscess or a chronic anal fistula. The majority of cases can be dealt with avoiding complication, but a small minority can present a major challenge to both sufferer and surgeon.

Although fistula-in-ano may be found in association with a variety of specific conditions, the current majority in the UK are classified as non-specific, idiopathic or cryptoglandular, their exact aetiology having not been fully proven, although the diseased anal gland in the intersphincteric space is considered central. Fistulas may be seen in association with Crohn's disease, tuberculosis, pilonidal disease, hidradenitis suppurativa, lymphogranuloma venereum, presacral dermoids, rectal duplication, actinomycosis, trauma and foreign bodies.[1] An important association is malignancy, which may manifest itself as a discharging opening on the perineum from a pelvic source, but which may also arise in long-standing fistulas, either cryptoglandular, as part of perianal Crohn's disease, or even in hidradenitis suppurativa.

The exact incidence of idiopathic anal fistula in the general population is not known, as most data come from hospital analysis in tertiary referral centres, which attract only the more difficult cases. Perhaps the most accurate information comes from Scandinavia, where incidences of between 8.6 and 10 per 10 000 have been reported.

All reported series have demonstrated a male predominance, most reporting a male to female ratio of between 2:1 and 4:1, for reasons that are unclear. McColl[2] found no sex differences in histology or distribution of anal glands in 50 normal human anal canals, and we have found no differences in circulating sex hormone concentrations between sufferers of either sex and healthy controls. Furthermore, the sex difference is not limited to humans. The German Shepherd dog is a breed particularly prone to the development of anal fistula compared with other breeds, and this is not due to any differences in anal crypt or gland anatomy. There is a 3:1 male to female ratio of the incidence of canine fistulas, compared to a 1:1 ratio for the whole dog population, and the incidence of fistula is much lower in neutered dogs and bitches compared with those that are sexually intact. Evidence supporting a hormonal explanation, via various mechanisms, for the observed gender difference has recently been published.[3]

Anal fistulas most commonly afflict people in their third, fourth or fifth decades.[4-6] There is little information on racial differences, although the peak incidence has been reported at a lower age in Nigerians and in African-Americans. Sedentary occupations cannot be implicated.[5] Whether bowel habit may be influential is unclear. Some authors take the view that diarrhoea may allow easier access of bacteria to the anal glands, especially in infants; others feel that hard stools are implicated by their abrasive passage through the anal canal.

The overall morbidity from fistula is difficult to assess in either individual or economic terms. For the majority of patients with simple fistulas, the time spent off work with the parent abscess and subsequent fistula management may be relatively short. However, it is not that uncommon for a patient with a complex fistula to have had multiple hospital admissions for attempted cure over several years, only to end up incontinent, or with a permanent stoma, and permanently incapacitated. For these patients in particular, tertiary referral centres that have gained the necessary expertise are essential, expertise lying in the hands not only of the surgeons, but also the nurses, radiologists, physiologists and psychologists, who all play an important part in management.

Aetiology

Anal glands and their link with anal fistulas have been recorded since the end of the 19th century. The function of the anal glands is uncertain. They have been shown to secrete mucin, but this has a different composition from that secreted by rectal mucosa. From comparative anatomical studies, McColl[2] showed that the anal glands are not vestigial remnants of sexual scent glands, and the suggestion that they are not true glands at all but rather vestigial epithelial remnants left after proctodeal invagination into the hindgut has not been substantiated.

Current thinking lays the blame at those anal glands situated in the intersphincteric space; these may constitute one-third to two-thirds of the total number of anal glands found in an anal canal.[5]

✅ Eisenhammer[7] considered all non-specific abscesses and fistulas to be the result of extension of sepsis from an intramuscular anal gland, the sepsis being unable to drain spontaneously into the anal lumen because of infective obstruction of its connecting duct across the internal sphincter.

Parks[8] proposed that, should the initial abscess in relation to the intersphincteric anal gland subside, the diseased gland might become the seat of chronic infection with subsequent fistula formation. The fistula is thus a granulation tissue-lined track kept open by the infective source, which is the abscess around a diseased anal gland deep to the internal sphincter. Parks[8] studied 30 consecutive cases of anal fistula and found cystic dilatation of anal glands in eight,

which he attributed to acquired duct dilatation or more probably a congenital abnormality, a precursor to infection within a mucin-filled cavity.

There have been few studies that have examined the cryptoglandular hypothesis. Goligher et al.[9] found intersphincteric space sepsis in only 8 of 28 cases of acute anorectal sepsis; of 32 cases of anal fistula, only 14 had evidence of either intersphincteric sepsis or the track travelling within (rather than simply across) the intersphincteric space. However, Goligher et al. failed to acknowledge that a proportion of cases of acute sepsis have nothing to do with fistula and that some common fistulas (e.g. superficial fistulas and those arising from a chronic anal fissure) have an aetiology separate from that postulated by Parks.

Another question arises from studies of the microbiology of fistula tissue. Although infection and its effective drainage are the primary problems in the acute stage, and although failure to treat secondary extensions and abscesses adequately will inevitably lead to recurrence, the possibility that the anal gland becomes the seat of chronic infection in the established fistula has found little support in the only two studies directed at this aspect of the hypothesis.[10,11] A more attractive theory as to why idiopathic fistulas persist is that they become (at least partly) epithelialised, a factor responsible for failure of healing of fistulas at other sites in the body. A histological study of the intersphincteric component of 18 consecutive idiopathic anal fistulas showed that although an association between anal gland and fistula may be demonstrated (as had been suggested by Gordon-Watson and Dodd[12] in 1935) in a minority of cases, epithelialisation from either or both ends of the fistula track is a more common finding.[13] Indeed, the presence of epithelium and local production of antimicrobial peptides may explain the relative paucity of organisms found in chronic fistulas.[14]

Spread of sepsis from an acutely infected anal gland may occur in any of the three planes, vertical, horizontal or circumferential. Caudal spread is the simplest and most usual way by which infection is thought to disseminate to present acutely as a perianal abscess (labelled **a** in **Fig. 14.1**). Cephalad extension in the same space will result in a high intermuscular abscess (**b** in Fig. 14.1) or a supralevator pararectal (syn. pelvirectal) abscess (**c** in Fig. 14.1), depending on the relation of the sepsis to

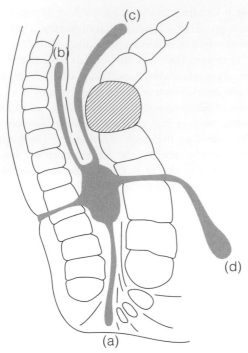

Figure 14.1 • The possible courses of spread of sepsis from the diseased anal gland in the intersphincteric space. See text for explanation. Reproduced from Parks AG. The pathogenesis and treatment of fistula-in-ano. Br Med J 1961; i:463–9. With permission from BMJ Publishing Group Ltd.

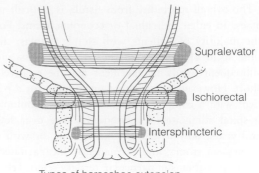

Types of horseshoe extension

Figure 14.2 • The three planes in which sepsis may spread circumferentially. Reproduced from Parks AG, Gordon PH, Hardcastle JD. A classification of fistula-in-ano. Br J Surg 1976; 63:1–12. © British Journal of Surgery Society Ltd. Permission is granted by John Wiley & Sons Ltd on behalf on the BJSS Ltd.

Management of acute sepsis

The majority of chronic anal fistulas are preceded by an episode of acute anorectal sepsis, although acute sepsis does not inevitably lead to fistula formation. The reported rates of recurrent abscess or fistula development following simple incision and drainage range from 17% to 87%. The optimal management of acute sepsis should reside in an understanding of aetiology. Pilonidal infection, hidradenitis and perianal Crohn's disease are usually fairly easy to recognise by history and examination. Pus in the perianal space may result from caudal spread of intersphincteric (cryptoglandular) infection or from simple skin appendage infection. Similarly, pus in the ischiorectal space may or may not be related to presumed anal gland disease.

Patients with acute anorectal sepsis usually present via the accident and emergency department rather than the outpatient clinic. Those with perianal sepsis tend to present early, 2 or 3 days after onset of symptoms, with pain and a palpable tender lump close to the anal margin, and usually with no constitutional symptoms. Patients with ischiorectal abscesses tend to present later with more vague discomfort, but because much more pus may accumulate in the large relatively avascular loose areolar tissue of the ischiorectal fossa, they often have fever and constitutional upset. Examination may reveal tender induration over the abscess rather than an exquisitely tender, well-defined lump as found when the sepsis is perianal.

the longitudinal muscle layer. Lateral spread across the external sphincter will reach the ischiorectal fossa (**d** in Fig. 14.1), where further caudal spread will result in the abscess pointing at the skin as an ischiorectal abscess; upward spread may penetrate the levators to reach the supralevator pararectal space. Circumferential spread (**Fig. 14.2**) may occur in any of the three planes, intermuscular (synonymous with intramuscular and equivalent to intersphincteric but with no restriction to a level beneath the anorectal ring), ischiorectal or supralevator. All those conditions that Eisenhammer[15] considered not to be of cryptoglandular origin he placed into the miscellaneous group of acute anorectal non-cryptoglandular non-fistulous abscesses (**Fig. 14.3**). These included the submucous abscess (arising from an infected haemorrhoid, sclerotherapy or trauma), the mucocutaneous or marginal abscess (infected haematoma), the perianal abscess (follicular skin infection), some ischiorectal abscesses (primary infection or foreign body) and the pelvirectal supralevator abscess originating from pelvic disease.

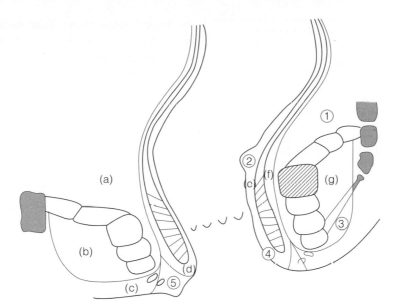

Figure 14.3 • The acute anorectal non-cryptoglandular non-fistulous abscesses of Eisenhammer: **(a)** pelvirectal supralevator space; **(b)** ischiorectal space; **(c)** perianal or superficial ischiorectal space; **(d)** marginal or mucocutaneous space; **(e)** submucous space; **(f)** intermuscular (syn. intersphincteric) space; **(g)** deep postanal space. 1, Pelvirectal supralevator abscess; 2, submucous abscess; 3, ischiorectal abscess; 4, mucocutaneous or marginal abscess; 5, perianal or subcutaneous abscess. Reproduced from Eisenhammer S. The final evaluation and classification of the surgical treatment of the primary anorectal cryptoglandular intermuscular (intersphincteric) fistulous abscess and fistula. Dis Colon Rectum 1978; 21:237–54. With permission from Lippincott, Williams & Wilkins.

Sepsis higher up in the sphincter complex may present with rectal pain, and possibly disturbance of micturition, and there may be no external signs of pathology. The rare submucosal abscess is revealed on digital examination of the anal canal as a distinct tender bulge, and the patient may have reported the passage of pus from the anal canal with relief of symptoms.

> ✔ Clues as to the aetiology of perineal sepsis may be gleaned from microbiology of the drained pus:[16,17] if skin organisms alone are cultured and the acute abscess is adequately drained, the patient may be told with confidence that recurrence should not occur and that a fistula will not result. If gut organisms are cultured, however, it is probable but not inevitable that there is an underlying fistula. The results of microbiology are therefore sensitive (100%) but not totally specific (60–80%), and of course are not available at the time of initial surgery.

Determination of the presence or absence of sepsis in the intersphincteric space (irrespective of the site of the main abscess or whether an internal opening is demonstrable) has been shown to be the most accurate way of determining the presence of an underlying fistula,[18] although it has been argued that such exploration is beyond the expertise of a general surgical trainee untrained in proctology for whom simple incision and drainage represents the safest option in the acute stage.

Those who advocate a more aggressive approach to acute sepsis do so on the basis that incision and drainage can only be effective if the abscess is not cryptoglandular,[15] that definitive treatment in the initial stage obviates further surgery, and that such a policy reduces the incidence of complex fistulas arising due to incompletely drained sepsis. Certainly, the reported recurrence/fistula rate following primary fistulotomy (0–7%) would support this. There are drawbacks, however: internal openings are evident in only about one-third of cases; the acute situation lends itself to the creation of false tracks and internal openings; and the unknown proportion of patients with cryptoglandular sepsis who might be cured by incision and drainage alone would not be well served by a procedure associated with a greater risk of flatus incontinence and soiling.

A prospective randomised trial involving 200 patients presenting with anal sepsis compared simple drainage to drainage plus primary fistulotomy, when the fistula was deemed low (subcutaneous, intersphincteric or low trans-sphincteric). This yielded recurrence rates of 36.7% in the drainage-alone group and 5% in those in whom the underlying fistula was laid open.[19] There was no reported incontinence following simple drainage, compared with 2.8% in the fistulotomy group. This was the largest of five randomised trials subjected to meta-analysis,[20] which concluded that fistulotomy resulted in 83% reduction in risk of recurrence at final follow-up (RR 0.17, 95% CI 0.09–0.32, $P < 0.001$), but was associated with a tendency to a higher risk of flatus incontinence and soiling (RR 2.46, 95% CI 0.75–8.06, $P = 0.140$).

A policy (in experienced hands) of simple incision when a fistula is not evident, and primary fistulotomy when a fistula is evident and low (or a draining loose seton placed if there is any doubt about the level, or concern about continence) is sensible, as long as the patient has been adequately counselled.

Patients with an established fistula usually give a history of intermittent pain and purulent discharge from an opening on the perineum, the pain building up until relief is felt when the pus escapes. Patients in whom the internal opening is rectal, and those with large internal openings irrespective of site, may pass flatus and stool through the external opening(s).

Classification of anal fistula

Successful surgical management of anal fistula depends upon accurate knowledge of anal sphincter anatomy and the fistula's course through it. Failure to understand either may result in fistula recurrence or incontinence. To this end, classification of pathology is extremely important.

The most comprehensive and practical classification, and the one most widely used presently, is that devised by Sir Alan Parks at St Mark's Hospital, based on a study of 400 fistulas treated there.[21]

The cryptoglandular hypothesis is central to this classification, which holds firstly that the majority of fistulas arise from an abscess in the intersphincteric plane and secondly that the relation of the primary track to the external sphincter is paramount in surgical management. Four main groups exist: intersphincteric, trans-sphincteric, suprasphincteric and extrasphincteric. These groups can be further subdivided according to the presence and course of any extensions or secondary tracks.

Intersphincteric fistulas (**Fig. 14.4**), constituting 45% of cases in the original St Mark's series, are usually simple; however, others have a high blind track, or a high opening into the rectum or no perineal opening, or even have pelvic extension, or arise from pelvic disease. Trans-sphincteric fistulas (**Fig. 14.5**; 29%) have a primary track that passes through the external sphincter at varying levels into the ischiorectal fossa. Such fistulas may be uncomplicated, consisting only of the primary track, or can have a high blind track that may terminate below or above the levator ani muscles. Suprasphincteric fistulas (**Fig. 14.6**; 20% in the 1976 series[21]) run up to a level above puborectalis and then curl down through the levators and ischiorectal fossa to reach the skin. Extrasphincteric fistulas (**Fig. 14.7**; 5%) run without relation to the sphincters and are classified according to their pathogenesis. In addition to horizontal and vertical spread, sepsis may spread circumferentially in any of the three spaces: intersphincteric, ischiorectal or pararectal.

The St Mark's classification does have a few drawbacks,[22] but these are of little clinical significance. Superficial fistulas and those associated with bridged

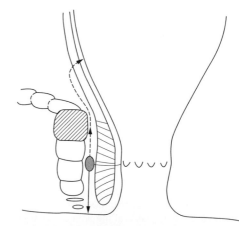

Figure 14.4 • The possible courses of an intersphincteric fistula. Reproduced from Marks CG, Ritchie JR. Anal fistulas at St Mark's Hospital. Br J Surg 1977; 64:84–91. © British Journal of Surgery Society Ltd. Permission is granted by John Wiley & Sons Ltd on behalf on the BJSS Ltd.

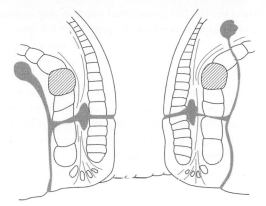

Figure 14.5 • A trans-sphincteric fistula with blind infralevator ischiorectal extension (left) and supralevator pararectal extension (right). Reproduced from Parks AG, Gordon PH, Hardcastle JD. A classification of fistula-in-ano. Br J Surg 1976; 63:1–12. © British Journal of Surgery Society Ltd. Permission is granted by John Wiley & Sons Ltd on behalf on the BJSS Ltd.

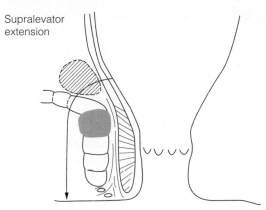

Supralevator extension

Figure 14.7 • Extrasphincteric fistula running without relation to the sphincter complex. Reproduced from Marks CG, Ritchie JK. Anal fistulas at St Mark's Hospital. Br J Surg 1977; 64:84–91. © British Journal of Surgery Society Ltd. Permission is granted by John Wiley & Sons Ltd on behalf on the BJSS Ltd.

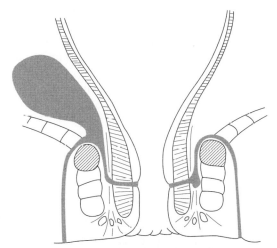

Figure 14.6 • Simple suprasphincteric fistula (right) and more complex form with associated secondary pelvic abscess (left). Reproduced from Parks AG, Gordon PH, Hardcastle JD. A classification of fistula-in-ano. Br J Surg 1976; 63:1–12. © British Journal of Surgery Society Ltd. Permission is granted by John Wiley & Sons Ltd on behalf on the BJSS Ltd.

pathology (arguing indeed that many are iatrogenic). The extreme rarity of suprasphincteric fistulas and the difficulty of distinguishing them from high trans-sphincteric tracks even raise doubts about their very existence. However, clinical differentiation from high trans-sphincteric fistulas is in most cases immaterial since the same methods of treatment would be employed.

Assessment

Clinical

A full history and examination including proctosigmoidoscopy are essential in all cases to exclude any associated conditions. Clinical assessment involves five essential points, enumerated by Goodsall and Miles at the end of the 19th century:

1. location of the internal opening;
2. location of the external opening;
3. course of the primary track;
4. presence of secondary extensions;
5. presence of other diseases complicating the fistula.

The relative positions of the external and internal openings will indicate the likely course of the primary track, and the presence of any palpable induration, especially supralevator, should alert the surgeon to a secondary track. The distance of the external opening from the anal verge may assist

fissures are not acknowledged by a classification whose emphasis is the intersphincteric space. There can be clinical difficulty in differentiating between a simple intersphincteric fistula and a very low trans-sphincteric fistula that crosses the lowermost fibres of the subcutaneous portion of the external sphincter. And some argue whether suprasphincteric tracks can be part of a classification based on cryptoglandular in differentiating an intersphincteric from a trans-sphincteric fistula; the greater the distance, the greater the likelihood of a complex cephalad extension.[5] Goodsall's rule generally applies in that the likely site of the internal opening can be predicted by the position around the anal circumference of the external opening. Exceptions to this rule include anteriorly located openings more than 3 cm from the anal verge (which may be anterior extensions of posterior horseshoe fistulas) and fistulas associated with other diseases, especially Crohn's and malignancy.

Thus, the first step in examining the anus is to identify the position of the external opening (or openings). Next, the perianal area should be carefully palpated with a well-lubricated finger to feel for the presence and direction of induration, which will indicate the course of the primary track (**Fig. 14.8**). If the track is not palpable, it is probable that the fistula is not intersphincteric or low trans-sphincteric. Digital examination within the anorectal lumen is then performed with the specific intention of feeling for any indentation/induration as the sign marking the site of the internal opening. Asking the patient to contract the anal sphincters allows an assessment of the position of the primary track in relation to the puborectalis sling (if posterior) or upper border of the external anal sphincter (if anterior), although it must be remembered that in trans-sphincteric

fistulas the level of the internal opening may not be the same as that at which the primary track crosses the external sphincter (which may be higher, especially if the internal opening is above the dentate line). The finger is then advanced into the rectum and any supralevator induration is sought (it feels like bone and is easier to notice when it is unilateral as there will be asymmetry; **Fig. 14.9**). Digital assessment of the primary track by an experienced coloproctologist has been shown to be 85% accurate.[23]

Examination under anaesthesia complements examination in the awake patient. The internal opening may be easily seen at proctoscopy, aided if necessary by gentle downward retraction of the dentate line, which may expose openings concealed by prominent valves or papillae. Lateral traction of an opened Eisenhammer proctoscope may reveal dimpling at the internal opening through its underlying fibrous inelasticity. Sometimes, the site of the responsible crypt may be seen only as scar tissue if the internal opening is not patent. Digital massage of the track may reveal the site of the internal opening as a bead of pus. If the track is simple, a probe may traverse its entire length, but if the probe comes to lie above or remote from the dentate line, a direct association between the track and the adjacent

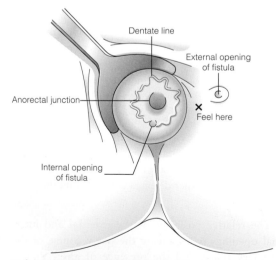

Figure 14.8 • Palpating for the direction and depth of the primary tract. Reproduced from Phillips RKS. Operative management of low cryptoglandular fistula-in-ano. Operat Tech Gen Surg 2001; 3(3):134–41. With permission from Elsevier.

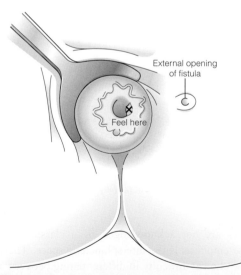

Figure 14.9 • Palpating for the presence of induration, indicating either a high primary tract or secondary extension in the roof of the ischiorectal fossa or supralevator space. Reproduced from Phillips RKS. Operative management of low cryptoglandular fistula-in-ano. Operat Tech Gen Surg 2001; 3(3):134–41. With permission from Elsevier.

anoderm cannot be assumed.[24] The instillation of various agents along the track via the external opening has also been advocated, including saline, hydrogen peroxide and dyes such as methylene blue and indigo carmine. In practical terms, instillation of dilute hydrogen peroxide is the easiest way of locating the internal opening, as staining is avoided.[24,25]

Careful probing can delineate primary and secondary tracks. If the internal and external openings are easily detected but the probe cannot easily traverse the path of the track, it is possible that there is a high extension, and a probe passed via each opening may then delineate the primary track. Failure to negotiate probes around a horseshoe posterior transsphincteric fistula suggests at least one acute bend in the track, within the intersphincteric space and crossing the external sphincter, or in the roof of the ischiorectal fossa, in which case anatomy will only be defined once surgery is under way (**Fig. 14.10**). Persistence of granulation tissue after curettage during the operation is an indication of a secondary extension.[25]

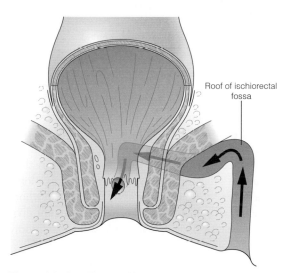

Roof of ischiorectal fossa

Figure 14.10 • Trans-sphincteric horseshoe fistulas may have several sharp bends along their course, preventing exact delineation unless the ischiorectal fossa is opened widely (to reach the acute bend in the roof of the ischiorectal fossa), and often necessitating dislocation of the posterior sphincter from its ligamentous attachments (to ascertain the site at which the tract crosses the external sphincter). Reproduced from Phillips RKS. Operative management of low cryptoglandular fistula-in-ano. Operat Tech Gen Surg 2001; 3(3):134–41. With permission from Elsevier.

Imaging

Careful examination of a fistula under anaesthesia has been considered the most important part of any assessment.[24] However, previous surgery leads to scarring and deformity, as well as the creation of unusual primary tracks, which can make clinical assessment extremely difficult. Until recently, techniques aimed at helping in fistula assessment have proved disappointing. The advent of endoanal ultrasound and magnetic resonance imaging (MRI), however, has resulted in a plethora of reports assessing and comparing imaging modalities, which have been comprehensively reviewed.[26]

In summary, the introduction of more accurate methods has rendered fistulography almost obsolete, but the technique should be considered if an extrasphincteric track is a possibility. Computed tomography suffers other disadvantages, and similarly is indicated only when there is suspicion that the fistula arises from an intra-abdominal or pelvic source.

Anal endosonography (AES) is relatively cheap and easy to perform, but is operator dependent and has limited focal range, which makes evaluation of pathology beyond the sphincters (either lateral to or above) difficult to assess, areas from which difficulty in clinical assessment often arises. Also, sepsis and scarring can confuse fistula assessment in those who have undergone previous surgery. Given the superiority of MRI, perhaps the main role of AES in patients with anal fistula is in the determination of internal and external sphincter integrity, although AES is superior to clinical evaluation.[27] Good agreement has been found between the newer imaging modalities of hydrogen peroxide-enhanced three-dimensional AES and endoanal MRI, but findings have not been compared to the best standard, i.e. healing after surgery, and neither technique is widely available.

The potential advantages of MRI include the lack of ionising radiation, the ability to image in any plane and the high soft-tissue resolution.

✅ Short tau inversion recovery (STIR) sequencing (a fat-suppression technique) to highlight the presence of pus and granulation tissue without the need for any contrast media[28] was used in a prospective study involving 35 patients at St Mark's Hospital that favourably compared MRI interpretations with the independently documented operative findings.[29]

Further prospective studies have confirmed that the technique certainly challenges operative assessment by an experienced coloproctologist as the 'gold standard'. A recent prospective study has demonstrated a therapeutic impact of MRI in the management of 10% of patients treated for primary anal fistulas,[30] although the therapeutic impact is much greater when used to assess recurrent fistulas.[31]

Perhaps a logical approach is that patients with (suspected) primary anal fistulas undergo AES, and those in whom there is clinical or sonographic suspicion of complexity go on to MRI. There is strong evidence that all recurrent fistulas should be examined using MRI preoperatively, and that the surgeon should use the scans to aid surgery. The accuracy of MRI also means that we are now able to refute or confirm the presence of sepsis in those patients with symptoms but in whom clinical examination is unrevealing, and in the prospective assessment of newer methods of attempted fistula eradication.

Physiological

The correlation between subjective assessment of an individual's continence and physiological static measurements recorded in a laboratory may be debatable, but the argument for physiological assessment (anal canal length, pressures along it, anorectal sensitivity, sphincter integrity and pudendal nerve conduction studies) in the clinical context of a patient with a complex fistula (or one deemed to have, or be at risk of, compromise in function) is nowadays strong. Continence may be regarded as a balance between rectal pressure and the power of the sphincters to overcome this, orchestrated by anorectal sensation.

✅ Milligan and Morgan[32] stressed the importance of the anorectal ring in fistula surgery: 'If this ring be cut, loss of control surely results, yet as long as the narrowest complete ring of muscle remains, control is preserved. All the anal sphincter muscles below this ring may be divided in any manner without harmful loss of control.'

Certainly, complete division of the puborectalis sling in suprasphincteric and extrasphincteric fistulas results in total incontinence to all rectal contents, but division of muscles below the ring may result in equally devastating consequences. It is reasonable to suppose that the higher the level at which the primary track crosses the sphincter complex, the greater the possibility of impaired function after fistulotomy, and the weaker the sphincters before surgical intervention, the greater the likelihood of such morbidity.

Traditionally, more importance has been apportioned to the external than to the internal anal sphincter in the context of muscle preservation in anal fistula surgery. Indeed, the importance of eradication of the presumed aetiological source, the diseased anal gland in the intersphincteric space, led Parks[8] to advocate internal sphincterectomy (excision of that segment of internal sphincter overlying the diseased gland) as an essential part of surgical management. Nowadays, most surgeons divide rather than excise the circular muscle, but the concept of getting rid of the intersphincteric source remains widely held.

To determine the physiological and functional effects of fistula surgery, we conducted a prospective study[33] of 37 patients successfully treated for either intersphincteric (15 patients) or trans-sphincteric fistulas. All patients underwent division of the internal anal sphincter and anoderm below the level of the primary track; 15 of the 22 patients with trans-sphincteric fistulas also underwent division of the external sphincter, at least to the level of the dentate line, whereas the remaining seven patients with trans-sphincteric fistulas were successfully treated without recourse to external sphincter division. As might be predicted, distal anal canal and maximum resting pressures were reduced in all patients after surgery, external sphincter division resulting in no greater reduction of maximum resting pressure than occurred after internal sphincter division alone. Squeeze pressures were unaffected in those in whom the external sphincter had been preserved, but division in the 15 patients who underwent fistulotomy of trans-sphincteric tracks resulted in significant reductions in distal anal canal squeeze pressures and maximum squeeze pressure.

However, functional outcome was not related to division of the external sphincter, with an equal incidence of minor disturbances of continence reported by those in whom it had been preserved (53% vs. 50%, respectively). Furthermore, the severity of postoperative symptoms was no different between the two groups, being related to reduced postoperative resting pressures, reduced maximum resting pressure and higher thresholds of anal electro-sensitivity in the sector of surgery, rather than to postoperative squeeze pressures.

It appears that total sphincter conservation would be optimal in terms of functional outcome, but the drawback is that no sphincter-preserving method heals the underlying fistula as surely as lay-open. This is important, because although this study revealed a relatively high incidence of functional disturbance, the vast majority of patients were satisfied with their management and tolerated a reduction in function as a reasonable price to pay in order to be rid of chronic anal sepsis. When asked prospectively, patients are frightened by the term 'incontinence' and would generally seek to avoid it.[34] It is important to outline the anticipated functional result and to be descriptive, while avoiding using emotive words such as 'incontinence'.

Principles of fistula surgery

Acute sepsis is an indication for early surgical intervention and drainage. However, in cases where a more complex procedure than lay-open is contemplated, acute sepsis should have been eradicated long before, leaving well-established chronic tracks. A loose seton may be required to achieve adequate drainage of the primary track. Secondary tracks should be either laid open, curetted or drained, according to their position in relation to the levators. Some authors advise bowel preparation before fistula surgery, although laid-open wounds in the perineum heal remarkably well despite the continual bacterial load. Most authors recommend parenteral antibiotics perioperatively and postoperatively for any of the more complex procedures.

In the UK, fistula surgery is usually performed under general anaesthesia, but in North America local or regional anaesthesia is more widely employed. Similarly, in the UK most anal fistula surgery is performed with the patient in the lithotomy position, although the prone jack-knife position is gaining in popularity, at least among some surgeons. Prophylaxis against development of venous thrombosis is advised, and in the UK is usually achieved with a combination of low-dose subcutaneous heparin and elasticated stockings. Finally, the operative findings and treatment should be recorded. The St Mark's Hospital

fistula operation sheet (**Fig. 14.11**) based on the Parks classification provides an excellent standardised format for documentation both by description and by illustration.

Surgical treatment

Lay-open remains the surest way of eliminating an anal fistula. The multiplicity of techniques designed to preserve sphincter function and at the same time eradicate fistula pathology reflects their relative lack of success. A degree of caution and scepticism may be appropriately apportioned when assessing reported results of the various approaches towards complex fistula, since:

1. patient populations may be markedly different;
2. fistula classification may be variable;
3. reports of successes may not be tempered by honest reporting of failures;
4. reports of success in terms of fistula cure have historically not always been accompanied by reports of changes in continence;
5. despite the increasing drive for evidence-based medicine, the use of adequately powered prospective randomised trials is perhaps unachievable, because of individual fistula (and sphincter) variability and individual surgeon preference and skill;
6. follow-up may be inadequate.

Fistulotomy

Fistulotomy means laying open and allowing to heal by secondary intention. Its application should, in the first instance, be restricted to situations where a significant degree of incontinence would not result. In principle, high trans-sphincteric (especially anterior tracks in women) and suprasphincteric tracks should not be treated by one-stage fistulotomy. Intersphincteric and low trans-sphincteric tracks are probably best treated by this method, but the decision whether to lay open rests on the skill and experience of the surgeon after informed advice to the patient.

Abcarian[35] recommends the following technique: after initial assessment of the track, a crypt hook is placed into the internal opening, which is laid open by diathermy cautery, the latter maintaining a dry operative field and thus allowing easy identification of granulation tissue. If examination with the crypt

ST. MARK'S HOSPITAL
FISTULA OPERATION NOTES

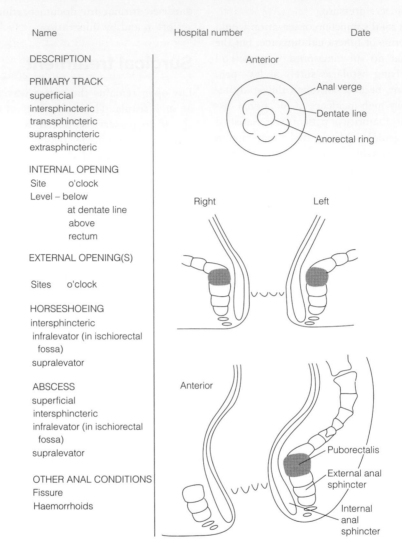

Name   Hospital number   Date

DESCRIPTION

PRIMARY TRACK
superficial
intersphincteric
transsphincteric
suprasphincteric
extrasphincteric

INTERNAL OPENING
Site   o'clock
Level – below
            at dentate line
            above
            rectum

EXTERNAL OPENING(S)

Sites   o'clock

HORSESHOEING
intersphincteric
infralevator (in ischiorectal
    fossa)
supralevator

ABSCESS
superficial
intersphincteric
infralevator (in ischiorectal
    fossa)
supralevator

OTHER ANAL CONDITIONS
Fissure
Haemorrhoids

Figure 14.11 • The St Mark's Hospital fistula operation sheet. Reproduced with thanks to Mr James P.S. Thomson, Emeritus Consultant Surgeon, St Mark's.

hook reveals the primary track to be intersphincteric or to involve only the lowermost fibres of the external anal sphincter, the tissue overlying the probe is divided along its length. If, however, the probe enters the depths outside the external sphincter, it is left in place and a second probe gently passed via the external opening, and the two probes manipulated until they can be felt or heard to touch. That portion of the track outside the external sphincter is laid open, and the internal sphincter divided over the crypt hook. An assessment is then made as to how much

voluntary muscle lies below the track and the decision is made either to lay the track open or to resort to a sphincter-saving procedure.

> ✔✔ Marsupialisation, i.e. suturing the divided wound edge to the edges of the curetted fibrous track, results in a smaller wound and faster healing.[36,37]

Secondary extensions from the primary track can be dealt with in two ways. The traditional method in the UK is to lay these open widely to allow maximal drainage, which is followed by healing by secondary intention. As long as the external sphincter is intact, the residual scarring after healing is remarkably little. In the USA, the use of incisions, counter-incisions and the placement of encircling drains is sometimes preferred; these drains are left in for 2–4 weeks, with more rapid healing and less deformity claimed.

Fistulotomy and immediate reconstitution

Parkash et al.[38] reported a series of 120 patients treated by fistulotomy and immediate reconstruction of the divided musculature, and with primary wound closure. The reported results were impressive: 88% of wounds had healed by 2 weeks, there was a 4% recurrence rate and all patients were satisfied with the functional outcome. However, 118 of the 120 fistulas were classified as low intersphincteric or simple trans-sphincteric, and the authors admitted that similar success would not be expected with more complex fistulas. The technique has been applied to a small cohort of patients with recurrent complex fistulas, not amenable to fistulotomy, with impressive results in terms of healing rates, manometric and functional outcomes, and with no report of dehiscence of the reconstituted sphincter.[39]

> ✔ A randomised trial of 55 patients with non-recurrent complex fistulas comparing fistulotomy combined with immediate sphincter reconstitution and advancement flap repair yielded equivalent results in respect to healing and functional outcomes.[40]

Fistulectomy

> ✔ The technique of fistulectomy, which excises rather than incises the fistula track, has been criticised on the basis that the greater tissue loss leads to delayed healing.[41]

However, Lewis[42] advocates fistulectomy, but by a core-out technique rather than excision of the track, because he claims that:

1. the precise course of the track is more accurately determined by core-out under direct vision, and does not involve the passage of probes along the track and thus creation of false tracks – a probe

is used only to open the external opening and assist in inserting a stay suture around it;
2. coring out the primary track reduces the risk of missing secondary tracks, which are seen as transected granulation tissue and which may be followed by the same technique;
3. the relation of the primary track to the external anal sphincter may be correctly ascertained before any sphincter muscle is divided;
4. a complete specimen is available for histology.

Once the track has been cored out, from the external towards the internal opening using either scissors or cautery dissection, the decision as to whether the tunnel left after the core-out can be safely laid open is made. For a non-recurrent single trans-sphincteric track, Lewis recommends simple anatomical closure of the cored-out tunnel, with mucosal closure and closure of the holes in the muscles. The wound outside the sphincters is lightly packed.

Of 67 low fistulas treated by Lewis[43] between 1985 and 1992 by coring out and laying open the resultant tunnel, there was one recurrence. Of 32 patients with high trans-sphincteric or suprasphincteric fistulas treated between 1972 and 1992 by core-out and simple anatomical closure, a temporary colostomy was raised in four and there were three recurrences. In the case of recurrent or more complex fistulas, Lewis recommends the adoption of other sphincter-conserving methods, since excessive scarring and the larger defect created by coring out this tissue make simple anatomical closure inappropriate.

Setons

The loose seton

Setons may be classified as loose, tight or chemical according to their different properties and modes of action. A thread, loosely tied, is often used as a marker of a fistula track when its exact position and level in relation to the external sphincter is unclear at surgery, perhaps because of scarring from previous surgery or because of the depth of sphincter muscle relaxation under anaesthesia. In such circumstances, the proportions of muscle above and below the fistula may be more accurately determined when the patient is awake and with the track palpably delineated by the thread. Similarly, a loosely tied thread can be used as a drain of acute sepsis, to allow subsidence of acute inflammatory changes and safer definitive fistula surgery.

More specifically in the field of sphincter and continence preservation, the loose seton can be used in three ways: to preserve the entire external sphincter; to preserve part of the voluntary muscle; or as part of a staged fistulotomy in order to reduce the consequences of division of large amounts of muscle in one procedure.

The key points of a staged fistulotomy are the amount of muscle divided at each stage and the time allowed for fibrosis to develop between the divided muscle edges before a further length of sphincter is divided.[44,45] Parks and Stitz[46] reported a series of 80 patients from St Mark's Hospital with trans-sphincteric and suprasphincteric fistulas in whom, at the first stage, the lower one-third to one-half of the sphincter was divided and at the second stage a few months later either the seton removed (if all had healed) or the seton-enclosed muscle divided (if there were high tracks or cavities that had failed to close in). About 38% of patients required division of the upper sphincter to achieve healing; unfortunately, the functional outcome in the two groups of patients was not clearly described.

Later at St Mark's the loose seton was used with the aim of entire external sphincter preservation. Tracks and extensions outside the sphincters were widely laid open, and in the past the internal sphincter was then divided to the level of the internal opening (or higher if there was a cephalad intersphincteric extension). Subsequently, attempts at internal sphincter conservation were made. In the case of the high posterior trans-sphincteric track, the passage of the primary track across the sphincter complex may sometimes be accurately judged only after division of the anococcygeal ligaments, thereby dislocating the posterior sphincter attachments but allowing access to the deep postanal space.[47] The seton, passed along the primary track across the external sphincter, is then tied loosely to encircle the denuded voluntary muscle. Postoperatively, the wounds are managed by daily digitation and irrigation rather than by tight packing, with a possible repeat examination under anaesthesia at 7–10 days to ensure that all tracks have been dealt with and that healing is progressing correctly. At outpatient review, if there is evidence of good healing both of the wounds and around the seton, the latter is removed at 2–3 months. Any suspicion of ongoing sepsis requires repeat examination under anaesthesia.

A series of 34 consecutive patients with complex idiopathic trans-sphincteric fistulas treated at St Mark's Hospital between 1977 and 1984 showed that cure of the fistula without recourse to external sphincter division occurred in 44%.[48] Of those in whom the method had been successful, 83% reported full continence compared with only 32% of those in whom the external sphincter had subsequently been divided. Of the 16 patients in whom the technique failed, nine reported some degree of incontinence to formed stool; none of the patients in whom the external sphincter had been preserved reported any such disturbance of sphincter function. Success rates of 67% and 78% have been reported from other centres.[47,49] The importance of adequate follow-up to determine long-term outcomes following a particular technique has been exemplified by Buchanan et al.,[50] who reviewed 20 patients treated by this method a minimum of 10 years following surgery. Although in the short term 13 of the 20 healed, by 10 years only four had remained so.

If the technique fails and it is certain that this is not due to any missed secondary extensions (detectable by MRI), untoward aetiology, etc., there are several options available: (i) the patient may be happy living with a 'controlled' fistula with a long-term draining seton [Editor's note: my own personal preference is for a permanent loose seton made of No. 1 Ethibond with just one knot to avoid bulkiness and to give comfort (nylon setons tend to be sharp, silastic setons to have bulky knots)]; (ii) the tight seton method may be employed; (iii) a fistulotomy may be performed and the functional results assessed postoperatively; or (iv) fistulotomy may be combined with the raising of a defunctioning colostomy, time allowed for full healing, before sphincter repair and then restoration of intestinal continuity at a final stage. The decision made must be between the individual patient and the surgeon.

The tight seton

The rationale of the tight or cutting seton is similar to that of the staged fistulotomy technique, in that the divided muscle is not allowed to spring apart but there is supposed to be gradual severance through the sphincter followed by fibrosis. Goldberg and Garcia-Aquilar[51] recommend the use of a tight seton whenever the fistula encircles more than 30% of the sphincter complex and when local sepsis or fibrosis precludes the raising of an advancement flap.

The portion of the track outside the sphincters is laid open, although others in the USA have recommended Penrose drainage of horseshoe limbs. The anoderm and perianal skin overlying that portion of the sphincter encircled by the seton are incised and the intersphincteric space drained by internal sphincterotomy, extended cephalad if necessary to drain any high intersphincteric (intermuscular) extension. Tightening of the seton (Goldberg uses a rubber band) does not commence until any suppuration has resolved, usually at 3 weeks postoperatively. Tightening is repeated every 2 weeks using a silk tie or Barron band until the seton has cut through.

Goldberg described the use of the cutting seton in 13 patients with trans-sphincteric fistulas between 1988 and 1992, and found that the average time for the seton to cut through was 16 weeks (range 8–36 weeks) with no recurrences at a median follow-up of 24 months (range 4–60 months). As might be expected, this cure rate was tempered by a relatively high incidence of functional morbidity: one patient suffered major incontinence, and a further seven patients (54%) complained of minor persistent loss of control to flatus or episodic loss of liquid stool.

The critical aspects of management by the cutting seton must be firstly the elimination of acute sepsis and secondary extensions before sphincter division, and secondly the speed with which the seton cuts through the sphincter. In a series of 24 patients with high trans-sphincteric fistulas, Christensen et al.[52] tightened the seton every second day; 62% of patients reported some degree of incontinence postoperatively, including 29% who wore a pad constantly. The 'snug' silastic (elastic) seton method, in which the muscle is cut through much more slowly but without the need for tightening, in the treatment of inter- and trans-sphincteric fistulas, was associated with healing in all cases, but with a 25% incidence of continence disturbance in the 16 patients followed up at a median 42 months after the seton had cut through.[53]

The chemical seton

This method, enjoying a resurgence in India where it is known as *Kshara sutra*, involves the weekly re-insertion of a specially prepared thread along the fistula track. The thread is prepared in a multistage process involving multiple layers of agents derived from plants. Apart from its antibacterial and anti-inflammatory properties, the alkalinity of the thread (about pH 9.5) would appear to be the means by which the thread slowly cuts through the tissues. Indeed, the chemical nature might be the reason behind the rather slow rate of cutting, about 1 cm of track every 6 days.

> ✔ In a prospective randomised trial involving 502 patients,[54] apart from a longer healing time (8 weeks vs. 4 weeks), the results of this outpatient treatment were comparable with fistulotomy (incontinence rate 5% vs. 9%; recurrence rate at 1 year 4% vs. 11%).

Recurrences usually occur for the same reasons as after conventional surgery, such as a missed secondary track or another internal opening, but the economic advantages of such a method in a less privileged country are obvious.

> ✔ For low fistulas, however, a more recent prospective randomised study from Singapore concluded that the method has no advantage over conventional fistulotomy.[55]

Advancement flaps

The use of an advancement flap was first proposed in 1902 for the repair of rectovaginal fistulas. Elting[56] described its use in managing anal fistula in 1912, supported by two principles: separation of the track from the communication with the bowel; and adequate closure of that communication with eradication of all diseased tissue in the anorectal wall. To Elting's principles, modern surgeons have added adequate flap vascularity and anastomosis of the flap to a site well distal to the site of the (previously excised) internal opening as important tenets. Modifications have included the use of full-thickness rectal flaps, partial-thickness flaps, curved incisions and rhomboid flaps, with or without closure of the defect in and outside the external sphincter,[57] and distally based (anocutaneous flaps transposed upwards) flaps. Most authors agree that the flap should include part if not all of the underlying internal sphincter in order to maintain vascularity. Apart from the presence of acute sepsis, large internal openings (>2.5 cm) would be considered a contraindication as the risks of anastomotic breakdown are high,[58] and a heavily scarred, indurated, wooden perineum precludes adequate exposure and flap mobilisation.

Although the technique has not enjoyed much popularity because of a low success rate at St Mark's Hospital, there are several studies that have reported excellent results, with cure rates of 90–100% for idiopathic anal fistulas and little in the way of functional morbidity. A review of the technique and its results has been published.[59] The report by Athanasiadis et al.[60] is interesting for several reasons. In the larger series of patients (n=224), internal sphincterotomy was performed aiming to eradicate the presumed aetiological source, but this led, as might be expected, to a much higher incidence of significant postoperative continence disorders than when internal sphincterotomy had not been performed. The persistence/recurrent fistula rate was 18% for trans-sphincteric fistulas and 40% for suprasphincteric fistulas. Preservation of the internal sphincter in a subsequent group of 55 patients resulted in a much lower incidence of functional morbidity, but unfortunately fistula persistence/recurrence was not reported. Physiological assessment has revealed that the technique may[57] or may not[61] be associated with preservation of resting and squeeze pressures, and success rates in terms of fistula healing decrease with time.[62]

Intersphincteric approaches

In 1993 the authors reported an intersphincteric approach with reasonable results.[63] The lift operation (ligation of the intersphincteric fistula tract) is similar and is quite popular at present, although longer-term results are awaited.[64–66] The addition of a bioprosthetic graft has been claimed to improve results, although follow-up is short.[67]

Plugs and glues (Table 14.1)

Enthusiastic initial reports have not always stood the test of time.[68] These approaches are highly attractive, as they require little innate surgical skill, but the Achilles heel is their uncertain success rate. They may be used as an adjunct to advancement flap surgery. There are many considerations: biocompatibility; rate of decomposition/integration with host tissues; and how to prepare the host environment

Table 14.1 • Biomaterials that have been used in the treatment of anal fistula

Autograft	Fibrin glue
	Fibroblasts
	Stem cells
Allograft	Fibrin glue
	Acellular dermal matrix plug
	Stem cells
Xenograft	Intestinal submucosal porcine collagen
	Dermal non-cross-linked porcine collagen
	Dermal cross-linked porcine collagen
Man made/hybrid	Bovine serum albumin/ glutaraldehyde
	Modified synthetic cyanoacrylic surgical glue
	Synthetic bioabsorbable polyglycolide–trimethylene carbonate copolymer
	Basic fibroblast growth factor

(drill/core-out/curette the tract or leave it alone, prior identification and drainage/eradication of secondary extensions, and so on).[69]

Fibrin glue

There have been three reviews.[70–72] Autologous glues have been largely replaced by commercially available virus-inactivated fibrinogen solution from donor plasma. The glue plugs the tract, promoting healing through fibroblast migration and activation and the formation of a collagen meshwork. Curettage to remove granulation tissue and debris (even employing a laser) is stressed. Difficulty with this and complete occlusion of secondary tracts may account for failure. Acute sepsis should first be managed with a loose draining seton. The internal opening itself is usually closed, either with direct sutures or an advancement flap.

> ✓ Poorer outcomes were observed following advancement flap repair of the internal opening and fibrin obliteration of the track than following advancement flap alone.[73]

Notwithstanding the various modifications employed, it is difficult to explain the highly variable reported success rates (0–100%). Paradoxically, treatment of short tracks appears less successful than longer ones. Postoperative MRI, despite clinical healing, has shown much lower true healing rates, of the order of 10–20%.[74]

> ✅ A randomised controlled trial demonstrated no benefit in terms of healing over fistulotomy in treating low fistulas, but for those fistulas deemed unsafe to lay open, a cumulative 69% success rate at 3 months[75] appears at least as good as other conserving techniques. Cutting remains more efficacious still, but there is a (usually small) functional price to pay.[76]

Being so simple, the attractions are self-evident. It may be that further developments will produce more effective glues, although success will need MRI validation of deeper healing.

Bioprosthetic plugs

More recently, reports of bioabsorbable xenografts that plug fistula tracks have usurped the popularity of fibrin glue in the literature, following a prospective non-randomised study that suggested that outcomes in the short term using lyophilised porcine intestinal submucosa were superior to those using fibrin glue[77] and that success was sustained at a median of 6 months in 38 of 46 (83%) patients,[78] with failure often attributed to plug extrusion. As with fibrin glue, MRI validation is needed.

> ✅ The plug has been compared with an advancement flap in two prospective randomised trials. One closed prematurely due to an unacceptable failure rate with the plug,[79] while in the other, recurrence with a plug was also higher.[80]

Management of the recurrent fistula

Failure of sphincter-preserving methods and persistent symptoms may make lay-open the most sensible option (although some patients may prefer to live with a long-term loose seton). After fistulotomy some patients are able to lead normal lives with the narrowest of (often fibrotic) anorectal rings, as Milligan and Morgan had stated in 1934.[32] However, some may request sphincter repair. MRI is a useful way of making sure that there is no covert pathology before embarking on repair. Over a 3-year period at St Mark's Hospital 20 patients underwent sphincteroplasty for incontinence after previous surgery for idiopathic fistulas. A good outcome (Parks' grade 1 or 2 continence score) was obtained in 13 (65%).[81]

It is important to consider the possibility of an extrasphincteric fistula arising from pelvic or abdominal disease or from a presacral dermoid cyst when a high 'blind' track is encountered. Failure to image (fistulography, barium studies or MRI) is a major reason for delayed diagnosis. If a track is truly high and blind, this might be because the internal opening has closed, or because surgery has dealt with the primary track and recurrence is because of an overlooked secondary extension.[82] In such cases, the component of the track outside the sphincters should be laid open and curetted. As the resulting wound may be large, it is often wise to make a circular rather than a radial incision to avoid sphincter damage. Following granulation tissue with curette and probe must be done extremely carefully if false tracks and iatrogenic openings are to be avoided. If the track peters out before reaching the intersphincteric space, it is safest to stop and come back another day. If the track enters the intersphincteric space but no internal opening can be identified, it is reasonable to assume that the opening has healed or is extremely small; internal sphincterectomy of that quadrant is then justified to try to prevent recurrence.

Key points

- A fistula has a primary track and may have secondary extensions.
- Complete eradication of both will lead to cure.
- All lay-open procedures divide some of the internal sphincter, so patients should be warned of a 1 in 3 chance of flatus incontinence and mild mucus leakage.
- Lay-open is the most certain treatment where it is possible and when the risks have been properly explained and accepted.

- Advancement flaps are intuitively attractive but practically uncertain.
- Glue is only rarely effective – bioprosthetic plugs are more attractive but long-term results of healing validated by MRI are awaited.
- In the balance between minor soiling with almost certain cure vs. potential recurrence with a less than certain technique, many patients allowed the choice will choose the former.
- Anterior fistulas in women are dangerous and should only rarely be laid open.
- STIR sequence MRI is the gold standard for imaging.
- A permanent, comfortable, loose seton will preserve continence and prevent much (but not all) future abscess formation, but continual discharge means all patients need continuing outpatient support and reassurance, and a minority find it unacceptable in the long term.

References

1. Phillips RKS, Lunniss PJ. Anorectal sepsis. In: Nicholls RJ, Dozois RR, editors. Surgery of the colon and rectum. New York: Churchill Livingstone; 1997. p. 255–84.
2. McColl I. The comparative anatomy and pathology of anal glands. Ann R Coll Surg Engl 1967;40:36–67.
3. El-Tawil AM. Mechanism of non-specific-fistula-in-ano: hormonal aspects – review. Pathophysiology 2011;http://dx.doi.org/10.1016/j.pathophys.2011.07.004.
4. Marks CG, Ritchie JK. Anal fistulas at St Mark's Hospital. Br J Surg 1977;64:1003–7.
5. Lilius HG. Fistula-in-ano: a clinical study of 150 patients. Acta Chir Scand 1968;383(Suppl.):3–88.
6. Sainio P. A manometric study of anorectal function after surgery for anal fistula, with special reference to incontinence. Acta Chir Scand 1985;151:695–700.
7. Eisenhammer S. The internal anal sphincter and the anorectal abscess. Surg Gynecol Obstet 1956;103:501–6.
8. Parks AG. The pathogenesis and treatment of fistula-in-ano. Br Med J 1961;1:463–9.
9. Goligher JC, Ellis M, Pissides AG. A critique of anal glandular infection in the aetiology and treatment of idiopathic anorectal abscesses and fistulae. Br J Surg 1967;54:977–83.
10. Seow-Choen F, Hay AJ, Heard S, et al. Bacteriology of anal fistulae. Br J Surg 1992;79:27–8.
11. Lunniss PJ, Faris B, Rees H, et al. Histological and microbiological assessment of the role of microorganisms in chronic anal fistulae. Br J Surg 1993;80:1072.
12. Gordon-Watson C, Dodd H. Observations on fistula in ano in relation to perianal intermuscular glands. Br J Surg 1935;22:703–9.
13. Lunniss PJ, Sheffield JP, Talbot IC, et al. Persistence of anal fistula may be related to epithelialization. Br J Surg 1995;82:32–3.
14. Kiehne K, Fincke A, Brunke G, et al. Antimicrobial peptides in chronic anal fistula epithelium. Scand J Gastroenterol 2007;42:1063–9.
15. Eisenhammer S. The final evaluation and classification of the surgical treatment of the primary anorectal, cryptoglandular intermuscular (intersphincteric) fistulous abscess and fistula. Dis Colon Rectum 1978;21:237–54.
16. Grace RH, Harper IA, Thompson RG. Anorectal sepsis: microbiology in relation to fistula-in-ano. Br J Surg 1982;69:401–3.
17. Toyonaga T, Matsushima M, Tanaka Y, et al. Microbiological analysis and endoanal ultrasonography for diagnosis of anal fistula in acute anorectal sepsis. Int J Colorectal Dis 2007;22:209–13.
18. Lunniss PJ, Phillips RKS. Surgical assessment of acute anorectal sepsis is a better predictor of fistula than microbiological analysis. Br J Surg 1994;81:368–9.
19. Oliver I, Lacueva FJ, Perez Vicente F, et al. Randomized clinical trial comparing simple drainage of anorectal abscess with and without fistula track treatment. Int J Colorectal Dis 2003;18:107–10.
Largest randomised trial of its kind.
20. Quah HM, Tang CL, Eu KW, et al. Meta-analysis of randomized clinical trials comparing drainage alone vs primary sphincter-cutting procedures for anorectal abscess-fistula. Int J Colorectal Dis 2006;21:602–9.
Primary fistulotomy in experienced hands is safe and effective.
21. Parks AG, Gordon PH, Hardcastle JD. A classification of fistula-in-ano. Br J Surg 1976;63:1–12.
22. Marks CG. Classification. In: Phillips RKS, Lunniss PJ, editors. Anal fistula. Surgical evaluation and management. London: Chapman & Hall; 1996. p. 33–46.
23. Choen S, Burnett S, Bartram CI, et al. Comparison between anal endosonography and digital examination in the evaluation of anal fistulae. Br J Surg 1991;78:445–7.
24. Fazio V. Complex anal fistulae. Gastroenterol Clin N Am 1987;16:93–114.
25. Seow-Choen F, Phillips RKS. Insights gained from the management of problematical anal fistulas at St. Mark's Hospital, 1984–88. Br J Surg 1991;78:539–41.
26. Halligan S, Stoker J. Imaging of fistula in ano. Radiology 2006;239:18–33.

27. Buchanan GN, Halligan S, Bartram CI, et al. Clinical evaluation, endosonography and MR imaging in preoperative assessment of fistula-in-ano: comparison with outcome derived gold standard. Radiology 2004;233:674–81.

28. Lunniss PJ, Armstrong P, Barker PG, et al. Magnetic resonance imaging of anal fistulae. Lancet 1992;340:394–6.

29. Lunniss PJ, Barker PG, Sultan AH, et al. Magnetic resonance imaging of fistula-in-ano. Dis Colon Rectum 1994;37:708–18.

30. Buchanan GN, Halligan S, Williams AB, et al. Magnetic resonance imaging for primary fistula in ano. Br J Surg 2003;90:877–81.

31. Buchanan G, Halligan S, Williams A, et al. Effect of MRI on clinical outcome of recurrent fistula-in-ano. Lancet 2003;360:1661–2.

32. Milligan ETC, Morgan CN. Surgical anatomy of the anal canal with special reference to anorectal fistulae. Lancet 1934;ii:1150–6, 1213–7.

33. Lunniss PJ, Kamm MA, Phillips RKS. Factors affecting continence after surgery for anal fistula. Br J Surg 1994;81:1382–5.

34. Ellis CN. Sphincter-preserving fistula management: what patients want. Dis Colon Rectum 2010;53:1652–5.

35. Abcarian H. The 'lay open' technique. In: Phillips RKS, Lunniss PJ, editors. Anal fistula. Surgical evaluation and management. London: Chapman & Hall; 1996. p. 73–80.

36. Ho YH, Tan M, Leong FPK, et al. Marsupialisation of fistulotomy wounds improves healing: a randomized controlled trial. Br J Surg 1998;85:105–7.

37. Pescatori M, Ayabaca SM, Cafaro D, et al. Marsupialization of fistulotomy and fistulectomy wounds improves healing and decreases bleeding: a randomized controlled trial. Colorectal Dis 2006;8:11–4. **Marsupialisation does have some advantages.**

38. Parkash S, Lakshmiratan V, Gajendran V. Fistula-in-ano: treatment by fistulectomy, primary closure and reconstitution. Aust N Z J Surg 1985;55:23–7.

39. Perez F, Arroyo A, Serrano P, et al. Prospective clinical and manometric study of fistulotomy with primary sphincter reconstruction in the management of recurrent complex fistula-in-ano. Int J Colorectal Dis 2006;21:522–6.

40. Perez F, Arroyo A, Serrano P, et al. Randomized clinical and manometric study of advancement flap versus fistulotomy with sphincter reconstruction in the management of complex fistula-in-ano. Am J Surg 2006;192:34–40.

41. Kronborg O. To lay open or excise a fistula-in-ano. A randomised trial. Br J Surg 1985;72:970.

42. Lewis A. Excision of fistula in ano. Int J Colorectal Dis 1986;1:265–7.

43. Lewis A. Core out. In: Phillips RKS, Lunniss PJ, editors. Anal fistula. Surgical evaluation and management. London: Chapman & Hall; 1996. p. 81–6.

44. Ramanujan PS, Prasad ML, Abcarian H. The role of seton in fistulotomy of the anus. Surg Gynecol Obstet 1983;157:419–22.

45. Kuypers HC. Use of the seton in the treatment of extrasphincteric anal fistula. Dis Colon Rectum 1984;27:109–10.

46. Parks AG, Stitz RW. The treatment of high fistula-in-ano. Dis Colon Rectum 1976;19:487–99.

47. Lunniss PJ, Thomson JPS. The loose seton. In: Phillips RKS, Lunniss PJ, editors. Anal fistula. Surgical evaluation and management. London: Chapman & Hall; 1996. p. 87–94.

48. Thomson JPS, Ross AHMcL. Can the external sphincter be preserved in the treatment of transsphincteric fistula-in-ano? Int J Colorectal Dis 1989;4:247–50.

49. Kennedy HL, Zegarra JP. Fistulotomy without external sphincter division for high anal fistula. Br J Surg 1990;77:898–901.

50. Buchanan GN, Owen HA, Torkington J, et al. Long-term outcome following loose-seton technique for external sphincter preservation in complex anal fistula. Br J Surg 2004;91:476–80.

51. Goldberg SM, Garcia-Aquilar J. The cutting seton. In: Phillips RKS, Lunniss PJ, editors. Anal fistula. Surgical evaluation and management. London: Chapman & Hall; 1996. p. 95–102.

52. Christensen A, Nilas L, Christiansen J. Treatment of transsphincteric anal fistulas by the seton technique. Dis Colon Rectum 1986;29:454–5.

53. Hammond TH, Knowles CH, Porrett T, et al. The snug seton: short and medium term results of slow fistulotomy for idiopathic anal fistulae. Colorectal Dis 2006;8:328–37.

54. Shukla NK, Narang R, Nair NG, et al. Multicentric randomized controlled clinical trial of Kshaarasootra (Ayurvedic medicated thread) in the management of fistula-in-ano. Ind J Med Res 1991;94:177–85.

55. Ho KS, Tsang C, Seoew-Choen F, et al. Prospective randomized trial comparing ayurvedic cutting seton and fistulotomy for low fistula-in-ano. Tech Coloproctol 2001;5:137–41.

56. Elting AW. The treatment of fistula in ano. Ann Surg 1912;56:744–52.

57. Finan PJ. Management by advancement flap technique. In: Phillips RKS, Lunniss PJ, editors. Anal fistula. Surgical evaluation and management. London: Chapman & Hall; 1996. p. 107–14.

58. Kodner IJ, Mazor A, Shemesh EL, et al. Endorectal advancement flap repair of rectovaginal and other complicated anorectal fistulas. Surgery 1993;114:682–90.

59. Lunniss PJ. The role of the advancement flap technique. Semin Colon Rectal Surg 1998;9:192–7.

60. Athanasiadis S, Kohler A, Nafe M. Treatment of high anal fistulae by primary occlusion of the internal ostium, drainage of the intersphincteric space,

and mucosal advancement flap. Int J Colorectal Dis 1994;9:153–7.

61. Uribe N, Millan M, Minguez M, et al. Clinical and manometric results of endorectal advancement flaps for complex anal fistula. Int J Colorectal Dis 2007;22:259–64.

62. van der Hagen SJ, Baeten CG, Soeters PB, et al. Long-term outcome following mucosal advancement flap for high perianal fistulas and fistulotomy for low perianal fistulas. Int J Colorectal Dis 2006;21:784–90.

63. Matos D, Lunniss PJ, Phillips RKS. Total sphincter conservation in high fistula in ano. Br J Surg 1993;80:802–4.

64. Rojanasakul A. LIFT procedure: a simplified technique for fistula-in-ano. Tech Coloproctol 2009;13:237–40.

65. Shanwani A, Nor AM, Amri N. Ligation of the intersphincteric fistula tract (LIFT): a sphincter-saving technique for fistula-in-ano. Dis Colon Rectum 2010;53:39–42.

66. Bleier JIS, Moloo H, Goldberg SM. Ligation of the intersphincteric fistula tract: an effective new technique for complex fistulas. Dis Colon Rectum 2010;53:43–6.

67. Ellis CN. Outcomes with use of bioprosthetic grafts to reinforce the ligation of the intersphincteric fistula tract (BIOLIFT procedure) for the management of complex anal fistulas. Dis Colon Rectum 2010;53:1361–4.

68. Christofiridis D. Who benefits from the anal fistula plug? Dis Colon Rectum 2010;53:1105–6.

69. Hammond TM, Porrett TR, Scott SM, et al. Management of idiopathic anal fistula using cross-linked collagen: a prospective phase I study. Colorectal Dis 2010;13:94–104.

70. Hammond TH, Grahn MF, Lunniss PJ. Fibrin glue in the management of anal fistulae. Colorectal Dis 2004;6:308–19.

71. Swinscoe MT, Ventakasubramaniam AK, Jayne DG. Fibrin glue for fistula-in-ano: the evidence reviewed. Tech Coloproctol 2005;9:89–94.

72. Cirocchi R, Farinella E, La Mura F, et al. Fibrin glue in the treatment of anal fistula: a systematic review. Ann Surg Innov Res 2009;3:12–9.

73. Ellis CN, Clark S. Fibrin glue as an adjunct to flap repair of anal fistulas: a randomized controlled study. Dis Colon Rectum 2006;49:1736–40.

74. Buchanan GN, Bartram CI, Phillips RKS, et al. Efficacy of fibrin sealant in the management of complex anal fistula. Dis Colon Rectum 2003;46:1167–74.

75. Lindsey I, Smilgin-Humphreys MM, Cunningham C, et al. A randomized, controlled trial of fibrin glue vs. conventional treatment for anal fistula. Dis Colon Rectum 2002;45:1608–15.

76. Altomare DF, Greco VJ, Tricomi N, et al. Seton or glue for trans-sphincteric anal fistulae: a prospective randomized crossover clinical trial. Colorectal Dis 2010;13:82–6.

77. Johnson EK, Gaw JU, Armstrong DN. Efficacy of anal fistula plug vs. fibrin glue in closure of anorectal fistulas. Dis Colon Rectum 2006;49:371–6.

78. Champagne BJ, O'Connor LM, Ferguson M, et al. Efficacy of anal fistula plug in closure of cryptoglandular fistulas: long-term follow-up. Dis Colon Rectum 2006;49:1817–21.

79. Ortiz H, Marzo J, Ciga MA, et al. Randomized clinical trial of anal fistula plug versus endorectal advancement flap for the treatment of high cryptoglandular fistula in ano. Br J Surg 2009;96:608–12.

80. van Koperen PJ, Bemelman WA, Gerhards MF, et al. The anal fistula plug treatment compared with the mucosal advancement flap for cryptoglandular high transsphincteric perianal fistula: a double-blinded multicenter randomized trial. Dis Colon Rectum 2011;54:387–93.

81. Engel AF, Lunniss PJ, Kamm MA, et al. Sphincteroplasty for incontinence after surgery for idiopathic fistula-in-ano. Int J Colorectal Dis 1997;12:323–5.

82. Phillips RKS, Lunniss PJ. Approach to the difficult fistula. In: Phillips RKS, Lunniss PJ, editors. Anal fistula. Surgical evaluation and management. London: Chapman & Hall; 1996. p. 177–82.

Minor anorectal conditions

Jit-Fong Lim
Francis Seow-Choen

Haemorrhoids

There is often considerable confusion in the nomenclature of haemorrhoids and haemorrhoidal disease. Internal haemorrhoids or the internal haemorrhoidal plexuses are normal arteriovenous plexuses or so-called anal cushions within the anal canal. Anal cushions are found in the upper anal canal above the dentate line, consisting of mucosa, submucosal fibroelastic connective tissues and smooth muscles in an arteriovenous channel system. Anal cushions complement anal sphincter function by providing fine control over the continence of liquid and gas. The external haemorrhoidal plexus is a venous plexus encircling the anal verge. When the anal cushions give rise to symptoms we call these symptomatic internal haemorrhoids and when these prolapse they result in external haemorrhoids. An external thrombosed varix occurs when a blood clot develops in the external haemorrhoidal plexus.

Pathogenesis and aetiology

The anal cushions function normally when they are fixed to their proper sites within the anal canal by fibromuscular ligaments, which are the anal remnants of the longitudinal layer of the muscularis propria from the rectum (Treitz's ligaments). When these submucosal fibres fragment, the anal cushions are no longer restrained from engorging excessively with blood and may result in bleeding and prolapse.

These fibres may be fragmented by prolonged and repeated downward stress related to straining during defecation. Veins that traverse the anal sphincter are blocked whereas arterial inflow continues, leading to increasing haemorrhoidal congestion. Defecation in the squatting position may also aggravate the tendency to prolapse as it increases perineal descent and pressure. Diarrhoea is also a risk factor for acute haemorrhoidal prolapse. Other factors that have been implicated are heredity, absence of valves within the haemorrhoidal plexus, as well as impedance of venous return from raised intra-abdominal pressure due to any cause, e.g. pregnancy. Portal hypertension may lead to engorgement of the haemorrhoidal plexus but this leads to anorectal varices not haemorrhoids.

Symptoms commonly seen among haemorrhoids sufferers are fresh bleeding associated with defecation, prolapse of haemorrhoidal tissue and pain from thrombosis of internal haemorrhoids as well as pruritis.

Thrombosed external varix, on the other hand, may have a slightly different aetiology and presentation. Bleeding is not usually the predominant complaint but severe pain can arise as a result of acute thrombosis with swelling and pain. Acute thrombosis results from sudden raised pressure causing rupture of the vascular plexus leading to a blood clot at the anal verge. Any activity requiring excessive abdominal straining such as over-exercising can cause this. However, many patients present with a thrombosed varix on waking up in the morning. If left untreated, the thrombosed external varix will shrivel and resorb but may leave a small skin tag.

Haemorrhoids may be divided into subcategories in order of severity, from first- to fourth-degree haemorrhoids. The definitions of each, as well as their management, are outlined in Box 15.1.

> ✓ Whilst haemorrhoids are often treated according to their stage, it is not often emphasised that at every stage haemorrhoids may be large or small. This size difference may alter dramatically the indication for the different procedures proposed for treatment at every stage, e.g. small fourth-degree haemorrhoids presenting with bleeding may be ligated but large first-degree haemorrhoids may need more drastic measures for effective cure.

Management

Firstly, it must be recognised that haemorrhoids may coexist with other conditions such as rectal cancer or inflammatory bowel disease. Patients who have symptoms including blood or mucus mixed in the stools, change in bowel habit, abdominal symptoms or family history of colorectal cancer should have further evaluation of the colon and rectum.

Box 15.1 • Management of internal haemorrhoids

First-degree haemorrhoids (bleeding but no prolapse)
- Stool softeners
- Local soothing creams or micronised flavonoids

Second-degree haemorrhoids (prolapse but spontaneously reducible)
- Rubber-band ligation
- Sclerotherapy
- Transanal haemorrhoidal dearterialisation
- (Haemorrhoidectomy)

Third-degree haemorrhoids (prolapse requiring manual reduction)
- Rubber-band ligation
- Sclerotherapy
- Transanal haemorrhoidal dearterialisation
- Either excisional or stapled haemorrhoidectomy

Fourth-degree haemorrhoids (irreducible prolapse)
- Either excisional or stapled haemorrhoidectomy (modified)

Secondly, the anal cushions are normal functional anatomical structures contributing to anal continence. Treatment should therefore be reserved for 'haemorrhoidal diseases' that result in symptoms that distress or disrupt patients from their normal lifestyle. Therapeutic strategies thus normally depend on the severity of symptoms and the amount of haemorrhoidal tissue prolapsing beyond the anal verge.

Non-prolapsing or mildly prolapsing haemorrhoids

If the piles are not permanently prolapsed, non-operative methods should be attempted first. The primary problems of constipation and straining at stool need to be addressed first. In some patients, improving bowel action with laxatives may help to control the symptoms.

Other forms of treatment that can give more immediate symptomatic relief include rubber-band ligation, injection sclerotherapy, medications such as micronised diosmin (currently not available in the UK), as well as toilet re-education. Topical applications are popular with many patients, who testify to relief from bleeding and pain. There are, however, no clinical trials to demonstrate any benefit from such applications.

Rubber-band ligation

In this technique, rubber bands are applied at the apex of (i.e. just above) the haemorrhoidal tissues. The strangulated tissue then becomes necrotic and sloughs off in a few days, after which the wound fibroses, resulting in fixation of the mucosa akin to forming new suspensory ligaments for the anal cushions. The haemorrhoidal tissue is thus prevented from engorging and prolapsing. Up to three haemorrhoids can be banded on the same occasion but we prefer to do one at a time as there is less immediate discomfort. This process is relatively painless if the bands are placed above the dentate line, but some patients may experience tenesmus for a day or two that is only partially relieved by analgesia. Banding is usually 60–80% effective, depending on proper selection of cases. There is a 2–5% risk of secondary haemorrhage.

> ✓✓ Rubber-band ligation is the treatment of choice for grade 2 haemorrhoids when compared with excisional haemorrhoidectomy. It achieved similar results but without the effects of surgery. Surgery should be reserved for grade 3 haemorrhoids or recurrent haemorrhoids after rubber-band ligation.[1]

Injection sclerotherapy

Sclerosant agents used include phenol (5%) in almond oil or sodium tetradecyl sulphate. These are injected into the submucosa around the pedicle of the pile, at the level of the anorectal ring. The sclerosant causes local inflammation, leading to reduced blood flow into the haemorrhoids. The sclerosant also causes fibrosis, which draws minor prolapse back into the anal canal. This technique is about 70% effective.

The correct plane is shown by elevation of the mucosa without blanching during injection. Inadvertently deep injections can cause perirectal fibrosis, infection and urethral irritation. Prostatic injection is intensely painful and the patient may develop an erection, a strong desire to void, haematuria or haemospermia. Severe sepsis is not uncommon and such patients should be admitted for antibiotics and observation until completely well.

Other methods

There are several available phlebotonics but Daflon 500® (Les Laboratoires Servier, France) is by far the best evaluated in the medical literature, and is widely used in Europe and the Far East as first-line treatment for piles.[2] Daflon 500, not currently available in the UK, is micronised diosmin and hesperidin, which belong to the hydroxyethylrutoside group of drugs.[3] Its pharmacological properties include noradrenaline-mediated venous contraction, reduction in blood extravasation from capillaries and inhibition of prostaglandin (PGE_2, PGF_2)-mediated inflammatory response.[4]

> ✔ Phlebotonics, although currently not available in the UK, have a proven therapeutic action in the symptomatic relief of haemorrhoidal symptoms with minimal adverse effects.[5,6]

Various other methods are also available. These include infrared photocoagulation, which requires additional equipment, and cryotherapy, which results in unpleasant and foul-smelling discharge. For such reasons, these methods have not been popular. Topical preparations that may contain local anaesthetics or steroids are also available, often without prescription. To date, there is no scientific evidence that such agents are any more effective than spontaneous remissions.

Irreducible prolapsed piles

The majority of patients are well treated by non-surgical methods. However, when anal cushions are prolapsed or thrombosed (**Fig. 15.1**), they no longer function effectively to maintain continence and surgery may be needed. In fact, sensory function may be impaired and this may partially account for the complaints of minor incontinence by some patients.

Traditionally, prolapsed piles are removed by excisional haemorrhoidectomy. Although there are variations to the technique,[7–10] the essential problems encountered remain similar. These are mainly postoperative pain,[8,11] anal incontinence[12] and haemorrhage. Some authors have described post-haemorrhoidectomy pain as being akin to passing pieces of sharp glass fragments, such that many patients would rather suffer the discomfort of large prolapsing haemorrhoids for years than submit to surgery.

Nonetheless, third- and fourth-degree haemorrhoids are more appropriately treated by surgery, which is conventionally performed by excision of the three primary piles. Minor variations in conventional excisional haemorrhoidectomy include whether the wounds are left to granulate or closed with sutures, whether the pedicle is ligated, or whether the piles are excised with scissors, laser or diathermy. More recently, closed excisional haemorrhoidectomy with energy devices has been used by surgeons with good results.

Severe circumferential prolapse with massive engorgement of both external and internal

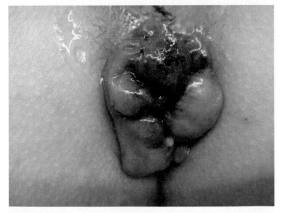

Figure 15.1 • Acute thrombosed haemorrhoids showing the classical bluish black coloration of the thrombus.

haemorrhoidal plexuses can be dealt with by either standard haemorrhoidectomy plus excision of the largest secondary pile with subsequent mucocutaneous reconstitution or a modification of the Whitehead or radical haemorrhoidectomy. In a study comparing Whitehead with four-pile haemorrhoidectomy, we concluded that four-pile haemorrhoidectomy was significantly easier to perform and, although residual tags and piles were left behind, the operation was preferred to radical haemorrhoidectomy.[13]

Currently, however, this discussion may be immaterial as stapled haemorrhoidectomy adequately addresses most circumferential prolapses.[14]

Stapled haemorrhoidectomy (haemorrhoidopexy)

Conventional surgical haemorrhoidectomy is not based on a correction of pathophysiology but on ablation of symptoms. Hence, if prolapsed piles are bleeding, painful or otherwise symptomatic, these piles are excised.

However, prolapsed haemorrhoids are not always symptomatic in the first instance. Once prolapse occurs, further engorgement of these vascular cushions leads to pain and an inflammatory response. Anal spasm then prevents reduction, and pathological changes such as thrombosis, oedema and inflammation occur.

Chronicity is caused by a vicious cycle of prolapse and congestion of these vascular cushions. The vascular cushions hence prolapse easily and engorge when the anal sphincters contract, resulting in further congestion, oedema and pain.

Conventional haemorrhoidectomy therefore deals with the symptoms alone without due regard to restoration of the normal physiology by re-fixation of the anal cushions. On the other hand, stapled haemorrhoidopexy tries to correct the primary pathology, theoretically resulting in resolution of haemorrhoidal symptoms.[15] After reduction of any prolapsed haemorrhoidal tissue, this technique then excises redundant lower rectal mucosa, fixing the prolapse back into its proper place on the wall of the anal canal. Once reduced, the engorged haemorrhoidal tissue will decongest and shrink. Our technique of stapled haemorrhoidectomy takes into account these pathophysiological changes and attempts to correct them all.[16] Although there

are concerns of long-term pain following stapled haemorrhoidectomy, this had not been seen in larger series.[17]

> ✓✓ In a recent meta-analysis of 12 randomised clinical trials comparing stapled versus conventional surgery for haemorrhoids, stapled haemorrhoidectomy is associated with a higher long-term risk of recurrence and the symptoms of prolapse. It is also likely to be associated with a higher likelihood of long-term symptom recurrence and the need for additional operations compared to conventional excisional haemorrhoidal surgery.[18]

However, stapled haemorrhoidectomy on its own may not deal adequately with the really massive haemorrhoidal prolapse. Massive haemorrhoids are prolapsed haemorrhoids more than 3–4 cm outside the anal verge. In this situation, there is not enough space within the staple housing to contain the massive redundant tissue of the prolapsed haemorrhoids. New stapler designs, however, may deal with these tissues more thoroughly and will deserve investigation when available.

An effective modified stapled haemorrhoidectomy technique where excess mucosa was first excised before the stapler was applied has been described to deal with such massive haemorrhoidal prolapse.[19] Another more expensive alternative might be to use two staplers at the same sitting.

Stapled haemorrhoidectomy has also been used for acutely thrombosed circumferentially prolapsed piles,[20] and was found not only to be feasible but also perhaps to result in less pain, a more rapid resolution of symptoms and an earlier return to work when compared with conventional Milligan–Morgan haemorrhoidectomy.

Stapled haemorrhoidectomy is a very surgeon-dependent operation with regard to immediate resolution of skin tags, as well as whether residual tags should be excised or left behind. We also believe that placement of the staple line and proper selection of patients are important factors in influencing long-term results with regard to pain and recurrence.

Transanal haemorrhoidal dearterialisation

In 1995, Morinaga et al.[21] introduced haemorrhoidal artery ligation (HAL) or transanal haemorrhoidal dearterialisation (THD). The definition of THD was preferred by Sohn et al.[22] in 2001. This technique consists of ligation of the terminal haemorrhoidal branches of the superior rectal artery using a specially designed proctoscope with a Doppler probe, resulting in reduction of blood flow to the haemorrhoidal plexus. Dal Monte et al.[23] reported more than 90% resolution of symptoms with minimal complications. This technique is nowadays usually combined with mucopexy, which increases efficacy.

Postoperative problems

Problems that occur after haemorrhoidectomy include severe pain, urinary retention, bleeding and faecal impaction. Compared to excisional surgery pain is significantly diminished after stapled haemorrhoidectomy and hence many more such procedures are treated in a day-surgery setting,[24,25] even though conventional haemorrhoidectomy may also be performed in a day-care setting with adequate patient satisfaction.

However, whichever technique is used, pain may still be significant in some patients in the postoperative period. Pain is multifactorial, spasm of the internal sphincter as well as the actual skin wound with its exposed nerves being the most significant factors.

✅ Use of botulinum toxin has been shown to reduce pain until the end of the first postoperative week.[26] The use of 0.2% glyceryl trinitrate (GTN) ointment is also associated with decreased postoperative pain, and contributes to more rapid healing of wounds after excisional haemorrhoidectomy.[27] Others have tried lateral sphincterotomy with haemorrhoidectomy with some success,[28] but we would not advocate this because of potential serious adverse effects.

The amount of pain after stapled haemorrhoidectomy is said to depend on the height of the anastomosis above the anal verge. Removal of squamous epithelium results in a greater intensity of postoperative pain and should be avoided. However, some patients with a staple line well above the dentate line have considerable pain as well. This situation may be caused by congestion of the haemorrhoidal plexuses, haemorrhoidal thrombosis or sepsis below the staple line. Another less frequent problem is postoperative haemorrhage. Bleeding in the immediate postoperative period is usually due to inadequate intraoperative haemostasis. Secondary bleeding is more often as a result of postoperative infection following surgery. Following stapled haemorrhoidectomy, bleeding may follow the rare staple-line dehiscence. Submucosal adrenaline (epinephrine) injection[29] has been shown to be effective for addressing bleeding after excisional haemorrhoidectomy.

Post-haemorrhoidectomy anal stricture is an uncommon occurrence seen in only 3.7% of haemorrhoidectomies.[30] The stricture usually presents 6 weeks postoperatively.

✅ Some surgeons believe that the use of the anal dilator/stapler in the course of stapled haemorrhoidectomy may be associated with a higher rate of anal sphincter damage. This has been shown to be the case in one randomised trial.[31] However, there were no differences in continence scores or anal pressures, the main difference being the persistence of internal anal sphincter fragmentation beyond 14 weeks postoperatively.[31]

For patients who have undergone stapled haemorrhoidectomy, we advise a review 3–4 weeks after surgery to detect early staple-line fibrosis, which is then still soft and can be easily dilated with digital rectal examination to prevent persistent stenosis.

Sepsis after treatment of haemorrhoids

Sepsis after either conservative or operative treatment is uncommon, but when it occurs, delay in treatment can be catastrophic. In one study, the incidence of transient bacteraemia from blood cultures after haemorrhoidectomy was 5–11%,[32] but this did not result in any cases of clinical sepsis.

Injection sclerotherapy has been reported very rarely to result in life-threatening retroperitoneal sepsis and rectal perforation.[33] Urological sepsis can result from a misplaced deep anterior injection with complications such as prostatic abscess, epididymitis, chronic cystitis, seminal vesicle abscess and urinary–perineal fistula. Pain and haemorrhage can occur in 14% of patients after rubber-band ligation.

> ✔ In a randomised trial by Carapeti et al.,[34] metronidazole was shown to reduce pain on days 5–7 after open, largely day-case, haemorrhoidectomy, resulting in a shorter time to normal activity and greater patient satisfaction. It was proposed that a reduction in bacterial colonisation was an important factor.

Secondary haemorrhage, often attributed to local infection, affects approximately 5% of patients undergoing haemorrhoidectomy. The advocated treatment is antibiotics; the incidence does not seem to be increased after emergency haemorrhoidectomy.

Following stapled haemorrhoidectomy, a very small number of patients develop a small perineal abscess, resulting in severe pain in the first or second week after surgery. This is especially seen after stapling large piles and may follow early oedema and thrombosis. Such oedema and thrombosis may obscure small abscesses, preventing correct diagnosis and treatment.

Conclusion

Anal cushions, which are normal structures, may result in symptomatic haemorrhoids following straining and other factors (**Fig. 15.2**).

Early and small prolapsing piles can be treated without surgery. Large prolapsed piles may be treated either by excisional haemorrhoidectomy or by stapled haemorrhoidectomy.

Anal fissure

An anal fissure is a linear ulcer in the squamous epithelium of the anal canal distal to the dentate line. It occurs equally in both sexes and can occur at any age (although the aetiology at different ages is not the same).

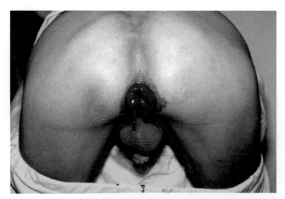

Figure 15.2 • Prolapsed bleeding haemorrhoids with bright red blood.

Clinical findings

Pain is usually the predominant symptom in anal fissures, but occasionally bleeding or the presence of a perianal skin tag may be more distressing to the patient. The pain classically presents during defecation and is described as excruciating, like 'a knife cutting'. This pain may last for several minutes or the entire day.

There may be associated fresh rectal bleeding, usually of a small amount. In rare cases, the predominant symptom is that of pruritus ani. Anal fissures can be visualised by gentle parting of the buttocks with eversion of the anal verge. Superficial anal fissures will show as a linear tear while deeper fissures may show the white transverse fibres of the internal anal sphincter. Deep fissures may also have fibrotic edges and are commonly associated with an external skin tag, often called a 'sentinel pile' (**Fig. 15.3**), and occasionally with a hypertrophic anal papilla (**Fig. 15.4**).

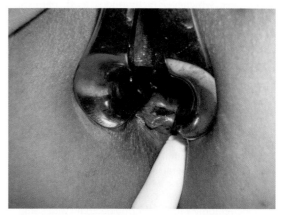

Figure 15.3 • Deep anal fissure with a sentinel skin tag at the posterior midline of the anal canal.

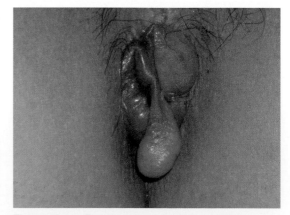

Figure 15.4 • Prolapsed hypertrophic anal papilla associated with a chronic anal fissure.

Intra-anal examinations should not be attempted in the clinic due to the severe pain thereby induced. Digital rectal and proctoscopic examinations should only be performed in the acute setting when there is a strong suspicion of a secondary pathology, in which case local, regional or general anaesthesia will be needed, or when surgery is being undertaken.

Although usually single and situated in the 6 o'clock position, some 2.5–10% may be sited in the 12 o'clock position.[35] When fissures are multiple or eccentrically located, inflammatory bowel disease, tuberculosis, syphilis or human immunodeficiency virus (HIV) infection must be considered. In older, particularly female patients, a ragged anus associated with a fissure may be a sign of anal digitation due to obstructed defecation. In patients with heart disease who are taking the drug Nicorandil, anal ulceration may be induced. Anal cancer can mimic a fissure. In some patients an intersphincteric abscess may drain into the base of a fissure.

Aetiology and classification

The aetiology of anal fissure is better understood under 'initiating' and 'perpetuating' factors and anal fissures better classified as 'superficial' or 'deep' anal fissures.

Initiating factors

Shafik[36] proposed a 'levator complex' theory of defecation in 1980, postulating that the levator ani contracted and shortened during defecation. However, the opposite has been shown on dynamic computer tomographic defecography. Li and Guo[37] demonstrated that the levator ani descended up to 20mm, changing from a funnel shape at rest to a deeper basin shape in normal individuals during defecation, the resultant force pushing the muscle downwards, which then widens the genital hiatus and opens the anus for the passage of stool (**Fig. 15.5**).

We believe this downward lengthening of the levator ani allows the excessive stretching of the overlying anoderm, making it more vulnerable to tearing by a hard faecal bolus or explosive diarrhoea. In particular, this overstretching tends to occur in the posterior midline due to shearing of loose anoderm over the relatively fixed anococcygeal ligament.[38,39] As less than 30% of patients admit to constipation prior to the anal fissure, excessive straining at defecation, even without hard faeces, can replicate the pathology (**Fig. 15.6**).

This posterior perineal descent coupled with excessive straining at defecation or extreme bowel pattern (hard constipated stools or explosive diarrhoea) is in our view the initiating factor in idiopathic anal fissure.

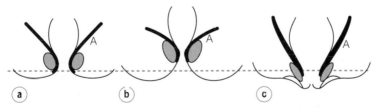

Figure 15.5 • Perineal descent. A = levator ani; B = anal sphincters. **(a)** shows the anal canal at rest with the levator ani being funnel shaped. **(b)** shows the levator ani being plate like in shape during squeezing of the anal canal. **(c)** shows the descent of the levator ani during defecation and becoming deeply basin shaped.

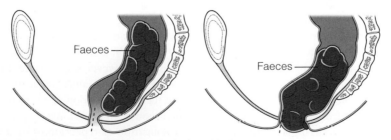

Figure 15.6 • Perineal descent during defecation without posterior perineal support causing an overstretching of the posterior anal margin.

More women are constipated compared with men, and childbirth with vaginal delivery is especially traumatic, resulting in more deep anal fissures.[40,41]

Perpetuating factors

After an initial tear, a vicious cycle of non-healing and repeated trauma can lead to development of deep fissures. Non-healing is a consequence of intrinsic anal sphincter hypertonia and relative tissue ischaemia associated with other unknown factors.

Nitric oxide (NO) relaxes smooth muscle. Reduced levels of nitric oxide synthase (NOS), the primary enzyme involved in NO synthesis, were demonstrated in the internal anal sphincter (IAS) of patients with anal fissures compared to controls, coupled with mean resting anal pressures noted to be often higher than 90 mmHg in patients with fissures.[42,43] The IAS alone appears to be responsible for the hypertonia.[44] This reduced production of NO provides a possible explanation for the high anal pressures seen in most affected patients and possibly explains why pressures return to pretreatment values in patients whose fissures have healed by non-surgical methods.

Post-mortem angiography of the inferior rectal artery revealed that 85% of anuses had a paucity of branches of the inferior rectal artery at the posterior commissure.[45] Morphometric studies of the capillaries further revealed them to be less dense in both the subanodermal space and within the IAS in the posterior midline in the majority of subjects. Hence, the relatively precarious blood flow of the posterior midline may explain the predilection of anal fissures at this position and the lack of granulation tissue seen at the base of a deep anal fissure.

Patients with deep fissures have significantly higher resting anal tone and decreased anodermal blood flow on Doppler flowmetry compared to healthy volunteers.[46] Following successful treatment by lateral sphincterotomy, a decreased anal tone and increased blood flow to the posterior midline of the anal canal has been observed.[46]

Posterior perineal descent is both an important initiating factor and a perpetuating factor, as the repeated perineal descent from each defecation continues to traumatise the anoderm, leading to deepening of the fissure and non-healing.

From 'acute vs. chronic' to 'superficial vs. deep' anal fissure

Anal fissures were historically classified as acute or chronic based on the duration of symptoms. Fissures of short duration were called 'acute' while those with symptoms of 6 weeks or more were 'chronic'. But if the duration turns out to be less than 6 weeks and yet examination shows features of chronicity, such as fibrosis, fibrotic edges, a perianal skin tag or a hypertrophic anal papilla, then surely such cases should also be classified as 'chronic'. The arbitrary timeline to us is misleading and creates confusion in patient treatment, and may account for the widely differing healing rates of various treatments in the literature.

In our view a complete name change based on morphology of the fissure is needed, as this aligns better with the treatment options available. Superficial fissures, as the name implies, involve only the superficial mucocutaneous layers of the anal canal. Symptoms of severe pain and bleeding may be present and the fissure shows up as a superficial separation of the anoderm with sharp edges. The base of the fissure does not reach the internal anal sphincter. The vast majority of superficial fissures will heal spontaneously within days or within a few weeks of appropriate conservative treatment. By contrast, deep fissures often persist and either tend not to heal without intervention or recur regularly.

Deep anal fissures are recognised by the deep, wide pear-shaped ulcer, often with visible fibres of the internal anal sphincter and minimal granulation tissue at the base. Other features of a deep anal fissure include the distinctive triad of indurated ulcer edges, a distal skin tag (sentinel pile) and a proximal hypertrophic anal papilla. The latter, however, is not universal.

Lindsey et al.[47] have proposed a definition based on the combination of chronology and morphology by describing a chronic anal fissure as 'the presence of visible transverse internal anal sphincter fibres at the base of an anal fissure of duration not less than 6 weeks'. However, such features can present within a week or less of painful defecation and/or bleeding and therefore duration seems to us irrelevant. Deep anal fissures, however, may result chronically from prolongation or repetition of the forces causing superficial anal fissures, or else they may arise de novo

Medical treatment

When managing anal fissures, the logical strategy is to treat both the initiating factors as well as the perpetuating factors concurrently. Any abnormal pattern of defecation (hard constipated stools or explosive diarrhoea) needs to be addressed by medication and appropriate dietary advice. Patients with relatively normal bowel function but excessive straining at defecation should have assessment for dyssynergic defecation and anorectal biofeedback to correct it.

In a study on dyssynergic defecation, some patients pressed on the posterior perineum as a form of 'manual perineal support' to overcome their difficulty defecating.[48] This technique is difficult to perform while sitting on the toilet seat and led to the development of a novel posterior perineal support device incorporated into a toilet seat.[49] The device is a form of 'manual perineal support' to counteract the downward perineal descent and overstretching of the anoderm (**Fig. 15.7**). In a study of 32 patients with deep anal fissures, there was a 97.5% improvement in pain relief, 84.4% improvement in constipation symptoms and 65.6% improvement in bleeding after using the device for 3 months.[49] This device is commercially available in the form of a modified toilet seat (Colorec Mecha-Medic Solution, Kuala Lumpur, Malaysia).

Other forms of medical treatment are aimed at treating intrinsic anal sphincter hypertonia or local tissue ischaemia, or both. Even in deep anal fissures, medical treatment should be attempted, although less likely to heal the fissure. In a recent review of the management of anal fissure, such medical modalities have been so popular and promising that surgery has been reserved for those who failed medical therapy.[50]

The recognition of NO as a neurotransmitter mediating the relaxation of the internal sphincter has led to many studies examining the use of isosorbide dinitrate and GTN to treat anal fissures.

> ✔✔ Different authors have tried oral, patch, sprayed and topical GTN, and 0.2% GTN topical ointment has become the standard as it achieves optimal healing in up to 70% of cases with minimal adverse effects (predominantly headaches).[51,52]

The enthusiasm for topical creams is mainly because of concerns about faecal incontinence, albeit usually mild, after sphincterotomy.

> ✔✔ Both 2% diltiazem and 0.2% GTN are equally effective in the treatment of chronic anal fissure, but GTN is associated with a higher rate of side-effects (headache or anal irritation). The recurrence rate of chronic anal fissure after the use of either GTN or a calcium channel blocker is equal.[53]

However, patients who are already on these drugs for hypertension and ischaemic heart disease may be unsuitable for this form of treatment, as the systemic use of these drugs suggests that the anal fissure is unlikely to respond to topical application of these drugs.

The parasympathomimetic bethanechol has been shown to lower resting anal pressure and may be useful in conjunction with other topical medications. Indoramin, an α-adrenoceptor blocker, and salbutamol, a β-adrenoceptor agonist, are further possible alternatives.

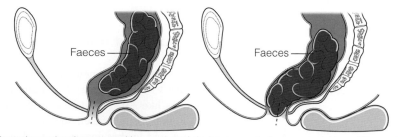

Figure 15.7 • Posterior perineal support with an external device prevents the overstretching of the anal verge preventing haemorrhoidal prolapse and tearing of the anus.[49]

Botulinum A toxin (Botox) reduces resting anal pressure and promotes healing of anal fissures in 70–96% of patients.[54]

> ✓✓ In a randomised clinical trial, injection of botulinum toxin resulted in healing of 46 (92%) of 50 patients compared with 35 (70%) of 50 patients receiving topical GTN. Those treated with botulinum toxin had mild incontinence to flatus that was short-lived and resolved spontaneously, while the GTN treatment was associated with transient moderate to severe headache.[55]

The mode of action remains unclear. The toxin binds to presynaptic cholinergic nerve terminals and inhibits the release of acetylcholine at the neuromuscular junction. This should lead to relaxation of the external sphincter but should have no corresponding effect on the internal sphincter. However, Brisinda et al.[56] have shown that maximal squeeze pressures were no different from pretreatment levels at 1–2 months after injection. The site of optimal injection is still unclear and complications include transient faecal incontinence, perianal haematoma, pain and sepsis.

> ✓✓ In a meta-analysis of 54 randomised clinical trials, medical therapy (Botox, calcium channel blocker, GTN) for chronic anal fissure is significantly better than placebo. These medications are safe and side-effects of therapy are not serious and are reversible with cessation of therapy. Surgery is then reserved for treatment failures. However, medications are not as effective as surgery and late recurrence is also higher with medical therapy.[57]

For all the advantages of medical treatment, there is still no answer for sentinel piles and fibrous polyps that often accompany deep fissures. These remain distressing to the patient as there may be associated pain and bleeding from trauma to sentinel piles or persistent tenesmus or soilage due to the presence of the fibrous polyp. Surgical excision at the time of lateral sphincterotomy offers not only good healing for the fissure but removes the sentinel pile and fibrous polyp at the same time.

Surgical treatment

> ✓ We believe that uncontrolled anal stretch or dilatation should no longer be performed.[58]

An uncontrolled fracturing of the internal sphincter by this method, although shown to have good rates of healing, nevertheless results in an unacceptably high incidence of incontinence with unknown long-term consequences. Posterior midline sphincterotomy is not favoured either; its results are not superior to lateral sphincterotomy and a gutter (keyhole) defect may lead to soiling.

> ✓ Patients who have failed medical treatment or who have features of chronicity such as sentinel piles should be offered lateral sphincterotomy. This may be performed by either an open or closed method, each showing similar results.[58]

One concern is the length of optimal internal sphincter division.[59] Classically, sphincterotomy was done with division of the internal sphincter up to the level of the dentate line. In a tailored sphincterotomy, the internal sphincter is divided up to the highest point of the fissure only. In practice this is gauged by eyeballing the distance between the top of the fissure and the dentate line and performing sphincterotomy accordingly. Most authors have described healing rates of 85–95%.

Sphincterotomy, by virtue of its division of the internal sphincter musculature, predisposes to incontinence to flatus and faecal soilage in up to 35% of patients (although the risk is usually far less than this).[59] Surgical removal of the fissure (fissurectomy) with subsequent use of isosorbide dinitrate cream or Botox injection has been shown to be promising, with no recurrence and no internal sphincter defects on postoperative endosonography.[60,61] This relatively new technique is as yet unverified by a randomised controlled trial. Other novel methods of treatment include bilateral sphincterotomy, anterior levatorplasty, sphincterolysis and controlled intermittent anal dilatation, but their results need to be verified by more research. In the latest meta-analysis by Nelson et al.,[58] lateral sphincterotomy is still the gold standard of surgical treatments.

Recurrent or atypical fissures

If the fissure is not in the anterior or posterior midline, then Crohn's disease or immunosuppressive conditions like AIDS must be considered. These patients should not be offered surgery at the first consultation and further investigations should be performed first. Even so, in their series Fleschner et al.[62] showed that 88% of patients with Crohn's-associated fissures healed after lateral sphincterotomy compared with only 49% on medical treatment. Furthermore, no significant increase in complications was noted in the sphincterotomy group.

Authors who believe in the ischaemic nature of chronic fissures cite this as the reason behind recurrences. Internal sphincter hypertonia leads to reduced blood flow, which in turn results in tissue hypoxia and consequent failure of healing. Hyperbaric oxygen therapy ostensibly provides increased oxygenation to hypoperfused tissue and induces neovascularisation, collagen synthesis and fibroblast replication, thus enhancing the repair process. In a study by Cundall et al.,[63] five of eight patients had healed fissures at the end of 3 months, and all showed symptomatic improvement with regard to pain and bleeding.

In patients with recurrence after lateral sphincterotomy, anal manometry and anal ultrasound are essential as they separate patients with low resting anal pressures from patients with persistently raised resting pressures and will identify those who might benefit from repeat lateral sphincterotomies in the opposite lateral quadrant.

Patients with low resting sphincter pressures may be helped by anal cutaneous advancement flaps along with fissurectomy. It is reasonable to believe that these patients will not experience improved blood flow to the fissure after sphincterotomy as sphincter hypertonia was probably not a causative factor in the first place. As such, further sphincterotomy will only increase the risk of incontinence. Island advancement flap healed most low-pressure fissures.[35,64]

Conclusion

Anal fissures are common and aetiology is multifactorial. Appreciating the aetiology in terms of initiating and perpetuating factors is important in directing management and future research. We believe a change in mindset from classifying anal fissures based on chronology (acute or chronic anal fissure) to morphology (superficial or deep anal fissure) would allow better comparison of the different methods of treatment in clinical trials. Lateral sphincterotomy remains the gold standard for deep anal fissures, but we believe posterior perineal support offers a new understanding of the aetiology of anal fissures and should be further investigated.

Pruritus ani

Pruritus ani is vexing to both surgeons and patients.

Aetiology and pathogenesis

There are numerous direct causes of perianal itch (Box 15.2). Clinically, however, idiopathic pruritus ani is most usually associated with a minor degree of faecal incontinence. The object of history taking and examination is to find the likely cause of faecal leakage. This may be due to local pathology permitting stool to leak to the outside or to difficulty with thorough anal cleansing, or to anal sphincteric dysfunction or other contributory causes such as irritative foods and, importantly, a high-fibre diet. In addition, applications of inappropriate topical creams and even excessive cleansing may further aggravate the situation.

Box 15.2 • Secondary causes of pruritis ani

Neoplasia
- Rectal adenoma
- Rectal adenocarcinoma
- Anal squamous cell carcinoma
- Malignant melanoma
- Bowen's disease
- Extramammary Paget's disease

Benign anorectal conditions
- Haemorrhoids
- Fistula-in-ano
- Anal fissure
- Rectal prolapse
- Anal sphincter injury or dysfunction
- Faecal incontinence
- Radiation proctitis
- Ulcerative colitis

Infections
- Condyloma acuminatum
- Herpes simplex virus
- *Candida albicans*
- Syphilis
- *Lymphogranuloma venereum*

Dermatological
- Neurogenic dermatitis
- Contact dermatitis
- Lichen simplex
- Lichen planus
- Lichen atrophicus

Chapter 15

Diagnosis

The diagnosis of causes of minor anal leakage is most often revealed by good history taking and physical examination.

Physical examination should include any evidence of skin disease. The perineum and underclothes should be carefully inspected for any reason for soilage.

Digital rectal examination may reveal anal sphincteric dysfunction or other reasons for the pruritus. Wiping with a moist gauze may confirm staining and thus anal leakage. Repeat examination after straining may be required to reveal a rectal prolapse. Endoscopy may be required in certain cases. Skin lesions may need to be biopsied and examined for fungus or other dermatological problems (this is very rare).

Another cause of pruritus ani is *Enterobius* or threadworm. These may be revealed by placing a piece of adhesive tape to the anus and then transferring to a microscopy slide. The presence of ova is indicative of infection.

Treatment

Treatment is dependent on the primary pathology. Advice should be cautious before any surgical intervention, as cure is not certain.

In primary pruritus ani, the aims of treatment are the reduction of leakage, maintenance of good personal hygiene and the prevention of further injury to the perianal skin. Soilage may be decreased by reducing flatulence by lowering dietary fibre and adding probiotics. Loose stools may also be solidified with antimotility medications. Small amounts of loose stool trapped within the anus may leak out and cause irritation later in the day long after the perineum had been cleaned.

Cleansing of the perineum using water with drying by gentle dabbing is preferred to vigorous rubbing with toilet paper. An anti-itch powder and the use of antihistamine medication may be useful to break the vicious cycle of itching and scratching. Loose underwear made of non-allergenic material may decrease the chance of contact dermatitis.

The desire to scratch may be due to fresh leakage and immediate flushing with water may obviate the desire to scratch, which otherwise may be well-nigh irresistible. Short-term use of a hydrocortisone cream may help to break the cycle, but steroid use should not be prolonged.

In a study by Lysy et al.,[65] topical capsaicin has been shown to be effective for idiopathic pruritus ani; 44 patients were randomised to topical capsaicin 0.006% or placebo (menthol 1%) and crossover was carried out after 4 weeks. Of these patients, 31 experienced relief with capsaicin but none with menthol.

> ✔ During defecation, the anus descends and the anoderm is exposed. The anoderm does not retract immediately after defecation and can be irritated by dry abrasive tissue on wiping. The irritation leads to premature retraction of the anoderm inward and traps stool that can seep out later. Use of water or wet wipes minimises stool trapping and may be helpful for patients with pruritis ani.

In patients with refractory pruritis ani, anal tattooing with methylene blue destroys the nerve endings around the anus, leading to hypo-aesthesia of perianal skin and relief from the annoying itch. We have used it to good effect and it has been reported to achieve good symptom control in up to 96% of patients.[66] Inappropriate dosing and injections may result in skin necrosis.

Conclusion

Pruritus ani remains a difficult problem to manage. Treatment is aimed at stopping anal leakage, whether from faecal soilage or flatulence. Avoiding a high-fibre diet helps. Good personal hygiene remains an important aspect of treatment and prevention of further irritation to the perianal skin.

Pilonidal sinus

The word 'pilonidal' is derived from the Latin words *pilus* meaning hair and *nidus* meaning nest, due to trapped hair found within the sinus. It usually affects hirsute young adults and males twice as often as females.[67]

Aetiology

Pilonidal sinus is an acquired disease resulting from a foreign body reaction to extruded hair in the skin. Keratin plugs and other debris may contribute further to the inflammation. This theory arose from the observation of pilonidal sinus appearing in the

242

hands of a barber.[68] Bascom postulated that the disease arose from infection of hair follicles in the natal cleft, which may have been occluded by keratin.[69] The infected hair follicle theory is supported by epidemiological findings that the age of presentation starts after puberty, affecting young adults. Obesity is another risk factor. Hormonal changes at puberty and obesity are closely linked to an increased incidence of infected pilosebaceous glands. Whether the cause is exclusive to either theory or a combination of both is unclear.

However, most authors agree that propagation of the inflammation to a chronic sinus is related to a foreign body reaction from a non-healing abscess. Loose hairs from the region tend to gather toward the natal cleft due to the anatomy and suction of the buttocks on movement. These hairs migrate into the sinus tip first and get trapped, aggravating the inflammatory process[70] (**Fig. 15.8**).

Clinical manifestation

Pilonidal disease often presents as an acute abscess in the midline of the sacrococcygeal region. Many patients will still develop a pilonidal sinus even if the abscess is treated. The primary tract may become epithelialised and form a small pit in the midline of the natal cleft. Curiously, this primary tract sometimes regresses and becomes asymptomatic.

However, some patients progress and develop a secondary tract that may run lateral and cephalad to the primary tract. This tract tends to persist as a discharging sinus lined by granulation tissue.

Hence, patients often present either in the acute abscess stage or with an off-midline discharging

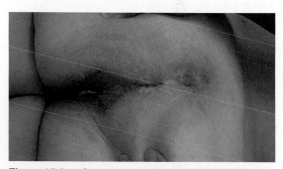

Figure 15.8 • Chronic pilonidal sinuses with inverted hair sticking out of the pits.

sinus. When they present with a chronic pilonidal sinus, it is common to note midline pits in the natal cleft that correspond to the healed primary tracts. In such cases, the pilonidal sinus would be situated slightly cephalad to the primary pit, 1–3 cm lateral to the midline, over the underlying sacrum.

If no primary pits are seen or if the sinus drains either lateral to the sacrum or appears caudal to the primary pits, other diagnoses should be considered. It is very unusual to find multiple sinuses that open into both buttocks simultaneously. In such a case, the differential diagnosis would include hydradenitis suppurativa, complex anal fistulas, osteomyelitis with draining sinuses to the skin, as well as infective conditions, such as tuberculosis or actinomycosis.

Treatment

Pilonidal abscess

Simple incision and drainage may be attempted if a small pilonidal abscess is initially diagnosed, with up to 58% of patients having complete healing.[71] Skin excision can futher reduce the recurrence rate to about 24%.[72] Meticulous skin care and good hygiene avoid skin maceration and regular hair shaving prevents hair from penetrating the healing scar. Such diligent wound care will further lower recurrence rates. As such, whichever surgical technique is used, careful attention to skin hygiene and hair exfoliation cannot be overemphasised.

Chronic pilonidal sinus

A chronic pilonidal sinus is a pilonidal sinus appearing after treatment of an acute pilonidal abscess. It is also used for patients who have a discharging sinus at first presentation with or without an abscess. The surgical management of a chronic pilonidal sinus aims to obliterate the epithelialised sinus tract and heal the wound.

Outpatient options

Simple outpatient options include phenol injection and excision and lay-open of the chronic tract. Phenol destroys the epithelium in the tract and sterilises the wound. An injection of 1–2 mL of 80% phenol is given into the tract, with great care taken to protect the surrounding skin with paraffin or other ointments. The surrounding hair is shaved off and wound dressing performed daily. The phenol injection can be repeated every 4–6 weeks till the wound has healed. This simple technique has the advantage of minimal time away from work, with a variable healing rate of 59–95%. However, the side-effects include skin necrosis and abscess formation in up to 22% of patients. Some authors have advocated a reduced strength of 40% phenol, with a reduced complication rate of 12% and a healing rate of 77%.[73]

Alternatively, the sinus tract can be laid open under local anaesthesia and dressed in the outpatient setting. Some authors have advocated using fibrin sealant or regular wound brushing to reduce the wound healing time or recurrence rate. However, whatever modifications are used, the recurrence rate is generally low, from 10% to 18%, with the added advantage of minimal complications or time away from work.

Inpatient options

Once a surgeon decides to perform a more complex procedure as an inpatient surgery, the options increase but the best method remains debatable. The principles of the operation are to eradicate the sinus tract, ensure complete healing of the overlying skin and prevent recurrence. The options include laying the wound open to heal by secondary intention or primary closure of the surgical wound. The techniques with primary closure are further categorised into midline closure or off-midline closure.

Lay-open methods include simple excision of subcutaneous tract, wide excision down to sacral periostium, brushing of sinus tract and marsupialisation of the wound. There may be long healing times. However, in a recent meta-analysis of techniques comparing open healing versus primary closure, techniques with open healing have a 58% lower risk of recurrence compared to primary closure techniques.[74]

Conversely, primary closure techniques have been adopted by many because the time to wound healing and return to work is shorter. In our opinion, midline closure should be abandoned in favour of off-midline techniques, there being fewer recurrences with off-midline closure (1.4% vs. 10.3% for midline closure) and wound infections (6.3% vs. 10.4% for midline closure).[74]

The theory behind off-midline techniques is that the natal cleft is an anatomical trough which loose hairs tend to gravitate toward. Negative pressure in the natal cleft produced by movement of the buttocks on sitting and walking also creates a suction effect attracting the tips of loose hair towards the natal cleft. Any wound in the midline will preferentially gather loose hairs in the wound, predisposing midline wounds to recurrence. Techniques of off-midline closure change the natal cleft contour and disperse suction pressure over a wider area, thereby reducing the likelihood of loose hair implanting in the healing wound.

> ✓✓ In a recent Cochrane Database Systematic Review, a meta-analysis of six studies comparing midline to off-midline closure for chronic pilonidal sinus found that off-midline wounds had faster healing times, lower wound infection rates and lower recurrence rates. The authors concluded that when closure of pilonidal sinuses was the desired surgical option, off-midline closure should be the standard management.[74]

The most established technique used in the UK is the Bascom operation,[75] where an incision is made lateral to the midline to curette the deep cavity free of loose hairs and granulation tissue, together with excision of the primary midline pits via small stab incisions of about 7mm. The midline incisions are closed primarily and the lateral wound left to heal by secondary intention. Some authors close the lateral wound over a drain to reduce the healing time, with good results.

Another popular technique is the Karydakis procedure.[76] A 'semilateral' 'D-shaped' incision is made incorporating the sinus tract down to the presacral fascia. The defect should be convex on one side and vertical (next to midline) on the other. The flap of tissue on the vertical wound side is mobilised down to the fascia to allow the flap to be brought over to the convex wound edge and sutured down in layers over a drain. Karydakis reported a recurrence rate of only 1%, with 8.5% wound complication rate.

Recurrent pilonidal sinus

Even with proper technique and meticulous wound care, a small group of patients develop recurrent pilonidal disease. In such cases, the local tissue scarring usually precludes the techniques mentioned above and rotational flap procedures are recommended. Z-plasty, modified Z-plasty, gluteus maximus myocutaneous flap, V-Y fasciocutaneous flap and rhomboid fasciocutaenous flap (Limberg/Dufourmentel) have all been described. The principles involved in this surgery are complete excision of the recurrent pilonidal sinus and scar tissue, mobilisation of a flap of adjacent healthy tissue down to fascia (at least) and tension-free repair of the flap. A review of the various rotational flap techniques showed no individual superiority.[77]

Our preference is for a modified Limberg flap procedure in such cases. The procedure is performed under general anaesthesia with the patient in prone jack-knife position. A large rhomboid-shaped excision incorporating the pilonidal sinuses is made, with care taken to place the cranial and caudal tips of the rhomboid away from the midline (**Fig. 15.9a**). The tissue is excised down to but preserving the presacral fascia. Next, an incision is made from the short diagonal of the rhomboid defect of length similar to any side of the rhomboid (**Fig. 15.9b**). A second line is then made at 90° to the lateral edge of the previous incision (**Fig. 15.9c**). This line is also of the same length as the previous one. In the classic Limberg flap procedure, this line is at 60°, but we feel that it creates a narrow tip under tension after repair and predisposes this 60° tip to necrosis and wound infection. The flap is mobilised down to and includes the fascia over the gluteus maximus on all edges of the wound and the flap is then secured over a suction drain (placed from the contralateral buttock), taking care to secure the flap at the levels of the fascia, subcutaneous tissue and skin (**Fig. 15.9d**). Patients are not given bowel preparation for this surgery and discharged after 2–3 days when the drain is removed. In our experience, we have had few wound infections and no recurrences so far (**Fig. 15.10**).

Conclusion

Pilonidal sinus disease can present as an acute abscess, a chronic pilonidal sinus or recurrent disease. Acute abscesses should be treated as simply as possible so as not to complicate treatment should the patient develop a chronic sinus. The choice of treatment in chronic pilonidal sinus is between delayed healing versus primary closure techniques. Whether one chooses

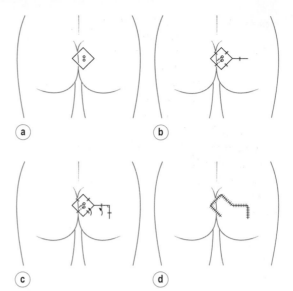

Figure 15.9 • Modified Limberg flap for recurrent pilonidal sinus showing: **(a)** off-midline rhomboid-shaped incision incorporating sinus tracts; **(b)** lateral extension of incision of length equal to the side of the rhomboid incision; **(c)** caudal extension perpendicular to lateral incision; and **(d)** securing rotated flap with sutures.

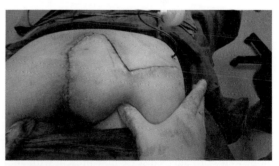

Figure 15.10 • End result of the modified off-centre Limberg flap after reconstruction.

an open healing or primary closure technique, lateralising the wound gives lower recurrences. In recurrent disease, a rotational flap procedure is the preferred method of treatment.

Anal stenosis

Anal stenosis is an abnormal narrowing of the anal canal with physical obstruction at that level. This is in contrast to anal canal spasm secondary to painful lesions or functional abnormalities where examination shows a supple and fully compliant anus.

Box 15.3 • Aetiology of anal stenosis

Congenital
- Imperforate anus
- Anal atresia

Acquired
- Irradiation
- Lacerations
- Following surgery of anal canal/low rectum (commonly anastomotic failure)

Neoplastic
- Perianal or anal cancers
- Leukaemia
- Bowen's disease
- Paget's disease

Inflammatory
- Crohn's disease
- Tuberculosis
- Amoebiasis
- *Lymphogranuloma venereum*
- Actinomycosis

Spastic
- Chronic anal fissure
- Ischaemic

Aetiology

The commonest cause is usually haemorrhoidectomy with excessive mucocutaneous excision. Other causes are listed in Box 15.3. Recurrent anal fissures, perianal abscesses with repeated surgical procedures and excessive excision of perianal skin in Bowen's or Paget's disease may present with anal canal stenosis.

Clinical presentation

A history of constipation, decreasing stool calibre, difficulty in voiding with the need to strain excessively, and tenesmus are usually the first symptoms of anal stenosis. Bleeding may occur from traumatic defecation or digitation. Scarring from previous anal surgery may be obvious. An index finger may not pass through the narrowing. If digitation is possible, the level of the stenosis relative to the dentate line as well as the length of the stenosis must be noted.

If digitation is possible the stenosis may be mild to moderate. Stapled haemorrhoidectomy can cause rectal obstruction, in which a digit can easily traverse the staple line but a prominent ridge of scar tissue is palpable circumferentially. A biopsy may be essential if no previous surgery or anal trauma was elicited. Anatomical findings may not correlate well with the magnitude of the obstructive symptoms.

Treatment

Treatment of anal stenosis depends on the severity and level of stenosis within the anal canal, as well as when it has arisen in relation to any prior anal operation. Anal stenosis below the dentate line is often related to previous anal surgery, such as excisional haemorrhoidectomy, or to inflammatory conditions, such as Crohn's disease. Anal stenosis above the dentate line may be secondary to stapled haemorrhoidectomy or low anterior resection. We need to distinguish between staple-line stenosis of the lower rectum, which usually is secondary to partial staple-line dehiscence or infection, and colonic stricture proximal to the staple line, which is usually secondary to ischaemia from reduced blood flow in the proximal colon.

Prevention

The key to treatment lies in its prevention. Good surgical judgment is the best mode of prevention. Excessive removal of the anoderm is often the cause of significant anal stenosis. Excessive excision of perianal skin during haemorrhoidectomy must be guarded against. Preserving a 'bridge' of anoderm at least 1 cm wide between wounds and limiting the distal extent of tissue resection to the anal verge may minimise anal stenosis. Preserving anodermal 'bridges' is crucial to all anal surgery and not haemorrhoidectomy alone.

Anal dilatation
Mild stenosis (tight anal canal but permitting the passage of the index finger) may be treated occasionally with bulk laxatives, but the recurrence rate is high. After initial manual dilatation, many surgeons have recommended regular dilatation with

the patient's own finger or an appropriately sized anal dilator (e.g. St Mark's anal dilator or Hagar dilators) to maintain the anal diameter. Good functional results may be achieved in this manner, particularly if a mild post-surgical stenosis is caught early. The patient should be guided to pass the dilator beyond the anal stricture twice daily for 2 months. The use of topical steroids has no documented additional benefit. Regular anal dilatation may not work if the scarring has already matured at the time of diagnosis. Further forceful dilatation at this stage may worsen the fibrosis and lead to more serious stenosis.

Severe anal stenosis, with inability to pass the index finger through the stenosis, will always require surgical intervention.

> ✔ Four-finger manual dilatation performed under anaesthesia should never be performed and is always unnecessary. The uncontrolled manner of anal tearing can lead to excessive anal sphincter damage and subsequent faecal incontinence.

A very scarred and stenotic anus, or one associated with Crohn's disease, may occasionally be self-maintained using Hagar dilators after initial Hagar graded dilatation under general anaesthesia if the patient is not keen on more complicated surgery. However, a worsening of scarring with time is inevitable. The principles of surgical treatment are outlined in Box 15.4.

Sphincterotomy

In the past, some surgeons believed that a hypertrophied internal anal sphincter could cause anal

Box 15.4 • Principles of surgical treatment for anal stenosis

- Stool bulking
- Anal dilatation
- Examination under anaesthesia with graded Hagar's dilator followed by postoperative self-maintenance
- Removal of cutaneous scarring
- Stricturoplasty for anal stenosis proximal to dentate line (worst cases may need an abdominal pull-through operation)
- Skin advancement (inwards)
- Mucosal advancement (outwards)
- Colostomy in desperate cases

stenosis and hence recommended anal sphincterotomy. However, there are no studies to verify this. These patients with so-called 'anal stenosis' actually have anismus or dyssynergic defecation. Anecdotal experience of sphincterotomy showing benefit is likely due to reduction of anal pressure in the short term. In the longer term, it could theoretically lead to faecal incontinence, though this is as yet unproven. These patients are better treated with biofeedback, a form of re-training of the various muscles involved to provide an appropriate coordination of defecation.

Stricturoplasty

In cases of anal stenosis proximal to the dentate line as in stapled haemorrhoidectomy, stricturoplasty has proved to be a simple and reliable method of treatment. The stricture along the anastomosis is palpated and two to four vertical incisions are made over the scar with a small narrow proctoscope. This incision is deepened until the entire thickness of the scar is incised without cutting the muscle layer of the rectal wall. The mucosa is approximated transversely with sutures and not left to heal by secondary intention. We prefer to make either two (anterior and posterior midline) or four (at 3, 6, 9, 12 o'clock positions) incisions across the stenosis based on the degree of stenosis. Special care must be taken not to cause full-thickness perforation to prevent septic and bleeding consequences. Adequacy of stricturoplasty is assessed by digital examination showing a supple and distensible anorectal wall at the level of the previous stenosis. In our experience, 1.2% of patients develop significant anal stenosis after stapled haemorrhoidectomy requiring strictureplasty. All of them derived good results with this procedure.[78]

Flap procedures
Mucosal advancement flap (above to down)

This involves the advancement of anal mucosa into the stenotic area by way of a vertical incision made in the stenotic area perpendicular to the dentate line in the lateral position. An excision of the scar tissue allows widening of the stenosis. The incision is then undermined for about 2 cm and closed in a transverse manner with vicryl 3/0, stitching the mucosal edge down onto the skin edge of the anoderm.

Y-V advancement flap (outside to in)

Originally described by Penn in 1948, a Y incision is made, with the vertical limb of the Y in the anal canal above the proximal level of the stenosis. The 'V' of the Y is drawn on the lateral perianal skin. The skin is incised and a V-shaped flap is raised; the length-to-breadth ratio must be less than 3. After excision of the underlying scar tissue in the anal canal with or without an additional lateral sphincterotomy, the flap can be mobilised into the anal canal and stitched into place. This may be done bilaterally with good results[79] and provides relief in 85–92% of cases. Tip necrosis occurs in 10–25% of cases and stenosis may recur.

V-Y advancement flap (outside to in)

Unlike the Y-V advancement flap, the V-Y flap has the advantage of bringing a wider piece of skin into the stenosis to keep it open. The V is drawn with the wide base parallel to the dentate line about 2 cm long. A similar length-to-base ratio as in the Y-V flap should be maintained. Marking the skin flap is followed by its mobilisation such that it may move without tension into the anal canal. Sufficient subcutaneous tissue must be mobilised with the flap, which derives its blood supply from the perforating vessels arising within the fat. The skin is then closed behind the flap to produce the limb of the Y. A treatment success rate of 96% has been reported with this flap.

Island advancement flap (outside to in)

First described in 1986 by Caplin and Kodner,[80] the island flap may be constructed in various shapes (e.g. diamond, house or U-shaped). The flap is mobilised from its lateral margins together with the subcutaneous fat after the scar tissue in the stenotic area has been excised. A lateral sphincterotomy may or may not be performed. A broad skin flap (up to 50% of the circumference) may be brought into the entire length of the anal canal and simultaneously allow for closure of the donor site. Improvement of symptoms may be as high as 91% at 3 years of follow-up; 18–50% suffer minor wound separation.[81,82]

S-anoplasty (outside to in)

This procedure mobilises bilateral gluteal skin into the entire anal canal after excision of the scar tissue up to the dentate line. The incision is designed in an S shape, hence the name of the flap. The breadth-to-length ratio must be more than 1, with the base of the S being about 7–10 cm. The skin is rotated to line the anal canal in a tension-free manner. This extensive procedure is rarely used.

Conclusion

The best form of treatment for anal stenosis remains prevention. Gentle and regular anal dilation can help mild stenosis but recurrent or severe cases require surgery. High stenosis above the dentate line is probably best treated by transanal stricturoplasty, or in the worst cases an abdominal pull-through operation.

Dietary fibre – more harm than good?

Advocating a high-fibre diet has been commonplace as part of the dietary advice given to patients suffering from haemorrhoids and anal fissures. However, this practice should be re-evaluated as many patients may not benefit but instead suffer further from the advice. The pathogenesis of frequent straining is multifactorial and differs among patients, even those suffering from haemorrhoids or anal fissures. Whilst dietary fibre is an essential part of our daily diet, its 'therapeutic' role remains controversial.

Insoluble fibre bulks stools, potentially leading to increased anal trauma and tearing. Soluble fibre ferments in the colon, leading to increased gas and flatulence. The more fibre ingested, the more stools will have to be passed. In addition, contrary to popular belief, we believe that the moisture content in stools is not increased following an increased intake of fibre, but rather increased water intake leads to an increase in urinary output and not softer stools. Increased straining due to the passage of large bulky stools due to increased dietary fibre leads to increased damage to the ligaments of Parks, trauma to the anal cushions and aggravates prolapsed haemorrhoids.[83] Also, passage of bulky stools causes more trauma or tearing of the anal mucosa, thus worsening anal tears and fissures.[83] Therefore, although dietary fibre may have other merits, its role in anal disorders should be re-evaluated and fibre should not be blindly used for all anorectal disorders.[84]

Key points

- Haemorrhoidal disease is common but other life-threatening diseases must first be excluded. Treatments by micronised flavonoids, submucosal injection, rubber-band ligation or transanal haemorrhoidal artery ligation allow for symptomatic relief. Consideration should be given either to stapled or excisional haemorrhoidectomy for severe degrees of prolapsing piles, depending on the sort of piles present and the expertise available.

- Anal fissures should be viewed as superficial or deep fissures ignoring duration. Their aetiology needs to be understood in terms of initiating and perpetuating factors. Treatment is based on addressing both initiating and perpetuating factors concurrently. Lateral sphincterotomy remains the gold standard for deep anal fissures but posterior perineal support warrants further investigation.

- Pruritus ani may result from many anorectal or dermatological conditions and remains a difficult problem to manage and treat. Reduction of anal leakage, reduction in fibre consumption and good personal hygiene remain important aspects of treatment.

- Treatment of pilonidal sinus depends upon presentation as well as patient preferences in terms of healing time, time off work and recurrence rates. Surgery should be combined with meticulous wound care and hair shaving to give best results. Off-midline wound closure is preferred to midline if primary wound closure is performed.

- Anal stenosis has many aetiologies but the commonest is a result of anal surgery. Treatments range from anal dilatation to flap procedures.

References

1. Shanmugam V, Thaha MA, Rabindranath KS, et al. Rubber band ligation versus excisional haemorrhoidectomy for haemorrhoids. Cochrane Database Syst Rev 2005;(1).
   Grade 2 haemorrhoids should be treated with rubber-band ligation while surgery is reserved for grade 3 haemorrhoids or recurrent haemorrhoids after rubber-band ligation.

2. Ho YH, Tan M, Seow-Choen F. Micronized purified flavonidic fraction compared favourably with rubber band ligation and fiber alone in the management of bleeding hemorrhoids. Dis Colon Rectum 2000;43:66–9.

3. Wadworth AN, Faulds D. Hydroxyethylrutosides. A review of its pharmacology and therapeutic efficacy in venous insufficiency and related disorders. Drugs 1992;44:1013–32.

4. Damon M. Effect of chronic treatment with purified flavonoid fraction on inflammatory granuloma in the rat. Study of prostaglandin E2 and F2 and thromboxane B2 release and histological changes. Arzneimittelforschung 1987;37:1149–53.

5. Cospite M. Double-blind versus placebo evaluation of clinical activity and safety of Daflon 500 mg in the treatment of acute haemorrhoids. Angiology 1994;6:566–73.

6. Ho YH, Foo CL, Seow-Choen F, et al. Prospective randomised controlled trial of micronised flavonidic fraction to reduce bleeding after haemorrhoidectomy. Br J Surg 1995;82:1034–5.

7. Ho YH, Seow-Choen F, Tan M, et al. Randomised trial of open and closed haemorrhoidectomy. Br J Surg 1997;84:1729–30.

8. Seow-Choen F, Ho YH, Ang HG, et al. Prospective, randomized trial comparing pain and clinical function after conventional scissor excision/ligation vs. diathermy excision without ligation of symptomatic prolapsed hemorrhoids. Dis Colon Rectum 1992;35:1165–9.

9. Ho KS, Eu KW, Heah SM, et al. Randomised clinical trial of haemorrhoidectomy under a mixture of local anaesthesia versus general anaesthesia. Br J Surg 2000;87(4):410–3.

10. Jane Tan JY, Seow-Choen F. Prospective randomized trial comparing diathermy and harmonic scalpel hemorrhoidectomy. Dis Colon Rectum 2001;44:677–9.

11. Ibrahim S, Tsang C, Lee YL, et al. Prospective, randomized trial comparing pain and complications between diathermy and scissors for closed hemorrhoidectomy. Dis Colon Rectum 1998;41:1418–20.

12. Ho YH, Tan M. Ambulatory anorectal manometric findings in patients before and after haemorrhoidectomy. Int J Colorectal Dis 1997;12(5):296–7.

13. Seow-Choen F, Low HC. Prospective randomised study of radical versus four piles haemorrhoidectomy for symptomatic large circumferential prolapsed piles. Br J Surg 1995;82:188–9.

14. Seow-Choen F. Stapled haemorrhoidectomy: pain or gain. Br J Surg 2000;88:1–3.

15. Seow-Choen F. Surgery for haemorrhoids: ablation or correction. Asian J Surg 2002;25:265–6.

16. Lloyd D, Ho KS, Seow-Choen F. Modified Longo's hemorrhoidectomy. Dis Colon Rectum 2002;45:416–7.

17. Cheetham MJ, Mortensen NJ, Nystrom PO, et al. Persistent pain and faecal urgency after stapled haemorrhoidectomy. Lancet 2000;356:730–3.

18. Jayaraman S, Colquhoun PHD, Malthaner RA. Stapled versus conventional surgery for haemorrhoids. Cochrane Database Syst Rev 2006;(4). Stapled haemorrhoidectomy is associated with higher risk of recurrence or symptoms of prolapse than excisional haemorrhoidectomy.

19. Jayne D, Seow-Choen F. Modified stapled haemorrhoidectomy for treatment of massive circumferentially prolapsing piles. Tech Coloproct 2002;6:191–3.

20. Brown SR, Ballan K, Ho E, et al. Stapled mucosectomy for acute thrombosed circumferentially prolapsed piles: a prospective randomised comparison with conventional haemorrhoidectomy. Colorectal Dis 2001;3:175–8.

21. Morinaga K, Hakuda K, Ikeada T. A novel therapy for internal haemorrhoids: ligation of the haemorrhoidal artery with a new devised instrument in conjunction with Doppler flow meter. Am J Gastroenterol 1995;90(4):610–3.

22. Sohn N, Aronoff JS, Cohen FS, et al. Transanal hemorrhoidal dearterialization is an alternative to operative haemorrhoidectomy. Am J Surg 2001;182:515–9.

23. Dal Monte PP, Tagariello C, Sarago M, et al. Transanal haemorrhoidal dearterialization: nonexcisional surgery for the treatment of haemorrhoidal disease. Tech Coloproctol 2007;11:333–9.

24. Guy RJ, Ng CE, Eu KW. Stapled anoplasty for haemorrhoids: a comparison of ambulatory vs. inpatient procedures. Colorectal Dis 2003;5:29–32.

25. Ho YH, Cheong WK, Tsang C, et al. Stapled hemorrhoidectomy: cost and effectiveness. Randomized, controlled trial including incontinence scoring, anorectal manometry, and endoanal ultrasound assessments at up to three months. Dis Colon Rectum 2000;43:1666–75.

26. Davies J, Duffy D, Boyt N, et al. Botulinum toxin (Botox) reduces pain after hemorrhoidectomy: results of a double-blind, randomized study. Dis Colon Rectum 2003;46:1097–102.

27. Hwang DY, Toon SG, Kim HS, et al. Effect of 0.2 percent glyceryl trinitrate ointment on wound healing after a hemorrhoidectomy: results of a randomized, prospective, double-blind, placebo-controlled trial. Dis Colon Rectum 2003;46:950–4.

28. Mathai V, Ong BC, Ho YH. Randomised controlled trial of lateral internal sphincterotomy with haemorrhoidectomy. Br J Surg 1996;83:380–2.

29. Nyam DCNK, Seow-Choen F, Ho YH. Submucosal adrenaline injection for post-hemorrhoidectomy hemorrhage. Dis Colon Rectum 1995;38:776–7.

30. Eu KW, Teoh TA, Seow-Choen F, et al. Anal stricture following haemorrhoidectomy: early diagnosis and treatment. Aust N Z J Surg 1995;65:101–3.

31. Ho YH, Seow-Choen F, Tsang C, et al. Randomised trial assessing anal sphincter injuries after stapled haemorrhoidectomy. Br J Surg 2001;88:1449–55.

32. Maw A, Concepcion R, Eu KW, et al. Prospective randomised study of bacteraemia in diathermy and stapled haemorrhoidectomy. Br J Surg 2003;90:222–6.

33. Guy RJ, Seow-Choen F. Septic complications after treatment of haemorrhoids. Br J Surg 2003;90:147–56.

34. Carapeti EA, Kamm MA, McDonald PJ, et al. Double-blind randomised controlled trial of effect of metronidazole on pain after day case haemorrhoidectomy. Lancet 1998;351:169–72.

35. Leong AFPK, Seow-Choen F. Lateral sphincterotomy compared with anal advancement flap for chronic anal fissure. Dis Colon Rectum 1995;38:69–71.

36. Shafik A. A new concept of the anal sphincter mechanism and physiology of defecation. IX. Single loop continence: a new theory of the mechanism of anal continence. Dis Colon Rectum 1980;23:37–46.

37. Li D, Guo M. Morphology of the levator ani muscle. Dis Colon Rectum 2007;50:1831–9.

38. Poh A, Tan KY, Seow-Choen F. Innovations in chronic anal fissure treatment: a systematic review. World J Gastroint Surg 2010;2:231–41.

39. Parks AG, Porter NH, Hardcastle J. The syndrome of the descending perineum. Proc R Soc Med 1966;59:477–82.

40. Lock MR, Thompson JP. Fissure in ano: the initial management and prognosis. Br J Surg 1977;64:355–8.

41. Corby H, Donnelly VS, O'Herlihy C, et al. Anal canal pressures are low in women with postpartum anal fissure. Br J Surg 1997;84:86–8.

42. Lund JN. Nitric oxide deficiency in the internal anal sphincter of patients with chronic anal fissure. Int J Colorectal Dis 2006;21:673–5.

43. Utzig MJ, Kroesen AJ, Buhr HJ. Concepts in pathogenesis and treatment of chronic anal fissure – a review of the literature. Am J Gastroenterol 2003;98:968–74.

44. Gibbons CP, Read NW. Anal hypertonia in fissures: cause or effect? Br J Surg 1986;73:443–5.

45. Klosterhalfen B, Vogel P, Rixen H, et al. Topography of the inferior rectal artery: a possible cause of chronic, primary anal fissure. Dis Colon Rectum 1989;32:43–52.

46. Schouten WR, Briel JW, Auwerda JJ. Relationship between anal pressure and anodermal blood flow. The vascular pathogenesis of anal fissures. Dis Colon Rectum 1994;37:664–9.

47. Lindsey I, Jones M, Cunningham C, et al. Chronic anal fissure. Br J Surg 2004;91:270–9.

48. D'Hoore A. Penninckx F. Obstructed defaecation. Colorectal Dis 2003;5:280–7.

49. Tan KY, Seow-Choen F, Hai CH, et al. Posterior perineal support as treatment for anal fissures – preliminary results with a new toilet seat device. Tech Coloproctol 2009;13:11–5.

50. Colins EE, Lund JN. A review of chronic anal fissure management. Tech Coloproctol 2007;11:209–23.

51. Lund JN, Scholefield JH. A randomised, prospective, double-blind, placebo-controlled trial of glyceryl trinitrate ointment in the treatment of anal fissure. Lancet 1997;349:11–4.
    Sustained relief of pain in patients with anal fissure was demonstrated. Over two-thirds of patients treated with topical GTN avoided surgery.

52. Carapeti EA, Kamm MA, McDonald PJ, et al. Randomised controlled trial shows that glyceryl trinitrate heals anal fissures, higher doses are not more effective, and there is a high recurrence rate. Gut 1999;44:727–30.

53. Sajid MS, Rimple J, Cheek E, et al. The efficacy of diltiazem and glyceryltrinitrate for the medical management of chronic anal fissure: a meta-analysis. Int J Colorectal Dis 2008;23:1–6.
    Diltiazem and GTN are effective in the treatment of anal fissures.

54. Maria G, Sganga G, Civello IM, et al. Botulinum neurotoxin and other treatments for fissure-in-ano and pelvic floor disorders. Br J Surg 2002;89:950–61.

55. Brisinda G, Cadeddu F, Brandara F, et al. Randomised clinical trial comparing botulinum toxin injections with 0.2 per cent nitroglycerin ointment for chronic anal fissure. Br J Surg 2007;94:162–7.
    In this study of medical treatment of chronic anal fissure, botulinum toxin was more effective than nitroglycerin ointment. Adverse effects in both treatments have been reported but are mild and self-limiting.

56. Brisinda G, Maria G, Bentivoglio AR, et al. A comparison of injections of botulinum toxin and topical nitroglycerin ointment for the treatment of chronic anal fissures. N Engl J Med 1999;341:65–9.

57. Nelson RL. Non-surgical therapy for anal fissure. Cochrane Database Syst Rev 2006;(4).
    Medical therapy can be used to treat anal fissure but is not as effective as surgery. The former is also associated with a higher rate of recurrence.

58. Nelson RL, Chattopadhyay A, Brooks W, et al. Operative procedures for fissure in ano (meta-analysis). Cochrane Database Syst Rev 2011;(11).

59. Littlejohn DR, Newstead GL. Tailored lateral sphincterotomy for anal fissure. Dis Colon Rectum 1997;40:1439–42.

60. Engel AF, Eijsbouts QAJ, Balk AG. Fissurectomy and isosorbide dinitrate for chronic fissure-in-ano not responding to conservative treatment. Br J Surg 2002;89:79–83.

61. Scholz TH, Hetzer FH, Dindo D, et al. Long-term follow-up after combined fissurectomy and Botox injection for chronic anal fissures. Int J Colorectal Dis 2007;22:1077–81.

62. Fleschner PR, Schoetz Jr DJ, Roberts PL, et al. Anal fissure in Crohn's disease: a plea for aggressive management. Dis Colon Rectum 1995;38:1137–43.

63. Cundall JD, Gardiner A, Laden G, et al. Use of hyperbaric oxygen to treat chronic anal fissure. Br J Surg 2003;90:452–3.

64. Nyam DCNK, Wilson RG, Stewart KJ, et al. Island advancement flaps in the management of anal fissures. Br J Surg 1995;82:326–8.

65. Lysy J, Sistiery-Ittah M, Israelit Y, et al. Topical capsaicin: a novel and effective treatment for idiopathic intractable pruritus ani. A randomised, placebo controlled, crossover study. Gut 2003;52:1323–6.

66. Sutherland AD, Faragher IG, Frizelle FA. Intradermal injection of methylene blue for the treatment of refractory pruritis ani. Colorectal Dis 2009;11:282–7.

67. Sondenaa K, Andersen E, Nesvik I, et al. Patient characteristics and symptoms in chronic pilonidal sinus disease. Int J Colorectal Dis 1995;10:39–42.

68. Patey DH, Scarff RW. Pilonidal sinus in a barber's hand: with observations on postanal pilonidal sinus. Lancet 1948;2:13.

69. Bascom J. Pilonidal disease: origin from follicles of hair and results of follicle removal as treatment. Surgery 1980;87:567–72.

70. Clothier PR, Haywood IR. The natural history of postanal (pilonidal) sinus. Ann R Coll Surg Engl 1984;66:201–3.

71. Jensen SL, Harling H. Prognosis after simple incision and drainage for a first-episode acute pilonidal abscess. Br J Surg 1988;75:60–1.

72. Vahedian J, Nabavizadeh F, Nakhaee N, et al. Comparison between drainage and curettage in the treatment of acute pilonidal abscess. Saudi Med J 2005;26:553–5.

73. Sakçak I, Avşar FM, Coşgun E. Comparison of the application of low concentration and 80% phenol solution in pilonidal sinus disease. JRSM Short Rep 2010;1:5.

74. Al-Khamis A, McCallum I, King PM, et al. Healing by primary closure versus open healing after surgery for pilonidal sinus. Cochrane Database Syst Rev 2010;(1).
    When closure of pilonidal sinuses was the desired surgical option, off-midline closure should be the standard management as it led to faster healing times and fewer recurrences compared to midline wounds.

75. Bascom J. Pilonidal disease: Origin from follicles of hair and results of follicle removal as treatment. Surgery 1980;87:567–72.

76. Karydakis GE. Easy and successful treatment of pilonidal sinus after explanation of its causative process. Aust N Z J Surg 1992;62:385–9.

77. Petersen S, Koch R, Stelzner S, et al. Primary closure techniques in chronic pilonidal sinus: a survey of the result of different surgical approaches. Dis Colon Rectum 2002;45:1458.

78. Kam MH, Ng KH, Lim JF, et al. Results of 7302 stapled haemorrhoidectomy operations in a single centre: a seven-year review and follow-up questionnaire survey. Aust N Z J Surg 2011;81:253–6.

79. Angelchik PD, Harms BA, Stanley JR. Repair of anal stricture and mucosal ectropion with YV or pedicle flap anoplasty. Am J Surg 1993;166:55–9.

80. Caplin DA, Kodner IJ. Repair of anal stricture and mucosal ectropion by single flap procedures. Dis Colon Rectum 1986;29:92.

81. Pidala MJ, Slezak FA, Porter JA. Island advancement anoplasty for anal canal stenosis and mucosal ectropion. Am Surg 1994;60:194–6.

82. Sentovich SM, Falk PM, Christensen MA, et al. Operative results of house advancement anoplasty. Br J Surg 1996;83:1242–4.

83. Tan KY, Seow-Choen F. Fibre and colorectal disease: separating fact from friction. World J Gastroenterol 2007;13(31):4161–7.

84. Chuwa EWL, Seow-Choen F. Dietary fibre. Br J Surg 2006;93:3–4.

16

Sexually transmitted diseases and the anorectum

Lester Gottesman
Josef A. Shehebar

Introduction

Sexually transmitted diseases (STDs) often present to colorectal surgeons. Signs and symptoms include diarrhoea, rectal bleeding, tenesmus, and ulcerative or fistulous lesions of the rectum, anus and perineum. The increased prevalence and variety of anorectal STDs have been attributed to greater use of the anorectum for sexual gratification, as well as human immunodeficiency virus (HIV) infection in men who have sex with men (MSM). All healthcare providers should be aware that high-risk behaviours, including unprotected sex, multiple partners and illicit drug use, can increase transmission of STDs as well, and HIV.[1,2] Females and heterosexual males can be affected by anorectal STDs as well, and a high index of suspicion is necessary. The presence of more than one infecting organism is not uncommon. For certain STDs, immunosuppression (including post-transplantation) plays a significant role.

There is a high prevalence of asymptomatic STDs among HIV-infected patients, especially MSM. There is 'epidemiological synergy' between HIV and both ulcerative and non-ulcerative STDs.[2] Genital ulcers facilitate shedding of HIV, and bleeding from them during intercourse can increase the potential for HIV infection due to mucosal trauma from anoreceptive intercourse. Non-ulcerative STDs can disrupt mucosal barriers by recruitment of HIV-susceptible inflammatory cells, further increasing the risk of HIV infection.

The commonest organisms causing STDs of the anorectum present in three symptom categories: suppurative, ulcerative and fistulous disease (Table 16.1).

The diseases presented in Table 16.2 are categorised by aetiological agent. Medications are suggested, but clinicians should consult full prescribing information before using them.

Viral

Human immunodeficiency virus

HIV is a RNA retrovirus that infects T lymphocytes. It is transmitted by mucosal contact with contaminated body fluids and, after a variable latent period of up to 2 years, it produces diminished immunological function, manifested as acquired immunodeficiency syndrome (AIDS). The incidence of HIV infection has levelled in the USA and Western Europe and the mortality has decreased as highly active antiretroviral therapy (HAART) has become available.[3]

Illnesses associated with immunosuppression include HIV anal ulceration, opportunistic infections, anal condyloma, Kaposi's sarcoma and lymphoma. Another concern is how HIV affects wound healing, especially for routine anorectal complaints (haemorrhoids, fissures, fistulas, etc.). It appears that patients who are HIV positive without AIDS have no increased risk of wound problems, while

Table 16.1 • Anorectal STDs categorised by predominant presentation

STDs with proctitis	STDs with ulcers	STDs with fistulas
• Gonorrhea • *Chlamydia* • Herpes simplex virus • Syphilis	• AIDS-associated anal ulcers • *Lymphogranuloma venereum* • Primary syphilis – chancre • Chancroid • Granuloma inguinale • Herpes simplex virus	• *Lymphogranuloma venereum* • Complex Bushke–Lowenstein tumours

those with AIDS and more advanced disease (CD4-positive count under 100, poor performance status) are more likely to have delayed healing.[4,5]

There are few data on the incidence of AIDS-associated anal ulcers. With HAART it is a less common problem because these ulcers mostly occur in patients with AIDS and low CD4-positive counts. This is a distinct disease process, different from typical anal fissures. Both result in pain with defecation, but AIDS-associated ulcers are more likely to cause disabling pain unrelated to defecation. AIDS ulcers are differentiated by their location proximal to the dentate line with a broad-based ulcer, which may dissect between tissue plains. The resulting

Table 16.2 • Sexually transmitted organisms that affect the anorectum

Organism	Symptoms	Anoscopy/ proctoscopy	Laboratory	Treatment
Viral				
HIV	Pain unrelated to defecation	Broad-based ulcers proximal to dentate line	Serology	HAART, debridement, unroofing cavities, intralesional steroid injection
Herpes simplex virus (HSV)	Anorectal pain, pruritus, rectal bleeding	Perianal erythema, vesicles, ulcers, diffusely inflamed and friable rectal mucosa	Cytological examination of scrapings or viral culture of vesicle fluid PCR	Aciclovir 400 mg p.o. three times daily × 7–10 days OR Aciclovir 200 mg p.o. five times daily × 7–10 days OR Famciclovir 250 mg p.o. three times daily × 7–10 days OR Valaciclovir 1 g p.o. twice daily × 7–10 days
Human papillomavirus (condylomata acuminatum)	Pruritus, bleeding, discharge, pain	Perianal warts	Excisional biopsy to determine serotype	Topical agents Excision or destruction (see text)
Molluscum contagiosum	Painless skin lesions	Flattened, round, umbilicated lesion	Excisional biopsy and staining for molluscum bodies	Expectant, excision or destruction
Bacterial				
Chlamydia trachomatis	Tenesmus, perianal pain	Friable, often ulcerated mucosa	Tissue culture, nucleic acid amplification, serological antibody titres	Azithromycin 1 g p.o. × one dose OR Doxycycline 100 mg p.o. twice daily × 7 days
Lymphogranuloma venereum	Systemic symptoms, inguinal adenopathy, anogenital ulceration	Friable ulcerated rectal mucosa	LGV serotyping with nucleic acid amplification, confirmation at specialty laboratories	Doxycycline 100 mg p.o. twice daily × 21 days OR Erythromycin base 500 mg p.o. four times daily × 21 days

Table 16.2 • (*cont.*) Sexually transmitted organisms that affect the anorectum

Organism	Symptoms	Anoscopy/ proctoscopy	Laboratory	Treatment
Haemophilus ducreyi (chancroid)	Anal pain	Anorectal abscesses and ulcers	Culture, Gram stain with 'school of fish' pattern, PCR	Azithromycin 1 g p.o. × one dose OR Ceftriaxone 250 mg i.m. × one dose OR Ciprofloxacin 500 mg p.o. twice daily × 3 days* OR Erythromycin 500 mg p.o. three times daily × 7 days
Neisseria gonorrhoeae (gonorrhoea)	Rectal discharge	Proctitis, mucopurulent discharge	Culture of discharge on Thayer–Martin or Modified New York City agar	Ceftriaxone 250 mg i.m. × one dose PLUS Treatment for *Chlamydia* if chlamydial infection is not ruled out **Alternative regimen** Spectinomycin 2 g i.m. × one dose
Calymmatobacterium granulomatis (granuloma inguinale)	Perianal mass, ulceration	Hard, shiny perianal masses	Smear or biopsy of mass or ulceration	Doxycycline 100 mg p.o. twice daily for at least 3 weeks* OR Azithromycin 1 g p.o. once weekly for at least 3 weeks* OR Ciprofloxicin 750 mg p.o. twice daily for at least 3 weeks* OR Erythromycin 500 mg p.o. four times daily for at least 3 weeks* OR Bactrim (trimethoprim-sulfamethoxazole) DS 160 mg/800 mg p.o. twice daily for at least 3 weeks* *Or Until all lesions have healed
Treponema pallidum (syphilis)	**Primary syphilis** Painful anal chancre, inguinal lymphadenopathy, lesions infected with spirochetes *Secondary syphilis* Condyloma lata, foul discharge, lesions infected with spirochetes **Tertiary syphilis** Rectal gumma, tabes dorsalis, severe perianal pain, paralysis of anal sphincters	See text	Dark-field microscopy of ulcer scrapings, immunostaining from biopsy, serology	**Treatment of primary and secondary syphilis** Benzathine penicillin G 2.4 million units i.m. × one dose **Early latent syphilis** Benzathine penicillin G 2.4 million units i.m. × one dose **Late latent syphilis** Benzathine penicillin G 7.2 million units administered as 3 doses of 2.4 million units at 1-week intervals **Tertiary syphilis** 7.2 million units administered as 3 doses of 2.4 million units at 1-week intervals

---

cavity contributes to stool and pus trapping, which may explain the severity of pain. Biopsy can exclude other treatable infective aetiologies.

> ✓ Treatment consists of debridement, unroofing and intralesional steroid injection (80–160 mg methylprednisolone acetate in 1 mL of 0.25% bupivacaine). The goal is pain relief, as ulcer healing is uncommon.[6,7]

Herpes simplex virus

Herpes simplex is a DNA virus of the Herpesviridae family that includes varicella zoster, Epstein–Barr and cytomegalovirus. Herpes simplex virus (HSV) is the most prevalent viral STD in the USA. Two serotypes exist. HSV-1 is usually associated with oral, labial or ocular lesions, but with increasing oral–genital contact the rate of HSV-1 genital infections has increased, accounting for 30% of genital infections.[8] HSV-1 also accounts for up to 13% of anorectal herpes infections. HSV-2 is more typically responsible for anogenital infections from direct anogenital contact, accounting for almost 90% of such infections.[9] The overall seroprevalence rate for HSV-2 is 10% in the UK and is estimated to be present in 20% of the general population in the USA.[9] A substantial percentage of MSM are HSV-2 seropositive and up to one-third of MSM with rectal symptoms are HSV-2 culture positive.[10] Recurrence and subclinical shedding is more frequent for genital HSV-2 infection. HSV infection increases the risk of acquiring and transmitting HIV threefold, and immunocompromised patients have a higher rate of recurrence and may have prolonged viral shedding.[11]

Transmission of HSV occurs by close contact with an individual shedding the virus. Direct inoculation may occur during anal receptive intercourse when the virus penetrates the mucosa or a break in the skin. The virus replicates within epithelial cells, resulting in cell death. Infection presents 4–21 days after inoculation with small painful vesicles (**Fig. 16.1**) affecting the perianal skin and anus with burning and pruritus, and may cause systemic symptoms such as fever, headache and myalgia. Patients may complain of mucoid or bloody faeces, tenesmus, constipation, and occasionally have inguinal lymphadenopathy.[12]

These herpetic lesions may manifest over the entire anogenital area and eventually ulcerate and coalesce. The vesicles and ulcers last for 2–3 weeks

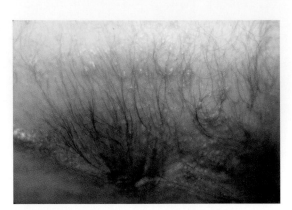

Figure 16.1 • Herpetic vesicles. Courtesy of L. Gottesman, MD.

and patients are highly contagious from their appearance until re-epithelialisation is complete. Secondary infection can occur, and often patients are treated with antibiotics as well as antivirals. Rectal involvement results in painful proctitis that on sigmoidoscopy demonstrates friable mucosa, diffuse ulcerations and occasionally intact vesicles or pustules affecting the distal 10 cm of the rectum.

Diagnosis is confirmed by viral culture or polymerase chain reaction (PCR) of ulcer swabs. Viral culture has a sensitivity of 50%, whereas PCR assays are more sensitive and specific.[13] The limiting factor for PCR as a primary diagnostic tool is cost, though several HSV serology tests are available with specificity and sensitivity greater than 90%.[3]

Symptomatic resolution of acute infection is frequently followed by a chronic relapsing course since the viral genome is maintained within the host nuclei. Prodromal symptoms of itching, burning or tingling can occur, followed by appearance of lesions that are usually in the same dermatomal distribution as the initial infection since HSV remains latent in the sensory ganglia of nerves innervating the infection site. Sacral paraethesias and perianal and buttock pain can precede recurrence of vesicles by several days.[14]

A sacral radiculitis can develop and last longer than the clinical infection. Symptoms include urinary retention, constipation, erectile dysfunction, paraesthesias and lower extremity weakness. Magnetic resonance imaging (MRI) reveals oedema of the spinal cord or roots and PCR of cerebrospinal fluid may aid diagnosis.[15]

Treatment is directed at two areas. The first is to provide symptomatic relief with measures such as analgesics, cool compresses, lidocaine oint-ment, sitz baths, etc. Hygiene is important to prevent bacterial superinfection. The second con-cern is direct antiviral treatment of patients with severe active infections and those with frequent reinfections.

> ✅✅ Antiviral therapy shortens the length of symptoms and decreases the time of infectivity. Pharmacotherapy of the initial presentation and of episodic recurrences of herpes proctitis or perianal ulcerations is with oral aciclovir for 7–10 days.[16]

Other antiviral agents such as valaciclovir and famciclovir that are used for genital herpes are probably effective for anorectal herpes, but evidence is lacking.[3] If a patient has severe mucocutaneous HSV infection and cannot tolerate oral medications, intravenous aciclovir should be administered. While this reduces the duration and severity of symptoms, it does not eradicate HSV or prevent recurrence or asymptomatic viral shedding.

Following initial infection and resolution most patients experience recurrences that tend to be shorter and milder than the initial episode and decrease in frequency. Viral shedding may occur during the prodrome, with active lesions, or in the asymptomatic.[17]

> ✅✅ Recurrent episodes should be treated with oral antivirals, though patients who experience several recurrences per year should have suppressive treatment.[18]

Rarely, perianal herpes (usually HSV-2) presents atypically with ulcerated, verrucous or vegeta-tive tumour-like masses that develop over a year. Biopsies reveal mild epithelial hyperplasia and ex-tensive and dense inflammation.[19]

Atypical herpes usually affects HIV-positive in-dividuals with a history of recurrent anogenital herpes. It frequently results in delayed diagnosis and/or unnecessary therapy, and a high level of suspicion is necessary. Diagnosis is confirmed with biopsy and immunohistochemical stain and/or viral culture.[20]

Treatment ranges from prolonged and high-dose antiviral therapy to excision. Surgery avoids po-tential toxicity from systemic agents, and exci-sion may be considered for refractory lesions. Additionally, the high likelihood of recurrence in

immunocompromised patients requires mainte-nance therapy with antiviral agents in addition to HAART.

The comprehensive treatment of HSV also in-cludes patient counselling on the risks of transmis-sion even in the absence of symptoms. Suppressive therapy does not eliminate latent infection and viral shedding. Abstinence is recommended while lesions are present and condoms are advised, although they provide incomplete protection. An HSV-2 vaccine has shown disappointing results.

Human papillomavirus

Human papillomaviruses (HPVs), which are small DNA viruses, cause benign and malignant changes to the epithelium of the anorectum and genitalia. It is likely the commonest STD worldwide, with an estimated incidence of over 6.2 million cases annu-ally in the USA.[21]

There are over 120 types of HPV and approxi-mately half are capable of anogenital infection.[22] Infections may remain subclinical or be active and induce benign, hyperproliferative lesions of the epi-thelia, called warts, papillomas, or condylomata.

The α-papillomavirus group of HPV types (com-prising 15 species distinguished to date) are those that typically infect the anogenital tract. These mucosotropic HPVs are further classified into non-oncogenic or low-risk (LR) types, such as HPV-6 and HPV-11, and potentially oncogenic or high-risk (HR) viruses, including HPV-16, HPV-18, HPV-51 and HPV-53. Lesions induced by the oncogenic types can progress to high-grade dysplasias and cancers. In contrast, the LR HPV-6 and HPV-11 are rarely found in anogenital cancers.[22]

The natural host tissue for the infection cycle of all HPVs is the squamous epithelium lining of body openings. A band of rapidly cycling and di-viding keratinocytes called the transformation zone establishes a squamo-columnar junction at each body opening.[22] Because this zone is particularly susceptible to papillomavirus infection, if the in-fecting strain is an HR genotype there is a risk of dysplasia and even progression to carcinoma. The ability to destabilise the tumour suppressors p53 and pRB, as well as other cellular proteins, is what largely accounts for the oncogenic potential of the HR HPVs.[22]

HPV infects the squamous epithelium when basal or parabasal cells are exposed by wounding and come into contact with infected skin, mucosa or fluid. Additionally, wounding of an infected surface may cause desquamation, releasing HPV virions and causing more infection. Transmission occurs most commonly via sexual contact with infected individuals, although perianal and genital involvement can occur without anal intercourse via skin-to-skin or skin-to-mucosa contact.[23]

Infection can be clinically silent or result in bleeding, pruritus, pain, wetness and/or the feeling of a lump. The lesions can range in appearance from a single, pinkish-white lesion, to multiple large cauliflower-like masses (**Fig. 16.2**).

✔ Diagnosis is primarily made on physical exam; anoscopy is necessary for complete evaluation because involvement within the anal canal can occur, although lesions above the dentate line are rare. Because associated genital lesions are common, patients with anal condyloma should undergo thorough physical examination, including a vaginal exam and Pap smear in women. Anal canal lesions that are missed on simple visual inspection with anoscopy can be detected with 5% aqueous acetic acid; regions of active HPV mucosal infection briefly turn cloudy white ('aceto-whitening'). Colposcopy of the anus (high-resolution anoscopy) can be used with acetic acid and Lugol's iodine to assess the presence of anal dysplasia and identify high-grade dysplasia from benign condyloma.

Lesions that are confused with anal condylomata include condyloma lata (syphilis), molluscum contagiosum and hypertrophied anal papillae. Histopathology will confirm the diagnosis. The goal of treatment is to destroy all visible disease while minimising morbidity. Because only gross lesions are treated, virus will remain in adjacent epithelium and can lead to recurrence.

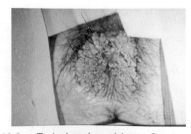

Figure 16.2 • Typical anal condyloma. Courtesy of L. Gottesman, MD.

✔ For small (1–3 mm) external and accessible lesions on the perianal skin, a topical patient-applied agent such as podofilox, imiquimod, cidofovir or green-tea extract (sinecatechins) is first-line therapy, although all have shown substantial failure and recurrence rates. The patient needs to be compliant and able to identify and reach all lesions. Patient-applied topical therapies are approved for external lesions only. If one type of topical therapy fails, another may be initiated.[3]

Podophyllin is a non-standardised resin from the may-apple plant (*Podophyllum peltatum*) that is cytotoxic. A 15–25% solution is applied once or twice weekly and washed off 4 hours later. It is not intended for use in the anal canal. Concerns about systemic side-effects when applied to larger lesions and inferior efficacy compared to podophyllotoxin have led experts to no longer recommend its use.[24]

Podofilox (podophyllotoxin) is the purified active antimitotic compound from *Podophyllum* spp., which is available as 0.5% solution or 0.15% cream. Both have demonstrated clinical superiority to podophyllin.[25] Podophyllotoxin can be self-administered twice daily for 3 days, followed by 4 days off, repeated for four cycles. The total volume used per day should not exceed 0.5 mL.[3] Resolution of warts has been reported in 20–50%, with recurrence rates of almost 50% at 1 year.[26] Ulceration occurs in 10–20% but other side-effects can occur if it is applied to areas greater than 10 cm² or to skin surfaces that allow systemic absorption, such as the mucosal surface of the anal canal.[27]

Imiquimod (Aldara) is an immune response modifier that induces α-interferon, tumour necrosis factor-α and other cytokines. It has the potential to eradicate HPV from mucocutaneous surfaces adjacent to gross lesions following excision/destruction; 5% cream is applied nightly three times a week and washed off after 8 hours. This can be continued for up to 16 weeks. Local skin reactions are common but only about 5% of patients cease treatment because of them. Complete resolution of external lesions occurs in over 50% and additional patients experience a substantial reduction of wart volume.[28,29] Recurrence rates have been reported to be between 19% and 23% at 3–6 months.[30] This agent is emerging as a safe, effective topical treatment, even in HIV-positive patients.

✅ Imiquimod can be used as initial treatment with electrodessication reserved for an incomplete response, although the authors use imiquimod to treat early recurrences after surgical treatment, or as adjuvant treatment after surgery in patients who have a tendency for recurrence.[30]

Cidofovir 1% gel is an acyclic nucleoside phosphonate with broad-spectrum antiviral activity. It has activity against vulval, vaginal and perianal intraepithelial neoplasia. When used for up to 6 weeks it has been shown to be more effective than electrosurgery in the treatment of anogenital warts in HIV-positive patients.[31] Cidofovir alone cleared all low-risk HPV and 57% of high-risk HPV, with a 35% relapse rate compared with 74% in the surgery-alone group at 6 months, although combined electrocautery and cidofovir gave the best results (100% complete response). While these studies are of great interest, the follow-up is short.[32]

A newer treatment for HPV is sinecatechin (Polyphenon E) ointment, a mixture of polyphenols from green-tea extracts, which has an antioxidative, anti-inflammatory and anti-cancer effect. Three trials have demonstrated eradication of anogenital warts in over 50% of patients using Polyphenon E ointment versus 35.4% using placebo. This ointment seems to be better tolerated than imiquimod. It is for external lesions only, and is applied by patients three times daily, for 16 weeks.[3] Sinecatechins are not recommended for immunocompromised patients or patients with genital herpes.[3]

Lesions inside the anal canal require provider-administered therapies including trichloracetic acid, cryotherapy and surgery. Trichloracetic acid as a 60–90% solution can be applied directly to perianal and anal canal lesions. Destruction of the lesion is by protein coagulation with tissue sloughing, so adjacent skin should be protected or cleaned immediately. Care is taken to apply the solution only on the warts and allow the solution to dry before the patient moves. It is applied weekly and numerous treatments are usually required. It is best reserved for lesions that are small (1–4 mm) and few. Multiple lesions can be treated simultaneously. The recurrence rate is about 25%.[33]

Cryotherapy is listed in the Centers for Disease Control (CDC) treatment guideline for anal warts.[3] Freeze–thaw cycles can be produced with a cryoprobe, application of liquid nitrogen with a cotton-tipped applicator or with aerosolised liquid nitrogen. The procedure is inexact and it is difficult to gauge depth of tissue destruction. Painful local reaction is common, and some may experience ulceration and foul-smelling discharge. The provider can repeat treatment of the warts every 1–2 weeks until the lesion has resolved. Studies have found the success rate to be about 75%, with a recurrence rate as high as 25–39%.[34]

Tangential excision or fulguration of small internal and external lesions (smaller than 5 mm) can be performed in the office with local anaesthetic after a circumferential anal block. Larger and broad-based lesions, which would require excision of a substantial portion of perianal skin, are treated by electrodessication, usually with a spinal anaesthetic, local anaesthetic, deep sedation or a combination thereof. The superficial-most layer of the condyloma is fulgurated with the cautery tip until it takes on a grey–white appearance. This is followed by curettage or simply abrading the fulgurated tissue with forceps or gauze. Treatment is repeated until the condylomata are completely removed without burning into the deep dermis. Pedunculated warts can be transected at their base. Tissue from HIV-positive patients, flat, recurrent or suspicious lesions that may be ulcerated, friable or hypervascular should be sent for histopathology, and it may be useful to send tissue for HPV typing too. Daily wound care with soap and water is usually adequate; however, in the USA mupirocin or sulfadiazine is given if evidence of infection develops.

✅✅ Compared to patient-applied and provider-applied therapies, surgical excision has the greatest success in treating anal condyloma, with clearance rates of 71–93%, and recurrence rates between 4% and 29%.[35,36]

Laser destruction has been advocated as less painful and associated with fewer recurrences than other destructive techniques. No prospective, randomised data support these claims. A risk of laser is the problem of aerosolised viral particles in the plume. Viable viral particles have been recovered from this smoke and cases of medical providers developing condylomata in their respiratory tract after using a laser to treat warts have been reported. Masks and smoke evacuators are recommended. Transmission of viral particles appears to be less of a problem with the larger-particle smoke from electrocautery. Finally, the laser is vastly more expensive than electrocautery and requires special training.

Intralesional interferon-α (IFN-α) has been used with good results in recurrent condyloma or condyloma that have been resistant to other therapy. It is administered as an injection of 1×10^6 IU under a maximum of five lesions, three times a week for 3–8 weeks.[32] IFN-α blocks viral reproduction and is an integral part of natural antiviral defences. Efficacy as primary treatment is no better than other modalities and systemic side-effects such as fever, myalgia, headache and leucopenia occur. When IFN-α is used in combination with surgery for resistant anal condyloma the recurrence rate is 12% at 4 months, compared with a 39% recurrence in a placebo group.[37,38]

Vaccination against HPV (Gardisil) was approved in the USA in 2006. The evidence for its use in preventing cervical intraepithelial neoplasia and cervical malignancies as part of a population immunisation programme is well established. The quadrivalent vaccine (against HPV-6, -11, -16 and -18) is delivered through a series of three intramuscular injections. Currently, the CDC recommends routine administration of the vaccine to girls and women from ages 9 to 26.[39] The vaccine has also shown efficacy against anogenital warts in Phase II/III trials. In a recent randomised trial performed on over 4000 healthy males aged 16–26, it was demonstrated to prevent infection with HPV-6, -11, -16 and -18 and the development of related external genital lesions with an efficacy of 65.5%.[40] A newer study has shown that the quadrivalent HPV vaccine is effective in preventing anal intraepithelial neoplasia (AIN) among MSM, although the study was limited to those who were HIV negative at enrolment.[41] Clarification of some uncertainties, notably vaccine efficacy in men and HIV-infected individuals, is required to establish the benefits of HPV vaccines for the prevention of malignant and premalignant anal lesions.[41] Although sexually active patients may have already been infected with one or more of the vaccine HPV serotypes, they may still derive partial benefit by getting vaccinated against those serotypes to which they have not yet been exposed.[42]

Immunotherapy with weekly injections of 0.5 mL of an autologous vaccine has been described,[43] with no adverse reactions. Disappearance of warts occurred in 84% of patients. Vaccine preparation and treatment time prevented this from more widespread use.

Buschke–Lowenstein tumour: giant anal condyloma

Buschke and Lowenstein described giant condyloma accuminata (GCA) in 1925 (**Fig. 16.3**). It is associated with low-risk HPV serotypes 6 and 11, but it does have histological differences from ordinary anal condyloma, such as marked papillomatosis, acanthosis, thickened rete ridges and increased mitotic activity. They have propensity for perianal fistula formation, infection and malignant transformation.[44] A large percentage of cases contain in situ or invasive squamous cell cancer. Wide local excision with a 1-cm margin is the treatment of choice. Local tissue flaps or grafted skin may be required. Disease within the anal canal but not invading the sphincters can be excised and the normal proximal mucosa can be brought down and tacked to the anoderm or anal sphincters similar to a rectal mucosal advancement flap. Temporary diversion may be needed for hygiene and wound healing. Abdominoperineal resection has been used for GCA if the anal sphincters are involved. Chemoradiation is an option, especially in those who are poor surgical candidates or when clear surgical margins are not attainable. Complete regression with chemoradiation has been reported.[45]

Molluscum contagiosum

Molluscum contagiosum is caused by a virus of the pox virus family and transmitted by direct contact.

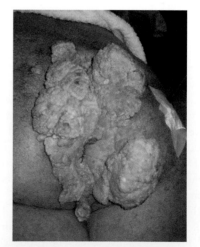

Figure 16.3 • Giant Buschke–Lowenstein tumour. Courtesy of N. Gandhi, MD.

It is a common cause of painless skin lesions at any site but can be spread to the anogenital region. The incubation period is 3–6 weeks, followed by the development of discrete 2–6 mm skin-coloured papules with central umbilication. Multiple lesions are common; however, immunocompromised patients can develop a severe form with hundreds of skin lesions. In immunocompetent patients, the papules often spontaneously resolve within 2–4 weeks. Although the diagnosis is clinical, biopsy and staining for molluscum bodies is recommended in patients with HIV as cutaneous cryptococcal infections appear.[46] Biopsy demonstrates enlarged epithelial cells with intracytoplasmic molluscum bodies.

While it is generally a self-limited disease, treatment can be used to prevent spread and for cosmetic purposes. Various treatments including curettage, cryotherapy, trichloracetic acid and electrocautery have been described but none have proven superior in trials.

Bacterial

Chlamydia trachomatis and *Lymphogranuloma venereum* (LGV)

Chlamydia trachomatis is the most frequently reported bacterial STD in western countries, and is the commonest in the USA, with an incidence of 1.2 million cases reported in 2008.[47] *Chlamydia* is an obligate intracellular bacterium that is sexually transmitted and can cause infections that resemble gonorrhoea. Anorectal transmission occurs primarily through anoreceptive intercourse, but can also occur via oral–anal transmission or as a late manifestation of a genital infection. Clinical syndromes resulting from chlamydial infection include cervicitis, pelvic inflammatory disease (PID), urethritis and proctitis.

Diagnosis is by culture, microimmunofluorescent antibody titres or PCR. The technique for transport of biopsies for culture is important and involves placing the biopsy in sucrose phosphate media on ice for immediate tissue culture inoculation. Recently, nucleic acid amplification tests (NAATs) have replaced *Chlamydia* cultures in most laboratories for endocervical and urethral specimens, and may become the test of choice in rectal specimens, as studies have suggested a sensitivity and specificity greater than 93% when comparing NAATs with culture.[3,48]

✅ In patients with a clinical presentation consistent with *Chlamydia* proctitis, a rectal Gram stain that shows polymorphonuclear leucocytes without visible gonococci can also make a presumptive diagnosis of *Chlamydia*.

Chlamydia has an incubation period of 5 days to 2 weeks and is broadly divided into two groups based on serotyping: non-LGV and LGV serotypes. Rectal infection with non-LGV serotypes (D–K) usually results in a milder form of proctitis, and some patients may be asymptomatic. Affected patients will experience non-specific symptoms of proctitis including tenesmus, urgency, bloody discharge and anorectal pain.

Infection with LGV serotypes (L1, L2, L3) has been endemic in the tropics, but in the past 5 years an increasing number of cases has been seen in western countries, almost exclusively in HIV-positive MSM.[49] In a recent study from the UK, 76% of patients diagnosed with LGV were also HIV positive.[50] Non-LGV serovar *Chlamydia* infection is limited to the mucosa and initial site of infection, whereas LGV serovars produce a lymphoproliferative reaction through direct extension from the primary infection site to draining lymph nodes. Areas of necrosis occur within the lymph nodes, which can then form abscesses, or a large matted mass with overlying erythema, mimicking syphilis. Small vesicles that become ulcerated are the initial signs of infection at the site of inoculation. After resolution of these an anogenitorectal syndrome occurs, with signs of systemic infection (fevers, myalgia) and a more aggressive infection involving the perianal, anal and rectal areas resulting in ulceration, rectal pain, discharge, bleeding and severe proctitis. On sigmoidoscopy, there is a severe, non-specific granular proctitis with mucosal erythema, friability and ulceration. Biopsies of the mucosa are consistent with infectious proctitis, including crypt abscesses, infectious granulomas and giant cells, and can be difficult to distinguish from Crohn's disease.[51] Long-term chronic inflammation from LGV results in stricture, fistulas, lymphoedema and in women can lead to the development of rectovaginal fistulas.

✅✅ Diagnosis is made by serotyping in patients determined to have *Chlamydia* by the methods listed above. Unfortunately, serotyping is neither rapid nor widely available. This has led to the recommendation to presumptively treat patients with anorectal *Chlamydia* who are at high risk of LGV (those with proctitis on proctoscopy, >10 white blood cells/high-power field on anorectal smear, or HIV positive).[52] Treatment is doxycycline for 3 weeks for LGV serotypes, with a shorter duration for non-LGV strains. Multiple other antibiotic regimens can be used for patients with allergies or resistant strains. Sexual contacts from the past 60 days should be treated, and patients should refrain from sexual activity for 7 days after completion of treatment. Because of the high co-infection rate of LGV and HIV in MSM, these patients should be tested for HIV and hepatitis C, as well as other STDs.

Chancroid

Haemophilus ducreyi is a Gram-negative coccobacillus that is a frequent cause of painful anogenital ulcerations in underdeveloped countries, but is uncommon in the USA and Western Europe, usually occurring in discrete outbreaks.[53] Transmission is via sexual intercourse, although some perianal ulcerations have developed in females without anal intercourse, occurring through breaks in the skin. Incubation is 4–10 days. Ulcers, which are frequently multiple, form hours to days after exposure, and present as infected, erythematous, tender papules, which turn into pustules that rupture and erode over days to weeks. In addition to ulceration, regional lymphadenopathy and bubo formation, frequently unilateral, may be noted. Buboes are fluctuant lymph nodes that arise 1–2 weeks after the primary ulcer. If left untreated, they can rupture and drain pus.

The definitive diagnosis of chancroid requires detection of *H. ducreyi* on Gram stain and culture. However, culture requires special laboratory techniques and at best is 80% sensitive. Gram stain is also unreliable (only 40–60% sensitive) and non-specific, but when detected these organisms clump into long parallel strands (a 'school of fish' pattern). PCR is more sensitive and is becoming more widely used at specialised labs.[54]

✔ The probable diagnosis of chancroid can be made in patients who have clinical findings suggestive of the disease, including painful ulcers and tender suppurative inguinal lymphadenopathy, plus negative tests for syphilis or other more common diseases. Patients should also be tested for HIV because of the high risk of co-infection.

Treatment consists of multiple antibiotic treatment regimens, including erythromycin, azithromycin, ceftriaxone or ciprofloxacin, with a combined 90–98% cure rate.[55] Fluctuant buboes associated with chancroid should be aspirated or incised and drained. If partners have had sexual contact with the patient within 10 days of presentation, they should be examined and treated as well.[3] Most patients will have symptomatic relief 48–72 hours after treatment is started and clinical improvement after 7 days.

Neisseria gonorrhoeae

Neisseria gonorrhoeae, a Gram-negative intracellular diplococcus, is the second most commonly reported infectious disease in the USA, but is likely the commonest bacterial STD involving the anorectum. It can infect the mucous lining of all body orifices with associated clinical syndromes consisting of urethritis, cervicitis, PID, pharyngitis, conjunctivitis and proctitis. Since 1997, the rate of gonorrhoea has plateaued, with 330 000–340 000 cases being reported in the USA yearly, although it is estimated that close to 700 000 people are infected annually.[47] The rates of gonorrhoea infection are highest for males and females in their teens and early twenties. The highest rate is among MSM and bisexual men, with 8% of this population having urethral swabs positive for gonorrhoea, most being asymptomatic.[47]

Transmission is by anal receptive intercourse; after an incubation period of 3 days to 2 weeks, proctitis or cryptitis results. In women it can also be spread by autoinoculation from gonococcal cervicitis. Oral–anal sex may be another route for the spread of anorectal gonococcal infection. Untreated infection can lead to disseminated gonorrhoea with symptoms of bacteraemia, arthritis (unilateral, migratory, purulent arthritis of large joints) or dermatitis.[14] Other rare consequences include endocarditis, pericarditis, meningitis or perihepatitis.

Symptoms of anorectal involvement include pruritus ani, bloody or mucoid discharge, tenesmus and anorectal pain. Mucopurulent discharge in combination with proctitis is the characteristic physical finding in gonococcal proctitis. On anoscopy, there is a thick, yellow mucopurulent discharge that can be expressed from anal crypts when pressure is applied. Even when the anal canal is spared, one may still see perianal erythema. The proctitis is non-specific and consists of oedema, friability and mucous discharge. While most genital gonococcal infections in men are symptomatic, a large percentage of patients who have positive cultures for rectal gonorrhoea will be asymptomatic – about 50% of males and 95% of females. Other causes of proctitis such as *Chlamydia trachomatis*, HSV and syphilis must also be excluded.

✔ Culture of the mucopurulent material is diagnostic, but lubricants other than water should be avoided during anoscopy as lubricant may introduce antibacterial agents and decrease diagnostic yield. If a lubricant has already been used prior to recognising an infection, multiple culture swabs should be taken. The diagnostic yield is highest when the mucopurulent discharge is swabbed under direct vision and immediately plated onto enriched medium. Culture is the 'gold standard' of diagnosis because it is easy to obtain and will allow antibiotic resistance testing. Gram staining from rectal samples has a low sensitivity but is rapid, inexpensive and highly specific.

Historically, penicillin G was the treatment of choice and was in widespread use until the 1970s, when penicillinase-producing *N. gonorrhoeae* emerged. More recently, high rates of quinolone-resistant *Neisseria gonorrhoeae* (QRNG) have been reported in Asia, the Pacific, the west coast of the USA and parts of Europe, including a rate of almost 10% in England and Wales.[3,56] Therefore, since 2007, the CDC no longer recommended quinolones for the treatment of gonorrhoea.[57] Obviously, local surveillance data will play an important role in therapeutic decisions. Cephalosporin resistance, particularly cefixime, has recently been reported, with the most current recommendation being a single intramuscular dose of ceftriaxone 250 mg plus treatment for chlamydia (i.e. azithromycin or doxycycline) as first-line therapy.[58] Alternative regimens include cefotaxime 500 mg i.m. or cefoxitin 2 g i.m. with probenecid 1 g orally. Spectinomycin can also be used.

✔ Because of the high rate of concomitant infection with *Chlamydia*, patients should be tested and treated for both infections at the same visit. As with all bacterial STDs, management of sexual partners is an integral part of decreasing disease spread and reinfection. Sexual partners from the past 60 days should be evaluated and treated, and patients should abstain from sexual activity until

treatment is completed and symptoms resolved. Routine testing after treatment is not indicated. Patients who remain symptomatic after treatment should undergo culture and antibiotic sensitivity testing for persistent infection, such as urethritis, cervicitis or proctitis.

Granuloma inguinale (Donovanosis)

Klebsiella granulomatis (formerly *Calymmatobacterium granulomatis*), a Gram-negative bacterium, is a rare cause of genital ulceration in western countries but is common in parts of Africa and South America. Transmission is mostly via sexual means but autoinoculation and faecal contamination may also play a role.[59]

Donovanosis is an ulcerating infection of the genitalia and anus. Initially, a firm papule appears and then ulcerates. Four morphological manifestations have been described, the commonest being the ulcerogranulomatous type marked by painless, fleshy and beefy-red ulcers. Less common types are hypertrophic or verrucous ulcers, necrotic ulcers, or the cicatricial or sclerotic form causing scarring without lymphadenopathy.[3] While genital involvement is the most common, anal involvement either alone or contiguous with the genitalia is seen (**Fig. 16.4**).

The diagnosis is made by tissue smear of a biopsy that reveals dark-staining Donovan bodies within macrophages. In endemic areas diagnosis may be made on clinical grounds alone. Treatment is with doxycycline for at least 3 weeks or Bactrim DS orally for 3 weeks or until all lesions have healed. An alternative is at least 3 weeks of ciprofloxacin, azithromycin or erythromycin, continued until all lesions have healed.[3]

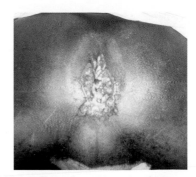

Figure 16.4 • Parianal granuloma inguinate.

Syphilis

Syphilis is a mucocutaneous STD caused by the spirochete *Treponema pallidum*. Recent surveillance suggests rates in the USA and UK are increasing, especially among MSM.[60,61] This is particularly concerning because syphilis facilitates HIV transmission and there is a high rate of HIV co-infection.[62] The incidence of syphilis previously peaked at 107 cases per 100 000 people in the USA in 1991, and decreased to 2.2 per 100 000 in 2001, when only 6103 cases were reported. However, since 2001, primary and secondary syphilis have risen, especially among men. In 2008, there were 13 500 cases.[3]

Syphilis can present in one of several progressive stages: primary (chancre or proctitis), secondary (condyloma lata) or tertiary (with involvement of the nervous and vascular systems). Anal syphilis occurs when the spirochete enters the anoderm and anal mucosa during anal receptive intercourse. The primary stage begins within 2–10 weeks of exposure with the appearance of an anal ulcer called a chancre. This is a raised, 1–2 cm lesion that begins as a small papule that progresses into an indurated, clean-based ulcer without exudates. Anal ulcers are frequently painful (in contrast to genital ulcers), they may be single or multiple, and can be located on the perianal skin, in the anal canal or in the distal rectum (**Fig. 16.5**). Differentiation from idiopathic anal fissure may be difficult. However, chancres are usually eccentrically located (off the midline), multiple and, if opposite each other, are known as 'kissing ulcers'. Painless but prominent lymphadenopathy is also common. If secondary bacterial infection occurs, patients can experience worsening anorectal pain. Rectal mucosal involvement results in tenesmus, rectal discharge or bleeding, though proctitis may occur with or without chancres.[45,63] Untreated lesions usually heal in 2–4 weeks.

If primary syphilis is untreated, haematogenous spread occurs 4–10 weeks after the primary lesions and leads to secondary syphilis. This presents with systemic symptoms including fever, malaise, arthralgia, weight loss, sore throat and headache, and as a non-pruritic macular rash on the trunk, limbs, palms and/or soles. Condyloma lata, a grey or whitish wart-like lesion teeming with spirochetes, may be found near the initial chancre. These lesions are moister and smoother than anal condyloma from HPV, are pruritic and have a foul discharge. Mucosal patches or ulcerations may appear in the rectum.[64] As with primary infection, this stage resolves after 3–12 weeks. About one-quarter of untreated patients relapse in the first year, termed early latent syphilis. Concomitant HIV infection may lead to more severe symptoms that take longer to resolve. Untreated for years, the tertiary stage can develop.

Tertiary syphilis is rare, but can present with the formation of chronic gummas, which are soft, tumour-like balls of inflammatory tissue surrounded by granulation tissue, which vary considerably in size. They typically affect the skin, bone and liver, but can occur anywhere, including the rectum, where a gumma can be confused with malignancy. Cardiac manifestations such as aortitis can occur. Patients may also develop tabes dorsalis, which causes severe perianal pain and functional problems due to paralysis of the anal sphincters.[14]

Treponema pallidum cannot be cultured. Darkfield microscopy of scrapings from chancres or lymph nodes is useful for diagnosis. The presence of commensal spirochetes in the rectum decreases the accuracy of dark-field microscopy. Specific immunofluorescent or silver staining of biopsy specimens can also diagnose *T. pallidum*.

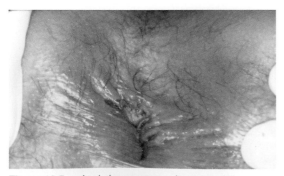

Figure 16.5 • Anal chancre secondary to syphilis. Courtesy of L. Gottesman, MD.

✓✓ Serology is useful and typically a two-stage process. The first is a non-treponemal test, which if positive is followed by a treponemal test. Non-treponemal tests are not specific for *T. pallidum* and include Venereal Disease Research Laboratory (VDRL) and rapid plasma reagin (RPR). Positive non-treponemal tests should be confirmed by a treponemal test, such as the enzyme immunoassay (EIA), the *T. pallidum* particle assay (TPPA) or the fluorescent treponemal antibody absorption test (FTA-ABS), which remains positive for life. EIA and TPPA can be used jointly as confirmatory tests. Qualitative VDRL/RPR assesses an appropriate response to treatment. PCR is available in some speciality labs.[65–67]

Primary and secondary syphilis are treated with benzathine penicillin G, 2.4 million units as a single intramuscular injection. Alternative regimens include doxycycline 100 mg orally twice a day for 2 weeks, and tetracycline 500 mg orally given four times a day for 2 weeks. Recommendations to sexual partners depend on the stage of diagnosis of the index case. In general, any sexual contact within 90 days of diagnosis is treated presumptively. Any sexual partners for the past 6 months are considered at risk for patients with secondary syphilis and those for the past year for early latent syphilis.[45] Follow-up RPR or VDRL confirming eradication of disease is performed at 6 months for HIV-negative patients and at 3 months for HIV-positive patients. Treatment failures are treated with 2.4 million units of penicillin at weekly intervals for a total of 3 weeks.

Empirical treatment

Several factors have led some authors to recommend treatment of STDs based on the clinical presenting syndrome: (1) point-of-care testing is not widely available for the pathogens discussed above; (2) the two common presenting complaints (proctitis or genital ulceration) are not specific to a particular organism; and (3) infection with multiple organisms is common. The approach to a patient with a presumed anorectal STD must be organised and standardised. Patients with proctitis or anogenital ulcers in whom an STD is suspected should undergo a thorough history and physical examination. Key pieces of information include the patient's symptoms, their onset and duration, and sexual history, including prior STDs, HIV status and any high-risk behaviours (multiple sexual partners, unprotected sex, illicit drug use). Recent travel history is also important to help exclude other infectious causes.

Physical exam must include inspection of the perianal skin, noting any masses, ulcers, abrasions, vesicles or fissures, and palpation for inguinal lymphadenopathy. Examiners should observe universal precautions. The base of the ulcers and vesicles and/or the anal canal should be gently swabbed circumferentially with laboratory-specific bacterial and viral culture swabs and sent to the microbiology lab for routine Gram stain and culture, and tested for all the common pathogens. Any mucopurulent or bloody drainage from the anus should be noted and cultured prior to digital rectal exam and anoscopy, as lubrication is bacteriostatic and may lower the yield of organisms on culture swabs.

Next, gentle digital rectal exam and anoscopy should be performed, again using water as the preferred lubricant. If the patient cannot tolerate this due to discomfort, lubrication jelly and anaesthetic cream may be used. The clinician should palpate the anal canal for masses, ulcers or fluctuance. This should be followed by anoscopy or rigid proctoscopy, again using water as the preferred lubricant, which will allow for better evaluation of the anorectal mucosa and any intra-anal lesions. Additional cultures can be obtained from the proximal anal canal and rectum if there is evidence of mucopurulent discharge. If the patient is too tender to be examined in the office, an exam under anaesthesia should be performed, with collection of both bacterial and viral cultures from external or internal lesions. If there are any masses or ulcers on the perianal skin or within the anal canal, these can be biopsied.

> ✔ It is rational to treat empirically for proctitis caused by gonorrhoea and *Chlamydia* (e.g. ceftriaxone and doxycycline) in these patients if anorectal exudate is noted or if polymorphonuclear leucocytes are seen on Gram stain. Additional treatment is determined by the results of testing for specific organisms, and once culture and laboratory results return, the antibiotic regimen can be tailored appropriately for the actual diagnosis.[3] The patient does not have to wait for treatment while a diagnosis is being made, and the possible transmission of an anogenital STD to another individual is limited.

Likewise, empirical management of ulcerative or vesicular anogenital diseases, even in the presence of HIV, can be successful. Again, thorough physical examination and appropriate testing for the most common causative organisms are performed, and empirical therapy should be initiated as well.[68]

Lastly, part of the complete treatment of STDs includes educating the patient as to the mode of transmission and on ways to avoid reinfection and the use of protection. This frequently includes treatment and counselling of sexual partners.

Key points

- Sexually transmitted diseases are common and increasing in frequency.
- A high index of suspicion and knowledge of lesions is required, and an appropriate sexual history is important in diagnosing these conditions.
- Empirical treatment of the most likely pathogen based on symptoms and examination is suggested.
- Patients and their partners must be treated.
- Excision has produced the best results for anal condylomata but imiquimod has shown promise.
- Quinolone-resistant *Neisseria gonorrhoeae* is becoming more common.
- Review of current testing and treatment recommendations is suggested when managing uncommon sexually transmitted infections.

References

1. Centers for Disease Control and Prevention (CDC). Increases in unsafe sex and rectal gonorrhea among men who have sex with men, San Francisco, California, 1994–1997. Morbidity Mortality Weekly Report (MMWR), 29 January 1999: Platinum Periodicals, ProQuest Web, 10 March 2010.

2. Fleming DT, Wasserheit JN. From epidemiological synergy to public health policy and practice: the contribution of other sexually transmitted diseases to sexual transmission of HIV infection. Sex Transm Infect 1999;75:3–17.

3. Centers for Disease Control and Prevention. Sexually transmitted diseases treatment guidelines. MMWR 2010;59(RR-121).

4. Centers for Disease Control. 1993 revised classification system for HIV infection and expanded surveillance case definition for AIDS among adolescents and adults. MMWR 1992;41(RR-17):1–19.

5. Moore BA, Fleshner PR. Rubber band ligation for hemorrhoidal disease can be safely performed in select HIV-positive patients. Dis Colon Rectum 2001;44:1079–82.

6. Brar HS, Gottesman L, Surawicz C. Anorectal pathology in AIDS. Gastrointest Endosc Clin N Am 1998;8:913–31.

7. Modesto VL, Gottesman L. Surgical debridement and intralesional steroid injection in the treatment of idiopathic AIDS-related anal ulcerations. Am J Surg 1997;174:439–41.

8. Edwards S, Carne C. Department of Health and Human Services, November 2009. Oral sex and the transmission of viral STIs. Sex Transm Infect 1998;74:6–10.

9. Jones DJ, Goorney BP. Sexually transmitted diseases and anal papillomas. Br Med J 1992;305:820–3.

10. Krone MR, Wald A, Tabet SR. Herpes simplex virus type 2 shedding in human immunodeficiency virus-negative men who have sex with men: frequency, patterns, and risk factors. Clin Infect Dis 2000;30:261–7.

11. Foley E. Treatment of genital herpes infections in HIV-infected patients. J HIV Ther 2004;9:14.

12. Goodell SE, Quinn TC, Mkritchian EE, et al. Herpes simplex virus: an important cause of acute proctitis in homosexual men (abstr). Gastroenterology 1981;80:1159.

13. Strick LB, Wald A. Diagnostics for herpes simplex virus: is PCR the new gold standard? Mol Diagn Ther 2006;10:17.

14. Wexner S. Sexually transmitted disease of the colon, rectum, and anus. The challenge of the nineties. Dis Colon Rectum 1990;33(12):1048–62.

15. Eberhardt O, Kuber W, Dichgans J, et al. HSV-2 sacral radiculitis (Elsberg syndrome). Neurology 2004;63:758–9.

16. Rompalo A, Mertz G, Davis G. Oral acyclovir for treatment of first episode herpes simplex virus proctitis. JAMA 1988;259:2879–81.
   A randomised controlled trial of oral aciclovir 400 mg five times per day versus placebo. The aciclovir group had significantly shorter duration of symptoms and viral excretion than those in the placebo group.

17. Kimberlin DW, Rouse DJ. Genital herpes. N Engl J Med 2004;350:1970–7.

18. Corey L, Wald A, Patel R. Once-daily valacyclovir to reduce the risk of transmission of genital herpes. N Engl J Med 2004;350:11–20.
   Oral valaciclovir taken by immunocompetent persons with recurrent genital HSV-2 infection significantly reduces the rates of HSV reactivation, subclinical shedding and transmission of genital herpes to a susceptible partner. A 500-mg dose of valaciclovir taken once daily reduced the risks by at least 50% in the acquisition of symptomatic genital herpes and acquisition of HSV-2 infection overall by susceptible, HSV-2-seronegative heterosexual partners when compared to placebo.

19. Chung V, Parker D. Surgical excision for vegetative herpes simplex virus infection. Dermatol Surg 2007;33:1374–9.

20. Nadal SR, Calore EE, Manzione CR, et al. Hypertrophic herpes simplex simulating anal neoplasia in AIDs patients: report of five cases. Dis Colon Rectum 2005;48:2289–93.

21. Weinstock H, Berman S, Cates Jr W. Sexually transmitted diseases among American youth: incidence and prevalence estimates, 2000. Perspect Sex Reprod Health 2004;36(1):6–10.

22. Chow LT, Broker TR, Steinberg BM. The natural history of human papillomavirus infections of the mucosal epithelia. APMIS 2010;118:422–49.

23. Hernandez BY, McDuffe K, Zhu X, et al. Anal human papillomavirus infection in women and its relationship with cervical infection. Cancer Epidemiol Biomarkers Prev 2005;14:2550–6.

24. von Krogh G, Longstaff E. Podophyllin office therapy against condyloma should be abandoned. Sex Transm Infect 2001;77:409–12.

25. Lacey CJ, Goodall RL, Tennvall GR, et al. Randomised controlled trial and economic evaluation of podophyllotoxin solution, podophyllotoxin cream, and podophyllin in the treatment of genital warts. Sex Transm Infect 2003;79:270–5.

26. Congilosi S, Madoff R. Current therapy for recurrent and extensive anal warts. Dis Colon Rectum 1995;38:1101–7.

27. Scheinfeld N, Lehman D. An evidence-based review of medical and surgical treatments of genital warts. Dermatol Online J 2006;12(3):5.

28. Beutner KR, Tyring SK, Tofatter KF, et al. Imiquimod, a patient-applied immune-response modifier for treatment of genital warts. Antimicrob Agents Chemother 1998;42:789–94.

29. Maitland JE, Maw R. An audit of patients who have received imiquimod cream 5% for the treatment of anogenital warts. Int J STD AIDS 2000;11:268–70.

30. Diamantis ML, Bartlett BL, Tyring SK. Safety, efficacy and recurrence rates of imiquimod cream 5% for treatment of anogenital warts. Skin Ther Lett 2009; 14(5)1–3, 5.

31. Scholefield JH, Harris D, Radcliffe A. Guidelines for management of anal intraepithelial neoplasia. Colorectal Dis 2011;13:3–10.

32. Trizna Z, Evans T, Bruce S, et al. A randomized Phase II study comparing four different interferon therapies in patients with recalcitrant condylomata acuminata. Sex Transm Dis 1998;25(7):361–5.

33. Swerdlow DB, Salvati EP. Condyloma acuminatum. Dis Colon Rectum 1971;14:226–9.

34. Beutner KR, Fernczy A. Therapeutic approaches to genital warts. Am J Med 1997;102(5A):28–37.

35. Jensen SL. Comparison of podophyllin application with simple surgical excision in clearance and recurrence of perianal condylomata acuminata. Lancet 1985;2:1146–8.

36. Beck DE, Jaso RG, Zajac RA. Surgical management of anal condylomata in the HIV-positive patient. Dis Colon Rectum 1990;33:180–3.
The recurrence rate for anal condylomata ranges from 26% to 43% after local treatment with podophyllin and from 4% to 29% after fulguration and excision, with few operative complications. Patients with HIV have been proven to tolerate surgical therapy with little added morbidity.

37. Baron S, Tyring SK, Fleischmann WR, et al. The interferons: mechanisms of actions and clinical applications. JAMA 1991;266:1375–83.

38. Fleshner PR, Freilich MI. Adjuvant interferon for anal condyloma: a prospective, randomized trial. Dis Colon Rectum 1994;37:1255–9.

39. CDC Media Relations. Media advisory: CDC's advisory committee recommends human papillomavirus vaccination. http://www.cdc.gov/media/pressrel/r060629.htm; 29 June 2006 [accessed 10.09.12].

40. Giuliano A, Palefsky J, Goldstone S, et al. Efficacy of quadrivalent HPV vaccine against HPV infection and disease in males. N Engl J Med 2011;364:401–11.

41. Palefsky J. Efficacy of the quadrivaent HPV vaccine to prevent anal intraepithelial neoplasia among young men who have sex with men. In: Proccedings of the 26th International Papillomavirus Conference. Montreal, 3–8 July2010, Abstract.

42. Markowitz L, Dunne E, Sariya M. Quadrivalent human papillomavirus vaccine: recommendations of the Advisory Committee on Immunization Practices (ACIP). MMWR 2007;56(RR02):1–24.

43. Abcarian H, Sharon N. Long-term effectiveness of the immunotherapy of anal condyloma acuminatum. Dis Colon Rectum 1982;25:648–51.

44. Yakan S, Cengiz F, et al. Rectal involvement of recurrent Buschke–Lowenstein tumor causing subileus: a case report. Gastroenterol Res 2011;4(4):177–9.

45. Beck D. The ASCRS textbook of colon and rectal surgery. 2nd ed. Springer Science and Business Media, LLC; 2011.

46. Murakawa GJ, Kerschmann R, Berger T. Cutaneous Cryptococcus infection and AIDS. Arch Dermatol 1996;132(5):545–8.

47. Centers for Disease Control, Prevention. Sexually transmitted disease surveillance, 2008. Atlanta, GA: US Department of Health and Human Services; November 2009.

48. Schachter J, Moncada J, Liska S, et al. Nucleic acid amplification tests in the diagnosis of chlamydial and gonococcal infections of the oropharynx and rectum in men who have sex with men. Sex Transm Dis 2008;35:637f.

49. White JA. Manifestations and management of Lymphogranuloma venereum. Curr Opin Infect Dis 2009;22:57–66.

50. Ward H, Martin I, Macdonald N, et al. Lymphogranuloma venereum in the United Kingdom. Clin Infect Dis 2007;44:26–32.

51. Martin IM, Alexander SA, Ison CA, et al. Diagnosis of Lymphogranuloma venereum from biopsy samples. Gut 2006;55:1522–3.

52. Van der Bij AK, Spaargearn J, Morre SA, et al. Diagnostic and clinical implications of anorectal Lymphogranuloma venereum in men who have sex

with men: a retrospective case–control study. Clin Infect Dis 2006;42:186–94.

> Use of proctoscopic findings and elevated white blood cell counts in anorectal smear specimens in addition to HIV infection status provided the highest diagnostic accuracy (in identifying the MSM who are most likely to have anorectal LGV results) with an overall sensitivity of 89% and specificity of 94%.

53. Marrazzo JM, Handsfield HH. Chancroid: new developments in an old disease. In: Remington JS, Swartz MN, editors. Current clinical topics in infectious diseases. Cambridge, MA: Blackwell Science; 1995. p. 129.

54. Alfa M. The laboratory diagnosis of *Haemophilus ducreyi*. Can J Infect Dis Med Microbiol 2005;16:31–4.

55. Lewis DA. Chancroid: clinical manifestations, diagnosis, and management. Sex Transm Infect 2003;79: 68–71.

56. Fenton KA, Ison C, Johnson AP, et al. Ciprofloxacin resistence in *Neisseria gonorrhoeae* in England and Wales in 2002. Lancet 2003;361:1867–9.

57. Centers for Disease Control. Update to CDC's sexually transmitted diseases treatment guidelines, 2006: Fluoroquinolones no longer recommended for treatment of gonococcal infections. MMWR 2007;56(14):332–6.

58. Centers for Disease Control and Prevention. Cephalosporin susceptibility among *Neisseria gonorrhoeae* isolates – United States, 2000–2010. MMWR 2011;60(26): 873–7.

59. O'Farrell N. Donovanosis. Sex Transm Infect 2002;78:452–7.

60. Centers for Disease Control. Trends in reportable sexually transmitted diseases in the United States, 2006. National surveillance data for Chlamydia, gonorrhoea, and syphilis. CDC; 2007. p. 1–7.

61. D'Souza G, Lee JH, Paffel JM. Outbreak of syphilis among men who have sex with men in Houston, Texas. Sex Transm Dis 2003;30:872–3.

62. Mindel A, Tovey SJ, Timmins DJ, et al. Primary and secondary syphilis, 20 years' experience. Clinical features. Genitourinary Med 1989;65:1–3.

63. Smith D. Infectious syphilis of the anal canal. Dis Colon Rectum 1963;6:7–10.

64. Rampalo AM. Diagnosis and treatment of sexually acquired proctitis and proctocolitis: an update. Clin Infect Dis 1999;28(Suppl. 1):S84–90.

65. Zetola NM, Engelmen J, Jensen TP, et al. Syphilis in the United States: an update for clinicians with an emphasis on HIV coinfection. Mayo Clin Proc 2007;82:1091–102.

66. Hamlyn E, Taylor C. Sexually transmitted proctitis. Postgrad Med J 2006;82:733–6.

67. Lewis DA, Young H. Syphilis. Sex Transm Infect 2006;82(Suppl. 4):S13–5.

> EIAs that detect both IgG and IgM are recommended as they tend to be more sensitive in primary infection. An EIA IgM test should be performed in addition to routine screening tests (i.e. VDRL/RPR) in all cases of genital ulceration as well as in those who are known contacts of syphilis. The rationale for this is that IgM becomes detectable in the serum 2–3 weeks after infection and IgG 4–5 weeks after infection. Therefore, there will be a window of 1–2 weeks when routine screening tests may be negative.

68. World Health Organisation. Guidelines for the management of sexually transmitted infections. 2003. p. 11–5.

17

Minimally invasive surgery and enhanced recovery programmes in colorectal disease

Ian Jenkins
Robin Kennedy

Introduction

Despite the introduction of laparoscopic colorectal surgery in the early 1990s, its adoption has been slow due to a difficult learning curve, the requirement for significant local service reconfiguration, and certain concerns. The influence on oncological outcome and the specific complication of port-site recurrence were concerns that have now been resolved. The technique's applicability in colorectal surgery is also clearer and there is more understanding regarding cost issues and when to convert to traditional open surgery.

When performed by surgeons with adequate experience and training, it is clear that laparoscopic colorectal surgery dramatically improves the functional outcome following bowel resection. In early 2000, Henrik Kehlet transformed the surgical landscape, introducing a multimodal approach to improve functional recovery after conventional surgery – the enhanced recovery programme (ERP) was born. The use of an ERP combined with laparoscopic colorectal surgery further improves results. We therefore anticipate that this combined approach in colorectal surgery will become the gold standard: after elective segmental colectomy, postoperative hospital stays of 3–4 days, with commensurate improvements in functional recovery, will become routine.

This chapter will discuss the main issues relevant to laparoscopic colorectal surgery and introduce the important areas in enhanced recovery (ER) care. Because of the considerable benefits to patients, we are seeing a transition from the utilisation of these approaches by a small minority of enthusiasts, to them becoming standard treatment in the vast majority of elective resections for benign and malignant disease.

Outcomes of laparoscopic colorectal surgery

The safety and advantages of laparoscopic colectomy for cancer have been much debated and several randomised controlled trials (RCTs) have clarified these issues. The published large RCTs comparing late cancer outcomes following open or laparoscopic resection of colonic cancer are from Spain,[1] North America[2] (COST trial – Comparison of Laparoscopically-assisted and Open Colectomy for Colon Cancer), Hong Kong,[3] the UK[4] (MRC CLASICC trial – Conventional versus Laparoscopic-Assisted Surgery In Colorectal Cancer) and Europe (CoLOR trial – Colon cancer Laparoscopic or Open Resection).[5] It is important to note that the only trial specifically addressing rectal cancer was the CLASICC trial. The ALCCaS trial from Australasia has replicated the short-term benefits for colon cancer reported in the other trials.[6]

Oncological outcomes

Initial fears regarding oncological outcomes after laparoscopic colorectal cancer resection, particularly port-site recurrence, resulted in its suspension outside trials in some countries. These concerns have now been dispelled and major RCTs report wound recurrence to be the same following either type of surgery: <1%. Short- and medium-term oncological outcomes are equivalent between open and laparoscopic groups, and in the highly cited study by Lacy et al., an improved cancer-specific survival for stage III disease was identified.[1] This improvement for the laparoscopic patients may be due to less postoperative immunosuppression and/or earlier initiation of adjuvant therapy. Critics have, however, attributed the difference to poor results in the open group.

Although oncological outcome is equivalent in the large multicentre studies, this is despite conversion rates of 17–29%, reflecting the relative inexperience of participating surgeons. In contrast, Lacy et al. reported a conversion rate of 11% and the largest reduction in hospital stay after laparoscopy, suggesting a smaller effect from the learning curve. If a difference in oncological outcome is not detected with conversion rates around 20%, then it is a tantalising prospect that once conversion rates decrease to single figures, due to increased expertise and appropriate case selection, an oncological benefit might be confirmed.

The CLASICC trial reported results at 3 and 5 years that showed no difference in overall survival between laparoscopic and open surgery.[7,8] Equivalence in oncological outcomes and the improvements in postoperative recovery after laparoscopy prompted the National Institute for Health and Clinical Excellence (NICE) in 2006 to endorse the use of laparoscopic surgery for colorectal cancer (www.nice.org.uk). NICE have provided the following guidance:

- Laparoscopic resection is recommended as an alternative to open resection for individuals with colorectal cancer in whom both laparoscopic and open surgery are considered suitable.
- It should only be performed by surgeons who have completed appropriate training in the technique and who perform this procedure often enough to maintain competence.
- The decision about which procedure (open or laparoscopic) is undertaken should be made after informed discussion between the patient and the surgeon.

At the time of initial guidance in 2006 it was recognised that the number of surgeons adequately trained in laparoscopy in the UK was insufficient and implemention of guidance was waived until October 2010 to permit appropriate training to be undertaken. Thereafter, all colorectal multidisciplinary teams should have ensured that every patient suitable for laparoscopic resection be given this choice of treatment and if laparoscopic surgery is not available, suitable onward referral arrangements be put in place.

The role of laparoscopy in the management of rectal cancer has been assessed in the CoLOR II trial, with 2:1 randomisation to laparoscopy or open surgery. Though operating times were longer, blood loss, hospital stay and time to first bowel movement were significantly improved in the laparoscopic group, with no difference in the anastomotic leak rate (7% laparoscopic vs. 6% open; $P = 0.6$), overall morbidity or mortality. Resection margin positivity for the laparoscopic and open groups was 9% and 10%, respectively, but for low rectal cancers a significant difference existed in the margin positivity rate, 9% versus 21% ($P = 0.013$) favouring the laparoscopic approach. Similar studies are being conducted in the USA (ACOSOG Z6051) and in Japan (JCOG 0404 trial).

Hospital stay and complications

The results of both RCTs and observational studies assessing laparoscopic colorectal surgery have been submitted to meta-analysis and have produced similar results.

> ✓✓ Following laparoscopic resection, operation times are longer, but benefits are a reduced wound infection rate, less pain and narcotic use, less overall morbidity and a shorter hospital stay.[9–11]

Compared to conventional surgery, minimal access surgery probably reduces the necessity for re-operation caused by adhesions or incisional hernias, although this has not yet been verified in prospective studies. A retrospective study of 716 patients by Duepree et al. identified a decreased rate in the laparoscopic group for both incisional hernia and small-bowel obstruction.[12] The overall re-operation rate in the open group was double that of the laparoscopic group (7.7% vs. 3.8%); however, further studies are required for confirmation.

Blood loss

A case–control study by Kiran et al. of 147 patients confirmed that the laparoscopic approach for colorectal surgery led to significantly less blood loss and blood usage than after open colectomy.[13]

Mortality

The major RCTs report no difference in the 30-day mortality, possibly reflecting their size and that they were not powered to detect differences in mortality, particularly when the surgeons had conversion rates of >20%. If laparoscopy reduces complications then it is likely to have a similar effect on mortality. Law et al. reported a reduced mortality with laparoscopic resection in a non-randomised study of 1134 colon and upper rectal resections (401 laparoscopic procedures), and in a meta-analysis of 17 RCTs assessing 4013 procedures by Tjandra and Chan, laparoscopic resection of colonic and rectosigmoid cancer had a significantly lower perioperative mortality (odds ratio 0.33, $P = 0.005$).[14,15]

Economic considerations

Although laparoscopic colectomy has demonstrated a variety of advantages, there was debate regarding whether reduced hospital stay and morbidity offset the potential cost increases resulting from increased operating time and the use of extra disposable instruments. Braga et al. assessed 517 patients undergoing laparoscopic colonic and rectal cancer resection, finding a slight increase in hospital costs.[16] Similarly, Murray et al. found laparoscopic techniques to be more costly overall.[17,18] This analysis informed the NICE assessment, estimating the difference in cost to be £265. This is a modest additional cost, considering the short-term benefits associated with a more rapid recovery. Conversely, King et al. found no cost difference and a systematic review by Dowson et al. reported cost equivalence between open and laparoscopic groups.[19,20] For resection of diverticular disease, Senagore et al. found laparoscopic surgery to be less costly.[21]

Operative times and conversion rates have decreased since the above studies were published and in the recent LAFA Trial.[22] Randomising between laparoscopic and open surgery within an ERP,

in-hospital costs were equivalent for the approximately 400 patients recruited to the trial. The length of hospital stay is an important element of the total cost and with laparoscopic surgery hospital stay is known to decrease. Although current evidence is limited, it seems likely that as operative times and conversion rates decrease, the total cost of laparoscopic surgery will be reduced.

Conversion to open surgery

The possibility of conversion is inherent in laparoscopic surgery. Reported conversion rates vary considerably in laparoscopic colorectal surgery, but it is important to emphasise that conversion to open surgery should not be regarded as a failure of the technique; it may be entirely appropriate. Problems arise as definitions of conversion are unclear and, when quoting rates, authors do not define the percentage of their population undergoing open surgery. The sum of three numbers – open interventions, operations attempted laparoscopically that are converted, and those completed laparoscopically – will be the denominator. Without defining this, quoted conversion rates are virtually impossible to interpret. Based upon appropriate experience and a suitable clinical workload, we believe laparoscopic resection can be attempted in over 90% of elective colorectal cancer patients, with a conversion rate of <10%.[23] In support of this, the laparoscopic unit in Brisbane reports a low conversion rate of 6.6%[24] and the authors' conversion rate in a recent RCT was 7.3%.[25]

The definition of conversion

To ensure an unambiguous definition, we regard conversion as the inability to complete specimen mobilisation laparoscopically, including vascular division, usually but not always resulting in a larger incision than would otherwise have been required for specimen removal. The emphasis on vascular division is because after bowel transection retrieval is possible through a very small incision such as 4–5 cm – provided vascular and mesenteric division has occurred – maximising the benefit from laparosopic surgery. Attempting to ligate vessels through the incision will invariably produce a larger incision than the anticipated 4–5 cm, or problematic ligation. Using this definition there will be patients in whom much of the mobilisation will have been undertaken laparoscopically and who will derive considerable benefit from this, even though conversion is required.

Predicting the risk of conversion

Defining the patient group most likely to be converted would be beneficial, yet this has proved difficult. A recent European Association of Endoscopic Surgeons (EAES) consensus statement on laparoscopic surgery for colonic cancer indicated the most common cause for conversion is the presence of a bulky or locally advanced tumour.[26] Obesity and previous abdominal operations were not considered absolute contraindications for laparoscopic colon cancer surgery, though most studies cite these factors as being risk factors for conversion.

Obese patients carry a higher risk of wound and cardiopulmonary complications in addition to a greater incidence of comorbidity, which has the potential to adversely affect outcome after surgery. This group may therefore achieve the greatest benefit from laparoscopic resection. Schwandner et al. assessed obesity (body mass index (BMI) >30 kg/m²) in 589 laparoscopic colorectal patients, finding no difference in conversion rates (7.3% vs. 9.5%) in 95 obese patients and 494 'non-obese' patients.[27] Overall complication rates were similar (23.3% in the obese group vs. 24.5% in the non-obese group). These results are perhaps a testament to the level of expertise exhibited by the surgeons treating these patients. Senagore et al. compared 59 obese (BMI >30 kg/m²) and 201 non-obese patients, identifying differences between the two groups: in the obese group significantly more conversions (23.7% vs. 10.9%), longer operations (109 vs. 94 minutes), higher morbidity (22% vs. 13%) and anastomotic leak rate (5.1% vs. 1.2%).[28] Buchanan et al. reported that a BMI ≥28 kg/m² increased conversions from 3% to 22% in colorectal cancer resection.[23] The results from these last two groups are perhaps more recognisable for most surgeons and reflect the degree of difficulty in obese patients.

Previous abdominal surgery has been considered a risk factor for conversion. Arteaga Gonzalez et al. found a higher conversion rate following previous abdominal surgery (26.1% vs. 5.1%),[29] but with increasing experience this effect seems to disappear.[23]

Tumour location also affects the likelihood of conversion. Buchanan et al. identified rectal cancer resections to have an increased conversion rate over colonic resections, but this decreased with experience. The difficulty in undertaking laparoscopic rectal resection derives from the location of the rectum within a confined space and the concern that the technique may compromise tumour clearance. In addition, the rectal dissection follows vascular ligation and bowel mobilisation, often involving splenic flexure mobilisation, so the novice laparoscopic colorectal surgeon may be challenged by a subsequent complex rectal mobilisation. Law et al. assessed the outcomes of 265 patients with upper and mid rectal cancers, of which 37% were performed laparoscopically, the latter group having less advanced disease. Cancer-specific survival and local recurrences rates, stratified by disease stage, were not compromised by the laparoscopic approach.[30] The CLASICC study did not demonstrate a significant worsening of oncological outcome following laparoscopic rectal cancer resection; however, it specifically noted that positive margin rates were non-significantly higher in laparoscopic resections (16/129 (12%) vs. 4/64 (6%), $P = 0.19$)[4], probably reflecting the learning curve.

Disease extent may also influence conversion rates and Buchanan et al. report that a magnetic resonance imaging (MRI)-predicted threatened resection margin in rectal cancer is associated with higher conversion rates.[23] Moloo et al. compared laparoscopic resection between stage IV colorectal cancer and stage I–III disease. Thirteen per cent of the 375 laparoscopic resections were with palliative intent yet no significant differences were found between the groups for intraoperative (4% vs. 9%) or postoperative complications (14% vs. 12%), perioperative mortality (8% vs. 4%), or length of hospital stay.[31] However, the conversion rate was increased in the palliative group (22% vs. 11%) owing to tumour fixation or bulk. These results support the view of many experienced surgeons that laparoscopic resection of contiguous involvement is technically possible and not contraindicated in certain patients.

High hospital case volume has been associated with improved outcome after open operation for colorectal malignancy and it is likely that the volume of laparoscopic surgery performed will impact upon outcomes such as conversion. Kuhry et al. assessed data from the CoLOR trial and stratified outcomes by low, medium and high case volumes, a high colorectal case load resulting in decreased conversions and improved short-term outcomes.[32]

✅ Tekkis et al. have developed a regression analysis model to predict the likelihood of conversion.[33] Predictors of conversion were BMI, ASA grade, type of resection, presence of intraoperative abscess or fistula, and surgeon seniority. Marusch et al. assessed results in a total of 1658 patients from the Laparoscopic Colorectal Surgery Study Group.[34] This group reported a low conversion rate of 5.2% and identified elevated BMI, rectal resection and intraoperative complications as predictors for conversion.

Outcome after conversion

Concerns remain that conversion is associated with increased morbidity and greater hospital costs. A case–control study by Casillas et al. with a conversion rate of 12% found conversion did not significantly increase operation time, morbidity, length of stay, cost or unplanned readmissions, compared with similar complex open surgery.[35] Marusch et al. found the opposite: after conversion, operation time increased and postoperative morbidity (47.7% vs. 26.1%), mortality (3.3% vs. 1.5%) and hospital stay were all negatively influenced.[34] Buchanan et al. observed similar outcomes and cautioned that although technically challenging resections may be attempted laparoscopically, when surgeons are sufficiently experienced, patients with a high chance of conversion represent the most challenging procedures and probably occur in a subset of people with the greatest comorbidity.

✅ The likelihood of conversion is greatest in patients undergoing rectal surgery, when there is an increased BMI, following previous major abdominal surgery, and in inflammatory bowel disease. Earlier rather than delayed conversion, especially when progress is not being made, is the authors' current policy. This will minimise errors due to tiredness or technical difficulties that might have been handled best by open resection.

Benign colorectal conditions suitable for laparoscopic surgery

The role of laparoscopic surgery for patients with ileocaecal Crohn's disease has been a contentious issue as adhesions secondary to inflammation or previous surgery increase technical difficulty. A key technical aspect of ileocolonic Crohn's resection is to mobilise fully the right colon, in order that when performing the anastomosis there is no restriction on the colon. A comparative study by Bemelman et al. found that laparoscopic resection for Crohn's disease was associated with similar morbidity rates to open surgery but a shorter hospital stay and improved cosmetic results.[36] The cosmetic aspect is relatively important as many Crohn's patients are young adults and also likely to require re-operation. Further studies confirm improvements in outcome with laparoscopic resection for this disease and some suggest that initial minimal access surgery increases the chance that future resections will be possible laparoscopically.[37,38] The first RCT assessing this subject demonstrated a benefit to laparoscopy with a decrease in complications and hospital stay.[39] Maartense et al. later randomised 60 patients with a conversion rate of 10%, demonstrating similar results but also a significant reduction in hospital costs.[40]

Schwandner et al. assessed the outcomes of laparoscopic resection for diverticulitis compared to non-diverticular disease and found a low conversion rate of ≈7% in both groups, with similarly low and comparable morbidity.[41] Purkayastha et al. performed a meta-analysis on 12 non-randomised studies, finding equivalent results for laparoscopic and open surgery in diverticular disease, with possible reductions in complications and hospital stay. However, significant study heterogeneity was identified, indicating likely bias.

To clarify the most appropriate technique for resection, the outcomes of open and laparoscopic total colectomy and ileoanal pouch surgery have been compared in several studies and feasibility confirmed. The laparoscopic approach should only be recommended when an experienced team is available. Studies confirm similar benefits to those reported for other indications.[42,43] Often there are marked variations in the reported 'laparoscopic' surgical approach. For example, some use a Pfannenstiel incision to permit completion of rectal dissection and/or transection of the rectum and, to some laparoscopic purists, this modification may reduce the benefit of a truly minimally invasive procedure. Study heterogeneity in the meta-analyses assessing these procedures underlines the fact that total colectomy and proctocolectomy are demanding procedures unsuitable for surgeons early in their experience of laparoscopic colorectal surgery. We would suggest that when experienced laparoscopic teams are available patients are likely to derive as much, if not more, benefit from this technique as patients undergoing laparoscopic segmental colectomy. Further randomised trial evidence is required.[44]

Laparoscopic colorectal technique

All patients considered for elective laparoscopic colorectal cancer resection will undergo preoperative staging by computed tomography (CT) of the abdomen, chest and pelvis, with MRI in addition for rectal cancer. This confirms tumour location, defines adjacent organ involvement that may pose technical problems, and excludes both synchronous pathology and widespread disease. Patients will undergo colonoscopy or virtual colonoscopy to evaluate the whole colon before surgery. Endoscopic India Ink marking techniques are used for the intraoperative identification of colonic polyps and early neoplasms in order to avoid on-table colonoscopy. Tumours are tattooed based on their location in the colon by an agreed protocol (**Fig. 17.1**), but rectal lesions below 15 cm from the anal verge are not tattooed to

---

Revised St Mark's Colonoscopic Tattooing Protocol 2011

Indications	Equipment	Procedure
• Prior to surgery to localise pathology • To mark lesions for endoscopic surveillance • **Do not tattoo rectal lesions** as they disrupt surgical planes • There is no need to tattoo lesions in the caecum, however, **if in doubt, then place a tattoo**	• Primed variceal injection needle with 10ml syringe filled with normal saline • 5ml syringe filled with Spot® (or 0.9ml sterilised Black (Indian) Ink made up to 5ml with normal saline)	• Direct needle at an angle to mucosa • Raise a bleb using 1-2ml of saline • Swap to syringe filled with Spot® or Indian Ink • Inject 1ml into the bleb to create tattoo • Swap to syringe filled with saline and flush ink out with 1ml saline before removing needle • Repeat process for 3 tattoos

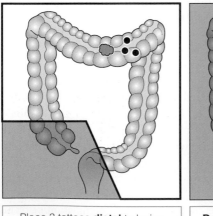

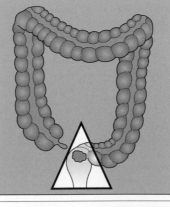

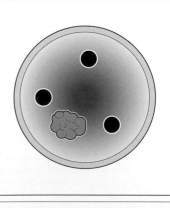

Place 3 tattoos **distal** to lesion	**Do not** place tattoo below 20cm but clearly record distance of LESION from anal verge	Place tattoos 120° apart **as close to lesion as possible** but separate from it

Remember: To document **how many** tattoos were placed and **the position relative to the lesion**

Figure 17.1 • Revised St Mark's colonoscopic tattooing protocol. Courtesy of Dr Adam Haycock and Mr Robin Kennedy, St Mark's Hospital.

avoid discolouring the fascia of Denonvillier. This approach has been found to be safe and effective in aiding lesion identification at laparoscopy.[45]

Patients undergoing laparoscopic colorectal resection are positioned using a modified Lloyd–Davies position, with shoulder and side restraints owing to the steep Trendelenburg and lateral tilt required for left-sided and rectal resections: care should be exercised, particularly in the morbidly obese, as bilateral brachial plexus injury has been reported.

For elective laparoscopic left colonic, sigmoid or rectal cancer resection, our approach is similar. Our favoured technique uses a four-port approach with an additional port added for low rectal dissection in laparoscopic total mesorectal excision (TME) (**Fig. 17.2**). A flexible-tipped zero-degree laparoscope is used for all resections, though a straight zero-degree laparoscope will suffice. Following identification of the relevant anatomy, an operative strategy is planned, skeletonising the vessels and proceeding to early vascular ligation using single clips or sutures (**Fig. 17.3a,b**). We generally mobilise the colon from medial to lateral using a harmonic scalpel, identifying the left ureter and gonadal vessels before the lateral peritoneal attachments are divided (**Fig. 17.4**). The splenic flexure mobilisation is performed as required, and when it is mobilised a medial to lateral approach is again favoured.[46] The distal end of the specimen is cross-stapled, divided

intracorporeally and the specimen extracted via a muscle-separating incision near the left groin. A stapled intracorporeal transanal anastomosis is then fashioned laparoscopically and leak-tested.

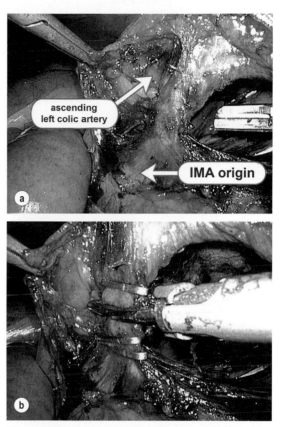

Figure 17.3 • Meticulous dissection is undertaken precisely to define the vascular anatomy at its origin before division between clips.

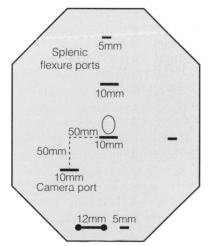

Figure 17.2 • Port positions for sigmoid colectomy, TME, rectopexy and left hemicolectomy.

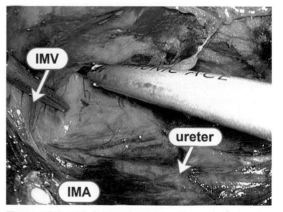

Figure 17.4 • Medial to lateral dissection exposing ureter and gonadal vessels maintaining an intact mesocolic package.

Right hemicolectomy

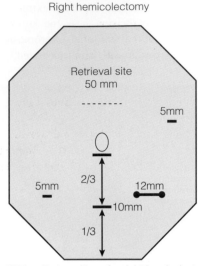

Retrieval site
50 mm

5mm

2/3

5mm 12mm

10mm

1/3

Figure 17.5 • Port positions for right hemicolectomy.

For resection of malignant right and right transverse colonic lesions we use a five-port technique (**Fig. 17.5**). Following an assessment of the anatomy and formulation of an operative strategy, we perform early vascular ligation of the ileocolic vessels near their origin, after identification of the superior mesenteric vein. Medial to lateral mobilisation is then performed before the middle colic vessels are identified and the right branch divided. Not only must surgeons be aware of the considerable variation in the vascular anatomy of this region, but also that the right gastroepiploic vessels consistently lie intimately opposed to the posterior aspect of the middle colic vessels. The 'right colic' artery is usually a branch of the middle colic vessel and its division allows further dissection of the transverse mesocolon from the pancreas. Having divided all vessels, the transverse colon and hepatic flexure are mobilised from medial to lateral, ensuring adequate clearance of the transverse colon distal to the proposed anastomosis. This allows the colon to be delivered via a 4–5 cm incision unimpeded by attached omentum. The operative site then moves to the pelvic brim, where the right ureter and gonadal vessels are identified. The peritoneum overlying these structures is incised, with dissection proceeding in the avascular plane anterior to the fascia of Toldt, to join the previous dissection. The resection and anastomosis is via a transverse, supraumbilical, muscle-separating incision and the mesenteric defect is closed laparoscopically.

Difficult aspects of laparoscopic resection

Laparoscopic colorectal resection can be made more difficult by the patient factors described above; however, certain technical aspects of laparoscopic resection require caution depending on the surgeon's experience.

Though a right hemicolectomy may be regarded as an initial stepping stone in open surgery, this is not always comparable for laparoscopic resection. In Crohn's disease, one should not hesitate to convert when there is extensive mesenteric thickening or difficult inflammatory adhesions. There is still likely to be benefit from bowel mobilisation even if conversion – using the strict definition provided above – occurs. Vascular control and dissection of the transverse colon can also be problematic for the novice.

Further technical issues relate to splenic flexure mobilisation and rectal dissection. Laparoscopic splenic flexure mobilisation by any approach can prove difficult. We would normally recommend a medial to lateral approach using dissection along the anterior surface of the pancreas, after proximal division of the inferior mesenteric vein (IMV). We would then separate the greater omentum from the superior surface of the transverse colon in a medial to lateral direction. This flexure can be challenging and the surgeon should be familiar with all approaches. Rectal dissection and particularly TME will continue to prove difficult in males with a narrow pelvis, irrespective of whether the procedure is open or laparoscopic. It is, however, a step too far for novices, even in women. The views obtained of the rectum at laparoscopy are unrivalled and with increasing experience laparoscopic TME is a satisfying procedure. Transection of the rectum at laparoscopic TME deserves special mention, as it can be difficult to ensure a straight staple line at a low level owing to access difficulties. To achieve this we routinely deploy the stapler through the 12-mm right suprapubic port and transect the rectum in the sagittal plane close to the pelvic floor. Prior to transection transanal palpation is performed by the surgeon in order to check the level of section in relation to the dentate line (one can place the transection within 1 cm of the dentate line) and that the staple line is perpendicular to the long axis of the rectum. This produces an anteroposterior orientation rather than the transverse staple line traditionally formed at open surgery. Two firings of a 45-mm stapler are usually all that is required and a portion of the cross-staple line is subsequently incorporated into the doughnuts from the circular staple line of the anastomosis.

Specific contraindications to laparoscopic resection are gross peritonitis, toxic megacolon and obstructing carcinoma. However, with the advent and improvement in colonic stenting it is not unusual for obstructed patients to undergo elective laparoscopic resection following successful stenting.[47] Cheung et al. randomised 48 patients with malignant left-sided large-bowel obstruction to stenting (with subsequent laparoscopic resection) or straight to open surgery, confirming stenting to offer a safe bridge to elective laparoscopic resection. Sixty-seven per cent of the group randomised to stenting underwent a successful single-stage laparoscopic resection without diversion, in comparison to 38% in the open group. No patients in the 'endolaparoscopic' group had a permanent stoma in comparison to 25% in the open group.[48]

Contiguous organ involvement may also be resected laparoscopically without conversion, when appropriate. For some large tumours, vascular ligation and the majority of mobilisation can be undertaken laparoscopically, in order to allow completion of the dissection through a smaller targeted incision than would otherwise have been possible using an open technique. This is often appropriate in TME when the rectal dissection may be completed through a much smaller incision than would otherwise have been possible. Some laparoscopic enthusiasts report small series when laparoscopic reintervention has been feasible in the setting of clinical anastomotic leakage, with improved subsequent outcomes compared to open re-operation.[49,50] However, such small studies have inherent biases and in the setting of gross peritonitis from a leak we would not advocate laparoscopy. We have employed laparoscopy with benefit when doubt remains regarding situations such as an internal hernia, a small leak or unexplained postoperative pain.

The learning curve and training in laparoscopic colorectal surgery

The laparoscopic learning curve is known to vary between surgeons and will be influenced by patient selection and operative complexity, with comparisons requiring appropriate case-mix adjustment.

Several authors have attempted to define a learning curve for laparoscopic colorectal resection. In one of the largest assessments to date, Tekkis et al. reported that more than 50 cases of each type of segmental colectomy were necessary to see a reduction in conversion rates.[51] Having adjusted for case mix, a learning curve of 55 cases for right-sided colonic resections versus 62 cases for left-sided resections was found. The reader should be aware that as experience builds surgeons will often attempt more complex cases, with inherently higher chances of conversion. This explains Tekkis et al.'s finding that a greater number of cases are necessary than was previously thought to be the case.

The measures upon which the learning curve has been assessed previously have relied upon outcomes including conversion and morbidity, but ideally there should be no deterioration in adverse outcomes during the learning process with mentored training. Alternative means to monitor training progression have been developed based upon task-specific operative checklists and global rating scales assessing surgical manoeuvres and behaviours, respectively.[52]

> ✅ In an excellent study, MacRae and colleagues reviewed conversion and outcome in ileocolonic resection for Crohn's, reporting that despite increasing case complexity outcome improved over time. This, like Buchanan et al.'s study on colorectal cancer, is one of the few that includes the totality of practice – thus conversion rates can be interpreted with respect to the proportion of patients undergoing open surgery.[53]

The appropriate method of imparting laparoscopic colorectal skills remains an area of debate and a full exploration is beyond the scope of this chapter. It is likely that the combination of teaching adjuncts and simultaneous clinical training will add value for trainees. Favourable reports have come from the use of virtual reality training[54,55] or videotaping and playback[56] for skills assessment. Video production by trainees may also prove useful in training. Our own approach is to separate components of each laparoscopic procedure into modules so that each module can be learned before the entire operation is attempted. In addition, each procedure is broken down into logical sequential steps, which are presented on a teaching video. The teaching video and recorded footage of the trainee are then used for regular review to optimise technique in training.

This standardised, didactic approach is taught along with the identification of predicted operative difficulty so that the surgeon can proceed to independent practice without the necessity to relearn unnecessary lessons. With this 'modular' approach we see proficiency gain as determined on a cumulative sum (CUSUM) chart after 35–40 cases when the totality of laparoscopic colorectal practice is considered.[57]

The most appropriate methods to optimise training in laparoscopic colorectal surgery remain unclear, although various systems have been initiated in the UK. These can be broadly categorised as preceptorship programmes for consultant surgeons, laparoscopic fellowships for senior trainees, animal and cadaver training courses, and the National Training Programme for consultant surgeons.

Future developments

It is clear that laparoscopic surgery is more technically demanding than conventional open surgery and this is in large part related to the two-dimensional views, limited dexterity of intruments within the confines of the abdomen, fixed instrument tips with only four degrees of freedom, and difficulty aligning hands and instruments. Robot-assisted surgery has been developed to counter some of these difficulties and offers three-dimensional images, a stable camera and operating platform, articulating instruments, seven degrees of freedom, potentially improved ergonomics, motion scaling and tremor-free movements. The theoretical benefits may, however, be outweighed by the loss of haptic feedback, restriction to a single quadrant in the abdomen, and increased operating times and cost.[58] Currently robotic colorectal resection is still in its infancy but appears to be feasible and safe when performed by experienced laparoscopic colorectal surgeons. Current reports comprise case series and small comparative studies, most studies employing a hybrid approach using the robot for the pelvic phase of surgery. A handful of studies report a fully robot-assisted approach. Although to date there are no results from RCTs of robotic rectal surgery, several studies demonstrate similar operation duration, intraoperative and postoperative complication rates, and short-term outcomes, when compared to laparoscopic controls.[59,60] The ROLARR trial (RObotic versus LAparoscopic Resection for Rectal cancer) will address the utility and efficacy of robotic

surgery and aims to recruit 400 patients overall using the conversion rate to open surgery as the primary outcome, with robotic surgery being required for only the mesorectal resection component of surgery (http://ctru.leeds.ac.uk/rolarr). The potential role of robotics in colonic surgery is even less clear as procedures such as right hemicolectomy and sigmoid resection can often be straightforward with conventional laparoscopy. Whether robotics might facilitate intracorporeal suturing of the anastomosis and natural orifice specimen retrieval remains to be determined.

Single incision laparoscopic surgery (SILS; or single port access (SPA) or single-port laparoscopic surgery (SPLS)) has been employed in many settings including appendicectomy, splenectomy, hernia repair and gynaecological procedures. To date only case series from enthusiastists are reported for colorectal resection, and these indicate its feasibility and safety in different colorectal resections. In case-matched comparisons, similar operation times, hospital stay, lymph node yields and complication rates are found.[61] As with robotics, more rigorous studies are still needed to determine the role of SILS. The University of Hong Kong is conducting a randomised clinical trial comparing conventional laparoscopic colectomy with single-port surgery (http://clinicaltrials.gov/ct2/show/study/NCT01101672), with postoperative pain as the primary outcome.

Transanal endoscopic surgery

The concept of local excision of a rectal lesion through the anus is not new but technological advances and modifications in technique have permitted expansion of the range of therapeutic opportunities for such lesions. True peranal or transanal resection is probably only safely feasible in a small proportion of lesions that are low in the rectum or near the anorectal junction. More proximal rectal access requires adequate visualisation and different systems have evolved to achieve successful and complete local excision. Transanal endoscopic microsurgery (TEMS) was introduced by Buess et al. in the early 1980s[62] and has since been employed in the management of large and sessile benign rectal polyps, small carcinoid tumours, early rectal cancers, palliating advanced rectal cancers and as an adjunct in natural orifice transluminal endoscopic surgery (NOTES), the rationale being, in part, that a patient may be spared the risks associated with major pelvic surgery (risk of temporary or permanent stoma formation, mortality, anastomotic leak, urogenital dysfunction, unfit patient, palliative intervention required) and organ preservation may maintain function and quality of life. TEMS is a minimally invasive surgical approach that uses a specialised magnifying rectoscope with a binocular viewing system with ports for insufflation, instrumentation and irrigation. TEMS has been proposed for use in local excision of rectal lesions that cannot be easily and directly visualised transanally, and as an alternative to open or laparoscopic rectal excision. Results indicate that the use of TEMS improves outcomes compared to traditional local excision. Further equipment modification has yielded transanal endoscopic operation (TEO), which uses existing laparoscopic visualisation and insufflation equipment and is perhaps ergonomically better. Both TEMS and TEO provide a stable operating platform for transanal resection. Both are potentially costly, with specific training being required owing to a steep learning curve and a relative dearth of suitable cases and expertise. More recently, novel adaptions of existing laparoscopic devices have offered unstable working platforms with encouraging initial reports on safety and feasibility, although overall current evidence is lacking. For example, an SILS port has replaced the rectoscope for rectal access in some case series.[63] A variety of inventive acronyms have also resulted, e.g. TAMIS (transanal minimally invasive surgery) and TEVA (transanal endoscopic video-assisted excision). Whether such modifications will encourage more widespread adoption of minimally invasive local excision remains to be established.

Of the indications stated above, few would doubt the utility of TEMS/TEO in the setting of large benign polyps, although randomised comparison with other endoscopic techniques such as endoscopic mucosal resection (EMR) is needed.[64] The greatest controversy currently lies with the application of local excision with TEMS/TEO in early rectal cancer treatment. This disease is regarded as likely to be cured with radical surgery; however, in a proportion of patients this is also likely to represent overtreatment as the risks of lymph node or microvascular involvement are so small that local excision alone would have been sufficient therapy. Unfortunately, it has been difficult to provide completely accurate preoperative predictions on the likelihood of extramural disease to guide decision-making, although a combination of MRI and endorectal ultrasound (ERUS) can optimise accuracy. As a general guide, small lesions of less than 3 cm that are well or moderately differentiated without lymphovascular invasion are the most suitable candidates. Moreover, historically, local excision for T1/T2 cancers has been beset with high local recurrence rates of 20–40% that when identified were frequently incurable or required extra-anatomical resection to offer clearance,[65,66] yet some groups report zero recurrences for T1 cancers at 5 years.[67] There are likely to be biases inherent in the many case series and cohort studies.

Of interest, in groups with fewer recurrences, TEMS procedures appeared to not only excise the full thickness of the affected rectal wall, but also the adjacent mesorectal tissue. In addition, where a local excision has identified adverse tumour histology then it appears that prior local excision does not add significant difficulty to subsequent radical surgery.[68]

More recently, a further treatment paradigm for early rectal cancer has been offered based upon the work of Habr-Gama, where up to a third of patients with resectable rectal cancer had a complete response to chemoradiotherapy, with 27% sustaining a complete clinical response such that radical surgery was avoided.[69] Furthermore, comparison of radical resection with local excision by TEMS after neoadjuvant chemoradiotherapy identified no difference in disease recurrence at a median follow-up of 56 months.[70] In the UK, these findings have prompted the phase II feasibility RCT TREC Trial (TEM and Radiotherapy in Early Rectal Cancer), where patients with T1/T2 N0 rectal cancers will be randomised between radical surgery and short-course radiotherapy followed by TEMS after 8–10 weeks.[71] The results will determine the suitability and design of a larger multicentre RCT.

Summary

The multiple benefits of laparoscopic colorectal surgery have been repeatedly proven in large studies. Consequently the laparoscopic approach has changed from being the preserve of a few enthusiasts, in a limited number of patients, to becoming the preferred approach. We anticipate a dramatic increase in the number of laparoscopic colorectal procedures performed in the UK, which will be fuelled by increasing patient awareness and demand. As NICE highlighted, further information is required on cost-effectiveness, late oncological results, postoperative incisional hernias, neuralgia and small-bowel obstruction.

Enhanced recovery programmes

Surgical injury induces a series of complex responses in endocrine/metabolic and humoral cascade systems that may subsequently pose a risk to the surgical patient, resulting in organ dysfunction and delayed recovery. By making many modifications to traditional perioperative care, enhanced recovery or 'fast-track' programmes (ERPs) are designed to reduce this surgical stress response and its consequences (**Fig. 17.6**). ERPs have evolved as a result of evidence-based advances, and important

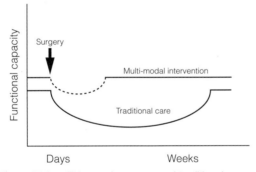
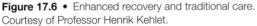

Figure 17.6 • Enhanced recovery and traditional care. Courtesy of Professor Henrik Kehlet.

aspects include patient education, physiological optimisation, improved anaesthetic and analgesic techniques, modifications in surgical technique, and an improved understanding of early feeding, fluid balance and mobilisation.

Traditional perioperative care

A hospital stay of 10–14 days following colorectal resection has been accepted as normal when accompanied by traditional perioperative care. Despite this, a postoperative stay of 2–3 days was first reported by Kehlet in Copenhagen and similar results have subsequently been achieved by other groups.[72–76] An understanding of what 'traditional' care means comes from Lassen et al.'s survey of colorectal surgeons in five Northern European countries.[77] This study highlighted the marked variation in practice between countries, suggesting that most surgeons have ignored evidence-based advances in perioperative care. Nygren et al. subsequently assessed these same five countries as part of the Enhanced Recovery After Surgery (ERAS) Group, comparing results in four centres with those from patients within an established ERP in Denmark.[78] This study was used to develop a consensus and a core protocol for ER care.[79] The core protocol was published by Fearon in 2005, key elements are summarised in **Fig. 17.7** and the subject has been more fully discussed in the recently published *Manual of Fast Track Recovery for Colorectal Surgery*.[80]

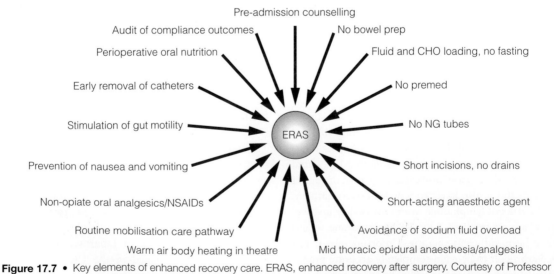

Figure 17.7 • Key elements of enhanced recovery care. ERAS, enhanced recovery after surgery. Courtesy of Professor Ken Fearon.

Perioperative interventions in enhanced recovery programmes

Reducing metabolic stress

To prevent aspiration, starvation for solids and fat is required for 6 hours before elective surgery, but for only 2 hours when considering liquids that do not contain fat or particulate matter (unless there has been previous gastric surgery or there is a known hiatus hernia). Evidence came initially from Ljungqvist's group in Stockholm that surgery is best conducted when the patient is in the fed state.[81–83] This can be achieved by the use of a 'complex carbohydrate' drink that, when taken 2 hours preoperatively, decreases postoperative insulin resistance. Traditional starvation, immobilisation and trauma increase insulin resistance and patients then behave more like type II diabetics, with a consequent increase in postoperative complications.

✓✓ Small detailed RCTs have also shown that protein balance is better maintained following preoperative carbohydrate loading.[84,85] Postoperative oral nutritional supplements significantly decrease postoperative complications and fatigue, maintaining nitrogen balance; hence early postoperative nutrition using supplements is encouraged.[85–87]

Preoperative bowel preparation

Systematic reviews and meta-analyses have assessed the role of preoperative bowel preparation in colorectal surgery and derived similar conclusions. A Cochrane Review by Guenaga et al. and two meta-analyses confirm that mechanical bowel preparation does not reduce anastomotic leakage and may even increase wound infections.[88–90] Two recent large RCTs assessing the role of mechanical bowel preparation have provided conflicting results.[91,92] Based on the existing evidence we now only use mechanical bowel preparation in patients undergoing TME. For other people who require left-sided colonic or high rectal resection we merely employ a preoperative enema in order to allow the anastomosis to be performed without gross faecal loading. A study from Sweden reported in 2007 that a defunctioning stoma decreases symptomatic anastomotic leakage following rectal surgery and has recommended it for all low anterior resections.[93] Our TME patients therefore receive bowel preparation, as it seems illogical to defunction them and leave faeces between the stoma and the defunctioned anastomosis.

Perioperative fluid balance

Perioperative fluid therapy is the subject of much controversy and clinical trials examining the influence of fluid therapy on outcome after surgery are contradictory. In the past evaporative loss from the abdominal cavity was often overestimated and assumptions regarding any third space loss may have been based on methodologically flawed studies. The fluid volume that actually accumulates in elective colorectal surgery is likely to be minimal and volume preloading following neuroaxial blockade causes postoperative overload.[94,95]

✓✓ Strong evidence from RCTs exists indicating that gut function, tissue healing, postoperative morbidity and hospital stay are adversely affected by the excessive prescription of perioperative fluid and sodium in elective surgery.[95,96]

Lobo et al. investigated the effect of fluid therapy on gastric emptying after colorectal surgery. In patients 'restricted' to <2 litres of crystalloid and 77 mmol of sodium per day gastric emptying significantly improved, compared to those given standard fluids of >3 litres and 154 mmol of sodium per day.[96] Bowel function and hospital stay were also significantly improved. Restriction of fluid and sodium was examined further by Brandstrup et al. in a multicentre RCT, which compared a traditional fluid replacement regimen with a restricted one. The latter aimed to maintain preoperative body weight and euvolaemia,[94] significantly reducing complications: cardiopulmonary (7% vs. 24%), tissue healing (16% vs. 31%) and overall complications (33% vs. 51%). Mortality was higher in the traditional group, though this difference was not statistically significant (0% vs. 4.7%, $P = 0.12$). In 2009 a consensus document on fluid management was produced – GIFTASUP guidelines – which provides an overview of the subject.[97]

Perioperative fluid administration also influences cardiac function, fluid overload producing a suboptimal right-shifted position on the Starling curve, and fluid deficit doing the opposite. Both situations increase the risk of perioperative cardiac morbidity. Intraoperative 'goal-directed' fluid therapy aims to optimise cardiac function, addressing these risks.[98,99] The timing of intraoperative fluid administration may also be important. Noblett et al. investigated the administration of colloid boluses, guided by oesophageal Doppler monitoring of cardiac function, in a double-blind RCT. The intervention group experienced a reduction in complications and hospital stay, largely resulting from the administration of relatively small amounts of colloid early in the intervention.[100]

Surgical technique and wound drainage

Transverse and smaller incisions have been encouraged within ERPs.[101] There is evidence that smaller incisions improve outcome, this being one important benefit of laparoscopic surgery. The direction of the incision is more contentious. A recent Cochrane Review found that although both analgesic use and pulmonary complications may be reduced with a transverse or oblique incision, this does not seem to be significant clinically as complication rates and recovery times are the same as with a midline incision.[102] Owing to heterogeneity in these studies the conclusions should be interpreted with caution.

The laparoscopic technique has been shown to decrease the stress response, with lower levels of interleukin-6 and C-reactive protein observed than after traditional open surgery, and better preservation of immune competence as measured by human leucocyte antigen expression on monocytes.[103]

The use of drains in elective colorectal surgery has been extensively studied in many RCTs. A Cochrane Review of 1140 patients from six such trials reported that 573 were allocated to drainage and 567 to no drainage.[104] No benefit was found for routine anastomotic drainage and we would regard drainage as unnecessary in most situations; in addition, it impairs patient mobility. In order to minimise pelvic haematoma formation after low rectal surgery, drainage for 12–18 hours may be appropriate. This is our current practice but it is unsupported by objective data.

Mobilisation

One of the central tenets of ER care is early mobilisation, with patients sitting out of bed on the day of surgery and walking regularly thereafter. Multiple attachments restrict mobilisation and we therefore aim to remove all tubes on the day after colonic

surgery – following a trial walk around the bed the urninary catheter will be removed on day 1. After low rectal surgery, due to the possibility of transient bladder dysfunction, this is delayed until day 2 or 3.

Pain control

There is consistent evidence from meta-analysis that epidural local anaesthetic, usually mixed with a low concentration of opiate, hastens return of postoperative gastrointestinal function after abdominal surgery by 24–37 hours and improves pain control.[105] It is not clear, however, that this technique reduces postoperative complications, other than pulmonary morbidity.[106] The epidural should be mid thoracic rather than lumbar to avoid lower limb motor paralysis and urinary retention. Compared to patient-controlled intravenous opiate analgesia (PCA), epidurals provide better analgesia, particularly during exercise, without the nausea and ileus incurred with opiates.[105] In addition, it has become routine to supplement analgesia with paracetamol and add another agent 2 hours before the epidural is stopped. Contrary views exist and Delaney et al. have routinely used PCA followed by multimodal oral analgesics with good results.[76,106] One of the critical factors in epidural analgesia is a low failure rate and if that is rising above 10–20% then the benefits of this technique become less clear. This is particularly true after laparoscopic surgery and many surgeons who have a low conversion rate have discontinued their usage. Rockall's group demonstrated that a one-shot spinal technique using bupivacaine and diamorphine, combined with postoperative PCA, seemed superior to either PCA or epidural alone in their hands.[107] With new modalities, such as longer acting epidural morphine formulations, wound local anaesthetic infusion catheters, transversus abdominis plane blocks and peripheral opioid antagonists, the choices are increasing.

Enhanced recovery trials

The principles of ER care have been applied in several RCTs, with favourable outcomes. These trials have been summarised in two recent meta-analyses in which hospital stay decreased by 2.5 days and complications were almost halved (relative risk 0.52; 95% confidence interval 0.36–0.73).[108,109] One of the initial concerns regarding ERPs related to an increased readmission rate. Proponents addressed this by changing the planned discharge date from 2 to 3 days, significantly reducing the readmission rate.[110] The meta-analyses above did not report increased readmission rates.

> ✅✅ Compared to traditional perioperative care, hospital stay and morbidity are significantly reduced in ERPs without significantly increasing readmission rates or mortality.[108–110]

Setting up RCTs to examine the effect of ER is difficult, as randomising patients to traditional care in an institution that has spent 1–2 years developing ER management seems counterintuitive. Consequently the RCTs to date have included small numbers and are weakened by the lack of blinding. In addition, analysing the relative contributions of individual ER components is also difficult and will require large numbers of patients for multivariate analysis.

The issue of whether ER care results in a transfer of cost to the community has been analysed in a carefully controlled study. Detailed cost and quality-of-life analyses were performed and did not demonstrate an increase in cost or deterioration in quality of life resulting from this change in care.[19]

ERPs applied to laparoscopic surgery

It is clear that with appropriate training the use of laparoscopy can considerably improve functional recovery after colorectal resection. The debate has therefore shifted to whether optimisation of the perioperative care associated with open surgery can produce similar outcomes. To date, three RCTs have examined this.[22,25,110] The first two trials were small single-centre studies, one showing a benefit from laparoscopic surgery while the other showed no influence on hospital stay. The recent LAFA Trial included 400 patients from nine hospitals in the Netherlands. The study randomised between laparoscopic or open surgery, and also ER and standard care. It demonstrated that laparoscopy was the only predictive factor having an effect on hospital stay and morbidity. It should be noted, however, that within the non-ER group only six of the predefined 15 ER elements were applied, as it was not felt appropriate to do this now.

Who should have ER care?

We currently use an ERP for all our patients undergoing elective colorectal surgery and it would seem logical that the more unfit a patient is, the greater the potential benefit of this perioperative optimisation. We would still recommend the use of mid thoracic epidurals after open surgery for postoperative analgesia, but have discontinued this after laparoscopic resection. We do not use non-steroidal anti-inflammatory drugs (NSAIDs) in people with known impairment of renal function and in all other patients we carefully monitor creatinine postoperatively to avoid adverse renal effects. Some data have been published on NSAIDs and anastomotic leakage but to date no conclusive evidence exists regarding this.

Starting an ERP

This development requires a multidisciplinary approach to perioperative care and extensive retraining of staff. Modest resource requirements are necessary, but a large change in the healthcare culture is essential. We use multidisciplinary courses directed at all key team members in order to start the training. A nurse facilitator to lead, teach and audit outcomes is also necessary to manage the process of change and maintain standards. The development requires many months to reach maximal effectiveness and will be aided by regular audit of compliance with the different interventions (Fig. 17.7). As the percentage compliance achieved for each ER intervention increases, patient recovery improves as monitored by complications and hospital stay.[111]

Summary

Enhanced recovery represents an evidence-based approach to perioperative care that reduces the stress response to surgery. Until recently, the surgical community has largely ignored this evidence. Interest is now increasing in the benefits of this approach. Colorectal surgeons should not restrict enhancement of recovery to unimodal interventions, such as laparoscopic surgery, but should offer it within the context of multimodal optimisation to obtain the best outcomes following colorectal surgery.

Key points

Laparoscopic colorectal surgery

- Though operation times may be slightly longer, laparoscopic colorectal surgery reduces wound infection rates, blood loss and postoperative pain, resulting in fewer complications, better recovery and a shorter hospital stay.
- Laparoscopic resection for colorectal cancer provides the same oncological outcome to open surgery. Future studies with potentially lower conversion rates may identify improved cancer outcomes.
- Although most authors report an increased cost associated with minimal access surgery, further experience and future decreases in instrument costs are likely to result in an economic benefit.
- The use of laparoscopy in rectal surgery, the obese patient and following previous major abdominal intervention has been associated with increased conversion rates. It is important to recognise the technical challenges accompanying laparoscopic resection in these situations, in order to minimise potential adverse outcomes.
- The most effective method of training in laparoscopic colorectal surgery is unclear but a structured, repetitive approach paying attention to operative complexity is essential.
- The role of robot-assisted colorectal resection and SILS remains to be established although early results are encouraging.

Enhanced recovery programmes

- Key components of an ERP include preoperative conditioning of expectations, reduction of metabolic stress and the avoidance of fluid overload, modifications of surgical and anaesthetic technique, improved postoperative analgesia allowing early mobilisation, reduction of ileus and early resumption of oral intake.
- This multimodal approach to rehabilitation improves recovery, reducing complications and hospital stay.
- The establishment of an ERP requires extensive and ongoing multidisciplinary training.

References

1. Lacy AM, Garcia-Valdecasas JC, Delgado S, et al. Laparoscopy-assisted colectomy versus open colectomy for treatment of non-metastatic colon cancer: a randomised trial. Lancet 2002;359(9325):2224–9.
2. Clinical Outcomes of Surgical Therapy Study Group. A comparison of laparoscopically assisted and open colectomy for colon cancer. N Engl J Med 2004;350(20):2050–9.
3. Leung KL, Kwok SP, Lam SC, et al. Laparoscopic resection of rectosigmoid carcinoma: prospective randomised trial. Lancet 2004;363(9416):1187–92.
4. Guillou PJ, Quirke P, Thorpe H, et al. Short-term endpoints of conventional versus laparoscopic-assisted surgery in patients with colorectal cancer (MRC CLASICC trial): multicentre, randomised controlled trial. Lancet 2005;365(9472):1718–26.
5. Veldkamp R, Kuhry E, Hop WC, et al. Laparoscopic surgery versus open surgery for colon cancer: short-term outcomes of a randomised trial. Lancet Oncol 2005;6(7):477–84.
6. Hewett PJ, Allardyce RA, Bagshaw PF, et al. Short-term outcomes of the Australasian randomised clinical study comparing laparoscopic and conventional open surgical treatments for colon cancer: the ALCCaS trial. Ann Surg 2008;248(5):728–38.
7. Jayne DG, Guillou PJ, Thorpe H, et al. Randomized trial of laparoscopic-assisted resection of colorectal carcinoma: 3 year results of the UK MRC CLASSIC Trial Group. J Clin Oncol 2007;25(21):3061–8.
8. Jayne DG, Thorpe HC, Copeland J, et al. Five year follow-up of the Medical Research Council CLASICC trial of laparoscopically-assisted versus open surgery for colorectal cancer. Br J Surg 2010;97(11):1638–45.
9. Abraham NS, Young JM, Solomon MJ. Meta-analysis of short-term outcomes after laparoscopic resection for colorectal cancer. Br J Surg 2004;91(9):1111–24.
10. Schwenk W, Haase O, Neudecker J, et al. Short term benefits for laparoscopic colorectal resection. Cochrane Database Syst Rev 2005;3:CD003145.
11. Abraham NS, Byrne CM, Young JM, et al. Meta-analysis of non-randomised comparative studies of the short-term outcomes of laparoscopic resection for colorectal cancer. Aust N Z J Surg 2007;77(7):508–16.

These meta-analyses assess the outcomes of randomised clinical trials and observational studies, and highlight the short-term benefits of laparoscopic resection of colorectal cancer over open surgery.

12. Duepree HJ, Senagore AJ, Delaney CP, et al. Does means of access affect the incidence of small bowel obstruction and ventral hernia after bowel resection? Laparoscopy versus laparotomy. J Am Coll Surg 2003;197(2):177–81.

13. Kiran RP, Delaney CP, Senagore AJ, et al. Operative blood loss and use of blood products after laparoscopic and conventional open colorectal operations. Arch Surg 2004;139(1):39–42.

14. Law WL, Lee YM, Choi HK, et al. Impact of laparoscopic resection for colorectal cancer on operative outcomes and survival. Ann Surg 2007;245(1):1–7.

15. Tjandra JJ, Chan MK. Systematic review on the short-term outcome of laparoscopic resection for colon and rectosigmoid cancer. Colorectal Dis 2006;8(5):375–88.

16. Braga M, Vignali A, Gianotti L, et al. Laparoscopic resection in rectal cancer patients: outcome and cost–benefit analysis. Dis Colon Rectum 2007;50:464–71.

17. Lourenco T, Murray A, Grant A, et al. Laparoscopic surgery for colorectal cancer: safe and effective? – A systematic review. Surg Endosc 2008;22(5):1146–60.

18. Murray A, Lourenco T, de Verteuil R, et al. Clinical effectiveness and cost-effectiveness of laparoscopic surgery for colorectal cancer: systematic reviews and economic evaluation. Health Technol Assess 2006;10(45):1–141, iii–iv.

19. King PM, Blazeby JM, Ewings P, et al. The influence of an enhanced recovery programme on clinical outcomes, costs and quality of life after surgery for colorectal cancer. Colorectal Dis 2006;8(6):506–13.

20. Dowson HM, Huang A, Soon Y, et al. Systematic review of the costs of laparoscopic colorectal surgery. Dis Colon Rectum 2007;50(6):908–19.

21. Senagore AJ, Duepree HJ, Delaney CP, et al. Cost structure of laparoscopic and open sigmoid colectomy for diverticular disease: similarities and differences. Dis Colon Rectum 2002;45(4):485–90.

22. Vlug MS, Wind J, Hollman MW, et al. Laparoscopy in combination with fast-track multimodal management is the perioperative strategy in patients undergoing colonic surgery: a randomised clinical trial (LAFA-study). Ann Surg 2011;254(6):868–75.

23. Buchanan GN, Malik A, Parvaiz A, et al. Laparoscopic resection for colorectal cancer. Br J Surg 2008;95(7):893–902.

24. Lumley J, Stitz R, Stevenson A, et al. Laparoscopic colorectal surgery for cancer: intermediate to long-term outcomes. Dis Colon Rectum 2002;45(7):867–75.

25. King PM, Blazeby JM, Ewings P, et al. Randomised clinical trial comparing laparoscopic and open surgery for colorectal cancer within an enhanced recovery programme. Br J Surg 2006;93(3):300–8.

26. Veldkamp R, Gholghesaei M, Bonjer IIJ, et al. Laparoscopic resection of colon cancer: consensus of the European Association of Endoscopic Surgery (EAES). Surg Endosc 2004;18(8):1163–85.

27. Schwandner O, Farke S, Schiedeck TH, et al. Laparoscopic colorectal surgery in obese and non-obese patients: do differences in body mass indices lead to different outcomes? Surg Endosc 2004;18(10):1452–6.

28. Senagore AJ, Delaney CP, Madboulay K, et al. Laparoscopic colectomy in obese and nonobese patients. J Gastrointest Surg 2003;7(4):558–61.

29. Arteaga Gonzalez I, Martin Malagon A, Lopez-Tomassetti Fernandez EM, et al. Impact of previous abdominal surgery on colorectal laparoscopy results: a comparative clinical study. Surg Laparosc Endosc Percutan Tech 2006;16(1):8–11.

30. Law WL, Choi HK, Ho JW, et al. Outcomes of surgery for mid and distal rectal cancer in the elderly. World J Surg 2006;30(4):598–604.

31. Moloo H, Bedard EL, Poulin EC, et al. Palliative laparoscopic resections for Stage IV colorectal cancer. Dis Colon Rectum 2006;49(2):213–8.

32. Kuhry E, Bonjer HJ, Haglind E, et al. Impact of hospital case volume on short-term outcome after laparoscopic operation for colonic cancer. Surg Endosc 2005;19(5):687–92.

33. Tekkis PP, Senagore AJ, Delaney CP. Conversion rates in laparoscopic colorectal surgery: a predictive model with 1253 patients. Surg Endosc 2005;19(1):47–54.

34. Marusch F, Gastinger I, Schneider C, et al. Importance of conversion for results obtained with laparoscopic colorectal surgery. Dis Colon Rectum 2001;44(2):207–16.

35. Casillas S, Delaney CP, Senagore AJ, et al. Does conversion of a laparoscopic colectomy adversely affect patient outcome? Dis Colon Rectum 2004;47(10):1680–5.

36. Bemelman WA, Slors JF, Dunker MS, et al. Laparoscopic-assisted vs. open ileocolic resection for Crohn's disease. A comparative study. Surg Endosc 2000;14(8):721–5.

37. Duepree HJ, Senagore AJ, Delaney CP, et al. Advantages of laparoscopic resection for ileocecal Crohn's disease. Dis Colon Rectum 2002; 45(5):605–10.

38. Lawes DA, Motson RW. Avoidance of laparotomy for recurrent disease is a long-term benefit of laparoscopic resection for Crohn's disease. Br J Surg 2006;93(5):607–8.

39. Milsom JW, Hammerhofer KA, Bohm B, et al. Prospective, randomised trial comparing laparoscopic vs. conventional surgery for refractory ileocolic Crohn's disease. Dis Colon Rectum 2001;44(1):1–9.

40. Maartense S, Dunker MS, Slors JF, et al. Laparoscopic-assisted versus open ileocolic resection

for Crohn's disease: a randomised trial. Ann Surg 2006;243(2):143–53.

41. Schwandner O, Farke S, Bruch HP. Laparoscopic colectomy for diverticulitis is not associated with increased morbidity when compared with non-diverticular disease. Int J Colorectal Dis 2005;20(2):165–72.

42. Pokala N, Delaney CP, Senagore AJ, et al. Laparoscopic vs open total colectomy: a case-matched comparative study. Surg Endosc 2005;19(4):531–5.

43. Tilney HS, Lovegrove RE, Heriot AG, et al. Comparison of short-term outcomes of laparoscopic vs open approaches to ileal pouch surgery. Int J Colorectal Dis 2007;22(5):531–42.

44. Antolovic D, Kienle P, Knaebel HP, et al. Totally laparoscopic versus conventional ileo-anal pouch procedure – design of a single-centre, expertise based randomised controlled trial to compare the laparoscopic and conventional surgical approach in patients undergoing primary elective restorative proctocolectomy – LapConPouch-Trial. BMC Surg 2006;6:13.

45. Arteaga-Gonzalez I, Martin-Malagon A, Fernandez EM, et al. The use of preoperative endoscopic tattooing in laparoscopic colorectal cancer surgery for endoscopically advanced tumors: a prospective comparative clinical study. World J Surg 2006;30(4):605–11.

46. Kennedy R, Jenkins I, Finan PJ. Controversial topics in surgery: Splenic flexure mobilization for anterior resection performed for sigmoid and rectal cancer. Ann R Coll Surg Engl 2008;90(8):638–42.

47. Law WL, Choi HK, Lee YM, et al. Laparoscopic colectomy for obstructing sigmoid cancer with prior insertion of an expandable metallic stent. Surg Laparosc Endosc Percutan Tech 2004;14(1):29–32.

48. Cheung HY, Chung CC, Tsang WW, et al. Endolaparoscopic approach vs conventional open surgery in the treatment of obstructing left-sided colon cancer: a randomised controlled trial. Arch Surg 2009;144(12):1127–32.

49. Pera M, Delgado S, Garcia-Valdecasas JC, et al. The management of leaking rectal anastomoses by minimally invasive techniques. Surg Endosc 2002;16(4):603–6.

50. Wind J, Koopman AG, van Berge Henegouwen MI, et al. Laparoscopic reintervention for anastomotic leakage after primary laparoscopic colorectal surgery. Br J Surg 2007;94(12):1562–6.

51. Tekkis PP, Senagore AJ, Delaney CP, et al. Evaluation of the learning curve in laparoscopic colorectal surgery: comparison of right-sided and left-sided resections. Ann Surg 2005;242(1):83–91.

52. Miskovic D, Wyles SM, Carter F, et al. Development, validation and implementation of a monitoring tool for training in laparoscopic colorectal surgery in the English National Training Program. Surg Endosc 2011;25:1136–42.

53. Evans J, Poritz L, MacRae H. Influence of experience on laparoscopic ileocolic resection for Crohn's disease. Dis Colon Rectum 2002;45(12):1595–600.

54. Aggarwal R, Grantcharov T, Moorthy K, et al. A competency-based virtual reality training curriculum for the acquisition of laparoscopic psychomotor skill. Am J Surg 2006;191(1):128–33.

55. Aggarwal R, Ward J, Balasundaram I, et al. Proving the effectiveness of virtual reality simulation for training in laparoscopic surgery. Ann Surg 2007;246(5):771–9.

56. Dath D, Regehr G, Birch D, et al. Toward reliable operative assessment: the reliability and feasibility of videotaped assessment of laparoscopic technical skills. Surg Endosc 2004;18(12):1800–4.

57. Sala S, Kennedy RH, Jenkins JT. Modular training in laparoscopic surgery accelerates proficiency gain. Colorectal Dis 2011;13(Suppl. 4):10.

58. Wexner SD, Bergamaschi R, Lacy A, et al. The current status of robotic pelvic surgery: results of a multinational interdisciplinary consensus conference. Surg Endosc 2009;23(2):438–43.

59. Pigazzi A, Luca A, Patriti A, et al. Multicentric study on robotic tumour-specific mesorectal excision for the treatment of rectal cancer. Ann Surg Oncol 2010;17(6):1614–20.

60. Zimmern A, Prasad L, Desouza A, et al. Robotic colon and rectal surgery: a series of 131 cases. World J Surg 2010;34(8):1954–8.

61. Adair J, Gromski MA, Lim RA, et al. Single incision laparoscopic right hemicolectomy: experience with 17 consecutive cases and comparison with multiport laparoscopic right hemicolectomy. Dis Colon Rectum 2010;53(11):1549–54.

62. Buess G, Hutterer F, Theiss J, et al. Das system fur die transanale rectum operation. Chirurg 1984;55:677–80.

63. van den Boezem PB, Kruyt PM, Stommel MWJ, et al. Transanal single-port surgery for the resection of large polyps. Dig Surg 2011;28:412–6.

64. van den Broek FJ, de Graaf EJ, Dijkgraaf MG, et al. Transanal endoscopic microsurgery versus endoscopic mucosal resection for large rectal adenomas (TREND-study). BMC Surg 2009;9:4.

65. Doornebosch PG, Ferenschild FT, de Wilt JH, et al. Treatment of recurrence after transanal endoscopic microsurgery (TEM) for T1 rectal cancer. Dis Colon Rectum 2005;48(6):1169–75.

66. Weiser MR, Landmann RG, Wong WD, et al. Surgical salvage of recurrent rectal cancer after transanal excision. Dis Colon Rectum 2005;48(6):1169–75.

67. Allaix ME, Arezzo A, Caldart M, et al. Transanal endoscopic microsurgery for rectal neoplasms: experience of 300 consecutive cases. Dis Colon Rectum 2009;52(11):1831–6.

68. Hahnloser D, Wolff BG, Larson DW, et al. Immediate radical resection after local excision of

rectal cancer: an oncologic compromise? Dis Colon Rectum 2005;48(3):429–37.

69. Habr-Gama A, Perez RO, Nadalin W, et al. Operative versus nonoperative treatment for stage 0 distal rectal cancer following chemoradiation therapy: long-term results. Ann Surg 2004;240(4):711–7.

70. Lezoche G, Baldarelli M, Guerrieri M, et al. A prospective randomized study with a 5-year minimum follow-up evaluation of transanal endoscopic microsurgery versus laparoscopic total mesorectal excision after neoadjuvant therapy. Surg Endosc 2008;22(2):352–8.

71. Birmingham Clinical Trials Unit. Transanal Endoscopic Microsurgery (TEM) and Radiotherapy in Early Rectal Cancer (TREC) Trial. Available at http://www.birmingham.ac.uk/research/activity/mds/trials/bctu/trials/coloproctology/trec/index.aspx; [accessed 6.09.12].

72. Basse L, Hjort Jakobsen D, Billesbolle P, et al. A clinical pathway to accelerate recovery after colonic resection. Ann Surg 2000;232(1):51–7.

73. Basse L, Raskov HH, Hjort Jakobsen D, et al. Accelerated postoperative recovery programme after colonic resection improves physical performance, pulmonary function and body composition. Br J Surg 2002;89(4):446–53.

74. Anderson AD, McNaught CE, MacFie J, et al. Randomised clinical trial of multimodal optimization and standard perioperative surgical care. Br J Surg 2003;90(12):1497–504.

75. Gatt M, Anderson AD, Reddy BS, et al. Randomised clinical trial of multimodal optimization of surgical care in patients undergoing major colonic resection. Br J Surg 2005;92(11):1354–62.

76. Delaney CP, Zutshi M, Senagore AJ, et al. Prospective, randomised, controlled trial between a pathway of controlled rehabilitation with early ambulation and diet and traditional postoperative care after laparotomy and intestinal resection. Dis Colon Rectum 2003;46(7):851–9.

77. Lassen K, Hannemann P, Ljungqvist O, et al. Patterns in current perioperative practice: survey of colorectal surgeons in five northern European countries. Br Med J 2005;330(7505):1420–1.

78. Nygren J, Hausel J, Kehlet H, et al. A comparison in five European Centres of case mix, clinical management and outcomes following either conventional or fast-track perioperative care in colorectal surgery. Clin Nutr 2005;24(3):455–61.

79. Fearon KC, Ljungqvist O, Von Meyenfeldt M, et al. Enhanced recovery after surgery: a consensus review of clinical care for patients undergoing colonic resection. Clin Nutr 2005;24(3):466–77.

80. Francis N, Kennedy RH, Ljungqvist O, et al. editors. Manual of fast track recovery for colorectal surgery. Springer; 2012.

81. Ljungqvist O, Soreide E. Preoperative fasting. Br J Surg 2003;90(4):400–6.

82. Soreide E, Ljungqvist O. Modern preoperative fasting guidelines: a summary of the present recommendations and remaining questions. Best Pract Res Clin Anaesthesiol 2006;20(3):483–91.

83. Soreide E, Ljungqvist O. Preoperative fasting. Can J Surg 2006;49(3):218–9; author reply 219.

84. Svanfeldt M, Thorell A, Hausel J, et al. Randomised clinical trial of the effect of preoperative oral carbohydrate treatment on postoperative whole-body protein and glucose kinetics. Br J Surg 2007;94(11):1342–50.

85. Soop M, Carlson GL, Hopkinson J, et al. Randomised clinical trial of the effects of immediate enteral nutrition on metabolic responses to major colorectal surgery in an enhanced recovery protocol. Br J Surg 2004;91(9):1138–45.
These elegant small RCTs assess the effect of perioperative feeding in attenuating the metabolic response. This group have identified benefits with this approach in maintaining whole-body protein balance and that the suppressive effects of endogenous glucose release are better maintained with preoperative carbohydrate loading and postoperative feeding.

86. Keele AM, Bray MJ, Emery PW, et al. Two phase randomised controlled clinical trial of postoperative oral dietary supplements in surgical patients. Gut 1997;40(3):393–9.

87. Rana SK, Bray J, Menzies-Gow N, et al. Short term benefits of post-operative oral dietary supplements in surgical patients. Clin Nutr 1992;11(6):337–44.

88. Guenaga KF, Matos D, Castro AA, et al. Mechanical bowel preparation for elective colorectal surgery. Cochrane Database Syst Rev 2005;1:CD001544.

89. Bucher P, Mermillod B, Gervaz P, et al. Mechanical bowel preparation for elective colorectal surgery: a meta-analysis. Arch Surg 2004;139(12):1359–65.

90. Slim K, Vicaut E, Panis Y, et al. Meta-analysis of randomised clinical trials of colorectal surgery with or without mechanical bowel preparation. Br J Surg 2004;91(9):1125–30.

91. Contant CM, Hop WC, van't Sant HP, et al. Mechanical bowel preparation for elective colorectal surgery: a multicentre randomised trial. Lancet 2007;370(9605):2112–7.

92. Platell C, Barwood N, Makin G. Randomised clinical trial of bowel preparation with a single phosphate enema or polyethylene glycol before elective colorectal surgery. Br J Surg 2006;93(4):427–33.

93. Matthiessen P, Hallbook O, Rutegard J, et al. Defunctioning stoma reduces symptomatic anastomotic leakage after low anterior resection of the rectum for cancer: a randomised multicenter trial. Ann Surg 2007;246(2):207–14.

94. Brandstrup B, Svensen C, Engquist A. Haemorrhage and operation cause a contraction of the extracellular space needing replacement – evidence and implications? A systematic review. Surgery 2006;139(3):419–32.

95. Brandstrup B, Tonnesen H, Beier-Holgersen R, et al. Effects of intravenous fluid restriction on postoperative complications: comparison of two perioperative fluid regimens: a randomised assessor-blinded multicenter trial. Ann Surg 2003;238(5):641–8.

96. Lobo DN, Bostock KA, Neal KR, et al. Effect of salt and water balance on recovery of gastrointestinal function after elective colonic resection: a randomised controlled trial. Lancet 2002;359(9320):1812–8. These studies have had a potent effect on our renewed interest in perioperative fluid management. Brandstrup et al.'s paper shows clear benefits to fluid restriction compared to traditional practice, with significantly elevated morbidity levels in the traditional group who received large fluid volumes in the perioperative period. Lobo et al.'s study on a small number of patients confirms the important effects of fluid management on gut function and recovery.

97. Powell-Tuck J, Gosling P, Lobo D, et al. British Consensus Guidelines on intravenous fluid therapy for adult surgical patients – GIFTASUP. JCIS 2009;10(1):13–5.

98. Walsh SR, Tang T, Bass S, et al. Doppler-guided intra-operative fluid management during major abdominal surgery: systematic review and meta-analysis. Int J Clin Pract 2008;62(3):466–70.

99. Pearse R, Dawson D, Fawcett J, et al. Early goal-directed therapy after major surgery reduces complications and duration of hospital stay. A randomised, controlled trial (ISRCTN38797445). Crit Care 2005; 9(6):R687–93.

100. Noblett SE, Snowden CP, Shenton BK, et al. Randomised clinical trial assessing the effect of Doppler-optimised fluid management on outcome after elective colorectal resection. Br J Surg 2006;93(9):1069–76.

101. O'Dwyer PJ, McGregor JR, McDermott EW, et al. Patient recovery following cholecystectomy through a 6 cm or 15 cm transverse subcostal incision: a prospective randomised clinical trial. Postgrad Med J 1992;68(804):817–9.

102. Brown SR, Goodfellow PB. Transverse versus midline incisions for abdominal surgery. Cochrane Database Syst Rev 2005;4:CD005199.

103. Veenhof AA, Vlug MS, van der Pas MH, et al. Surgical stress response and postoperative immune function after laparoscopy or open surgery with fast track or standard perioperative care: a randomised trial. Ann Surg 2012;255(2):216–21.

104. Jesus EC, Karliczek A, Matos D, et al. Prophylactic anastomotic drainage for colorectal surgery. Cochrane Database Syst Rev 2004;4:CD002100.

105. Gendall KA, Kennedy RR, Watson AJ, et al. The effect of epidural analgesia on postoperative outcome after colorectal surgery. Colorectal Dis 2007;9(7):584–600.

106. Liu SS, Wu CL. Effect of postoperative analgesia on major postoperative complications: a systematic update of the evidence. Anesth Analg 2007;104(3):689–702.

107. Levy BF, Scott MJ, Fawcett W, et al. Randomised clinical trial of epidural, spinal or patient-controlled analgesia for patients undergoing laparoscopic colorectal surgery. Br J Surg 2011;98(8):1068–78.

108. Varadhan KK, Neal KR, Dejong CH, et al. The enhanced recovery after surgery (ERAS) pathway for patients undergoing major elective open colorectal surgery: a meta-analysis of randomised controlled trials. Clin Nutr 2010;29(4):434–40.

109. Adamina M, Kehlet H, Tomlinson GA, et al. Enhanced recovery pathways optimise health outcomes and resource utilisation: a meta-analysis of randomised controlled trials in colorectal surgery. Surgery 2011;149(6):830–40.

110. Basse L, Jakobsen DH, Bardram L, et al. Functional recovery after open versus laparoscopic colonic resection: a randomised, blinded study. Ann Surg 2005;241(3):416–23.

111. Gustafsson UO, Hausel J, Thorell A, et al. Adherence to the enhanced recovery after surgery protocol and outcomes after colorectal cancer surgery. Arch Surg 2011;146(5):571–7.

18

Intestinal failure

Carolynne Vaizey
Janindra Warusavitarne

Introduction

The term intestinal failure (IF) encompasses a spectrum of conditions that manifests itself as an inability to maintain adequate nutritional, fluid and electrolyte homeostasis without supportive therapy.[1] The vast majority of cases are transient, without significant gut pathology, and are routinely managed in general surgical units. They frequently occur secondary to postoperative ileus. However, there is a group of cases distinguished by loss of functional gut that results in prolonged intestinal failure lasting from months to years, some patients requiring permanent parenteral nutrition. These cases may be due to massive gut loss following surgery, or loss of functioning intestine available for absorption, as occurs after enterocutaneous fistula formation.

Management of these cases may be complex, prolonged and expensive, in terms of both financial cost and clinical input. Care may be optimised by involvement of a multidisciplinary unit devoted to the management of IF. This unit will include a nutrition support team with the capacity to facilitate the transition of the patient's care from a hospital environment to a home environment. The care of patients with IF is prolonged and involves specialist gastroenterological, surgical and nursing input. Surgical treatment is generally the last of many steps in the management but accounts for an important part of the workload of specialised IF units.[1]

The nursing staff on the ward and in clinic, specialist nutrition nurses and the home parenteral nutrition (PN) team are the backbone of delivery of care to these patients and their families. The different functions of each of these groups and their separate locations make it imperative that all are coordinated in their approach to each patient. Failure to achieve this results in confusion and demoralisation of this psychologically vulnerable group of patients, who are faced with prolonged hospital admission, a debilitating illness, the prospect of no longer being able to eat normally (or at all) and the likelihood of incomplete functional recovery. Those who do survive find it difficult to accept the major limitations to their opportunities in life, especially in the case of young adults who constitute a significant proportion of these patients. A high level of technical training of the carers is required, which necessitates a specialist centre to maintain the technical base to these skills.

In addition, congenial working conditions will help prevent high staff turnover and consequent loss of skills. Coordination is achieved by a sense of team purpose and familiarity, consultant-led weekly multidisciplinary rounds, and a consensus approach to patient management that is explicitly stated in a protocol, but which allows flexibility for medical and social demands.

The British Government has set up and funded two supraregional units in England through the National Specialist Commissioning Advisory Body. One is at St Mark's Hospital in London (Watford Road,

Harrow, Middlesex HA1 3UJ), the other is at Hope Hospital in Salford (Stott Lane, Salford, Manchester M6 8HD).

Intestinal failure: criteria for referral

The following criteria[2] are an indication of the type of cases that warrant referral to a nationally designated intestinal failure unit:

1. Persistence of intestinal failure beyond 6 weeks, without any evidence of resolution and/or complicated by venous access problems.
2. Multiple intestinal fistulation in a totally dehisced abdominal wound.
3. An intestinal fistula outside the expertise of the referring unit (e.g. recurrent in a non-specialist unit) or second and third recurrences in a colorectal centre.
4. Total or near-total small-bowel enterectomy, resulting in less than 30 cm of residual small bowel.
5. Recurrent venous access problems in patients needing sustained parenteral nutrition. This definition includes recurrent severe infections and recurrent venous thrombosis, where all upper limb and cervical venous access routes have become obliterated.
6. Persistent intra-abdominal sepsis, complicated by severe metabolic derangement (characterised by hypoalbuminaemia), that is not responding to radiological/surgical drainage of sepsis and provision of nutritional support.
7. Metabolic complications relating to high-output fistulas and stomas and to prolonged intravenous feeding, not responsive to medication and adjustment of the feeding regimen. Disorders of hepatic and renal function associated with intravenous nutrition that are resistant to metabolic and nutritional supplementation.
8. Chronic intestinal failure (from whatever cause) in a hospital without adequate experience/expertise to manage the medical/surgical and nutritional requirements of such patients.

Epidemiology

The prevalence of IF is unknown, but estimates can be made by considering those who require home PN. The incidence of home PN in Europe is estimated to be 3 per million population and the prevalence at 4 per million population, of whom 35% have short bowel syndrome (SBS).[3] In the USA the use of home PN is estimated to be 120 per million population, of whom approximately 25% have SBS.[4] Such data do not include the patients who have not required home PN or those who have been successfully weaned off home PN. In the UK the estimated incidence of IF requiring treatment at a specialised unit is 5.5 per million population.[1]

As SBS is an uncommon condition, specialised centres with expertise in SBS have been created.[1,5,6] A recent study showed an overall survival rate of 86% in patients undergoing autologous surgical reconstruction at a median follow-up period of 2 years in a specialised unit.[7] Similar results have been achieved in other units and highlight the importance of multidisciplinary care.[1,8]

Causes

The causes of IF are multifactorial but can be categorised into four broad areas:

1. loss of intestinal length;
2. loss of functional intestinal length;
3. loss of intestinal absorptive capacity;
4. loss of intestinal function.

Loss of intestinal length

In the adult population IF is most commonly related to a loss of intestinal length as a result of multiple or one massive intestinal resection.[9,10] Multiple resections are most common in recurrent Crohn's disease; an isolated massive enterectomy usually follows a vascular catastrophe, such as mesenteric arterial thrombosis or embolism or a venous thrombosis. Massive resection can also be necessary in cases of volvulus, trauma or, in the case of children, necrotising enterocolitis or gastroschisis.

The relation between the amount of bowel removed and the degree of IF is variable, influenced by the age of the patient, the site of resection and the presence or absence of colon. The normal small bowel is around 600 cm in length but may range between 300 and 800 cm. The important figure is not how much small bowel is removed but how much remains. An approximate figure of less than 100 cm in the presence of an ileostomy or less than 50 cm with colon present is likely to result in dependence on PN at 3 months. Children may function with shorter bowel as small-bowel adaptation (see below) can be very dramatic. The function of the remaining bowel may also be influenced by the presence of active Crohn's disease as well as the presence or absence of colon, as this may have a significant absorptive function.

Loss of functional absorptive capacity

Enterocutaneous fistula (ECF) is the commonest cause of IF where the mechanism is loss of functional absorptive capacity. Fistulous disease commonly bypasses otherwise normal functional small intestine. This is usually the result of an ECF, but hidden internal fistulas may also be responsible.

At a specialised IF unit, 42% of patients had Crohn's disease and the commonest complication necessitating admission was formation of ECFs.[1] The second most common cause of fistulas is abdominal surgery. The majority of fistulas occuring in postoperative patients[11,12] are the consequence of anastomotic breakdown. Risks for this include the age of the patient, the state of the bowel undergoing anastomosis, preoperative nutritional status and the site of anastomosis.[11] When associated with malignancy, factors including tumour fixity, presence of obstruction, previous radiotherapy, associated abscess and surgical technique all affect the risk. Non-absorbable mesh can erode into the bowel and cause fistula, particularly where there is fragile postoperative or diseased bowel. The use of vacuum-assisted closure (VAC) systems in the open abdomen can result in fistula when applied next to the bowel wall. In patients with intestinal or peritoneal inflammation and/or multi-organ failure there is a 20% rate of intestinal fistulisation associated with the use of a VAC system.[13] Newer VAC systems designed to prevent the sponge from making direct contact with the bowel have yet to be evaluated.

Other causes of fistulas include colorectal cancer, diverticular disease and radiation. Fistulas resulting from radiation damage are usually complex and carry a high mortality. Rarer conditions include trauma and congenital fistulas, such as a patent vitello-intestinal tract. Tuberculosis may fistulate as a complication of an ileal mass, and actinomycosis is an alternative possibility. Ulcerative colitis may fistulate, but this is more commonly postoperatively, and occasionally the diagnosis needs reviewing as to the possibility of Crohn's disease.

Loss of intestinal absorptive capacity

Inflammatory conditions of the small bowel can result in non-functioning enterocytes that reduce absorptive capacity. Such conditions include inflammatory bowel disease, sprue, scleroderma, amyloid, coeliac disease and radiation enteritis.

Loss of intestinal function

In the acute setting, postoperative ileus is the commonest reason for a loss of intestinal function, but this is usually self-limiting and does not require more than short-term supportive treatment. More chronic conditions such as pseudo-obstruction, visceral myopathy or autonomic neuropathy can result in functional disability and present a significant challenge for management.

Pathophysiology

The three stages of intestinal failure

Following the initiating event, intestinal 'recovery' results in three recognisable phases that have implications for management.

Stage I: hypersecretory phase
Of the 7 litres secreted daily by the duodenum, stomach, small intestine, pancreas and liver, about 6 litres are reabsorbed proximal to the ileocaecal valve. A further 800 mL are reabsorbed in the colon, leaving just 200 mL of water in the faeces.

Lack of absorption results in large volume losses. This phase can last 1–2 months and is characterised by copious diarrhoea and/or high stoma or fistula outputs. The main focus of treatment is on fluid and electrolyte replacement while PN may be required to maintain nutrition.

Stage II: adaptation phase

The process of intestinal adaptation involves a series of histological changes in the intestinal mucosa that permit enhanced mucosal absorption within the residual intestine. The triggers for adaptation are the maintenance of fluid and electrolyte balance and the gradual introduction of enteral feeding. The process of adaptation takes 3–12 months and the degree of adaptation varies with age (more adaptation occurs in the paediatric population), underlying disease extent, and the site of resection (ileum has better capacity for adaptation than jejunum).

Stage III: stabilisation phase

Maximum intestinal adaptation may take up to 1–2 years and the extent and route of nutritional support will vary. The overall goal for the patient is to achieve as normal a lifestyle as possible, which means achieving stability at home.

Normal physiological functioning of the intestine involves complex fluid, electrolyte and nutrient exchanges to maintain homeostasis. Interruption of this arrangement can result in gross imbalances that require supplementation enterally or parenterally. The normal physiology of the intestine is discussed below.

Fluid and electrolytes

Sodium absorption in the small bowel is actively linked to the absorption of glucose and certain amino acids. Water absorption is passive and follows the sodium. The jejunum is freely permeable to water, so the contents remain isotonic.

> ✔✔ Movement of sodium into the lumen occurs if luminal sodium concentration is low, and absorption of sodium, and hence water, occurs only when the concentration is greater than 100 mmol/L.[14]

Sodium absorption normally occurs in the ileum and colon. In the absence of the absorptive capacity of the ileum and colon the net sodium losses are expectedly high. This occurs in the presence of a high fistula or jejunostomy. If there is a high fistula or jejunostomy, the daily net loss of sodium and net loss of water from the body will be approximately 300–400 mmol and 3–4 L, respectively. This highlights the importance of sodium replacement when there is a high jejunostomy or fistula. Oral fluid concentrated in sodium will help reduce enteric fluid losses. The minimum required daily oral sodium replacement is 100 mmol. The sodium concentration that is absorbable is limited by palatability.[15]

The colon has a significant absorptive capacity, amounting to 6–7 L of water, up to 700 mmol of sodium and 40 mmol of potassium per day. Connection of colon in continuity with the residual small bowel will significantly reduce water and sodium losses.

Potassium absorption is usually adequate unless there is less than 60 cm of small bowel. In this scenario, standard daily intravenous requirements of 60–100 mmol of potassium are required. Magnesium is usually absorbed in the distal jejunum and ileum. Loss of these will result in significant magnesium loss and deficiency. Magnesium deficiency may precipitate calcium deficiency because hypomagnesaemia impairs the release of parathyroid hormone.

Nutrients

Carbohydrates, proteins and water-soluble vitamins

The upper 200 cm of jejunum absorbs most carbohydrates, protein and water-soluble vitamins. Nitrogen is the macronutrient least affected by a decrease in the absorptive surface and utilisation of peptide-based diets rather than protein-based ones has demonstrated no benefit.[15] Water-soluble vitamin deficiencies are rare in patients with SBS, although thiamine deficiency has been reported.[16]

Fat, bile salts and fat-soluble vitamins

Fat and the fat-soluble vitamins (A, D, E and K) are absorbed over the length of the small intestine.[17] Hence loss of ileum will impair absorption. Bile salts are also reabsorbed in the ileum and bile salt deficiency will contribute to reduced fat absorption. However, bile salt supplements such as cholestyramine have shown no benefit and may worsen steatorrhoea due to binding of dietary lipid[18] and may also worsen fat-soluble vitamin deficiency. In view of multifactorial metabolic bone disease, vitamin D_2 supplements are often given empirically along with calcium supplements. Vitamin A and E deficiencies have been reported, but usually an awareness that visual or neurological symptoms may indicate deficiency combined with infrequent monitoring of serum levels are all that is necessary. If the patient is wholly dependent on PN, then replacement along with vitamin K injections is required. Most patients have lost their terminal ileum and so require vitamin B_{12} replacement. Trace elements appear not to be a problem, with normal levels being found in patients on long-term PN.

Loss of bowel results not only in decreased absorptive capacity but also rapid transit. Reduced time for absorption will exacerbate nutritional deficiencies.

Adaptation

Following massive small-bowel resection there are changes in the mucosal surface of the remaining small intestine. Most experimental work has been in small animals such as rats. It appears that adaptation will occur only if there is enteral feeding. Patients who are wholly dependent on PN have mucosal atrophy, which is reversed on refeeding enterally. The mechanism for this is at present unknown, but various trophic factors have been proposed. Current theory is that increased crypt cell proliferation leads to lengthening of villi and deepening of crypts, so resulting in increased surface area. Because the ileum has shorter villi it is able to adapt further, but is unfortunately more frequently resected. The stimulation to adapt appears to be threefold: (i) direct absorption of enteral nutrients leading to local mucosal hyperplasia; (ii) enteral nutrition resulting in the release of trophic hormones and a paracrine effect; and (iii) increased fluid and protein secretion with subsequent resorption, leading to increased enterocyte workload and adaptation.[17]

Another form of adaptation occurs in neonates, infants and young children, where continued developmental growth of the small intestine may make the difference between dependence on PN and managing with an enteral diet.[18]

Role of the colon in SBS

The colon has significant absorptive capacity, not only for fluid and electrolytes as described above, but also for short-chain fatty acids.[19,20] These are an energy substrate and in the region of 500 kcal may be derived in this way. It is estimated that having a colon is the equivalent of approximately 50 cm of small bowel for energy purposes.[21] The colon will also slow intestinal transit, particularly if the ileocaecal valve is present, which will improve absorption.

Having overcome the immediate problems of fluid balance and nutritional replacement, a frequent problem for those patients who still have their large bowel in continuity is diarrhoea. Excessive carbohydrate entry into the colon may result in osmotic diarrhoea.[22,23] Alternatively, choleric diarrhoea may be brought on by failure to reabsorb bile salts completely. Colonic bacteria deconjugate and dehydroxylate these into bile acids, which stimulate water and electrolyte secretion. In the more extreme cases of SBS, bile salt depletion may occur that will then give rise to steatorrhoea from incompletely digested long-chain fatty acids. Bile salts increase colonic permeability to oxalate. As the undigested fatty acids bind calcium in preference to oxalate, there is a resultant increase in enteric oxalate uptake and hence increased renal stone formation.[23]

✔✔ There is also an increased frequency of mixed gallstones, possibly because of interruption of the enterohepatic circulation.[24]

Lastly, D-lactate acidosis[25] is a rare syndrome that comprises headache, drowsiness, stupor, confusion, behavioural disturbance, ataxia, blurred vision, ophthalmoplegia and/or nystagmus. The exact mechanism is unknown. It may be provoked by a carbohydrate load and is relieved by antibiotics. Whether it is a direct result of D-lactate or whether this is a marker for some other substance is unclear. There is anecdotal evidence that neomycin or vancomycin has led to improvements.

Surgical catastrophe and management

The management of IF and ECF can present a paradigm of multidisciplinary care. In those patients who fail to heal spontaneously, surgical treatment is generally one of the last of many steps in treatment. Owing to the heterogeneity of this condition, randomised controlled trials have not been performed in patients and most recommendations are based on expert opinion. The multidisciplinary approach to management involves initial 'damage control' and medical management followed by definitive surgical management. It is vitally important to initiate wound and psychological management early in order to prevent and reduce effluent-associated excoriation and prepare the patient mentally for what may be at least a few months of therapy.

Resuscitation

As discussed above, the scenarios in which patients usually develop IF are often acute catastrophes, and the very nature of IF is such that patients are often severely fluid and electrolyte depleted. In the light of this, urgent fluid and electrolyte replacement is vital. This will often have been undertaken when the patient was first admitted to hospital, before transfer to a specialist intestinal failure centre.

Restitution

The key components of restitution may be summarised by the acronym SNAPP, representing sepsis, nutrition, anatomy, protection of skin and planned surgery.

Sepsis

Sepsis is often present in patients who have developed intestinal failure and adversely influences outcome.

> ✅ In a study of patients with enterocutaneous fistulas, Reber et al.[11] reported an overall mortality of 11%, with 65% of these associated with sepsis. In patients who had their sepsis controlled within 1 month the mortality was 8%, with spontaneous closure of the fistula in 48%. In those where sepsis remained uncontrolled the mortality was 85%, with a spontaneous closure rate of 6%.

Awareness of the high probability of associated sepsis is vital, and if the suspicion arises patients should be thoroughly investigated. Currently the optimum tool to identify collections is computed tomography (CT). Management includes appropriate antibiotics and drainage of sepsis. This is usually possible and successful radiologically, and is the preferred option where possible. Surgical drainage carries a high risk of further bowel damage.

Nutrition

Sepsis and inflammatory bowel disease can add to patients' state of malnutrition. Replacement of fluid, electrolytes and nutrients, including carbohydrate,

protein, fat and vitamins, is vital. Monitoring fluid and electrolyte replacement is a key part of nutritional support and involves serum electrolyte measurements and regular weight measurements. Hiram Studley in 1936 commented that 'Weight loss is a basic indicator of surgical risk' and this still remains true today.

Fluid and electrolytes

Following resuscitation, fluid and electrolyte requirements will depend on the patient's losses. As described above, the first stage of IF is a hypersecretory phase, with high outputs and gastric hypersecretion. Fluid and electrolyte replacement should be by the intravenous route, with the following requirements:

- Water: losses + 1 L
- Na^+: losses (100 mmol/L effluent) + 80 mmol
- K^+: 80 mmol/day
- Mg^{2+}: 10 mmol/day.

Nutritional support

Early return to enteral nutrition should be the aim as soon as the patient is haemodynamically stable and fluid and electrolyte replacement complete. Parenteral nutrition should be regarded as a support mechanism rather than the main source of calories. Overall energy requirements depend on the size and weight of the patient, activity levels and metabolic status, with sepsis increasing demand. The rule of thumb is that males require 25–30 kcal/kg/day and females 20–25 kcal/kg/day of non-protein energy. For research purposes, more exact estimates can be made using the Harris–Benedict equation:

$$\text{Male energy expenditure} = [66 + (13.7 + W) + (5 + H) - (6.8 + A)] + SF$$

$$\text{Female energy expenditure} = [665 + (9.6 + W) + (1.7 + H) - (4.7 + A)] + SF$$

where W represents weight (kg), H height (cm), A age (years) and SF stress factor.

However, the Harris–Benedict equation is inconvenient for daily use. Replacement should also include 1.0–1.5 kg/day of protein.

Daily requirements from the American Gastroenterological Association[26] for patients with SBS are recorded in Table 18.1.

Parenteral nutrition will provide calories (carbohydrate and fat), protein (amino acids), vitamins

Table 18.1 • Dietary macronutrient recommendations for short bowel syndrome

	Colon present	Colon absent
Carbohydrate	Complex carbohydrate, 30–35 kcal/kg daily soluble fibre	Variable, 30–35 kcal/kg daily
Fat	MCT/LCT, 20–30% of caloric intake, with or without low fat/high fat	LCT, 20–30% of caloric intake, with or without low fat/high fat
Protein	Intact protein, 1.0–1.5 g/kg daily, with or without peptide-based formula	Intact protein, 1.0–1.5 g/kg daily, with or without peptide-based formula

LCT, long-chain triglyceride; MCT, medium-chain triglyceride.
Reproduced from Buchman AL, Scolapio J, Fryer J. AGA technical review on short bowel syndrome and intestinal transplantation. Gastroenterology 2003; 124:1111–34. With permission from Elsevier.

and trace elements. The volume should also be considered as part of the daily fluid requirement, with additional fluid requirements given as normal saline.

Reduction of output

Losses from stomas, fistulas or the anus may be very substantial, making replacement and simple management difficult. A number of strategies should be introduced to reduce these losses. Although they should be allowed to eat solids, patients should be restricted to around 500 mL of water orally per day, as hypotonic drinks will increase output in patients with SBS as described above. They should be cautioned against consumption of plain water and be given electrolyte solution, which will reduce intestinal fluid and electrolyte losses. There are several commercially available formulas. The St Mark's electrolyte solution is made from 1 L of water to which is added 20 g of glucose (six tablespoons), 3.5 g of sodium chloride (one level 5-mL teaspoon) and 2.5 g of sodium bicarbonate (one heaped 2.5-mL teaspoon). This provides 100 mmol of sodium per litre. The problem is palatability, although this may be improved by the addition of orange squash or similar flavourings. Patients at home can make up this solution themselves. The World Health Organisation recommendations are similar but also contain 20 mmol of potassium chloride.[27]

Medication is also given to reduce gastric hypersecretion. H_2-receptor blockers can reduce gastric hypersecretion,[28] as can proton-pump inhibitors, but not always enough to obviate the need for parenteral fluid supplements.[29,30]

Patients are routinely started on omeprazole to reduce gastric output. Octreotide produces a similar action but is more expensive and has been shown to be of little benefit to patients except in the first 2 weeks.

A review of all controlled studies evaluating the effects of somatostatin or octeotride showed that none demonstrated a significant increase in the rate of fistula closure.[31] Medication to slow intestinal transit or gastric emptying should in theory improve absorption,[28] so both codeine phosphate and loperamide[32,33] are used on an empirical basis. They are given before meals and often at higher doses than normal, frequently crushed. However, codeine runs the risk of addiction and clinical trials are equivocal as to the benefit of both,[34] so monitoring the effluent and weighing patients daily are essential for individual assessment. Bulking agents have shown no benefit in reducing stomal effluent. Cholestyramine may be used to treat hyperoxaluria, but it has no place in those with a jejunostomy, and in those with a colon in continuity it may reduce jejunal bile salt concentration to a level below the minimal micellar concentration for absorption of fat, resulting in steatorrhoea. A review of long-term medication is always useful, paying particular heed to site of uptake. Enteric-coated tablets are unlikely to be useful.

Dietary modification

Oral feeding should be introduced gradually with additions made one at a time and assessed. Patients should remain fluid restricted and continue on oral rehydration solution, gastric antisecretory drugs and antidiarrhoeal medication, the latter taken 30–60 minutes before meals. Drinking should be avoided during meals as this increases losses. It is important to continue intravenous maintenance therapy during this time as this will reduce the pressure on the patient to drink. In the early part of the second clinical stage it may be necessary to feed the patient wholly using PN, as gastric hypersecretion in response to even the smallest volume of enteral feeding can prejudice newly stabilised fluid balance.

A change of eating pattern to one of 'grazing' or 'little and often' increases the absorption window for the small intestine. Alternatively, overnight nasogastric tube or percutaneous endoscopic gastrostomy feeding can utilise otherwise unproductive absorption time.[35]

Oral magnesium oxide capsules, 12–16 mmol daily, are started and intravenous therapy is gradually withdrawn. Magnesium replacement may need to remain intravenous, albeit intermittent.

The precise balance between oral and parenteral requirements will vary between patients. As a rule of thumb, daily stoma/fistula losses below 1500 mL may be managed with oral replacement alone; losses between 1500 and 2000 mL require sodium and water replacement, usually as subcutaneous or intravenous fluids, but no parenteral nutrition; and losses of more than 2000 mL per day require parenteral nutrition. Requirements will change over time as adaptation occurs; this can continue for up to 2 years and in the case of children can be very dramatic.

Outcome aims and monitoring

Clinically, the aim is for the patient to have no thirst or signs of dehydration, with acceptable strength, energy and appearance. Biochemical targets should include the following:

- Gut loss: <2 L/day
- Urine: >1 L/day
- Urine Na^+: >20 mmol/L
- Serum Mg^{2+}: >0.7 mmol/L
- Body weight within 10% of normal.

The mainstays of monitoring in the first stage are those used in the normal postoperative patient (temperature, pulse, blood pressure, postural hypotension, urinary output, and daily urea and electrolytes), combined with random estimations of urinary sodium osmolality. If urinary sodium content falls below 20 mmol/L, then deficiency is likely. As the patient stabilises, fluid balance is monitored with daily weight estimation and the acute observations are reduced in frequency. A meticulous watch is kept on the input/output volumes, with specifically designed charts for ease and clarity of recording. With the fluid balance under control and the eradication of any associated septic foci, reassessment of the underlying trend of the patient's nutritional status is performed. This is done by calculating body mass indices, skinfold thickness and serum albumin, and by making an estimate of likely return to normal activities. As the patient moves into the third stage of maximum adaptation, the common nutrient deficiencies are assessed (Table 18.2) and the rarer complications are clinically looked for (Box 18.1).

Table 18.2 • Supplementation required in patients with intestinal failure depending on whether the patient needs partly enteral or wholly parenteral feeding

Nutrient	Parenteral	Partly enteral	Route
Potassium	Yes	If <60 cm and a jejunostomy	In PN or oral supplement
Magnesium	Common with a jejunostomy Uncommon with a colon		Magnesium oxide 12–24 mmol daily
Calcium	Uncertain	Vitamin D_2 400–900 IU daily	
Vitamin D	Uncertain		
Vitamin A	Uncommon		Watch for visual and neurological symptoms and monitor levels 3-yearly
Vitamin E	Uncommon		
Vitamin K	Yes	Normal	Monthly injections
Vitamin B complex	Yes	Normal	In PN
Vitamin C	Yes	Normal	In PN
Vitamin B_{12}	If terminal ileum lost (most patients)	Bimonthly hydroxycobalamin 1000 µg	
Iron	Yes	Normal	In PN
Zinc	Yes	Normal	In PN
Copper	Yes	Normal	In PN

PN, parenteral nutrition.

Box 18.1 • Complications of intestinal failure

Early
- Dehydration
- Hyponatraemia
- Shock
- Hypokalaemia

Intermediate
- Morale
- Weight loss
- Immune compromise
- Peptic ulcers
- Gastro-oesophageal reflux disease
- Proximal small-bowel inflammation
- Diarrhoea
- Bacterial overgrowth
- Peristomal excoriation

Late
- Vitamin deficiency syndromes
- Growth retardation in children
- Depression
- PN-induced liver disease
- Recurrent sepsis
- Intravenous line-related complications
- Cholelithiasis
- D-lactate acidosis
- Urolithiasis

Total parenteral nutrition

PN is used either as a temporary measure to maintain fluid and energy intake while the remaining small bowel undergoes adaptation or as definitive treatment in itself. It may also be used as non-total parenteral nutrition in the third clinical stage. The advantages of maintaining some enteral nutrition, even if unable to be totally sufficient in terms of energy needs, include maintenance of normal gut flora, increased gastrointestinal adaptation and prevention of biliary sludge accumulation. With better understanding has come a willingness to maintain patients at home on PN. This is a great advantage for those who are dependent on PN and who have not otherwise responded to medical therapy. The benefits of the home environment cannot be overestimated in terms of morale and psychological well-being in an otherwise chronically hospitalised patient.[36] Home PN depends upon a stable physiological condition, other medical pathology, a suitable social set-up and good patient education, coupled with a dedicated PN team providing technical support and advice. Even then, it is not without complications, the chief among them being catheter sepsis.[37,38] Meticulous aseptic technique on the part of the team and patient is essential if this is to be avoided. It takes about 3 weeks as an inpatient for the nursing staff to teach sufficiently rigorous self-care of the feeding line. Other complications, such as catheter occlusion, hepatic dysfunction, gallstones and bone disease, may occur.[39] Guidelines to its use are well established.[40]

Anatomy (mapping)

Defining the anatomy is important in terms of both planned management and prediction of long-term outcome. This may vary from determining how much small bowel remains, which may give an indication as to the likely necessity for permanent PN, to defining the anatomy of ECFs that will enable planned surgery later. The key facts to identify therefore are small-bowel anatomy, site of origin of a fistula (if present) and the anatomy of fistulous tracts.

Radiological contrast studies are the investigations of choice for assessing remaining bowel length and may include small-bowel follow-through or enema, and fistulograms. CT enteroclysis and magnetic resonance (MR) enteroclysis can also be very useful in examining pathological bowel and areas of other pathology, such as areas of ongoing obstruction or septic collections.[41–43] CT scanning can also provide valuable information, such as safe sites of entry into the abdominal cavity. Active discussion between the IF team and the radiologists is essential as each case is unique and poses different questions.

Protection of skin

Protection of the skin is an essential component of management of patients with intestinal failure. Small-bowel output is caustic and excoriation of skin around a stoma or fistula is a painful, demoralising and highly visible immediate complication. The extent of the problem will vary, ranging from a standard end ileostomy, through patients with an ECF, to those with a laparostomy and multiple open loops of small bowel visible in the wound. This requires specialist stoma care from highly skilled nurses who will use a wide variety of shaped appliances, wide-necked bags, and protective dressings and pastes to protect the skin and contain the small bowel contents. In rare situations, emergency surgery is indicated to either refashion a stoma or construct a controlled proximal stoma in the presence of a more distal fistula. An example of the need for this may be an enterovaginal fistula, where a proximal stoma is the only means of control possible.

The resolution of wounds over time may be very significant. This is usually a factor of time, nutrition and skin protection. In the case of patients with laparostomy, there is usually significant reduction in the diameter of the wound and bowel loops become indistinguishable following growth of granulation tissue over them.

Planned surgery

Surgical intervention should be planned and frequently delayed. In the case of IF associated with ECF, early operative intervention to close the fistula is contraindicated by the associated high mortality due to re-fistulisation, sepsis, malnutrition and difficulties with fluid balance.[44] Indications for early surgery may include the following:[45]

1. drainage of pus when this cannot be achieved percutaneously;
2. excision of ischaemic bowel;
3. laying open of abscess cavities in the abdominal wall;
4. construction of a controlled proximal stoma;
5. catastrophic anastomotic failure, by exteriorisation of proximal and distal bowel ends.

These are usually the most septic patients and there is an associated high mortality with these procedures. Only in life-threatening situations should surgery be undertaken early in these patients and the decision should not be taken lightly as early surgery can result directly in multiple complications.

Patients managed with an open abdomen have a higher mortality and ECF rate when compared with historical case-matched controls with a closed abdomen,[46] patients with an open abdomen having a mortality rate of 25% and fistula formation rate of 14.8%.

Reconstruction

When considering reconstructive surgery, the aim is to have a well patient, with no signs of dehydration or evidence of sepsis and with a good nutritional status. The aim of the management described above

is to produce this scenario, such that surgery can be undertaken as safely as possible. The decisions then concern when to operate and what to do.

The decision about when to operate is vital. In the 1960s, Edmunds et al. proposed that early intervention using a conservative approach was associated with 80% mortality compared with 6% mortality for an operative approach. Supportive care has changed significantly since that time, however, particularly the use of PN. In 1978, Reber et al.[11] proposed planned intervention following eradication of sepsis. In the case of ECF, they reported a proportion of spontaneous closures, of which 90% occurred within 1 month, 10% within the next 2 months and none thereafter.

As discussed above, early surgery is made extremely difficult by the severity of the adhesions. It is important to delay surgery until these adhesions have softened, thereby reducing the risk of iatrogenic complications. This will often necessitate a delay of 5–6 months following the patient's previous surgical intervention. Clinically, this may be indicated by the identification of prolapse of stomas or fistulas, and by the impression, on examination, that the abdominal wall is moving separately to the underlying bowel (**Fig. 18.1**).

The second decision is what definitive reconstruction to undertake and this must be individualised. It may range from connecting an end ileostomy to the remaining colon, with the aim of bringing the colon into continuity, to closure of multiple complex fistulas in a hostile abdomen full of severe adhesions.

Surgery to increase nutrient and fluid absorption by either slowing intestinal transit or increasing

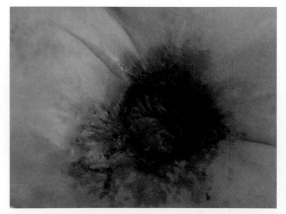

Figure 18.1 • Intestinal fistula with prolapsing bowel indicating correct time for surgery.

intestinal surface area is not commonly undertaken in the adult population. The operations include reversed small-bowel segments,[47–49] colonic interposition and tapering with small-bowel lengthening.[50–52] The first two attempt to slow the transit of luminal contents by antiperistaltic activity or interposition of colonic tissue. They have achieved some clinical success but run the risk of further sacrifice of small bowel, obstruction or anastomotic leakage. Tapering with small-bowel lengthening (the Bianchi technique) has been applied in children with some success.[53] It involves dividing the dilated adapted bowel in two longitudinally, while maintaining mesenteric blood supply via careful dissection in the axis of the mesentery, allocating vessels to either segment. The bowel is then tubularised and joined sequentially.[54–56] However, no new mucosa is formed and there are risks of multiple adhesions and leakage or stenosis from the long anastomotic line.

The serial transverse enteroplasty (STEP) procedure involves serially stapling the dilated short bowel, leaving a lumen of 1–2 cm. The staple direction is alternated between the mesenteric and antimesenteric borders and the bowel length (but not overall surface area) is increased. Sudan et al. describe their experience with both the Bianchi and STEP procedures. In a combined analysis incorporating both children and adults 69% of patients were off PN after intestinal lengthening. The exact benefit of intestinal lengthening procedures in the adult population is unclear in this analysis.[57]

Artificial valves, recirculation loops, electrical pacing,[58–60] tapering and plication, growth of neomucosa and mechanical tissue expansion[61] are all experimental techniques that are either untried in clinical practice or limited to case reports only.

Enterocutaneous fistula

High-output proximal small-bowel fistulas are associated with IF by producing functionally short bowel, and are often associated with significant problems with sepsis, malnutrition and difficulties with fluid balance.[44] Initial management is as described above.

Natural resolution of the fistula depends on the underlying pathology. Postoperative fistulas heal in around 70% of cases,[62] usually within the first 6 weeks of starting PN. Factors preventing healing may be specific to the fistula itself, as indicated in Table 18.3, or general, including ongoing sepsis,

Table 18.3 • Factors influencing spontaneous fistula closure

	Unfavourable	Favourable
Anatomy	Jejunum	Ileum
	Short and wide fistula	Long and narrow fistula
	Mucocutaneous continuity	Mucocutaneous discontinuity
	Discontinuity of the bowel	Continuity of the bowel
Small bowel	Active disease	No active disease
	Distal obstruction	No distal obstruction

nutritional deficiency, or infiltration of the tract by underlying disease such as malignancy, Crohn's or tuberculosis.

Surgical intervention tends to be somewhat 'freestyle' as, despite detailed investigations, findings at surgery may be unexpected. General principles are well described.[63] The abdominal cavity is entered and the small bowel mobilised carefully as the adhesions are usually considerable. The fistula-bearing segment(s) of bowel is resected en bloc and the remaining ends of bowel re-anastomosed. This includes resection of any cutaneous abdominal wall component of the fistulous tract. If an anastomosis is likely to be in an area of residual sepsis, a stoma is usually advisable. Abdominal wall closure may be problematic and may necessitate a component separation abdominoplasty in order to obtain fascial closure due to tissue loss from the abdominal wall or the use of Vicryl mesh.

Rehabilitation

The goal of therapy is for the patient to resume work and a normal lifestyle, or as normal a one as possible. This can be a considerable undertaking as the patient will generally have spent a prolonged period of time in hospital, sometimes up to 6 months. Sending patients home on PN whilst they await surgery can reduce the time to long-term rehabilitation.

Rehabilitation must be multidisciplinary, involving stoma care, physiotherapy, dietetics and occupational health. There needs to be detailed stoma care for patients with high-output stomas and referral to a community continence service for patients with intestinal continuity and incontinence due to liquid stools.

Referral to a medical social worker for assistance with social security benefits is important. A proportion of patients will need to remain on intravenous therapy, either saline or PN. Patients must be taught how to manage their tunnelled feeding lines appropriately in order to allow them to move from a hospital environment to home.

Considerable psychological support may be required and patients should be put in contact with supporting organisations. Long-term sequelae must also be considered. This may involve long-term home PN or recurrence of the underlying disease. Long-term care will include regular monitoring and review of therapy, vitamin B_{12} replacement if more than 1 m of terminal ileum has been resected, and review of other nutrients such as zinc, iron, folic acid and fat-soluble vitamins.

Transplantation

Around two patients per million commence home PN and 50% are suitable for consideration of small-bowel transplantation. In the UK this results in a possible 50 cases per year (50% children). A study of 124 consecutive adult SBS patients with non-malignant disease at two centres in France reported survival of 86% at 2 years and 75% at 5 years.[64] Dependence on PN was 49% at 2 years and 45% at 5 years. Small-bowel transplantation remains an experimental procedure. At the last update of the international registry (www.intestinaltransplant.org), 1292 intestinal transplants had been performed on 1210 patients in 64 different centres. This included intestine-only transplants (45%), combined intestine/liver transplants (40%) and multivisceral transplants (15%). The majority have been performed in patients under the age of 16 years (62%).[65]

The most recent evaluation has reported 1-year patient and graft survival of 79% and 64%, respectively, for intestine-only transplants, and 50% and 49%, respectively, for intestine/liver transplants. Long-term patient and graft survival for intestine-only transplants is 62% and 49%, respectively, at 3 years, and 50% and 38% at 5 years.[66] Because survival is poorer than that of patients on home PN, the indication for transplantation is SBS not maintainable on dietary supplements, and in whom PN is no longer possible due to severe complications. These usually include lack of access sites because of central venous occlusion, or cholestatic liver disease progressing to fibrosis and cirrhosis. The possibility of gut-lengthening operations must be considered first. The portal vein must be patent and should be checked by Doppler studies, as should the other great veins, in a search for vascular access for the perioperative period.

Complications are chiefly due to graft rejection and immunosuppression. Rejection leads to bacterial translocation and sepsis in an immunosuppressed patient who is often already malnourished. Current immunosuppressives such as tacrolimus have been paramount in reducing graft sepsis but have adverse effects of neurotoxicity, nephrotoxicity and glucose intolerance. The antiproliferative agents may cause bone marrow suppression. The consequences of chronic steroid use are osteoporosis, cataracts and diabetes, and growth retardation in children. Opportunistic infections are a major problem, particularly cytomegalovirus.[67]

Recently, a report of an experimental procedure in beagles described the transplantation of ileal mucosa to the colonic lumen. This raises the possibility of autogenic allotropic small-bowel mucosa transplantation.

Supporting organisations

Like most chronic conditions, a supporting structure has evolved to assist in overall management. The patient support group is Patients on Intravenous and Nasogastric Nutrition Therapy (PINNT, 258 Wennington Road, Rainham, Essex RM13 9UU). The paediatric version is called half-PINNT. Apart from the functions of providing advice and understanding from patients in a similar condition, the association also enables the borrowing of portable equipment to allow holidays away from home.

The professional supporting body is the British Association of Parenteral and Enteral Nutrition (BAPEN, PO Box 922, Maidenhead, Berkshire SL6 4SH). Keeping an overall view of intestinal failure is the British Artificial Nutritional Survey (BANS, 4 Low Moor Road, Lincoln LN 3JY), which maintains a census of patients on long-term nutritional support. Most importantly, the pharmaceutical firms that supply the various nutritional mixtures are also involved in providing and delivering the bags to patients at home; this also includes maintenance contracts that ensure continued functioning of the necessary fridges and emergency back-up in case of failure.

Summary

Recent developments in IF, including home PN and a greater understanding of the pathophysiology of massive intestinal resection, have allowed clinicians to treat and maintain such patients, resulting in long-term survival. The complex medical and surgical management is prolonged and multidisciplinary. It is summarised in Box 18.2.

Box 18.2 • St Mark's intestinal failure protocol

Stage 1: Establish stability

Restrict oral fluids to 500 mL daily

Achieve and maintain reliable venous access

Administer intravenous sodium chloride 0.9% until the concentration of sodium in the urine is greater than 20 mmol/L

Maintain equilibrium by infusing:

1. Fluid: calculated from the previous day's losses and daily body weight records
2. Sodium: 100 mmol/L for every litre of previous days' intestinal loss plus 80 mmol (more if the intestinal loss is excessive)
3. Potassium: 60–80 mmol daily
4. Magnesium: 8–14 mmol daily
5. Calories, protein, vitamins, trace elements: only if enteral absorption is inadequate

Stage 2: Transfer to oral intake

1. Continue intravenous maintenance therapy
2. Start low-fibre meals
3. Start antidiarrhoeal medication 30–60 minutes before meals
4. Start gastric antisecretory drugs
5. Start oral rehydration solution. Discourage drinking around meal times
6. Restrict the intake of non-electrolyte drinks to 1 L daily
7. Encourage snacks and supplementary nourishing drinks, within above limits

Consider the need for enteral tube feeding

1. Start oral magnesium oxide capsules 12–16 mmol daily
2. If intestinal losses remain high, start octreotide 50–100 mg s.c. t.d.s.
3. Gradually withdraw intravenous therapy

Stage 3: Rehabilitation

1. The patient and family should by now understand the physiological changes that have occurred and the rationale for treatment
2. There needs to be detailed stoma care for patients with high-output stomas
3. Referral to community continence service for patients with intestinal continuity and incontinence due to liquid stools
4. Referral to medical social worker for assistance with social security benefits
5. If intravenous therapy cannot be withdrawn because of continuing intestinal losses (>2 L/day), teach the patient/family to perform intravenous therapy at home

Stage 4: Long-term care

1. Regular monitoring and review of therapy
2. Vitamin B_{12} replacement if more than 1 m of terminal ileum resected
3. Review other nutrients such as zinc, iron and folic acid and also fat-soluble vitamins

Key points

- Intestinal failure is a multifactorial entity with improved long-term outcome with developments in nutritional and specialised care.
- Nutritional requirements will vary according to phase of IF. In the hypersecretory phase the aim is to maintain fluid balance and reduce stoma output, and TPN may be required. In the adaptation and stabilisation phases enteral nutrition is encouraged and TPN requirements may be reduced or weaned.

- A clear understanding of normal intestinal physiology is required to understand the pathophysiology of IF.
- Prevention of IF is important and involves meticulous attention to anastomotic technique and techniques to preserve intestinal length in conditions such as Crohn's disease. The use of non-absorbable mesh and VAC dressings should be avoided in the setting of intestinal inflammation.
- A staged approach to management will ensure good long-term outcome. Nutritional management, defining the anatomy by radiological means, and skin protection should be the initial steps in management. Any definitive surgery should be deferred till nutritional optimisation has been achieved, all sepsis is eradicated and maturation of adhesions has occurred.
- The multidisciplinary team approach to management of IF is the standard of care and consideration should be given to referring these patients to a centre dedicated to the management of IF.
- Intestinal transplantation is a valuable addition to the armentarium of treatments available for IF.

References

1. Scott NA, Leinhardt DJ, O'Hanrahan T, et al. Spectrum of intestinal failure in a specialised unit. Lancet 1991;337(8739):471–3.

2. Anonymous. Intestinal failure: criteria for referral. London: St Marks Hospital; 1999(internal).

3. Bakker H, Bozzetti F, Staun M, et al. Home parenteral nutrition in adults: a European multicentre survey in 1997. ESPEN-Home Artificial Nutrition Working Group. Clin Nutr 1999;18(3):135–40.

4. Howard L, Ament ME, Fleming CR. Current use and clinical outcome of home parenteral and enteral nutrition therapies in the United States. Gastroenterology 1995;109:355–65.

5. Carlson GL. Surgical management of intestinal failure. Proc Nutr Soc 2003;62(3):711–8.

6. Nightingale JM. Parenteral nutrition: multidisciplinary management. Hosp Med 2005;66(3):147–51.

7. Sudan D, DiBaise J, Torres C, et al. A multidisciplinary approach to the treatment of intestinal failure. J Gastrointest Surg 2005;9(2):165–76.

8. DiBaise JK, Young RJ, Vanderhoof JA. Intestinal rehabilitation and the short bowel syndrome: part 2. Am J Gastroenterol 2004;99(9):1823–32.

9. Buchman AL. Etiology and initial management of short bowel syndrome. Gastroenterology 2006; 130(2, Suppl. 1):S5–15.

10. DiBaise JK, Young RJ, Vanderhoof JA. Intestinal rehabilitation and the short bowel syndrome: part 1. Am J Gastroenterol 2004;99(7):1386–95.

11. Reber H, Roberts C, Way L, et al. Management of external gastrointestinal fistulas. Ann Surg 1978;188:460–7.

12. McIntyre P, Ritchie J, Hawley P, et al. Management of enterocutaneous fistulas: a review of 132 cases. Br J Surg 1984;71:293–6.

13. Rao M, Burke D, Finan PJ, et al. The use of vacuum-assisted closure of abdominal wounds: a word of caution. Colorectal Dis 2007;9(3):266–8.

14. Spiller RC, Jones BJ, Silk DB. Jejunal water and electrolyte absorption from two proprietary enteral feeds in man: importance of sodium content. Gut 1987;28:681–7.
This highlights the importance of sodium concentration in water reabsorption in the intestinal lumen.

15. Lennard-Jones J. Oral rehydration solutions in short bowel syndrome. Clin Ther 1990;12(Suppl. A):129–37.

16. Allou M, Ehrinpreis M. Shortage of intravenous multivitamin solution in the United States. N Engl J Med 1997;337:54–5.

17. Vanderhoof JA, Young RJ, Thompson JS. New and emerging therapies for short bowel syndrome in children. Paediatr Drugs 2003;5(8):525–31.

18. Kurkchubasche A, Rowe M, Smith S. Adaptation in short-bowel syndrome: reassessing old limits. J Pediatr Surg 1997;28:1069–71.

19. Hoffman A, Poley R. Role of bile acid malabsorption in pathogenesis of diarrhoea and steatorrhea in patients with ileal resection. Gastroenterology 1972;62:918–34.

20. Gouttebel MC, Saint-Aubert B, Astre C, et al. Total parenteral nutrition needs in different types of short bowel syndrome. Dig Dis Sci 1986;31(7):718–23.

21. Jeppesen P, Mortensen P. Significance of a preserved colon for parenteral energy requirements in patients receiving home parenteral nutrition. Scand J Gastroenterol 1998;33:1175–9.

22. Spiller R, Brown M, Phillips P. Decreased fluid tolerance, accelerated transit, and abnormal motility of the human colon induced by oleic acid. Gastroenterology 1986;91:100–7.

23. Ammon H, Phillips S. Inhibition of colonic water and electrolyte absorption by fatty acids in man. Gastroenterology 1973;65:744–9.

24. Nightingale JM, Lennard-Jones JE, Gertner DJ, et al. Colonic preservation reduces need for parenteral therapy, increases incidence of renal stones, but does not change high prevalence of gall stones in patients with a short bowel. Gut 1992;33(11):1493–7.
Seminal paper on the role of the colon in reducing extraintestinal manifestations of intestinal failure.

25. Oh M, Phelps K, Traube M, et al. D-Lactic acidosis in a man with the short bowel syndrome. N Engl J Med 1979;301(5):1493–7.

26. Buchman AL, Scolapio J, Fryer J. AGA technical review on short bowel syndrome and intestinal transplantation. Gastroenterology 2003;124:1111–34.

27. WHO. Treatment and prevention of dehydration in diarrhea diseases: a guide for use at the primary level. Geneva: World Health Organisation; 1976.

28. Nightingale JM, Kamm MA, van der Sijp JR, et al. Disturbed gastric emptying in the short bowel syndrome. Evidence for a 'colonic brake'. Gut 1993; 34(9):1171–6.

29. Goldman C, Rudloff M, Ternberg J. Cimetidine and neonatal small bowel adaptation: an experimental study. J Pediatr Surg 1987;22:484–7.

30. Jacobsen O, Ladefoged K, Stage J, et al. Effects of cimetidine on jejunostomy effluents in patients with severe short-bowel syndrome. Scand J Gastroenterol 1986;21(7):824–8.

31. Hesse U, Ysebaert D, de Hemptinne B. Role of somatostatin-14 and its analogues in the management of gastrointestinal fistulae: clinical data. Gut 2001;49(Suppl. 4):iv11–21.

32. Schlemminger R, Lottermoser S, Sostmann H, et al. Metabolic parameters and neurotensin liberation after resection of the small intestine, syngeneic and allogeneic segment transplantation in the rat. Langenbecks Arch Chir 1993;378:265–72.

33. Farthing M. Octreotide in dumping and short bowel syndromes. Digestion 1993;54(Suppl. 1):47–52.

34. Rodrigues C, Lennard-Jones J, Thompson D, et al. The effects of octreotide, soy polysaccharide, codeine and loperamide on nutrient, fluid and electrolyte absorption in the short-bowel syndrome. Aliment Pharmacol Ther 1989;3:159–69.

35. McIntyre P, Wood S, Powell-Tuck J, et al. Nocturnal nasogastric tube feeding at home. Postgrad Med J 1983;59:767–9.

36. Gulledge A, Gipson W, Steiger E, et al. Home parenteral nutrition for the short bowel syndrome. Psychological issues. Gen Hosp Psychiatry 1980;2:271–81.

37. Lake A, Kleinman R, Walker W. Enteric alimentation in specialized gastrointestinal problems: an alternative to total parenteral nutrition. Adv Pediatr 1981;28:319–39.

38. Kurkchubasche A, Smith S, Rowe M. Catheter sepsis in short-bowel syndrome. Arch Surg 1992;127:21–4.

39. Foldes J, Rimon B, Muggia-Sullam M. Progressive bone loss during long-term home total parenteral nutrition. JPEN J Parenter Enteral Nutr 1990;14:139–42.

40. Anonymous. Guidelines in the use of total parenteral nutrition in hospital patients. JPEN J Parenter Enteral Nutr 1987;10:441–5.

41. Lappas JC. Imaging of the postsurgical small bowel. Radiol Clin North Am 2003;41(2):305–26.

42. Umschaden HW, Gasser J. MR enteroclysis. Radiol Clin North Am 2003;41(2):231–48.

43. Wiarda BM, Kuipers EJ, Houdijk LP, et al. MR enteroclysis: imaging technique of choice in diagnosis of small bowel diseases. Dig Dis Sci 2005;50(6):1036–40.

44. Chapman R, Foran R, Dunphrey J. Management of intestinal fistulas. Am J Surg 1964;108:157–64.

45. Keighley MR. Intestinal fistula. In: Keighley MR, Williams N, editors. Surgery of the anus, rectum and colon. London: WB Saunders; 1993. p. 2014–43.

46. Adkins AL, Robbins J, Villalba M, et al. Open abdomen management of intra-abdominal sepsis. Am Surg 2004;70(2):137–40.

47. Pigot F, Messing B, Chaussade S, et al. Severe short bowel syndrome with a surgically reversed small bowel segment. Dig Dis Sci 1990;35(1):137–44.

48. Panis Y, Messing B, Rivet P, et al. Segmental reversal of the small bowel as an alternative to intestinal transplantation in patients with short bowel syndrome. Ann Surg 1997;225(4):401–7.

49. Hennessy K. Nutritional support and gastrointestinal disease. Nurs Clin North Am 1989;24:373–82.

50. Thompson J, Pinch L, Murray N, et al. Experience with intestinal lengthening for the short-bowel syndrome. J Pediatr Surg 1991;26:721–4.

51. Thompson J, Vanderhoof J, Antonson D. Intestinal tapering and lengthening for short bowel syndrome. J Pediatr Gastroenterol Nutr 1985;4:495–7.

52. Weinberg G, Matalon T, Brunner M, et al. Bleeding stomal varices: treatment with a transjugular intrahepatic portosystemic shunt in two pediatric patients. J Vasc Interv Radiol 1995;6:233–6.

53. Bianchi A. Longitudinal intestinal lengthening and tailoring: results in 20 children. J R Soc Med 1997;90:429–32.

54. Pokorny WJ, Fowler CL. Isoperistaltic intestinal lengthening for short bowel syndrome. Surg Gynecol Obstet 1991;172(1):39–43.

55. Boeckman C, Traylor R. Bowel lengthening for short gut syndrome. J Pediatr Surg 1981;16:996–7.

56. Dionig IP, Spada M, Alessiani M. Potential small bowel transplant recipients in Italy. Italian National Register of Home Parenteral Nutrition. Transplant Proc 1994;26:1444–5.

57. Sudan D, Thompson J, Botha J, et al. Comparison of intestinal lengthening procedures for patients with short bowel syndrome. Ann Surg 2007;246(4): 593–601.

58. Cullen J, Kelly K. The future of intestinal pacing. Gastroenterol Clin North Am 1994;23:391–402.

59. Gladen HE, Kelly KA. Electrical pacing for short bowel syndrome. Surg Gynecol Obstet 1981;153(5):697–700.

60. Brousse N, Canioni D, Rambaud C. Small bowel transplant cyclosporine-related lymphoproliferative disorder: report of a case. Transplant Proc 1994; 26:1424–5.

61. Stark GB, Dorer A, Walgenbach KJ, et al. The creation of a small bowel pouch by tissue expansion – an experimental study in pigs. Langenbecks Arch Chir 1990;375(3):145–50.

62. Levy E, Frileux P, Sandrucci S. Continuous enteral nutrition during the early adaptive stage of the short bowel syndrome. Br J Surg 1988;75:549–53.

63. Fazio V. Intestinal fistulas. In: Keighley M, Pemberton J, Fazio V, Parc R, editors. Atlas of colorectal surgery. New York: Churchill Livingstone; 1996. p. 363–71.

64. Carbonnel F, Cosnes J, Chevret S, et al. The role of anatomic factors in nutritional autonomy after extensive small bowel resection. JPEN J Parenter Enteral Nutr 1996;20(4):275–80.

65. Grant D. Intestinal transplantation: 1997 report of the international registry. Transplantation 2000;69:555–9.

66. US Scientific 2000 Registry of Transplant Recipients and the Organ Procurement and Transplantation Network. 2000 Annual Report. Transplant data 1990–1999. Rockville, MD and United Network of Organ Sharing, Richmond, VA: US Department of Health and Human Services, Health Resources and Services Administration, Office of Special Programs, Division of Transplantation.

67. Pirenne J. Short-bowel syndrome. Medical aspects and prospects of intestinal transplantation. Acta Chir Belg 1996;96(4):150–4.

Index

NB: Page numbers followed by *f* indicate figures, *t* indicate tables and *b* indicate boxes.

A

Abdominal hand pressure 19
Abdominoperineal excision (APE) 75
Abscesses
    perianal 161, 161*f*
    pilonidal 243
    surgery 156–158
ACCENT I/II study 152*b*
Acquired immunodeficiency syndrome (AIDS) 253–254
Acticon Neosphincter™ 175, 175*f*, 176*f*
Active Ulcerative Colitis Trial 1/2 (ACT1/2) 126*b*
Activity Index 124–125
Acute anorectal non-cryptoglandular non-fistulous abscesses 213–214, 215*f*
Acute complicated diverticulitis 112*f*
Acute sepsis 214–216
Adalimumab 149–150, 151–152, 152*b*, 161
Adenocarcinoma, anal 101
Adenomatous polyps 49, 54
Advancement flaps 225–226
Age factors, diverticular disease 104
Agency for Medical Innovations (AMI) 175
ALCCaS (Australasian Laparoscopic Colon Cancer Study) trial 269
Altemeier's procedure 185, 186*t*, 187*f*
Ambulatory manometry 5
American College of Surgeons Oncology Group (ACOSOG), Z6051 study 270
American Gastroenterological Association 7*b*, 124, 294
American Medical Systems (AMS) 175
    Acticon Neosphincter™ 175, 175*f*, 176*f*
    AMS 800 artificial urinary sphincter 175
American Society of Clinical Oncology (ASCO) 85
American Society of Colon and Rectal Surgeons (ASCRS) 175
5-Aminosalicylic acid (5-ASA) 125–126
    colitis 126
    Crohn's disease 149–150, 151*b*, 153
Amitryptilline 203*b*
Amsterdam criteria (HNPCC) 35, 35*b*
Amyloidosis 145
Anal canal
    anatomy/physiology 1–3
    sensation 5–6
Anal cancer 95–102
    adenocarcinoma 101
    malignant melanoma 102
    tumours *see* Epidermoid tumours, anal
Anal condyloma 258*f*
    giant condyloma accuminata (GCA) 260, 260*f*
Anal dilatation 247, 247*b*
Anal endosonography (AES) 9, 10*f*, 219

Anal fissure 161, 236–241
    aetiology 237
    classification 237, 238–239
    clinical findings 236*f*, 241
    initiating factors 237–238, 237*f*
    perpetuating factors 238
    recurrent/atypical 240–241
    treatment
        medical 239–240, 239*f*
        surgical 240
Anal fistula 161–162, 212–230
    aetiology 213–214, 214*f*, 215*f*
    assessment 217–221
        clinical 217–219, 218*f*, 219*f*
        imaging 219–220
        physiological 220–221
    classification 216–217, 216*f*, 217*f*, 219–220
    imaging 11, 12*f*
    management 214–216
    recurrent 227–228
    surgery
        principles 221, 222*f*
        treatment 221–227
Anal function, quality 76
Anal intraepithelial neoplasia (AIN) 96, 97, 101, 260
Anal papillomavirus-associated lesions 96*b*
Anal plug 173
Anal sphincteroplasty 173–174, 173*f*
Anal sphincters
    artificial 174
    imaging 9–13
    magnetic (MAS) 176, 176*f*, 177*f*
    reconstruction 174
Anal stenosis 245–248
    aetiology 246, 246*b*
    clinical presentation 246
    prevention 246–248
    treatment 246
Anastomosis
    appositional serosubmucosal 58–59, 58*f*, 59*f*
    colonic cancer 58–60
    end-to-end 77
    end-to-side 77
    hand-sewn 130–133, 134*f*, 135*f*
    ileorectal (IRA) 128, 129
    results 59–60
    stapled 59, 59*f*
        double 130–133, 132*f*, 133*f*
Anastomotic strictures 134
Anatomy (mapping) 297
Anorectal investigation 1–16
    anatomy/physiology 1–3
        rectoanal inhibitory reflex 2–3, 3*f*
    defecography/evacuation proctography 8
        dynamic pelvic magnetic resonance imaging (MRI) 8, 8*f*
        dynamic transperineal/three-dimensional pelvic floor ultrasound 8